MW00559629

DISCARDED
Worthington Libraries

the
PRACTICE
of
NATURAL
MOVEMENT

RECLAIM POWER, HEALTH, AND FREEDOM

By **ERWAN LE CORRE**, *Creator of* **MOVNAT**

VICTORY BELT PUBLISHING INC.

First Published in 2019 by Victory Belt Publishing Inc.

Copyright © 2019 by Erwan Le Corre

All rights reserved

No part of this publication may be reproduced or distributed in any form or by any means, electronic or mechanical, or stored in a database or retrieval system, without prior written permission from the publisher.

ISBN-13: 978-1-628602-83-8

The information included in this book is for educational purposes only. It is not intended or implied to be a substitute for professional medical advice. The reader should always consult his or her healthcare provider to determine the appropriateness of the information for his or her own situation or if he or she has any questions regarding a medical condition or treatment plan. Reading the information in this book does not constitute a patient-physician relationship.

The author/owner claims no responsibility to any person or entity for any liability, loss, or damage caused or alleged to be caused directly or indirectly as a result of the use, application, or interpretation of the information presented herein.

Cover and Interior photography by Anton Brkic
Author Photo by Erik Tranberg
Page 39 photo by Christopher Baker

Cover design by Erwan Le Corre and Dylan Chatain
Interior design by Charisse Reyes and Elita San Juan

Printed in Canada
TC 0118

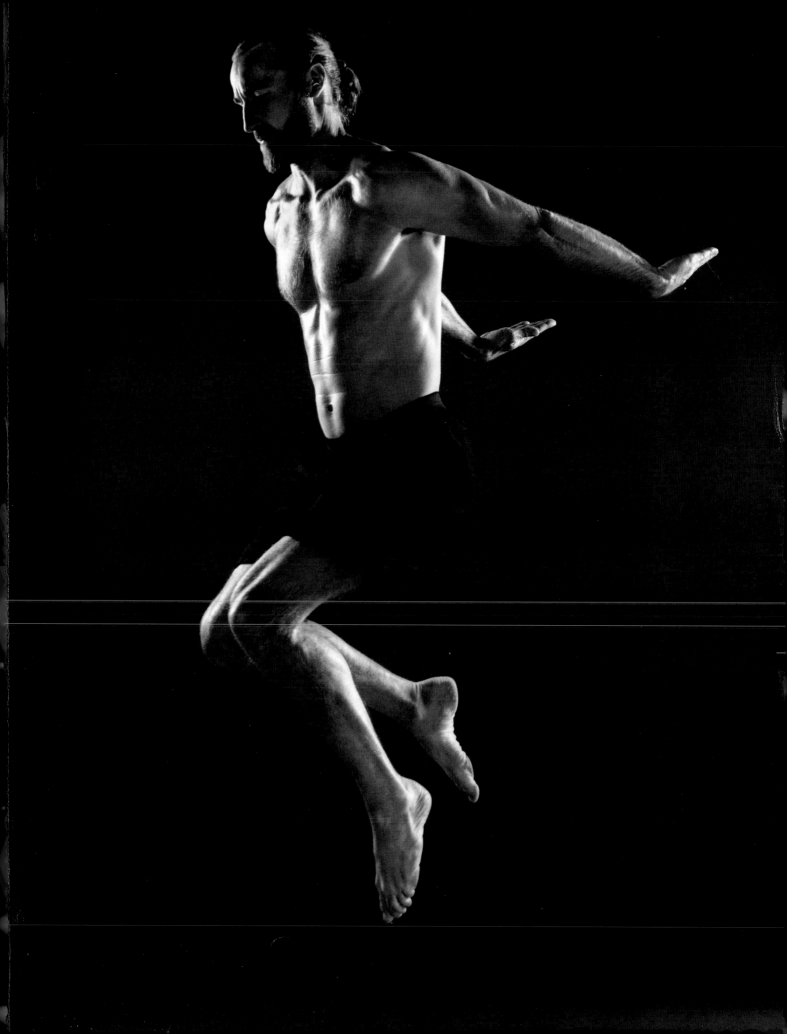

Contents

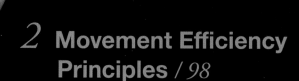

Preface

"See that bump on the trunk? Put your foot right there." My dad was talking to me as he helped me climb an apple tree. I was barely four—and a little afraid—but I was willing to follow and trust his guidance; I was willing to show ability and strength; I was willing to learn.

Did I have a choice? Could I step down and quit? It didn't seem like it. My father wasn't beneath me to catch me if something went wrong; instead, he was right above me. I was six feet off the ground, which seemed like a deadly height to me. This exercise was way beyond what I had ever attempted on my own. My older brother Yann was next to my father and already confident in his own ability, which just added to my desire not to disappoint my dad. I wanted to succeed. I wanted to be proud of myself, and I wanted my father and brother to be proud of me, too.

It's a natural instinct in young children to seek peer validation through their achievements. At the time, I was too young to think of the situation in those exact terms, but I had the intuition of the practical, real value the challenge held. I knew it in my gut.

I remember this first big tree-climbing experience very well, but that's not really when my Natural Movement training had started. My dad told me about another situation that I have no memory of, which proved to be a pivotal experience for me. He had climbed to the top of a steep muddy hill as I struggled along behind him. I was quite young—only about two years old. My father said I called for help, but he wouldn't come back down to assist me. I tried to climb but kept sliding down and back. After a few attempts, I started weeping in frustration and again called for help. My dad kept asking me to try again; he was not going to come to my rescue, and I had to make it on my own.

Because I had no choice, I stopped fussing and fought to make it to the top, where he cheered me and explained what the lesson had been about: You are capable of more than you think. My dad recalled feeling a little bad about refusing to help me, but he also wanted to teach me at a young age about self-reliance, which is a timeless lesson about a necessity that must be trained.

By the age of six, I was hanging from a metal rail outside my bedroom window—my whole body in the void 15 feet above ground. I wasn't showing off; there was no one around. I just wanted to see if I could do the maneuver with self-control. Instinctively, I was replicating what my dad had taught me four years before. Now I was training it on my own.

Apart from his long daily walks, my dad never had a healthy lifestyle, and consequently his health slowly but surely deteriorated over the years. On the other hand, I was growing up fast, but I wasn't particularly tall, strong, or athletic. In fact, I just looked like a regular teenager. I was looking for a direction in life, and I knew I didn't want to follow in my father's footsteps from a lifestyle perspective. I had a vision of being strong, healthy, happy, and free, and he was none of those things.

By age 15, I had taken up karate and started to practice with great commitment. I loved the combination of physical and mental strength the practice required. The Japanese martial art taught me a lot about precise movement, efficiency, and methodical practice. I was an addict; I trained every day—sometimes twice a day—and added daily supplemental training in the form of running, swimming, stretching, and even weightlifting. I started competing—first at the local level and then at the national level. It felt as if karate was the be-all and end-all.

When I was 19, I began to study at the university, but after a few weeks I gave up out of utter boredom. However, I was a young adult now, and things were a bit more complicated than they had been when I was younger. What was I supposed to do with my life? How could I make myself strong, healthy, happy, and free in this world? I didn't expect anything conventional would make me feel that way, and I questioned every single aspect of what's called a "normal" life.

Then I met someone who understood me. "Don" was my dad's age and a charismatic character who was known for being something of a nature stuntman and natural-lifestyle guru. He had once jumped off a helicopter into the freezing waters of Greenland. He was near an iceberg and equipped with only a pair of shorts from the company he was promoting. I was fascinated by everything I heard and saw about this man. In many ways, Don embodied what I was looking for.

I reached out to him and started training with him the day we met. I immediately became a follower of his philosophy and practice. While other young people were still studying or starting a career and family (living "normal" lives), I was running barefoot in the streets of Paris by night, climbing bridges, balancing at great heights, diving in dark and icy waters wearing only swim trunks, jumping from rooftop to rooftop without safety equipment, practicing Thai boxing moves in forbidden areas of the Paris underground, and doing breathing drills at the crack of dawn to draw energy from the "elements." I was doing 15 hours of fasting (only drinking water) daily, and once each week I'd fast for a stretch of 24 to 36 hours.

I had ditched conventional forms of entertainment to dedicate all my energies to this lifestyle and to getting as healthy, strong, and free as I could through my daily practice. The Internet was still new to most people, and smartphones didn't exist. I didn't own a TV and couldn't have cared less about not having one. I was running barefoot long before it became a thing. I was training "wild" or "primal" long before it was a thing. I was doing "intermittent fasting" and cold plunges before both were trendy—before digital cameras and social media. I was doing all of it almost 20 years ago, when I was only 19.

I was immersed in an atypical existential quest. I learned a lot in the process—so much that I could write a whole book about that period of my life.

During these years of consistent lifestyle practice, I often got to train outside in the streets, in parks, and in nature—anywhere, anytime. People often looked at me as if I was weird, and I couldn't have cared less. Sometimes they pointed at me. Sometimes they laughed or smiled in a sarcastic manner. Some people would ask me what I was doing because they were puzzled that I was barefoot, long-haired, and dressed in ninja-like black clothes as I did some kind of mysterious practice they couldn't identify. The way I described my approach didn't seem to enlighten anyone. They'd say, "If you want to be 'strong,' why not just do bodybuilding?" There seemed to be a thick wall separating my perception, behavior, and lifestyle from a normal one, but I had to follow my innate drive. It felt vital to me, although I recognized the evident mismatch between what I was doing and the behavior society normally expects from a young man. I wasn't practicing conventional fitness; I wasn't doing military training; and I wasn't involved in a sport or a known physical discipline. So, what was I doing? Training to be a stuntman? Thinking I was some sort of Rambo? Even when I tried to explain, nobody would really get it.

I started to understand that what was missing and what I had intuitively been looking for all my life was that I wanted to develop and maintain the most timeless skills in human beings.

You could go to a park and identify physical activities that you spot people doing. Someone holding a pose, maybe upside down? Yoga, of course. Someone doing slow, controlled, mindful movements? Tai chi or qi gong. Someone stretching? Well...that's stretching. Someone doing handstands or acrobatics? Gymnastics or calisthenics. Someone doing push-ups and sit-ups? General conditioning. You get the point. You can identify when someone is doing capoeira or hip hop, karate or judo. Most people can even identify diverse styles of dance. You don't even have to be a practitioner to recognize when other people are doing those activities.

Now imagine an adult man or woman climbing a tree, jumping off a branch, and landing in a roll before immediately transitioning to a crawl, then to a sprint, then to a jump before eventually throwing something to another person or maybe even carrying another person. What would you think? What is that activity? Are these people sane? Is it something new?

I started my Natural Movement practice as a young child, without knowing it by that name or that it was a very ancient practice. Only later in my life did I realize that the very idea of having a physical practice or activity entirely based on the full range of movements that are natural to humans was novel to most people. I came to the realization that many physical activities or disciplines had a name and were recognized by all, but this ancient movement practice didn't have a name. Without a name, it had no identity; without an identity, it had no recognition; without recognition, it had no value; and without value, it had no place in our modern world and lives.

In studying the history of physical training, I learned that others had attempted to champion this type of physical practice, with mixed results. My new heroes became Girolamo Mercuriale, Johann Heinrich Pestolazzi, Francisco Amorós, Johann GutsMuths, Friedrich Jahn, and Georges Hébert, to name the most important innovators. I realized that a long line of people had been exploring this area of physical training, and I was its new thought-leader and spearhead.

NOTE

If you'd like to learn more about the history behind MovNat, read "The Roots of 'Methode Naturelle'" on the MovNat journal (www.movnat.com/the-roots-of-methode-naturelle/).

I decided that my mission would be to first give the practice a name, and then develop a rationale or concept to explain it in a straightforward, intelligible manner so that I could bring the idea to mainstream awareness and share the practice on a worldwide scale. How ambitious! My vision was to bring the benefits of this practice and lifestyle to as many other people as I could in order to benefit them as much as possible; I hoped to help improve many lives. This is the intention behind this book, and it has been my life's work for many years through the MovNat method I created a decade ago.

More and more people are becoming aware that "Natural Movement" involves the skills of crawling, walking, running, balancing, jumping, and so forth, but that has not always been the case. Do you remember the first time you heard about Natural Movement as a discipline or physical practice rather than as a mere anecdotal way to describe a movement using the "natural" label? Today, after I have spent a whole decade dedicated to continuously and systematically promoting the Natural Movement term and concept through countless magazine articles, podcasts, blog entries, interviews, videos, and finally this book, the concept is finally on the verge of reaching mainstream awareness.

Humans, just like other animals, have been moving naturally since the dawn of our species, but Natural Movement as a clearly, objectively defined and delineated concept with a set of detailed principles has existed only since I created it and made it popular. Whereas a small handful of individuals may have used the same term in the past—for instance, as a book title or descriptor—they used it to describe something entirely different and did so without drawing any real attention to the subject.

When I began to design and talk about the MovNat method and people would ask me what it was about, I was surprised that, regardless of what country people came from, the most frequent reactions were, "Natural Movement? What is it?" or, "You mean it's yoga or some kind of tai chi?" Not a single fitness professional I talked to even knew what I meant by this term. This made me quickly understand three things:

- The idea of Natural Movement was unknown to most people.

- The term I had chosen to quickly explain MovNat required an explanation and a definition of its own.

- Even by giving the practice a name, I still would have to work hard until the day would come where people would respond, "Natural Movement? You mean crawling, balancing, running, jumping, climbing, lifting, and so on?"

The process of defining the concept had to be more thorough than simply enunciating the diverse movement skills involved in the practice. It had to rely on fundamental principles that make it a solid, rational concept rather than a relatively vague notion. As a result, I have determined the twelve principles of Natural Movement that I outline in Part 1 and that constitute the "Natural Movement Manifesto." Although I could simplify each principle to a single sentence, I have taken the time to provide in-depth insights for all of them. You will see how interrelated these principles are and how they work together. Reading and understanding each principle will provide answers to most of the questions you might have about what is—or isn't—Natural Movement.

The many insights I share with you in the manifesto might rock the conventional idea of "exercise." You should know that my opinion is that mainstream, machine-based fitness is a dying experiment—an industrial approach that has overwhelmingly failed people more than it has helped them. The manifesto contains elements of critique of the modern approach to fitness—as well as a critique of the unhealthy aspects of modern lifestyle—that I believe are reasonable and objective. In defying conventional wisdom, I buck convention while doing my best to extract and retain wisdom from those who have come before me. My motivation for sharing these insights and principles is a deeply rooted desire to help people. The positive insights and few elements of constructive critique in the manifesto are designed to inform and inspire you. And the manifesto is immediately followed by pages of practical information that address the issues that I expose in my discussion of the principles.

To me, if you are a physically active person, you are a hero of modern times regardless of which modality you have chosen for exercising and moving your body. If you are one of the lucky ones who has figured out the best way, or at least your preferred way, to exercise, and it is helping you physically and mentally, you deserve nothing but a mother lode of thumbs-ups and cheers. If you haven't figured it out yet, it doesn't mean that you have never tried; it probably means that, among other obstacles placed in your way by modern life, you have never been convinced by any particular system or program. Perhaps after reading this book, you'll discover that you've finally found a movement approach that works for you.

For most people looking for a way to get back into shape, there is no simple answer to the question "What is the best way for me to become fit?" The fitness industry offers so many options that it has become quite confusing for the average person to choose which exercise program might be best for them. I have a simple question for you; although it might amuse you, it also might help you answer the "which program is best for me?" dilemma. Here's the question: What is the best fitness regimen for a tiger?

Does the question make you smile? Does it sound irrelevant or silly? Most importantly, what's the answer? How would you train a wild tiger to be fit? Would you tell the tiger to sit on an exercise machine and run on a treadmill? Would you instruct the tiger to jump on a BOSU and focus on activating its core because it's functional? Can you imagine our tiger sweating on an elliptical and frequently checking its pulse rate? Or could it be that a tiger doesn't need to exercise at all because it's naturally or genetically fit?

Here's my answer: To become fit and remain optimally healthy, a tiger needs to move the way tigers move for their day-to-day survival within their natural biome. It's that simple. Tigers move naturally when they're free to live the natural life every tiger should live—as will all wild animals. Throughout their lives, wild animals move the way nature and evolution intend them to move simply because, in nature, moving naturally and staying fit is a matter of survival and being able to reproduce, so life goes on and the species doesn't disappear from the Earth. Every newborn animal starts developing its species-specific movement aptitudes early on for this very reason. If wild animals maintain optimal fitness in this natural way, why on Earth should it be any different for humans? Because we're not "animals"? Because we're smart and they're not? Because we're advanced and they're unevolved? Or because we know better thanks to science? Isn't it logical to consider that human beings could attain incredible fitness by following a species-specific approach to movement and conditioning that is methodical, scalable, progressive, and safe?

Gray Cook, a renowned physical therapist and functional movement expert, once said: "We are made to grow strong and to age gracefully. Reclamation of authentic movement is the starting point." So maybe it is high time for a healthy and meaningful paradigm shift in the way we approach exercise.

After you've read this entire book, the idea of Natural Movement might seem very simple. That's my hope. You might discover that Natural Movement is a truth that you've been familiar with even though it's been somewhat absent from your life. You just needed someone else to point it out for it to become obvious again.

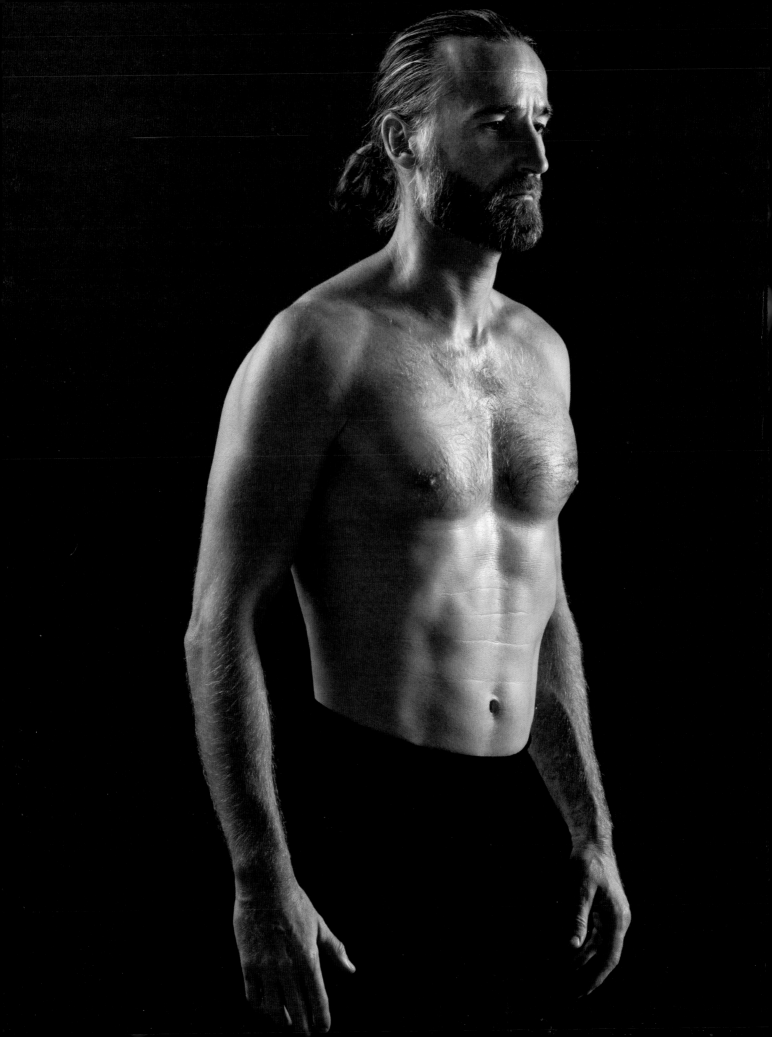

1
Manifesto

1. Evolutionary: **Natural Movement stems from the way our species has adapted to life in nature since the dawn of mankind.**

2. Instinctual: **We start developing fundamental Natural Movement patterns as infants without needing instruction.**

3. Universal: **Natural Movement is everyone's birthright regardless of ethnicity, gender, or age.**

4. Practical: **The primary purpose of Natural Movement is to be useful at ensuring basic physiological needs.**

5. Vital: **Natural Movement supports survival in life-threatening circumstances and ultimately serves biological fitness.**

6. Unspecialized: **Natural Movement skills are interrelated and work symbiotically.**

7. Adaptable: **Natural Movement adjusts to the diverse contextual variables and demands of the real world.**

8. Environmental: **Natural Movement originally developed as adaptive behavior for the diverse natural environments in which early humans lived.**

9. Progressive: **Natural Movement capability is developed and should be maintained over time.**

10. Efficient: **Natural Movement tends to meet the level of performance necessary for maximum effectiveness, energy conservation, and safety.**

11. Mindful: **Attention ensures efficiency in Natural Movement.**

12. Cooperative: **Humans use Natural Movement primarily for the benefit of the group or community they belong to.**

1
Evolutionary

"There is more in us than we know. If we can be made to see it, perhaps, for the rest of our lives, we will be unwilling to settle for less."

—Kurt Hahn

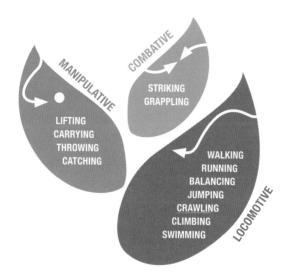

Evolutionary Background

Imagine yourself going for a walk in nature, maybe with a small group of close relatives and friends, except the time is 50,000 years ago. Your body structure is not different than today, but the world around you is completely wild—no roads, cars, cities, restaurants, or malls, and no planes in the sky. You are a hunter-gatherer, occasionally a scavenger, and your hungry band is on its way to procure the most nutritious food in the greatest amount it can find.

You're equipped with only primitive tools, although your body is in itself a remarkable piece of biological technology. It might or might not look muscular, lean, or "fit" by modern standards, but it is certainly strong, nimble, agile, and resilient. On top of these highly desirable physical qualities and physiological adaptations, you also possess very sharp senses, acute alertness, and mental fortitude. Lastly, you have wit and experience, which are indispensable for planning effective survival strategies in a way that raw strength and brute thinking could never match. You might have to explore a broad territory, encountering diverse environments and varied weather conditions, so you can hunt or gather what is necessary for your group to survive. Whatever your survival strategies are, effective natural movements are what you need to be opportunistic, adaptable, and, most importantly, successful.

Your way of life demands frequent, varied, and sometimes intense physical action. While long periods of rest and recovery are a vital component of survival, there is no room for perpetual slackers in this wild era and world. Your band is made up of untamed, wild, primal individuals. In other words, you are a natural human, and performing Natural Movement is a daily necessity and reality. This is what the situation was for humans and early hominids for roughly three million years.

Then something happened about 12,000 years ago—a dramatic change in survival strategy that eventually profoundly affected the life of most human beings on Earth: the advent of agriculture. Although producing our own food was an undeniable survival advantage when it was combined with fishing, hunting, and harvesting wild foods, as it progressively became the main method of supplying food—along with raising animals—it started to cause problems from a physical and movement perspective.

Humans didn't need to wait until the advent of the information age—or even until the advent of the industrial age—to undergo a dramatic change in physical behavior; the change started with the agricultural age. Choosing to tend fields, crops, and domesticated animals that mostly didn't wander over large areas meant that the distances humans needed to cover were immediately reduced by a considerable amount. There was no need to "commute to work" by walking or running for miles and miles. The change went beyond the distances covered in a day, though; it also radically altered the diversity of movements we once performed routinely. Fields, which had been cleared of as many natural variables as possible, were artificial environments; trees (live or dead), stumps, unwanted vegetation, large rocks, and even bumps and depressions in the ground were cleared so land could be fully controlled and farmed. Fields were flat, linear, and predictable with little to no environmental complexity and diversity. Drastically altering the terrain also drastically modified our Natural Movement behavior.

Activities that were formerly necessary for daily living—running, jumping, balancing, crawling, and climbing—had become rare occurrences. This is not to say that these movement patterns became totally absent—young children kept practicing them instinctually—but they were not the norm any longer. It also doesn't mean that physical effort was eliminated; in fact, physicality might have become even more necessary than ever because old-school farm work required almost constant physical effort. However, in comparison to the movement of the hunter-gatherer, the movement variety of the farmer had been extraordinarily reduced because of the changes to the environment where humans moved and procured food.

If we look at the overall movement behavior of contemporary, yet still technologically primitive, hunter-gatherers, we observe that they have maintained, by necessity, a broad movement repertoire—the full range of Natural Movement aptitudes including running, crawling, jumping, balancing, climbing, throwing, catching, lifting, carrying, and occasionally swimming. They may not perform all these movements with the same frequency and intensity—because those qualities depend on individual roles and ability and the environment in which a given human group lives—but, overall, we can observe a greater diversity of natural movements than in agricultural populations.

Clearly, there is a phenomenal mismatch between today's physical behaviors and those of our faraway ancestors and contemporary hunter-gatherer relatives. Having been physically and physiologically shaped by millions of years of Natural Movement in wild environments, a few millennia did not give our bodies enough time to genetically adapt to the circumstances of our modern way of life. This evolutionary mismatch is affecting our bodies, our health, our psychological states, and our lives. Evolution—or, if you prefer, millions of years of life in nature—has not only determined what we are capable of but also what our biology expects from us physically and mentally. Humans may not be completely out of place in the modern world we have created, but some of our evolutionary behaviors sure are.

Evolutionary Mismatch: *The* Zoo-Human Predicament

Let's look at the typical physical behavior and movement habits in modern, civilized humans. For now, I'm not addressing the artificiality of modern living environments, which is also part of the evolutionary mismatch and what is sometimes called our "zoo-human" condition. At this point, I'm considering how we move, or don't move, within modern environments.

What do we do when we wake up? We get out of bed and walk a few steps to the kitchen, where we sit for breakfast, or we go to the bathroom where we stand for a shower. Soon it is time to go to either school or work. We might have to walk a short distance to the car, the bus stop, or the train station. A minority of physically active people choose to take their bikes; yet even those who do travel by bike sit as they're riding.

At school or work we immediately take a seat and start studying or working. At lunch time, we might stand up and walk a few steps to sit somewhere else until we return to work. Throughout the day, we might take a few breaks from sitting; at those times, we stand up and walk a few steps to go to the coffee machine (where we might stand and chat for a moment) or the bathroom (where we sit for a moment).

We return home the same way we traveled to school or work—probably sitting. We feel tired at the end of the day and need to sit on a couch to relax and entertain ourselves, or we might sit on a chair for more computer time, be it for extra work hours or to connect with other people on social media. Physically active people, which are a minority in today's society, might go to a gym after work—traveling there by sitting in private or public transportation—and they work out while mostly sitting at exercise machines. Then we sit for dinner.

Eventually, we walk a few more steps to go to bed, sleep, and probably repeat the same pattern the next day. Apart from sitting, rising to a standing position, walking a few steps, and making some hand gestures for communication, what other movements have we performed?

> ❝ **With human nature caged in a narrow space, whipped daily into submission, how can we speak of its potentialities?"**
>
> *—Emma Goldman*

When your main, if not exclusive, form of day-to-day natural locomotion is to slowly walk very short distances on flat surfaces and to be physically idle by sitting the rest of the day, from a biological perspective you're in a state of movement poverty. Where is the diversity, the variability, the frequency, the intensity, the efficiency, and the adaptability in movement that we're evolutionarily capable of? Nowhere. It's nowhere to be observed in the typical physical behavior of modern humans. Although this deficit of activity is viewed as "normal," does that mean it is? Does it mean it's natural? Is it healthy or desirable?

Evolutionary science, or the simple observation of how most wild animals behave, indicates that physical idleness is not "laziness"; it's a necessary adaptation for successful survival. If you want to last, you can't exhaust all your energy; you must conserve energy for a time when you really need it, and you expend it only when necessary. It's a similar survival instinct to overeating in a situation where food procurement is unsure, intermittent, and scarce. Nonetheless, we have become "bio-slackers"—people who have neglected their biological nature to such an extent that we have become, in many ways, alien to our own bodies—starting with their need for movement.

I call physical idleness *movement poverty*. Movement poverty leads to physical weakness, diminished health, and depression. Movement poverty is a self-inflicted condition no one can biologically afford.

We are far away from the physical capability and day-to-day movement frequency and variety of our ancestors. Instead we see our bodies as hassles or even burdens that we try to ignore yet must put up with almost as if they are something separate from us. Movement has become one of those inconveniences that stems from having a body, and we try to avoid it as much as we possibly can. However, nearly complete and constant physical idleness is nothing but a biological anomaly, a behavioral void that is shrinking our physiological health to the point of slowly but surely deteriorating our bodies over time. There's no need to be launched into space to spend time in a zero-gravity field to suffer loss of muscle mass and bone density; a physically idle lifestyle on Earth will do.

There are possible adverse consequences of movement practice—although for the most part those adverse consequences are only minor and temporary—but the silent damaging of physical inertia over time is guaranteed. Such damage can be very hard to reverse—or even become completely irreversible—and often people have no idea what caused it. (Lack of movement isn't the only reason, but it's one of the main ones.)

In a documentary I once watched, a hunter-gatherer from the Amazon visited the United States and was following his host to a supermarket. He was absolutely baffled when he saw that his host was trading a small piece of plastic—a credit card—in exchange for all this food. The hunter-gatherer was extremely perplexed when, after the transaction had been completed, the cashier gave the piece of plastic back to the host. How is it possible to procure food that you neither move and hunt for nor trade anything for?

Originally, food procurement wasn't possible without Natural Movement activity. Today, however, in just a few clicks and while using only our brains, eyes, and our index fingers, we can conveniently order a whole meal of our choice to be delivered to us at any time we want. Don't get me wrong, such convenience does come at some cost and efforts, but it's not the same as going out to move in nature for hours. If Natural Movement was mandatory for modern humans to procure food, physical health and vitality levels would rapidly skyrocket, but that imperative is gone.

Although we laugh at a movie like *WALL-E*, in which humans of the future are unable to stand up and walk, we are not realizing that walking already has practically become an optional component of modern life. If walking is an option today, it might become nothing but a notion in the world of tomorrow—if not a memory of the past. (Someday we might hear someone say, "You're telling me people had to MOVE with their body before? No way!") A person who's defined as being in "decent shape," by modern civilized-world standards, might soon mean nothing more than that a person can achieve the extraordinary feat of standing up without technological assistance.

When young people are growing up and observe everywhere around them mostly out-of-condition adults who perform clumsy, troublesome movements and have a reluctance to engage in physical effort, and when every day at school physical stillness is an obligation, and students who want to move are labeled "agitated" or "hyperactive," then what happens? Those children will subconsciously accept the idea that an inept, out-of-condition, or even dysfunctional body is the body we are supposed to have, and they also will think that physical idleness is the default, normal physical behavior to have in life. Despite Natural Movement being a potent behavioral drive and need in children, a majority of us have been taught from a young age to repress, distrust, neglect, and sometimes even ridicule it. Hanging is for monkeys, crawling for crocodiles, jumping for kangaroos—the movements are all some kind of strange animal behavior that we are supposed to outgrow so we can finally become "serious" about life and exercise one day. The truth is that—except for people born with limiting conditions—people aren't born as "bad" movers, and they're certainly not born as "non-movers." You don't even *become* a mover; you were born one.

> **Those who do not move do not notice their chains."**
> —*Rosa Luxemburg*

Alejandro Jodorowsky once wrote "Birds born in cages think that flying is an illness." Why are people concerned about potentially harming their bodies by being physically active, yet they never seem to understand how much deterioration occurs in their bodies by being physically idle?

Have you been led to believe that movement is an option, or even a chore? Motion is not a sickness; however, no motion is *loco*. Most of us are stuck in a self-imposed "movement coma," which has also become one of the most common self-prejudices of modern times. Not having to be physically active is no longer a luxury that only wealthy people can financially afford. It is an impoverishment of life that no one—rich or poor—can biologically afford. Physical sedentariness is a biological anomaly, an artificial behavior, a culture-inflicted imprisonment, and a destructive habit. A deficit of movement is not just a deficit of health and strength in our lives; it's a deficit of *life* in our lives. We have to literally move our way out of it.

The Meaning *of* Naturalness

Theodosius Dobzhansky, a famous geneticist, once stated "Nothing in biology makes sense except in the light of evolution." Biology is the study of living organisms, divided into specialized fields covering their morphology, physiology, anatomy, behavior, origin, and distribution. As living beings, our human morphology, physiology, and anatomy are elements of our biology that come from our common past as an animal species. Likewise, human movement behavior, comprising our fundamental movement reflexes, movement aptitudes, and movement needs, is a component of our biology so significant that it greatly affects our physiological functions, physical appearance as humans, and—originally at least—our chances of survival. As such, Natural Movement is the outcome of evolution or, in other words, of life and survival in nature over an extended period of time. Socially, culturally, and creatively influenced movement behaviors certainly add a superficial layer of movement diversity to the overall human movement repertoire, but they neither constitute the foundation of human movement behavior nor are they a fully satisfactory substitute.

If we're looking for a method of exercise that would be relevant to our biology, we need to look into the collective movement past of our species. In other words, the primary principle that qualifies a physical activity as "natural" is to be evolutionarily natural; simply put, it should be the natural outcome of evolution. In this regard, a lack of relevance to evolution would be a lack of relevance to naturalness. To paraphrase Dobzhansky, we could say that "Nothing natural makes sense except in the light of evolution." Evolution is the foundation of naturalness and as such is a foundational principle of Natural Movement.

Indeed, what is natural movement to a tiger, eagle, or dolphin? It is to be moving like a wild tiger, eagle, or dolphin moves in nature, right? Where do the movement patterns and skills they use come from? From the evolution of their very own species. To become and stay optimally fit to life or survival in nature, tigers don't need to do burpees, jumping jacks, or crunches, use exercise machines, or dissociate strength drills from mobility drills (which isn't to say that humans cannot benefit from these methods). They just need to move like tigers do. They need to practice "Tiger Natural Movement" behavior. Tigers don't need to do the "crocodile," "crab," or "bear" crawl do they? They move like a tiger because they have evolved to be tigers, not some other animal species, and they don't need to imitate other species to figure out what is their own movement naturalness.

Animals' natural movement aptitudes are specific to the species they belong to, and they have been doing these movements forever, which explains why tigers can't fly high in the sky, why eagles can't swim across oceans, and why dolphins are in real trouble when trying to climb up trees. We may minimize, dismiss, and neglect our biology, yet a person can't biologically reinvent him- or herself. If we decide to adopt or conserve the most biologically inadequate lifestyle, we must prepare for a fight we'll lose. Whereas we can alter human rules, we can't alter natural laws. Nobody fools biology; we only fool ourselves. Biology: Either you're with it or against it.

Modern fitness programs that stem from concepts, theories, conventions, or even creativity but not from millions of years of human natural physical activity in the wild are not the outcome of evolution; they're the outcome of concepts, theories, conventions, or creativity. They might involve elements of naturalness, but they are not what I define as Natural Movement. It should be hopefully understood that questioning naturalness is in no way, shape, or form a denial of the intrinsic value or benefits of different physical practices; it simply means that you can't call them "natural" or "Natural Movement." I elaborate even more on this idea when I discuss other principles.

To be relevant to the notion of evolution-based naturalness, you must be able to trace the origin of the movement aptitudes practiced within such a program to our most ancient past—not 1,000 years ago, and not even 10,000 years ago; you have to go back 100,000 or millions of years ago.

Since the time of our early Homo ancestors, we've amassed close to three million years of experience in Natural Movement skills. Not bad, is it? Some movements have been practiced for so long that they have shaped our very anatomy, morphology, and physiology, but they've also influenced fundamental behaviors, reflexes, and even our brain structure and psychology. This significant difference in time frame proportionally makes even a 5,000-year-old "ancient" practice almost look like it's the latest craze. Natural Movement has been a fitness "fad" since the dawn of humankind.

Being "fit" is the prerequisite to any physical activity, but it is actually maintaining physical activity that builds up the fitness you need for physical activity. You don't need to be "fit" for Natural Movement; you need Natural Movement to become and stay fit. Movement is the prerequisite. Trust me, you are not going to "die" if you engage in Natural Movement practice; it might actually revive you beyond expectations.

Exercising should not be a task, a chore, a punishment, or a coping mechanism. It should be liberating, energizing, and empowering, which it can be if the approach, modality, equipment, and facilities would evolve toward more naturalness rather than toward artificiality and technology. We have almost reached a point where people are under the impression that sports and fitness systems are the origin of our movements, whereas it actually is our evolutionarily natural movements that make all sports and fitness practice possible.

Sport and exercise are not the reason why you can move naturally; moving naturally is the reason why you can do sports and exercise. Nonetheless, it is not at the gym but rather on the sports fields that some elements of Natural Movement find their most direct and relevant expression. Walking, running, jumping, balancing, climbing, throwing, catching, or lifting are Natural Movement skills commonly used in regulated sports. I explain why these skills are not considered to be "Natural Movement" as stand-alone physical training when I discuss principle 6, "Unspecialized."

It isn't politically correct to state that our modern society is overall physically degenerated, even when it is clearly so. Just look at the alarming health statistics, which are trending further away from health.

How has modern comfort become so incredibly stressful and ill-adapted to our evolutionary background? A society with increasing medical technology yet declining health is still a society that merely survives. Living healthily is not just a biological necessity or a simple individual option anymore. It is a personal and social duty.

" Before beginning a program of physical inactivity, see your doctor. Sedentary living is abnormal and dangerous to your health."

—*Frank Forencich*

Physical activity has well-documented health benefits, and any type of physical activity is better than complete physical idleness. But that is a backward statement. It should read, "Chronic physical idleness has well-documented health consequences."

To temporarily alleviate, or even mask, physical and mental deficiency or suffering that has been caused by the mismatch between our ancestral and modern lifeways, we humans have invented a variety of coping mechanisms, and fitness training in its modern and most conventional forms is one of them. We are losing physical function not because we don't know conditioning drills or corrective exercise, and not even because we don't participate in sports, but because our lives lack the Natural Movement behavior we need.

The solution to the adverse health effects of poor lifestyle behaviors isn't more medication and medical technology; it's better behaviors, starting with, or at least including, how we move. The *cause* of most physical dysfunctions is movement behavior, but the *solution* to most physical dysfunctions also is movement behavior. Within us, there is an ancestral memory of movement that longs to be reawakened. We modern humans can learn to master again the ancient biotechnology that our bodies represent.

Although a truly natural approach to fitness comes from an evolutionary perspective, a true "evolutionary fitness" approach should involve practicing the full range of human movement skills that are evolutionarily natural. Evolution and biology should determine what you train, whereas observation, experimentation, and optionally science should determine how you train. Natural Movement is to fitness what organic and wild is to food.

But if getting people to move naturally was as simple as telling them to "go climb a tree" then millions would be at it already. Of course, the solution is not in a radical refusal of modern comforts and conveniences, in a "re-enactment" of the caveman lifestyle, or in a "primitive," brutish way of exercising. The repackaging of a selection of so-called "functional," conventional drills, even when wrapped with a trendy evolutionary rationale and primal-sounding name, is also irrelevant and gimmicky. Our evolutionary movement and physical potential is not an unevolved, outdated phenomenon that should stay stuck in the past. It's still natural and relevant to us. Natural Movement has always been and will always be a timeless biological necessity. What we need is a well-thought-out, effective, systematic fitness method based on and involving the training of all evolutionarily natural movement aptitudes that also judiciously draws from exercise science to devise the most effective programs. Natural Movement is timeless, yet it has been ignored from modern fitness for way too long.

> ❝ **Natural Movement has always been and will always be a timeless biological necessity.**❞
>
> —*Erwan Le Corre*

2
Instinctual

"The very essence of instinct is that it's followed independently of reason."

—*Charles Darwin*

Through evolution, biological features—including Natural Movement behavior and abilities—are transmitted from generation to generation within a given species. Evolution in that sense is not something that happened a long time ago; it is an ongoing process from the past to the present time, and you are part of it.

Do you remember the very first moment when you started moving? You probably can't because it was at such an early stage in your life. (As a matter of fact, you already moved to some extent in your mother's womb before you were born.) Experts call the early stage of a child's motor development the "developmental stage," and it involves not just the physiological aspects of a child's physical growth but also his or her fundamental motor skills, ability to move around, and ability to manipulate the environment. This is the early development stage of our Natural Movement. The acquisition of movement skills is so important to your future life and survival ability that your movement-development journey begins before you can even form a thought or articulate a word. Because it is a foundational component of your biological survival agenda, Natural Movement is a powerful, evolutionary drive that is an instinctual, innate behavior.

For this reason, infants start moving naturally without the need for any instruction or even visual demonstration. They follow a species-specific developmental sequence and hierarchy of movement patterns that takes place almost totally similarly in every child. It is species-specific because it has to do with the evolutionary make up and movement aptitudes of our human species: You won't see young children consistently flapping their arms as young birds instinctively do with their wings as a preparation for flying. Flying is part of the Natural Movement of most birds, but it's not part of Natural Movement for humans. Kids may later pretend they are birds for fun, but at the stage I'm talking about they are not pretending to move like other animals, and they're not "pretending" to move like humans, either; they're just instinctively starting to move like humans.

During the first months of their lives and before they can even walk, infants learn to keep their heads erect when they're upright, to roll from the side to their backs, to raise their positions with their arms when lying on their bellies, to grasp objects with their hands and arms, to sit alone, to crawl on their knees and hands, and then to pull themselves to a standing position and so forth until they can walk on their own. While many parents pride themselves on thinking that they "taught" their children to walk, the truth is that they merely assisted them. As for the acquisition of all those other diverse ground movement patterns during the child's first months, it definitely took place without any intervention from the parents, and those movements are not necessarily less complex or

 There is a voice that doesn't use words. Listen."

—*Jalal ad-Din Rumi*

difficult to acquire than walking. I'm not saying that verbal instruction or visual example cannot play a part in a child's movement development at a later stage, but at that very early stage they are superfluous.

I'm also not saying that children and adults could unveil their whole Natural Movement potential solely through instinct without any kind of guidance. For instance, whereas the most basic grappling, kicking, or punching patterns are innate in young children, one must learn and drill techniques to channel, enhance, and extend a basic instinctive ability to fight into an advanced fighting capability and skill.

> ## " Don't you dare underestimate the power of your own instinct."
>
> —*Barbara Corcoran*

Even at that later stage and while learning techniques through self-teaching or someone's instruction, instinct—or a genetic program that is deeply rooted in our brains and cellular memory—keeps playing a major role in the continuous development of greater movement skills. Similarly, despite their total lack of conceptual or scientific knowledge relating to the proper ways to exercise or become fit, our ancestors were unquestionably physically strong, agile, capable, and resistant enough to survive some of the harshest circumstances of wild life. In other words, if modern fitness equipment and methods of exercise had been necessary for early human beings to develop themselves physically, and if we had had to wait until science had defined the laws of and programs for optimal physical development, our ancestors wouldn't have survived, and we wouldn't be here today to discuss the subject. Furthermore, we still would have to send fitness experts—along with exercise equipment—to some the most remote areas of the planet to instruct hunter-gatherer tribes in how to be "in shape" so they can survive.

Over the years, I have taught many fitness coaches who spend their time indoors, doing muscle-isolation exercises and working on fitness machines, and although their muscles have looked good on paper,

their ability to run, jump, balance, climb, and so forth in natural environments were questionable at best. Mainstream fitness and Natural Movement are not the same at all; they don't have the same purpose or method, and they logically produce incredibly different results. Instinct, necessity, observation, common sense, practice, and real-world experience was all our ancestors had to work with, and it is all that the millions of people who still live close to nature have as well. Their physical development took place organically, symbiotically, experientially—in other words, naturally. It worked thousands of years ago, and it still works quite well.

Would you ever imagine that young children would spontaneously do segmental, mechanistic, simplistic, repetitive exercise drills such as biceps curls or "crunches" to get fit and start their physical development as prerequisite strength training and conditioning before they could perform actual natural movements? Of course not. That's because such a conventional approach to physical fitness is in no way a part of our instinctual, natural process for movement and physical development. No science-based training protocol could replace, or even improve, the evolutionary "program" that is naturally built in to all of us. Instead, children develop the full range of human Natural Movement aptitudes through instinctual practice. It is a drive so strong they cannot resist, and it pushes them to be moving almost continuously during their wake time, even when adults around them aren't remotely as physically active in terms of variety, frequency, volume, intensity, or complexity of activity. Although adults mostly sit on elevated surfaces without much movement or variety in their positions, young children sit on the floor in many different ways, always transitioning and constantly in motion; they won't stop crawling, rolling, turning, twisting, pushing, pulling, reaching, grasping, throwing, and manipulating, even before they can kneel, stand up, walk, balance, run, jump, climb, and so on. Do not mistake my meaning: Ground movements are not "simple" movements. They are sophisticated patterns and skills that many adults are surprised to discover that they need to remember how to do properly. However, children are still able to do complex ground movements because of their instinctive drive to move.

Young children, fortunately, have no concept of social convention or other restrictions that might inhibit their instinctive exuberance for movement. Any environment presents itself as an opportunity to explore, practice, and develop their innate movement abilities. It is not something children consciously plan to do at a certain time, in a certain place, in a certain way, and for a certain outcome (or to show off on social media). It is a subconscious impulse—a pure expression of who they are as young human animals. They cannot help it: They are growing!

Deep inside of them, children know that they must move to grow strong, and any environmental context will do, whether it's an outdoor, natural space or an indoor, man-made, artificial one. Children crawl under a table like they crawl under a fallen tree or climb on top of a couch like they climb on top of a small boulder. They don't expect and don't really need a special place to express their instinctual movement agenda; they practice opportunistically. Although adults and experts are quick to label such activity as "creative," in fact it's a tremendously pragmatic and practical approach. Children explore nearly limitless variations of movements, most of which are fundamentally useful and others that might look "crazy" to the reasonable grown-up who has culturally and socially formatted movement behaviors. Are children really creating new movements, or are they simply replicating the movements that every other child of their age is doing somewhere else on the planet, and that generation after generation of young children have also done since the dawn of mankind?

We like to believe that children are only playing. Indeed, they are at play, but that kind of play is not purely about fun. The way children play can be risky, or even aggressive and brutal. They instinctively push their limits. They challenge themselves and take risks. If we were to have adults participate in similar activities, most of us would likely drop out quickly, finding this kind of "child's play" too hard, too difficult, or too dangerous. Our so-called "grown-up" bodies would most certainly not be able to keep up, as if they weren't even built for such Natural Movement activity.

However, without any teaching or consideration for subjective rules and conventions, kids spontaneously express their splendid human physicality through energetic movement with incredibly effective simplicity and total freedom.

Yet their explorative practice is not just random. The "program" within each and every one of their cells demands certain results and the development of particular skills, at a certain level of performance. There is nothing random about it. When you notice a child repeating the exact same movement—such as a jump—many times in a row, it is not only because of the pure enjoyment they get from that action but also because repetition is the key to acquisition. I have observed my own young children joyfully exploring almost every variation possible of swinging, spinning, and hanging from an adult-size gymnastic ring, and I have also witnessed them repeating the exact same move time after time after time with total focus just a moment later; they don't smile, they aren't seeking approval, and they don't get distracted at all. To them it's both fun and serious, both free and dedicated—a thoughtless yet mindful practice.

My point is that it would be a mistake to label children's movement activity as "play" only. Although it looks random, it actually is purposeful; although it looks exploratory, it is often systematic and repetitive; although it looks only playful, it actually can be hard, challenging, and risky. Children are instinctually practicing the very skills that are, from an evolutionary perspective at least, supposed to ensure their survival, and it takes both playful, and sometimes serious and not-so-playful practice. Play is one of the components of an overall instinctive strategy for optimum physical development. Such "work" is never boring or a chore to them. Most often it provides tremendous enjoyment and great satisfaction even when their so-called play gets tough and scary.

The **Physical Idleness Predicament**

Unfortunately, under constant pressure of social conventions and the irresistible comforts and distractions of modern life and technologies, this instinctual drive for moving might, in most cases, seemingly disappear or significantly decrease in intensity. Even though the example set by parents, or the lack thereof, will rarely dissuade very young children from moving intensely within the safe environment where they're usually confined, as the children grow older their drive for movement is often greatly influenced by the example of their parents and other adult associates. When the adults whom children look at every day of their lives are never physically active, sit all day, and can't kneel without pain or squat without falling backward, children may subconsciously assume that this is a normal condition and that Natural Movement is superfluous, limited to what adults can do, a behavior that is not "appropriate" in most social situations, and even something one must avoid engaging in because it is too dangerous.

" The pursuit of normality is the ultimate sacrifice of potential."

—Faith Jegede

The number-one reason why some children lose their instinctual drive to move the way they're naturally designed to isn't just the lack of example of healthy, vibrant adults—or other children—who are physically active daily, but the ubiquitous presence of the exact opposite example: adults and/or other children who limit themselves to standing up and walking a few steps to the next seat. Next to the strength of instinct, mimicry is the most potent behavioral instinct that shapes who we become. (As the saying goes, monkey see, monkey do.) This is because humans are highly intelligent, social animals who learn a lot through direct observation of older humans. If a young child's adult role models for movement behavior provide poor examples, it is likely that the child's movement behavior will not be as "rich" as it should be.

I was personally blessed to have parents who not only encouraged me to go outside and move but who would also show me diverse examples, though only partially, of what Natural Movement is. My parents frequently would take me and my brothers and sisters in the woods, where we would hike for miles regardless of weather conditions. We also climbed boulders and trees, jumped off rocks to the ground or to the next rock, balanced on fallen trees, crawled through dense vegetation, slid down slopes, and so on. The proximity of such a natural "playground" was a blessing, but I was also fortunate to be shown such an example and pushed beyond my physical and mental limitations while participating in such healthy physical behavior with my family. How many modern children have seen their own parents climbing trees and have been encouraged to do so themselves, rather than being told by their parents to never climb a tree so they don't hurt themselves?

" It is impossible to overlook the extent to which civilization is built upon a renunciation of instinct."

—Sigmund Freud

My siblings and I were, to use a current term, "free-range" children. I was free to go solo anywhere I wanted, especially in the woods. I actually wanted to be there as often as I could, first because I just felt great in nature, but also because I wanted to keep expanding my "range." Would it have been the same if my parents had spent all their time in front of a TV screen and told me to not go outside or do "crazy things" such as jumping and climbing? My natural instinct for Natural Movement was fully supported both verbally and by tangible example—as I strongly believe it should be for all children. My parents were not "bad," careless, or negligent; they trusted us and didn't need to supervise us constantly in an overprotective manner. Yes, we took risks—a lot—but those risks were never unreasonable because we had experientially and progressively learned to be realistic about what we could do safely. Nothing bad ever happened.

Sadly, most children today are not only deprived of having a sound Natural Movement example, but they are literally prevented from going outside and taking the physical risks necessary for their optimal physical, psychological, and emotional development. Instead they are told to stay still, to stay put, to just sit, and to entertain themselves mostly through electronics. The message that movement gets you hurt, gets you dirty, and gets you in trouble is very loud, clear, and omnipresent. Which is more criminal: letting kids climb trees on their own and play outside in nature as often as they want, or keeping them indoors to watch TV and play with electronics on the couch when they're not in school?

Those children who are lucky enough to at least play through free movement on playgrounds made for them show the way to adults, but those adults often won't listen. The adults sit on benches and chat or are glued to their smartphones and never physically engage with their children. Every time I have been at a park, alone or with my children, I've been moving naturally. Children stop and watch, baffled to witness an adult who "speaks their language"—the language of human Natural Movement. Then they often try to follow me and do the same; they're excited to be shown the example they've been secretly looking for.

We are collectively dealing with a modern health predicament. Lack of movement is a *major* part of the issue—in addition to unhealthy nutrition, stress, and sleep deprivation—and it's causing an important diminution of our movement instinct and a shrinkage of our movement variability, frequency, and intensity. With this lack of movement comes an erosion of physical function in millions and millions of humans across the planet. Even though many modern sports or hobbies provide an outlet for each of our natural movement skills—for instance, playing Frisbee involves running, catching, and throwing—what proportion of people actually engage in such activities? It's alarmingly low. Clearly, this is not just a childhood issue; it's also an adulthood issue because either you might have lost your movement instinct as an adult, or you might be one of the unfortunate children who never got a chance to fully develop their Natural Movement potential. Regardless of the reason, you are suffering the adverse consequences of it, and as you become a parent yourself, you might not realize how this issue is passed on to your own children.

In principle 1, "Evolutionary," I explained that in our modern, civilized, convenient lives, Natural Movement is no longer a survival necessity. It's been relegated to a mere option—an accessory element of a so-called "healthy lifestyle." There is close to no variability, no intensity, and no adaptability involved in our day-to-day movement.

What about fitness remedies or "solutions"? Most of us have at least one experience with the tremendous boredom incurred by conventional muscle-isolation or machine-based exercises at a local gym. We've never felt that those programs were based on our Natural Movement instinct, or satisfying to them, and the truth is that the overwhelming majority of people consider these programs to be a chore, or worse, a punishment for being out of shape. They are linear, predictable, mechanistic, reductionist, and sterile. They look and feel like factory labor. They are an extension of work.

However, remember the "Evolutionary" principle: Our bodies—and minds, for that matter—are designed for Natural Movement in nature, and both expect us to move and physically behave like our wild ancestors did. Although it is socially acceptable for an adult to "work out" on an exercise machine, it would be considered strange for an adult to move like children do, to move like wild humans do—that is, to run, jump, balance, crawl, climb, and so on—especially in places that are not "officially" designed for fitness activities. We have become, to a significant degree, domesticated creatures. Unfortunately, the process of domestication involves repression, diversion, distraction, subversion, and suppression of important natural behaviors. Our dysfunctional, limited movement patterns and activities reflect the effects of this process. It's no surprise our instinct to move is gone in most of us! Neither is it a surprise that modern humans may "instinctually" attempt ineffective movements when they're forced to physically respond to unexpected real-world situations. Instinct, in the absence of consistent practice and an overall healthy lifestyle, can take you only so far.

We need to stop tormenting our innate nature and begin nurturing it instead. Normalcy is not our friend; it's a silent killer. Conventional wisdom is too often all convention and little wisdom. It's time to make the physical expression of our Natural Movement instinct an intentional, constructive, beneficial act. Pay a visit to the playground and watch how children move. Young children truly lead by example because they have not yet been influenced by the fitness machines and trainers at the big-box fitness centers, and they are still free enough to follow their instinct to move.

Children haven't fully developed their Natural Movement potential yet, but they are actively establishing the foundation for potential future excellence. They trust their human animal instincts, whereas adults are busy "teaching" them not to. We need to start seeing our own animality not as a "lower" plane of behavior in life, but as the manifestation of our biological foundation and essential biological needs that we should not deny. Are you hungry; thirsty; tired; sexually aroused; anxious to get outside; about to yawn, sneeze, take a deep breath, scratch your scalp, or smell your own armpits? Hello,

Human Animal! There's nothing to worry about; you are a biologically alive and active animal. Does it make you a "lesser" person to acknowledge this reality? Does it take away from your superb abstract intelligence, moral integrity, or even spiritual elevation? Not at all.

Spontaneous, explorative, instinctual reconnection to Natural Movement is the first phase of your journey to future Natural Movement mastery, and it enables you to rewire the entire system of your human body so that it goes back to its original mode and function. After you realize again the powerful simplicity and amazing potential that moving naturally holds for your health and fitness goals, it will be time to consider effective methods and guidance to bring your Natural Movement potential to the level it deserves (see principle 10, "Efficient").

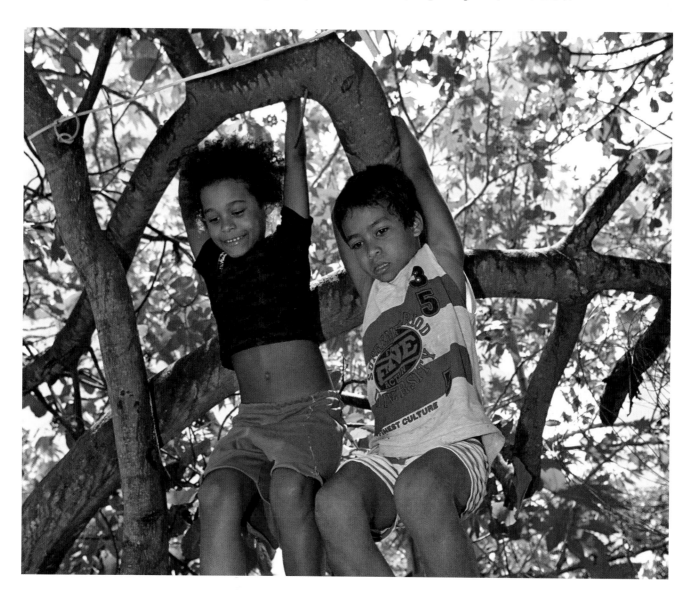

3

Universal

"There is something in every creature born that transcends its time and place of birth."

—Marty Rubin

We all look different, yet we also all look the same, right? Our phenotype, or the observable characteristics that are physically expressed in an individual (such as stature and eye color) and that are the outcome of both genetic makeup and environmental influences, differs with every person, but we all share a set of similar anatomical and physiognomic characteristics that make us look like a human being. We also all move differently, yet we also all move the same.

Human phylogenetic motor skills—meaning those skills related to evolutionary development and diversification—are common among all cultures. Since Natural Movement abilities are shaped by our common biology, which is shaped by our common evolution as a species, it is a biological heritage that all humans share in common regardless of gender, ethnicity, or cultural or religious background. Not everyone may be in great shape, naturally skilled, proficient, or even avid at performing those evolutionary, instinctual movement patterns—especially in modern, civilized populations—but at least no one really starts from scratch. Absolutely everyone possesses minimal Natural Movement abilities, as well as dormant potential for even greater levels of capability.

Moving naturally is not a matter of theory, style, traditions, conventions, invention, or creativity. The Natural Movement of the African or the European, of the Japanese or the American, of the Christian or the Buddhist, of the rich or the poor, of the man or the woman, of the young or the old is not determined by the superficial aspects that define their individual identities. If you are human, you fundamentally move like all other humans do, just like a tiger fundamentally moves like all other tigers.

So, if tigers should move like tigers, can we simply say that we should "move like humans"? That would work only if humans had not imagined close to limitless ways to move beyond Natural Movement that are not universally shared. People skateboarding, breakdancing, dancing the tango, or performing pantomime all move like humans, but those movements are significantly different from each other. All creative, folkloric, choreographic, traditional movement styles are human as well, but they're not universal to all people.

People's movement and physical habits and abilities are influenced by their culture, origin, religion, social status, gender, or age to some extent. For instance, in some countries people mostly kneel or sit on the floor rather than on seats. In some cultures, everyone dances spontaneously and freely, whereas in other cultures people tend to be shy and stiff, and dancing patterns can differ significantly depending on local folklore and customs. However, whenever people do move naturally, such as walking or jumping when navigating through a natural environment, the fundamental patterns they use are biomechanically similar regardless of identity. Moving naturally is truly universal. It is a birthright that belongs to all of us—whoever we are and wherever we come from.

Think about it. In every corner of the world, on every continent and in every country, when given the freedom to do so, children cycle through and master the same species-specific movement stages as they develop; they're driven by nothing but instinctual curiosity and determination. Therefore, you would be hard-pressed to find a single human group that does not possess a potential for the full-range of the human Natural Movement skills. You could certainly find human groups where a particular Natural Movement skill—such as running, carrying, diving, or climbing—is a forte and other groups in which that same skill could be relatively underdeveloped because of the environment in which the people have lived and the survival strategies they've been relying on.

No human group on Earth needs to be taught Natural Movement as if it was something alien to their own culture. If you were to visit the most remote village of the world and ask the people living there if they know what running, crawling, balancing, jumping, and so on are, everyone would nod affirmatively while wondering how you could ask such a ridiculous question. Conversely, if you were to ask them about bodybuilding, tai chi, yoga, or even waltzing, it is likely that they would have no idea what you are talking about. This is not because you are using a different name than the one they're familiar with; it's because they would have literally no knowledge of what you are talking about. They could not join you in these activities without first seeing some demonstrations and having some lessons, because the movement would be something entirely new to them. Why is that? Because those disciplines, which are influenced by culture or individual creativity, are extremely recent with regard to evolution, they're not instinctual to all humans; consequently, they aren't universal. All humans could learn these forms of movement if they were taught, but that doesn't make the movements automatically "universal." Movement patterns or skills that are innate in all humans around the planet without instruction are what we consider *universal*.

But again, you can go anywhere in the world and see people move naturally, or ask them if they could jump, climb, carry, throw, or defend themselves, and they will know what to do immediately. They might be in poor physical shape, they might be clumsy or frail, and they might possess limited proficiency, but—barring any severe physical disability—they will still possess basic ability in all these movement aptitudes. No explanation, no initiation, no instruction is needed. Everyone knows and can perform these fundamental human movements. Our evolution didn't reserve specific natural movements for elite athletes and some others for everyday people. All natural movements are for everyone regardless of individual level of performance.

We may have different eye and hair color, skin tones, voices, personalities, morphologies, past experiences, and views on life, but our human anatomy, its biomechanical function, and its physiological function are the same, and they respond to the same biological and natural laws. Our common ancestors were the same people, and our universal Natural Movement potential was forged in the same evolutionary cradle. We are the outcome of a long, long line of people, and so are our fundamental movements.

Cultural, social, religious, and traditional conventions can seem like boundaries that differentiate us, and we have to look past the many differences to finally be able to see what is universal to all. For instance, dance seems to be quite an evolutionary drive and behavior common to all cultures, but contrary to Natural Movement abilities, it is not universally expressed in the same way. Styles of dance vary enormously from one culture to another (or even from one individual to another). The same goes for body language and hand gestures, which are common to all humans but heavily influenced by cultural background.

Yet, if you were to visit playgrounds and villages around the world and observe children at play, you would see the same thing—children using Natural Movement. All children, given the freedom to do so, move, play, and laugh—these are universal languages. Our Natural Movement commonalities connect us and can bring us together. The universality of Natural Movement is responsible for a lot of its beauty. Natural Movement is the physical behavior all modern humans should culturally embrace, with "human" being the only "kind" and identity that matters.

In the meantime, we observe the emergence of a global culture of physical disempowerment. Our universal birthright of Natural Movement is becoming almost universally ignored, and therefore it's becoming culturally endangered. It's not the future of Natural Movement that is at stake but our future as humans. The philosopher Jiddu Krishnamurti once wrote, "It is a not measure of health to be well-adjusted to a profoundly sick society." Culture should always be countered when it is dysfunctional and unhealthy. To rise above an unhealthy mainstream culture is not a new form of elitism; it's plain common sense and biological wisdom. One should always counter unhealthy cultural patterns with healthy individual habits. Within a culture of unconscious physical disempowerment, you have to cultivate voluntary self-empowerment.

If you agree with the motto "think globally, act locally" and consider how it applies to your physical life, then the most evident way to act locally is to take good care of your own body—its biological needs and real-world capability—and to hope that the human community worldwide will do the same as a whole, before we end up in a *WALL-E* kind of world.

Instead of getting confused by the plethora of fitness programs available, open yourself to the "new" experience, which is our original, universal human movement mode. You are born to move naturally. A vast number of natural movements are available to us! How many do you know? How many do you practice and master? Make authentic, Natural Movement your primary feel-good reflex. Move because you want, move whenever you can, and move as long as you possibly can...before you can't. Ancient moves never get old because they are timeless. The most ancient form of physical training becomes revolutionary. Your body is the technology you need to connect to, and Natural Movement is the universal workout the world has forgotten.

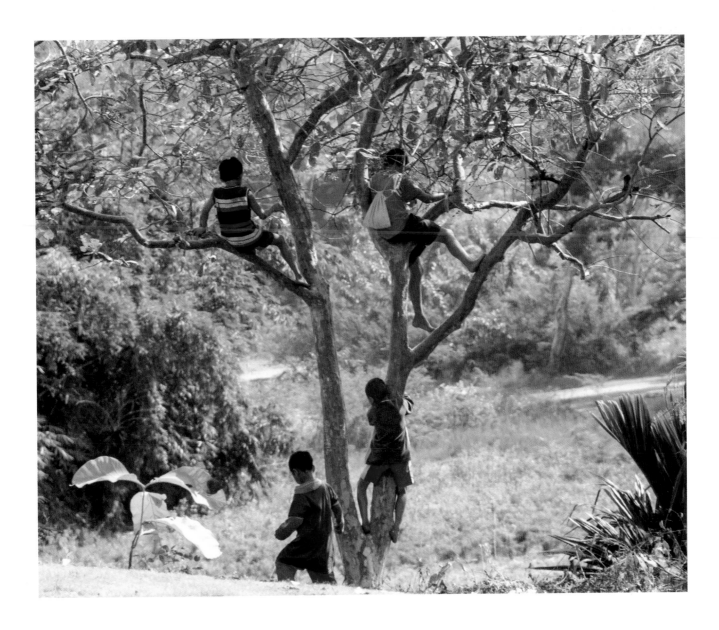

4

Practical

"The essential is always threatened by the insignificant."

—René Char

When I discuss principle 11, "Mindful," I explain that movement is more than a physical drive; it is an agenda. The primary motive for movement comes not from muscles but from an intention in the brain, conscious or not, with the nervous system commanding to the body. But what is the intention? What are you trying to achieve?

The fundamental purpose of Natural Movement lies not just in the vital ability to effectively respond to the challenging circumstances of the real world and stay safe, which is the premise of principle 5, "Vital," but also to ensure day-to-day needs are satisfied through physical performance of diverse difficulty or intensity levels. Natural Movement has an applicability with outcomes or rewards that are both immediate and useful in an obvious, tangible way. Natural Movement is about real-world capability, which itself results from both movement competency and physical capacity. Natural Movement competency spans the whole range of evolutionary movement skills, such as jumping, climbing, lifting, and so on, which require motor-control qualities such as coordination, balance, or accuracy. On the other hand, physical capacity involves diverse physiological adaptations such as strength, power, endurance, or resiliency.

In that sense, Natural Movement it is not just effectively taking place for no obvious reason or for the sake of "freedom of movement." It has a practical purpose. Originally, squatting was not done for the sake of gaining mobility but to enable people to cook, rest, work, poop, or give birth, and mobility was maintained in the process of performing these activities. Lifting and carrying heavy loads weren't about strength; those skills were used to move children around, bring fresh game or water to camp, and

build a shelter; strength grew in the process of performing these tasks. Jumping was not done for plyometrics and stamina, and balancing was not done just for the sake of balance; those skills were used to clear obstacles as one traveled from one place to another. Crawling was not done to imitate animal species, but to move as humans must move when they stalk, hide, or find themselves in confined environments.

Practicality is the primary motive for Natural Movement. The bulk of the physical activity of hunter-gatherers is made of practical physical actions. Regardless of whether a movement is low or high intensity, almost every movement is necessary rather than optional. In Natural Movement, you don't have to guess or imagine whether any movement is easy or hard, simple or complex, safe or risky: It is evident.

Even in history from the ancient civilizations—Assyrians, Egyptians, Greeks, Romans—to the medieval times to during and after the Industrial Revolution, physical training was based on Natural Movement (even though people in those times did not use this particular term). The goal was to form physically capable soldiers who were able to defend the land or conquer more. Beyond the obvious weaponry practice, soldiers' training heavily relied on walking, running, jumping, climbing, lifting, carrying, throwing, catching, and barehand fighting in close-quarter combat, which are all movement skills necessary to fight wars. The original Olympic Games and the diverse physical education methods that emerged in Europe in the nineteenth century involved the same skills.

An old-school gym is not like a bodybuilding gym from the 1980s that's filled with vintage barbells. A gym from the nineteenth or early twentieth century was filled with horizontal bars, ropes, poles, maces, obstacles, and other apparatus designed to train practical physical competency through jumping, running, balancing, climbing, combating, or manipulating objects. Earlier civilizations were practicing Natural Movement intuitively. They didn't know kinesiology, and they didn't know exercise science. In short, they didn't know "better." What those people did in those gyms was all about practicality and being ready for physical performance by training practical movements and scenarios. People understood the practical principle intuitively because they also understood the vital principle: Real-world physical capability can prove vital for saving lives; lack thereof could be fatal.

The degree of usefulness of a movement in a real-world context is ultimately how the practicality of any movement can be assessed. For instance, balancing on a single arm and balancing on a single leg are both physiologically useful, but you would be hard-pressed to imagine any realistic real-world scenario that would demand that you balance on a single arm, whereas the ability to balance on a single leg is fundamental to day-to-day life. Similarly, it is biomechanically possible to train a young elephant to balance on its hind legs for a circus show, but what that elephant primarily needs is to be free to move through the savanna and develop the Natural Movement skills required to stay alive in the wild. Anything beyond those vital movements are optional tricks for fun or show rather than fundamental movement skills.

My philosophy is that it is the practical actions to be performed and the practical goals to be reached that justify movement; the by-products that movement generates are secondary. "Training with purpose" is a no-brainer, but it is also not enough because different people have differing purposes.

There's an agenda behind everything we do. Bodybuilding isn't purposeless, is it? The goal of having a bulky muscular physique is a perfectly valid purpose to those who value or prioritize that body style. The question is, how much clarity do we have about our own agendas when it comes to exercise?

In Natural Movement and the MovNat method, the core purpose is "Practical Physical Capability." This purpose might not seem to be a timeless or universal endeavor, but it unquestionably remains a timeless necessity. Very clear end-goals facilitate defining effective strategies to achieve them. Otherwise, we easily get confused by the plethora of diverse modalities available when we're not absolutely sure of the end result that we are pursuing. A clear goal precedes effective methods and programs. The inverse statement isn't necessarily true. If we agree on specific goals to be attained, we can constructively debate the methods required to achieve the goals. If we pursue different end results, comparing methods is totally irrelevant. Even the notion of "movement-based" fitness programs isn't sufficient to address the issue of lack of practicality. Remember, movement can be anything, including absolutely nonpractical movements. However, although practicing some form of movement activity is commendable, its effect on our physical ability to perform when confronting real-world demands (its practicality) is what's most important.

Modern society has reached a point where little of what we see being done in schools for physical education or at commercial gyms for fitness is actually practical. There is widespread physical ineptness throughout society. Most of us can operate electronic technologies more effectively than we can operate our own bodies beyond standing and walking short distances. Such physical lack of capability is no longer an embarrassment. Normalcy not only makes it socially acceptable that kids spend significantly more time playing video games than playing on the playground but also that they become experts at virtually "killing" characters in those games with their thumbs on the game controller although their bodies are clumsy on the playground.

What's worse is that a new norm has emerged in which physical inability is not even part of a debate: We don't question it simply because we don't realize there is an issue. In today's society, being able to do things that once were normal activities for all people is now considered something almost incredible. In a world crippled by physical degeneration, those people who have great movement skills seem like they are endowed with some kind of superpower. But they're not. They're just physically capable individuals, and their skill shouldn't be seen as anything special.

Everyone expects children to get out of school with basic knowledge that makes it possible for them to perform professionally in the real world. If young people were to leave school without knowing how to read or write, it obviously would be scandalous. Yet every year millions of young people leave school physically uneducated and inept. Physical education programs are ineffective at producing physically capable young adults, which is not the fault of physical-education teachers but an issue with the way PE programs are designed. The result is that it leaves generations and millions of people close to being physically helpless. If you haven't built a body that is strong, reliable, competent, and capable, can you actually call yourself a "grown-up" just because you've naturally grown in size over the years? Regardless of one's muscle size and shape, strength, mobility, and stability, a body and mind that cannot effectively respond to the practical physical demands of the real world in every way necessary hasn't been fully built. You get what you train for...or don't train for as the case may be.

Except in rare cases, the current fitness industry, which predominantly emphasizes physical appearance rather than practicality and real-world capability, falls short of solving the issue. It is as if the commercial fitness technocracy wants to maintain everyone in a state of physical ineptness by promoting physical-conditioning programs that have almost no practical application so that participants come away from the program with nothing other than the facade of fitness rather than building a foundation of physical capability. Fitness is the mere replacement of a biological necessity for physical activity that has ceased to exist, except that the substitute is irrelevant to how we are naturally built to behave physically. The original purpose of movement is gone, and our original movement behavior has gone with it, as if nobody can even remember why we ever had to move in the first place. Practicality is absent from most fitness programs. This is not to say that they aren't effective, which is a different thing. Effectiveness has to do with reaching particular objectives, but those objectives aren't necessarily about developing practical physical capability.

> **Few people actually want to be fit; most just want to *look* fit."**
>
> *—Erwan Le Corre*

The tragedy of conventional fitness is seeing people led to pursue goals that will never make them fit from a real-life practical standpoint even if they achieve all the goals of the program. Few people actually want to be fit; most just want to *look* fit. Many people want the image but not the function.

The notion of "functional exercise" was born as a result of trying to steer the industry back toward more realistic practices and goals, and it has had mixed results. For most people, stepping into any fitness program is a big step out of their comfort zones, so movement-based approaches to exercise—where one mostly stands on one's feet rather than sitting and where one performs full-body movements rather than doing isolated movements—feels revolutionary. Despite being a commendable step toward healthy movement behavior, the conceptual notion of "function" supersedes that of empirical practicality.

Whereas muscle-isolation is rejected as part of these functional fitness programs, functional movement is still practiced mostly in isolation of context (which is something I discuss in detail in principle 7, "Adaptable"). The extraordinarily rich scope of Natural Movement is reduced to a few "functional" movement patterns (squat, lunge, pull, push, twist, bend, and so on), and performing the movement is divorced from the specific demands of the environments or situations in which they normally take place. The result is that there's no possibility of genuinely understanding the practicality of the movements and assessing the results in real time, which is something you can do with Natural Movement because it is mostly contextual.

These "functional movement patterns" are treated as if they're the be-all and end-all of functional performance, whereas the fantastically wide range of actual natural movements is viewed as merely "supplemental." Experts even talk about "transitional movements" when they mention the movements required to switch from one of those "fundamental" patterns to another without considering that all natural movements are fundamental and that all movements are, in essence, "transitional." The reality is that no set of specific movements can constitute a substitute for the full Natural Movement spectrum. By emphasizing a small selection of movements, you are excluding a great variety of equally important practical movements. The problem—which I address in principle 6, "Unspecialized"—is that all those many other natural movements that are discarded are equally functional and demanding, and without training them specifically you can't be competent at them regardless of how much "functional training" you do.

By discarding a significant number of practical movements, you shrink your overall practical physical capability. Conversely, by training such a diversity of natural movements, you will actually improve in those particular functional patterns on top of becoming skilled at a much more diverse set of practical movements and skills.

Gray Cook, a highly respected and well-known physical therapist, lecturer, and author, wrote an article entitled "Function?" in which he said, "The sad truth is most exercise and rehabilitation professionals believe in the functional value of an exercise by what it looks like and not by what it produces."*

It doesn't matter how adept you think you are at particular functional movement patterns, until you submit them to real-world demands, you just don't know what your actual practical movement competency is. Permanently insulating fitness training from the reality of the real world unfortunately produces unrealistically "fit" people. By avoiding the test of reality or leaving it to the individual to figure out—if they want to—physical practice becomes an intellectual pursuit whereby movements must fit theory. If you want to realistically know how functional your body is, go run on natural terrains; jump and climb obstacles; and lift, carry, throw, and catch uneven objects and loads on uneven terrains and you will discover how functional your fitness is.

Is it beneficial to break down complex natural movements into smaller patterns and to isolate such patterns from external demands? Yes, it may be; we use that strategy in the MovNat method, and I give you examples in this book. However, you have to rapidly get past the stage of separating movements from their practical purposes and gradually educate people in practical physical capability—that is, techniques, skills, strength, and physiological adaptations that are appropriate to the diversity and complexity of environmental and situational demands. Keep it practical all the way.

Unfortunately, too many by-the-book fitness experts often turn themselves into pseudoscientists who reject any practice protocol that isn't considered "science-based." The tragedy is that exercise science overwhelmingly addresses the diverse physiological adaptations that stem from particular training protocols because it can be measured relatively easily, whereas very little scientific literature discusses the effects of training on practical capability. Yet there is a difference between being smart about movement and being movement-smart; there's also a difference between intellectual or conceptual knowledge of exercise physiology and biomechanics and having a personal experiential knowledge and competency in movement.

Practical training immediately shows you whether you're effective and efficient. It's not about proving a theory; it's about assessing one's movement capability because it can meet a variety of contextual demands. It's an observation that cannot be denied. Either it works, or it doesn't. "Results" in that sense, or lack thereof, are based on tangible practical consequences rather than theoretical outcomes. Someone once said, "paralysis by analysis," and I want to give that person's hand a warm handshake. The dismissal of real-world context is a rejection of realism, which confines practice to a certain level of artificiality. In truth, by carefully avoiding any confrontation with real-world demands, you are conveniently avoiding the ugly little facts of lack of capability to be exposed so they won't ruin the grand theories you've been cherishing. Theories always need a reality check.

Whereas functional exercise *tries* to replicate a (limited) scope of real-life movement patterns and the practicality is unclear, Natural Movement actually performs them all as they're used in the real world. If the practicality of your exercise isn't clear, it is very likely that it is because it is not even that practical in the first place. Functional maybe, but not practical. Once you've realized the power and specificity of contextual demands and the necessity of matching and confronting them as closely as possible, functional isn't enough and practical becomes the end goal.

---

*Gray Cook, "Function?" Gray Cook website, accessed April 18, 2018, http://graycook.com/?p=922.

When he was about two my younger son saw me do a reaching movement from a Tall Half-Kneeling position I had assumed while waiting for him to take a bath. In the absence of context, I was indeed simulating reaching out to something. He looked at me and simply said "catch." Not "mobilizing," "mobility," "stability," "functional," or even "practical" for that matter. He actually did not even ask what I was doing, he just stated what he saw, and what he saw was a practical catching movement. Daddy was trying to reach and get something invisible. He had not studied fitness theory, so he went straight to the point based on his age-appropriate vocabulary. He recognized a practical movement because he does it every day of his life, empirically and experientially. Fitness experts would see a bird flapping his wings while in a standing position and would think "upper-body mobilization." A child would see the same thing and recognize that the bird is about to take off and fly.

A pragmatic approach to physical exercise starts with a context-oriented mindset. It aims at practical goals, and the relevance of the movement is validated by such goals. This is Natural Movement. It is not about having your body do anything you want but about having it do anything that is or could be necessary in a wide range of environments or situations that necessitate a physical response.

Natural Movement doesn't necessarily demand that you must always train in real environments or situations; the only demand is that you train in sufficiently realistic environments to develop practical mind-body capability.

You might be wondering how play factors into movement behavior because of the emphasis on practicality in Natural Movement. It might seem that play is movement without having any useful value. Wrong! For one thing, utility movement doesn't necessarily mean *work* in the same way play does not necessarily mean *fun*. Play often uses movement, but movements—at least large ones—are not necessarily required to engage in play, as you can "play" while sitting and using only your arms or even fingers. Many games are played mentally rather than physically, which also means that players are not just experiencing fun but can also experience tension, frustration, or even anger. In fact, even when it involves a physical aspect, play is a mindset more than anything: One might have no fun participating in some games, whereas one might find ways to have some fun while performing a chore many other people find boring or arduous.

Playfulness is one of the mindsets that can be employed to achieve utility actions, the same way utility actions can be employed to have fun. Having fun serves the purpose of experiencing fun and ultimately creating happiness, and that is an important purpose. Having fun can make practice more enjoyable and productive, but not always.

In the case of Natural Movement, playful exploration is certainly not devoid of practical purpose. It is an innate strategy employed by most baby animals to develop and refine fundamental movement skills that are vital. Play is the strategy for achieving capability. Even when kids play through movement, the biological, evolutionary purpose is to enhance function and develop greater levels of competency through play and not for the sake of fun.

Coincidentally, once skills have been acquired and a youth has become an adult, the drive to play doesn't fully disappear, but it does diminish very significantly. When hunter-gathers play, it is often based on Natural Movement, such as running, jumping, balancing, or throwing for friendly competition, show, and amusement. That type of play might look like it's just for fun, but the point is also to keep practicing movement competency and for everyone to show that they are still physically capable and adept at supporting the group. However, it is very natural that adults who have been deprived since late childhood of Natural Movement activity and then were led to machine-based and muscle-isolation types of exercise in their teen and adult years would first experience Natural Movement practice as pure "play" because they finally are being liberated from rules, conventions, programs, and artificial environments and equipment that have been limiting their natural physical expression.

Again, play is one of the mindsets that can be part of your practice as well as a modality of training when Natural Movement is occasionally expressed in the form of a game such as tag that would involve many Natural Movement skills, but it's not a finality or what Natural Movement is. It doesn't matter whether you call it play, work, or practice; Natural Movement is not monodimensional in how you choose to experience it. Are you having fun? Are you working hard? Are you exploring on your own or following someone's guidance? Are you remembering and rediscovering? Are you learning something new? Are you growing or

PRACTICAL VERSUS NONPRACTICAL MOVEMENT

I am not in any way being dismissive of forms of movement training that don't aim at real-world practicality. Fortunately for us, our minds are creative enough and our bodies are adaptable enough to enable a diversity of positions and movements. The exploration and practice of nonpractical movement types can be enjoyable and expand our movement horizon very beneficially.

Again, nonpractical doesn't mean useless or devoid of benefits and value. For instance, elite gymnasts display exceptional levels of body control, strength, and agility through the pursuit of acrobatic skills and performance. However, if you can balance on your hands better than you can balance on your feet, then from a Natural Movement perspective you have your priorities wrong. The ability to perform impressive physical tricks or beautiful choreography is part of the amazing human movement potential, but if you can't run fast or long, can't jump or climb, can't lift and carry heavy loads, and can't fight to defend yourself, you are necessarily entertaining enormous deficiencies in your real-world physical capability, which is massively problematic.

There is no opposition between practical and nonpractical movement skills; they are not mutually exclusive, and both have their benefits. You must simply decide which of the two is the priority. Understanding principle 5, "Vital," which I cover next, might be a great help in helping you decide which of the two matters the most to you.

fine-tuning? All of it is a possible part of your Natural Movement practice and experience as long as you never lose sight of the practical finality of movement.

In the same way that trying to match the conventional image of a fit body will always keep you unsatisfied, not having a clear sense of the usefulness of your physical practice leaves you unsatisfied as well. A lot of people are looking for a fitness program that quickly brings results, in the shortest amount of time and for the least time spent exercising. The reason is that they just detest exercising. They see it as a chore and want to spare the amount of time and energy dedicated to that chore. Most often we need motivation not because exercise programs are too challenging but simply because they are overly boring, and they are boring because we are missing the original practical point of being fit or because the point is not that desirable after all. When you're given the chance to see that training for real-world capability and actually testing such capability—so you can see what it does, what you can do with it, and what you're capable of thanks to it—might be the point you've been consciously or unconsciously looking for.

Exercising is a lifestyle option with no social consequences for not doing it. Among those who exercise, training with the intention of acquiring a base-line of practical physical capability is itself an option. Yet since modern lifestyles rarely involve practical movement demands that are challenging, it becomes our choice and responsibility to place those demands upon ourselves and to aim at such a level of capability. It is about adopting a down-to-earth, pragmatic, realistic mindset and objectives. You want to think about real-life situations, the possible challenges you might face that would demand a physical response from you, and how well you want to perform. You want to train real movements with imaginary situations in mind, so you don't find yourself responding to real situations with imaginary movements later.

The first step in becoming capable is deciding that you *are* capable and re-acquiring the most ancient movement skill set—not for a romantic reason but for its practical value. Knowing that your goal is to clear an obstacle or carry a person over a distance is a powerful source of motivation. You never know when people around you might need your physical assistance. Are you prepared? Are you physically helpful or helpless? Physical empowerment is not about physically prevailing over others; it's about being strong to never be helpless for oneself and to always be potentially helpful to others. False physical capability is the belief that you would be able to perform any physical task, including those you've never before experienced. With Natural Movement, you can experience many diverse movements, efforts, environments, and situations in a way that is progressive. You can acquire a realistic knowledge of your ability; you won't have to guess what your level of ability is. Trust and belief come through practice...of the practical!

You don't build a body just by growing the size of its muscles the same way you don't build a human being just by building the body. There are many ways to be helpful to others in practical ways, such as teaching or encouraging others, that do not involve physicality. Yet possessing Natural Movement skills is a great start as they're a form of "equipment" that is available at any time and in any place. You don't even need to imagine having to face any life-threatening situation outside your house: Can you get down to the ground and back up smoothly, pain-free without using your hands, in several ways? If that isn't the case, it already indicates that your practical movement capability is considerably diminished. If the word *practical* that I've been using repeatedly seems a little abstract, you could replace it with *freedom of movement.* How much freedom of movement do you have? How much do you want in your life?

The benefits of a practical approach to physical exercise expand beyond the training itself. You will love the serene self-esteem and self-confidence that acquiring real-world movement and physical competency will bring to your life. If looking fit can boost your self-confidence, think of what having actual real-world physical capability could do it?

Self-entitled people expect everything from others. Self-empowered people expect everything from themselves. Ultimately, we are not dealing with issues of physical strength versus weakness or physical adeptness versus ineptness; it's an issue of self-limitation versus self-actualization. Forming yourself into a physically capable human being to the greatest extent you can—which extends to thriving mentally and why not spiritually at the highest level you can—is not just a lifestyle option; it's a duty to yourself, your family, and your community.

Get your power back for yourself and others. Because if you can't empower yourself, who will do it for you?

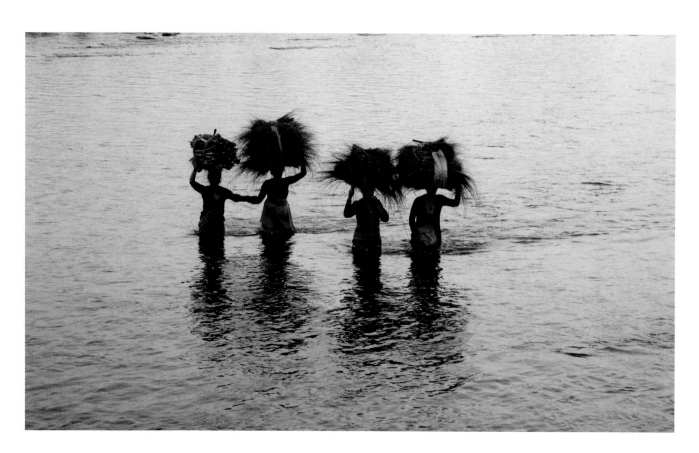

5
Vital

"We don't even know how strong we are until we are forced to bring that hidden strength forward. In times of tragedy, of war, of necessity, people do amazing things. The human capacity for survival and renewal is awesome."

—*Isabel Allende*

While humans may occasionally reflect about the purpose of their lives, the fundamental biological agenda of all animals is not only survival but also reproduction, which ensures that their genetic pool is transmitted to their offspring and therefore perpetuates itself. Even to those of us who are seeking a higher purpose in life, the primary concern of any human being is first to stay alive as long as possible and, for most of us, to eventually have children.

Fitness, from a biological standpoint, is nothing but the ability to reproduce successfully, which first requires that we are healthy enough to remain alive long enough to become fertile in the first place. In that sense, fitness is survivability.

While we definitely tend to take fitness for granted or choose to see it as optional in our lives, that has not always been the case throughout the history of mankind. Even by today's standards of relative peace and safety, life—and successful reproduction, for that matter—is in no way guaranteed for anyone. Movement may have become almost optional, but staying alive as long as biologically possible is mandatory.

So, what is the relation between the agenda of life, biological fitness, and Natural Movement? It is an essential one. Boiled down to its two fundamental aspects, survival is the vital ability to find and seize opportunities while avoiding threats or danger so one can stay alive until one reproduces and until the off-spring becomes autonomous. Whether you are predator or prey, both aspects are ensured by the alertness of our senses, acute observation, situational awareness, experience, what we could simply call "instinct," and also species-specific Natural Movement. In short, the better you can move, the better you are at survival in the wild. Even the most alert prey cannot escape predators if the prey is unable to move, and even the hungriest predator cannot catch prey if the predator is unable to move. The loss (even if only partial loss) of Natural Movement ability would be the predictor of an imminent death. Having the ability to engage in Natural Movement is ultimately what ensures survival, at least within the original conditions of life in nature.

By logical extension, the vital principle makes the case for high levels of physical and mental vitality and health, which effective Natural Movement obviously demands. You are supposed to be optimally healthy

Survival, in the cool economics of biology, means simply the persistence of one's own genes in the generations to follow."

—*Lewis Thomas*

and highly energetic by biological design rather than unhealthy and physically apathetic by cultural influence.

Despite continuous advancement in medical technology, global health levels are declining. What this indicates is that humankind is still in a state of survival, but today that survival is dependent on technology. The "health" industry is not actually making us healthy; it's simply managing our unhealthiness, and for that reason it could easily be renamed "sickness industry." Medication and medical technology enables you to keep holding on to a deleterious lifestyle, but it doesn't make you robust; only a healthy lifestyle can make you that.

Make no mistake, by today's lifestyle standards, if you do nothing deliberately healthy, then it is very likely that you are doing something unhealthy without being aware of it, even if you're not deliberately doing something you know to be unhealthy. In this case, doing "nothing" is the same as doing "something." Episodic resolutions or challenges that do not fundamentally question overall unhealthy lifestyles are smoke screens. Consistently choosing to stay away from lifestyle habits or choices that you know are harming you in both the short and the long run is not just a genuine form of courage; it has become a vital imperative.

In times when physical neglect has become an acceptable state and the accepted norm, those who strive to be their healthiest and fittest instead of being unconcerned and apathetic about the issue are like modern heroes. The most cynical among us are quick at stating that such efforts are useless and doomed because everyone will age and die. But those who do something intentional about preserving high levels of health and energy are not trying to be healthy because physical activity supports longevity alone. Of course, we all age and eventually die, but exercising may not exactly have any antiaging property; it only prevents the abnormally fast aging that a lifetime of physical inactivity guarantees. The point is not to prevent aging, which is impossible, but to prevent our biological age from advancing much faster than our chronological age. Have you ever met a person in his or her forties who physically looked and moved as if he or she had already turned fifty or sixty? That's a mismatch between the two types of age, chronological and biological. Aging is unavoidable, but some people will go

through the years like a good wine; they will age beautifully and gracefully and live as healthily and with as much vitality as possible. Consequently, they will enjoy the greatest life possible for as long as possible. Dismissing any effort to become healthier and stronger on the basis that one is not "naturally" healthy or strong is another very cheap yet very common excuse.

> " **Resilience is all about being able to overcome the unexpected. Sustainability is about survival. The goal of resilience is to thrive."**
>
> —*Jamais Cascio*

Vitality and survival are closely related. The truth is that, while having at least minimal levels of physical and mental strength, energy, and vitality may be the prerequisite for moving your body, moving your body frequently and vigorously is one of the major prerequisites for having physical and mental strength, energy, and vitality. Energy drinks are temporary, artificial energy boosters. Natural Movement helps you generate organic, clean, renewable, sustainable energy. This deliberately healthy behavior is often not just physical but also psychological and promotes positive thinking. We know that our thoughts affect our bodies, but we too often forget that our bodies affect our thoughts. It is not a surprise that the most physically thriving individuals are often those who are the most mentally positive, energetic, or "life-affirming."

Along with healthy nutrition, deeply restorative sleep, and frequent contact with nature, movement is one the easiest, most underrated, and most underutilized forms of health practice you can access.

We must understand that we have been led to see this type of healthy physical behavior as "medicine" only because unhealthy lifestyles have become the norm, and any improvement and return to natural healthy habits necessarily become a beneficial "antidote" or "cure." Healthy behaviors should be the norm, so we shouldn't think of them as being beneficial or healing. Instead, we really should be regarding unhealthy behaviors as being detrimental and deleterious.

The primary focus of the vital principle—the ability to effectively perform natural movements—starts with the simplest, most practical physical actions that take place in the easiest circumstances and ends with extreme, life-threatening circumstances: Natural Movement will potentially save your life and the lives of others. In times of danger, you will never hear, "Play ping-pong for your life!" Instead, you're likely to hear, "Run for your life!"

> ❝ **Luck is a very thin wire between survival and disaster, and not many people can keep their balance on it."**
>
> —*Hunter S. Thompson*

You might very well have to jump, climb, crawl, or swim for your life; you even might have to fight for your life. Or you might have to perform those same movements and physical actions to help save someone else's life. In any case, in a life-threatening situation, you might have to hold an awkward position for some time until you are rescued, but it might not be remotely as fancy and awkward as some of the most intricate yoga poses; it'll be whatever position will ensure that you stay alive until help shows up, and "perfect form" will have no influence whatsoever. Whatever you must physically do in a survival situation has nothing to do with culture, tradition, style, sports, or exercise-science protocols. It has to do with the tangibly useful physical performance that will serve the highest practical purpose, which is keeping you or someone else alive. The vital value of Natural Movement physical competency is timeless.

In a world where modern comforts have come, slowly but surely, to the point of making walking an accessory activity, you might wonder why on Earth you should practice these timeless skills. In a modern context that's seemingly devoid of danger, it is a very common thing to regard our Natural Movement capacities as optional leisure and our evolutionary movement skills as complete anachronisms. We barely need them anymore, right? Wrong. Even a highly technological world like ours is not devoid of dangers. Some are different, and some are new. Dangers are out there, and everyone and anyone can be confronted by them at any time, be it in the form of an accident, an explosion, an aggression, a shooting, a flooding, a storm, and many other potential scenarios. In any of these scenarios, your immediate reaction will be to physically respond in the form of some Natural Movement. Real-world physical capability only seems optional as long as you don't need it and until challenging circumstances make you realize it is indispensable. You could say, "It will never happen to me." My reply would be, "How do you know?"

In that sense, the evolutionary nature of our natural movements, while remaining relevant, becomes almost inconsequential: I am not romantically trying to replicate how my ancestors moved, I am moving the way that makes me and keeps me physically capable in today's world.

From a modern standpoint, fitness is mostly about looks, hence the term *physical fitness* as opposed to *biological fitness*. There is certainly a close link between how physically active you are and how good you physically look as well as between physical attractiveness and mating (and ultimately reproduction).

We tend to obsess about what our bodies look like in the mirror rather than focusing on what we can physically do with a fit body in the real world. When it comes to physical fitness, most people simply want to be "beach ready," which means having a body that looks good enough to impress others in the summertime. From a Natural Movement standpoint, you are not "beach ready" just because your body shape looks good; you also need to be capable of swimming without endangering yourself or capable of sprinting, swimming, and diving to reach someone who's drowning and then swimming back to shore while dragging the victim and keeping them afloat and able to breathe. You also might need to be able to lift and carry that person on land to get help. You can, of course, apply the same idea to other types of life-threatening situations. You might not become a first responder, but you should be able to respond first in the absence of assistance.

Look at firefighters and other rescuers; they might use equipment and technological tools, but do they solely rely on them, or do they also have to physically intervene? When they do intervene physically, what movements are they using? They run, climb, jump, balance, crawl, swim, throw and catch equipment, and lift and carry victims. That all sounds like Natural Movement to me, and it sounds like those capabilities are a much more realistic assessment of fitness than anything else. It's definitely more accurate than looking at the size of someone's biceps.

Could you sprint fast or run over a long distance if it was necessary? Could you jump over a large gap and land skillfully on the other side? Could you swim underwater and hold your breath for at least two minutes if you had to? Could you hang from a ledge and be able to climb to the top of the surface? Could you lift and carry someone that is your weight, or maybe heavier, over a mile or more? You can imagine a variety of physical demands and mentally assess how well you would do. In fact, you should.

To be fit doesn't necessarily mean possessing a good-looking body; it means being physically ready for demanding real-world situations. In fact, authentic self-confidence even stems from knowing that you possess such vital, real-world movement competency and physical preparedness. Fitness isn't for the show-off; it's for real life. Not so long ago, actual physical capability was more impressive than looks. I'm not saying that we should get back to rough times where such capability was a daily necessity, but it doesn't hurt to realize that, in many parts of the world, it is still the case.

66 I have an instinct for survival, for self-preservation."

—Julian Barnes

The point of the vital principle is not to alarm and scare you but to remind you that life is not guaranteed. It's a precious gift we owe to ourselves to preserve in every way we can, and Natural Movement is an important part of this ability. There is neither a guarantee that you will ever find yourself in such a situation nor a guarantee that even if you trained physically that your physical competency and preparedness would be sufficient. However, you are pretty much guaranteed to find yourself in trouble, if not totally helpless, if you are in a life-threatening situation and you aren't trained, competent, and prepared. By being helpless to yourself, you also become helpless to assist anyone else. As a matter of fact, one of the most potent ways to never find yourself helpless is to learn and train to become physically helpful.

We ideally want to be strong physically and mentally, to be physically competent and prepared, and to possess mental qualities for action—including alertness, responsiveness, self-control, courage, and willingness to help. In that regard, we need to embrace a realistic, no-nonsense, situational mindset in the way we approach physical training. No matter whether you call it exercise, working out, or fitness training, it has a higher, more meaningful, and nobler purpose than helping you look better or do more push-ups in a row. Ultimately, physical training is all about being life-fit (or life-ready); the upside is that physically training to be capable is very likely to improve your looks and increase your attractiveness in the process.

If you do some research, you will find countless examples of survival stories that involve individuals or groups of people who are struggling for their lives, as well as stories of people saving other people's lives in harsh, extreme conditions. Some of these individuals may have been physically trained, but most often they aren't. That's not the point; what's important is the thing that all these stories have in common: Natural Movement was the key to staying alive or saving a life. The survivors had to walk, run, crawl, jump, climb, lift, carry, and so on.

Therefore, it is essential to evaluate the practical value of any fitness regimen not just in terms of health, well-being, or cosmetic satisfaction but also in terms of contribution to the preservation of life when needed. You might be wondering what essential techniques or benchmarks you should possess to make it out of any challenging situation. As I describe in principle 6, "Unspecialized," you never know which Natural Movement skill will be the potential lifesaver or at what level you will need to perform any movement in difficult circumstances. Aren't all movements potentially vital?

For instance, I've often met guys would could do many Pull-Ups in a row but who were unable to actually mount the top of the bar they were pulling from.

In a realistic scenario, you won't need to pull yourself to the level of the surface you hang from twenty times in a row, but you might need to mount the top of that surface one time, with a tragic consequence if you can't. This is what happens when the only goal of exercise is to develop muscle mass or strength: Realistic capability goes unchecked, and lots of energy is spent on efforts that do not contribute anything to actual real-world competency. Again, strength does matter, and muscle mass may support greater levels of strength. There is nothing wrong at all with either of those things, just as there is nothing wrong with having a great-looking body. However, the vital aspect of physical training should be the priority, starting with the practical nature of it.

By extension, a real-world, vital approach to physical fitness should do more than involve the training of Natural Movement skills. It should occasionally simulate the scenarios, environments, or context in which those skills must be performed, which helps train situational awareness. Even though a familiar motto to all those concerned with real-life preparedness is to "expect the unexpected," you want to start preparing for what you can realistically expect, especially for those situations that are statistically likely to happen. Nobody is ready for everything, but we can most cer-

tainly prepare for many things, and such preparation begins with equipping ourselves with a baseline physical capability.

With the near complete disappearance of the necessity for movement and the erosion of our movement instincts, we are left with no choice but to embrace a *mindset* and create a *strategy* that enables us to not only get "some" physical activity but to restore our original, Natural Movement behavior. While the intellectual notion that Natural Movement should be practiced because it's evolutionary, universal, and instinctual is already very useful, such notions may not be sufficiently motivating to prompt us to train. But if we understand and take the vital principle to heart, we can start training today with a new powerful motivation: purposeful, useful, helpful, real-world physical training, competency, and preparedness.

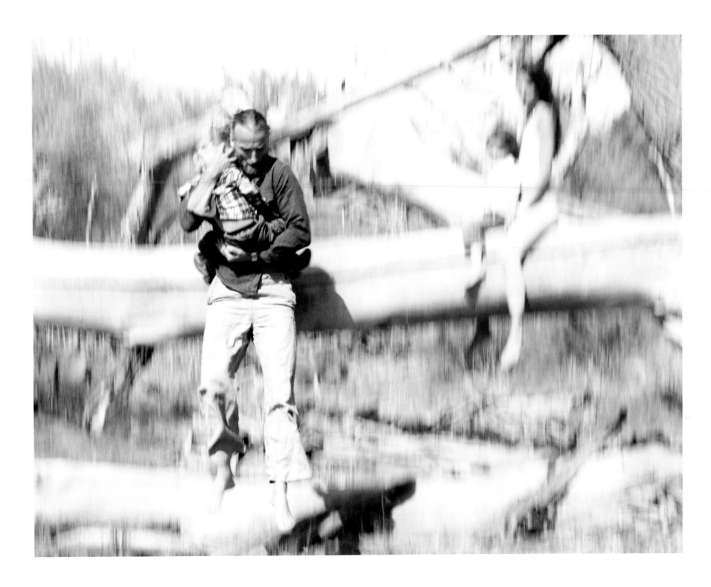

6
Unspecialized

> "We are in an age that assumes the narrowing trends of specialization to be logical, natural, and desirable."
>
> —R. Buckminster Fuller

Natural Movement is unspecialized so that the practice can be both practical and vital. Being unspecialized makes Natural Movement practical because human beings have evolved as "movement generalists," so we could survive not only a variety of environments but also so we could use a variety of survival strategies that require diverse movement skills. As a result, human beings are, from a movement perspective, extremely versatile compared to most other animal species. However, because humans are generalists, we might not really excel at any particular movement skill compared to other animal species: A regular goat easily leaves behind the fastest human on Earth; the weakest gorilla will prevail over the strongest MMA fighter; and many other animal species will effortlessly surpass humans in terms of jumping, balancing, climbing, swimming, or diving. Other species have developed movement strategies for their locomotion that humans cannot perform, such as slithering or flying in the air.

However, from the same movement perspective, what animal species on Earth is as versatile as humans? Our natural movements for the purpose of locomotion are quite diverse, and we also excel at manipulating external bodies by the means of lifting and carrying loads long distances or throwing and catching with amazing dexterity and precision. Such versatility is obviously extremely practical when it comes to real-world movement adaptability.

Natural Movement is also unspecialized from a vital standpoint. Just as you never know when you might have to run for your life, you also cannot possibly know if you'll have to run, jump, crawl, or swim for your life, or lift and carry someone else to save his or her life. To be prepared to meet real-world demands effectively, you need to be well versed in all movement skills because none are optional. How could you respond to life-threatening situations with only a single specialized skill? You would have to be extremely lucky that the physical response required is made of the single skill which happens to be what you are trained for.

Similarly, you cannot afford to be physiologically ready only for endurance efforts or only for short bouts of high intensity. This is because real-world capability is made of the combination of movement competency (the Natural Movement skills) and physical capacity (the physiological adaptation we develop through the practice of said skills). From the vital principle standpoint, deficiencies in competency and capacity are unforgivable, which dramatically highlights the evident importance of the unspecialized principle.

If you can lift heavy, but you can't run fast or long in a situation that only demands that you run, how fit are you? Conversely, if you can run fast and long but can't lift or carry anything heavy in a situation that requires zero running, how fit are you? In those cases, you are "specific-fit," not real-world fit; when you're exposed to contextual demands you do not train for, you're immediately in trouble. I have encountered countless fit, athletic people like that. These people are so accustomed to their specialized exercise regimens that they aren't able to rapidly transition to other movement skills and different types of physical effort without immediately going outside their comfort zones, and their performance suffers for it.

Sports Specialization

Even within a movement skill, the problem of specialization arises often. Say you are a great runner on pavement but you slow down significantly and are fearful of running on natural, uneven terrains; if that's the case, are you really a great runner? Your running performance depends on a type of terrain you have specialized on. If you have interest in real-world physical performance, this simple example of "specialized specialization" and how it affects broad capability should profoundly transform your perspective of what it means to be fit, or simply able and ready. Life includes both predictable and unpredictable events. The predictable events require us to be *adapted*, and the unpredictable events require us to be *adaptable*. Although it is usually relatively easy to manage preparation for predictable events, it can be seriously challenging to handle the unpredictable events because it might require instant situational decision-making that implies appropriate movement in relation to unfamiliar parameters. The more contextual parameters you are familiar with, the better off you are, and vice versa.

The implications of specialization aren't limited to a lack of overall real-world physical capability. Evidently, specialized sports coaches often obsess over highly specific movement patterns while overlooking general functional deficiencies that can actually weaken performance in the specific skills while inducing chronic injury of the body parts that are consistently stressed. Overuse injury rates are extremely common in specialized athletes; stress and burnout also are problems. Training more holistically through Natural Movement could reduce such risks. It could also potentially increase performance in a given specific skill as deficiencies and inefficiencies in overall fundamental movement function are addressed.

Movement specialization is a cultural luxury of modern times. The versatility of our Natural Movement is one of the main reasons humans have been so successful as a species; why should we limit ourselves? What else but culture compels us to see such specialization as something both normal and desirable, to the point of even pursuing specialization within a given physical specialty—for example, to swim using a certain technique but not others, or to never swim underwater, dive deep, or train to water rescue? Or to lift very specific heavy objects but not others, or to lift objects without ever carrying those objects over diverse distances and terrains? In short, what's up with our modern obsession for specialization? Is it because the whole culture around us is systematically pointing us in that direction from a young age?

As a matter of fact, physical education programs in schools are far from addressing the complete range of Natural Movement skills our children should practice—and certainly would love to be free to practice; instead they have them compete in specialized sports from a young age. Sometimes parents also push their children to become the next champion at a given sport. Children aren't given a Natural-Movement-based physical education; they are episodically kept busy with highly regulated sports activities.

The sad reality is that generations of children forced to sports specialization at a young age often end up physically deficient and imbalanced. While a minority may develop a taste for a particular sport or for sports in general, the majority develop an aversion to physical activity.

> **The future belongs to those who learn more skills and combine them in creative ways."**
> —*Robert Greene*

> **A specialist's mind is a slave to his specialization."**
> —*Mokokoma Mokhonoana*

Those children who are intensively trained to become the future champions often end up psychologically broken, and all the childhood years of joy and innocence are lost because they were forced to embrace the mindset of an adult Olympian when they were just kids longing to just have fun. In this case, I'm talking only about those few naturally gifted children who draw most of the attention, but we have to also talk about the majority of children who apparently don't have a special gift; haven't been deemed future champions; don't get much attention, guidance, or praise; and end up disheartened and believing that they aren't "made" for a physical activity. Those children are condemned to experience sports only when watching TV. How unfair and messed up is that?

Specialized Fitness

Even the modern industry we know as the fitness industry is for the most part into specialization. It starts with specialized exercise machines: one for the calves, one for the quadriceps, one for the biceps, those for strength, those for cardio, and so on. Technically speaking, muscle-isolation has never been achieved in a gym; it happens only on dissection tables.

Muscles are designed to work synergistically for movement effectiveness and adaptability; attempting to isolate them is a biological heresy and a falsified physical behavior. The only "full-body workout" I know is that which covers the full range of human Natural Movement. Conventional fitness programs based on muscle isolation reflect a shockingly profound dismissal of the original way humans are designed to physically perform; those programs ignore the Natural Movement potential in us.

Rather than focusing on the lower body one day and the upper body the next day, which is indeed effective for bodybuilding, shouldn't most people simply move their whole body every day? Rather than artificially isolating body parts to bulk them up, shouldn't we mostly make sure that we become skilled and strong at operating our whole body through complete practical movements? The answer is a clear "No" if your goal is limited to growing your muscles for an aesthetic purpose regardless of what you can do with them. The answer is "Yes" if your goal is practical performance in the real world. Methods are only relevant in relation to the goal they pursue, and muscle isolation is highly effective for bodybuilding goals.

A "movement-based" rather than "muscle-based" approach is certainly more natural, but only to a limited extent as "movement" may entail pretty much anything. If you are to move your whole body vigorously while techno music is playing loudly, you could say that it's a movement-based program even though you're not training Natural Movement and certainly not getting ready for the highly diverse physical demands of the real world. You're not even getting ready for a zombie apocalypse; you're still specializing.

Compartmentalized Fitness

Among the more functional fitness modalities that reject muscle isolation, most inherently maintain an isolation approach in the sense that they systematically dissociate, isolate, and target strength, power, endurance, mobility, balance, or coordination with specific drills and programs as if they couldn't or shouldn't ever be addressed symbiotically the way it's been done by all humans until only recently. This is not to say that compartmentalized training can't be used on occasion to achieve specific benefits; compartmentalized training is used in the MovNat method as well, but it is not the priority or the main method.

Is a fully compartmentalized approach—separating mobility, strength, and metabolic conditioning—to physiological functions and adaptations the best way to approach human physical performance, especially in nonathletes? Such compartmentalization can certainly be helpful and effective in particular cases, but why would you systematically compartmentalize each of those components and forget the big picture and the fact that all these "systems" are designed to work synergistically? The common denominator of all those physical attributes and physiological adaptations, and the original "glue" between them, is a Natural Movement behavior.

By evolutionary design, our brain is masterful at connecting and synchronizing what our modern analytical minds are so eager to intellectually disconnect and subjectively separate. Mobility, strength, cardioconditioning, coordination, balance, and so on were neither finalities in themselves nor able to operate in isolation; those tasks were designed to serve Natural Movement, which itself was designed to serve *life*. Wild predators don't train mobility, power, or coordination in isolation before they become able to use their movement skills to catch prey because they would starve to death; instead, they move naturally to perform practical, adaptable actions, which develops and maintains those physical attributes they need to use their skills at the highest level of effectiveness.

In that sense, Natural Movement is not a "cross-training type of fitness." We only need to "cross-train" diverse fitness modalities when we have isolated them and have become specialized in the process. When you are a sport or a fitness specialist, it's very likely that you need supplemental training to cope with the deficiencies of your preferred (or exclusive) physical activity. Such supplemental exercise, which may be called "physical preparation," is an attempt to address the physical deficiencies, lack of aptitude, or even chronic injuries caused by specialization. Ironically, physical preparation to the weight lifter might be to do running for cardio, whereas to the runner conditioning could be lifting weights to gain strength. Were it not for such benefits to their activity, the lifter wouldn't run for the sake of his or her actual running ability, and the runner wouldn't lift for the sake of developing actual lifting ability and practical strength.

We have seen that Natural Movement skills are no longer practiced for what they are—that is, for their practical applications. Instead, they are used for indirect, sometimes ultra-specific outcomes. I have explained this already in my explanation of principle 4, "Practical," but the point is that if we were to seek real-world practicality, we would broaden and tend to equalize our physical capability more. The results would be that we would avoid ending up with massive deficits in our physical competency. If you value being "ready for whatever life throws at you," you had better hone broad movement skills rather than specialized ones.

> ❝ **No single exercise can represent the full spectrum of human movement.**❞
>
> —*Gray Cook*

Even a set of twenty fundamental functional movements—based on the concept of General Physical Preparation (GPP, which is general conditioning to improve strength, speed, endurance, and flexibility to support specific movement skills and performance)—are extraordinarily better than most other approaches in terms of overall physical preparation, but they're still significantly limited and limiting when compared with the broad scope of Natural Movement training. Most fitness professionals and aficionados love the convenient idea that a handful of movement drills is sufficient to keep them "in shape" without realizing that to maintain optimum levels of function, competency, and preparedness, dozens of techniques and hundreds of movement variations must be regularly practiced.

You want to be a well-rounded, unspecialized movement athlete who is physically and mentally conditioned in a "broadly specific" manner. Let me explain. "Broadly specific" means that you're specifically adapted—note that this is about specificity, not specialization—to a broad variety of motor skills and physiological adaptations that stem from exposure to a broad variety of specific practical demands, and that makes you unspecialized and highly adaptable. A single movement variation alone isn't the practice of an entire movement skill, is it? For instance, a Pull-Up is a climbing movement pattern, yet it clearly doesn't represent the full scope of climbing movements. In short, being strong at Pull-Ups may help your climbing ability to some degree, but in the absence of actual climbing techniques and the diverse physiological adaptations that stem from them, you are not at all ready to climb diverse surfaces. "Conditioning" your legs in a general way through specific drills doesn't make you instantly skilled at running, jumping, and landing. Such general physical preparation isn't specific enough; for that reason, it's actually also a specialized approach. Natural Movement training is general yet highly specific. There is no dissociation between strength and other physiological adaptations and specific motor skills, and strength doesn't precede development of motor skills. They both happen symbiotically (for the most part). In short, even though it sounds like an oxymoron, training that's too general is also inherently overly specific. Strength and conditioning is not the be-all and end-all. Technique is not everything, either. Physical capability not only requires both, but it needs both to work synergistically, which is mostly achieved by training synergistically. The real world is way too complex to realistically expect any general physical preparation program to prepare you for absolutely anything.

> **In sports, to be declared an individual of superior physical value, it is enough to carry out an exceptional performance, even if that person is hopeless in other kinds of exercises. The records established by the specialists thus distort the outlook on the value of the individual who is capable in a complete and practical way. The latter, being capable of all kinds of exercises, yet cannot reach the performances of the specialists."**
>
> —*Georges Hébert*

Equalization

Natural Movement is a naturally integrated system in which a fundamental level of capability in each Natural Movement skill—including both the skills and physiological adaptations associated with them—is established in an "equalized" fashion. This is especially true for the beginner, who should absolutely embrace a practice of Natural Movement that's as inclusive as possible. Whereas you might have a liking for or possess strengths in one or several skills and might even occasionally emphasize a particular skill and enjoy the specific benefits of temporary specialization, the necessity of overall real-world capability doesn't really leave you with the option to become a pure or permanent specialist. No natural capacity of movement should ever be totally neglected. The goal is to be well-rounded, maybe with a few sharp edges.

I want to emphasize that this principle does not, in any way, undervalue some of the great benefits of specialization; it also does not negate precious advancements brought by sport specialization over the last decades in terms of technique, training protocols, or scientific data. Sport specialization has proved to contribute to understanding and, in many aspects, to improving physical performance. But such achievements or benefits are not collectively shared. Millions of us aren't pursuing gold medals, breaking world records, or into any kind of sport specialization. Shouldn't we simply aim at achieving our Natural Movement potential and be equipped with the baseline levels of movement skills and physical preparedness required by the real world, while also enjoying a healthy body and life for as long as possible?

> ❝ **There is also hope that even in these days of increasing specialization there is a unity in the human experience.**❞
> *—Allan McLeod Cormack*

Unless you are a pure specialist at heart or a high-level sport practitioner and competitor, you have everything to gain by practicing evolutionarily natural skills in an equalized way; you'll be rewarded health-wise, fun-wise, and satisfaction-wise. Natural Movement is everything our human biology needs in terms of physical behavior. In that regard, any other physical activity is either incomplete or optional.

The bulk of Natural Movement skill acquisition to quite decent levels of effectiveness and efficiency takes place in significantly much less time required than to reach competitive levels in specialized sports. Why pick one skill when you could simultaneously develop many at once without having to isolate them in practice? It is said that thousands of hours of practice are required to master a single skill, yet the progress that you can achieve in many diverse skills in just dozens of hours of dedicated Natural Movement practice is breathtaking. It is often much easier to specialize in a given skill after you have equalized your overall skills than to equalize your capability after you have become specialized; therefore, you should equalize before you specialize.

An unspecialized Natural Movement approach to training can even tremendously benefit the sport specialist from many aspects—in skill acquisition, physically and physiologically, and even psychologically.

As you begin, I strongly encourage you to first address your deficiencies and weak points rather than persist in reinforcing your fortes. At a minimum, before you reinforce your strengths, you should enrich and broaden the practical movement scope you can perform with a decent level of efficiency, even if the movements don't feel quite "natural" to you at first and you're out of your comfort zone. Exposing your weaknesses is definitely being honest with yourself, and it also demonstrates courage.

Lifestyle Specialization

No human is born a specialized athlete or a specialized mover. We are natural "polymovers," not "monomovers." Hamsters run endlessly in a wheel not by choice but because they're caged. Humans run endlessly on treadmills pretty much for the same reason; they limit themselves to a single physical activity because of their culturally induced, self-imposed limitations. They don't know different because everyone around them does the same.

The behavior and mindset involved in specialization isn't even limited to sports or the fitness world. It starts at home in the scope of movement we do—and in the wide range of movements we rarely or never do but that all our ancestors did daily. For most modern humans, sitting, working, eating, and playing on surfaces raised above ground level occupies 90 percent of our wake time; the other 10 percent of time is spent either standing or walking short distances on flat, linear, stable, predictable surfaces. How would you describe such a movement behavior and pattern in a straightforward way? *Specialization.* It is not a "hidden" form of movement specialization but simply a form we no longer notice. For instance, sitting for hours each day is clearly a form of physical specialization that stems from our modern "movement poverty" issue.

Except in rare and very unfortunate cases, we're all born with incredible mobility. Yet how do you explain that millions of "modern"—which is not to say "advanced"—humans cannot Deep Squat any longer? Is it because they don't do yoga, stretching, or mobility drills? Is it because they have opted out of whichever compartmentalized, specialized physical practice would help with the issue? Or is it simply because they never, or too rarely, use the essential natural movement that is the Deep Squat, and as a result they have lost the range of motion needed for it? Mobility is a built-in physical quality, yet it has become supplemental training because lifestyles have become significantly deficient in fundamental natural movements. This is just one example. If you feel that your muscles get weaker over time, there's a special fitness compartment to address just that. If you feel that you get stiffer over time, do yoga. If you feel that you get out of breath easily, you need cardio-training.

If you feel that a "compartment" of your body is deficient, then you turn to a series of drills, an accessory training, a necessary chore, a temporary program or therapy until it feels better. You might have been thinking, "I have a specific issue; therefore, I need a specialized solution," but in doing that, you have separated and isolated one of the diverse physiological functions that's necessary for movement.

Maybe you even have multiple issues that stem from poor movement behavior. Instead of needing a specific remedy for each issue that stems from a lack of Natural Movement behavior in your life, maybe you just need to use Natural Movement to globally address all your functional issues.

Doing compartmentalized, specific training a little every day or a few times a week can certainly be helpful (and yes, it *is* better than nothing), but that practice is a supplemental approach to "fixing" an overall impoverished movement behavior. Can you compensate for the adverse effects of a highly processed industrial diet just by swallowing supplements every day? No. The supplementation of a deficient, unhealthy diet is not as effective as a healthy diet without supplementation. By the same token, supplementing a deficient, unhealthy movement behavior with a compartmentalized solution is not as effective as a healthy, complete movement behavior without specific drill supplementation.

Again, specific strategies or therapies can be extremely helpful. However, they will fail to last for the long term in the absence of healthy, consistent movement behavior. We keep looking at the tiny percentage of deliberate movement activity we could add in our life and that could make a bit of difference, but we are still failing to understand that it is the overwhelming percentage of our unconscious movement behavior—which mostly consists of sitting and standing and that cruelly lacks diversity, variability, frequency, and consistency—that is causing the problems we need supplemental exercises for.

When you think of specialization, you normally think of how it makes you so skilled at one thing you do the most. For 95 percent or more of our wake time, most of us are simply sitting and not moving. When we do move, we are probably just walking very short distances. That is a specialized movement be- havior even though it isn't "training." Does that mean that people today are amazing at walking? Not in the least. First off, most people cannot walk very far, or very fast, without being quickly out of breath. Second, they become even slower and look very clumsy the moment they have to walk on uneven terrain. Last, if you remove a person's protective footwear and have him or her walk on a rocky terrain, they start look- ing absolutely ridiculous, with their arms flailing all over; they move very slowly and grimace a lot. Clearly this kind of "specialization" has not made people into walking experts. The only thing we're specialized in is being physically idle.

But what did we expect? We can't diminish and neglect our original Natural Movement behavior that much and expect to become magically adept at it in time of need. What people need is not some kind of "bio-hack" to help them "break in" their bodies as if they're alien things. People don't need temporary quick fixes; instead they need long-term behaviors. The magic potion you have to drink frequently—every day—is a Natural Movement lifestyle that reintroduc- es a significant number of lost, forgotten, and natu- ral movement patterns. It is not, and can never be, a quick fix. You can't trick, fool, or hack your biology. You can only understand, respect, and nurture it.

The silver bullet you need is the one that shoots dead the perception that "a little movement is good for you (especially if 'science-based')." Let me reverse-engineer this idea: The truth is that "very little movement is terrible for you," and very little movement is probably the reality of your daily life. A lot of movement is your default biological duty. If you approach Natural Movement in the conventional three-times-a-week way, you are still specializing in the sense that for the majority of time, your physical behavior remains very limited movement.

An unspecialized approach means that your prac- tice is not limited to the "special" moment of practice that must take place at a certain time or place or with particular clothing or gear. Not all movements are "ex- ercise," but you can turn every movement into a prac- tice, as well as add many movements to your practice throughout the day. Don't just ask yourself how many times a week you should exercise; instead ask how many times a day you should practice *movement*.

The beauty of Natural Movement lies in the fact that your drive to become better will be so strong that you will stop looking at the clock, you might want to stop counting repetitions, and, last but not least, you might want to prolong your movement sessions rath- er than shrink and expedite them. Rather than avoid- ing extra exercise, you will be seizing every opportu- nity you can find to practice extra movement. You will devise strategies to create opportunities for practice. You will brush your teeth in a Deep Squat, work on your laptop while kneeling, read a book while sitting on the floor, tiptoe when you wait in line, practice po- sition and breathing while sitting, walk or jump up the stairs rather than choosing escalators, hang from that tree branch for a few seconds every time you walk under one, and so on. You will fall in love with move- ment again, and you will want to move all the time.

You are not switching to a different body or be- coming a different person the moment you stop exer- cising. Your activity may change, but the person you are and the biology that is alive in you won't change. Just like anything else that you do, movement exercise is not solely something you do; it's an expression of who you are. Experiencing and manifesting who you are is never compartmentalized; it's an uninterrupted process. The you who is exercising and the you who is physically inactive are the same person. The more you realize this continuum, the more the illusion of a separation between the different activities and occu- pations in your life becomes clear. Only the activities differ; the person is the same.

Depart from your physically idle self and reunite with the physically live one by reconnecting with the original, diverse Natural Movement behaviors all hu- mans once practiced.

7
Adaptable

"Adaptability is the simple secret of survival."

—*Jessica Hagedorn*

Contextual Demands
environment and situation create contextual demands

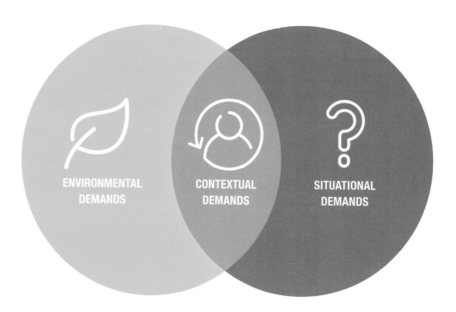

Adaptability is the essence of evolution. Evolutionarily and biologically speaking, the fundamental reason why animals—including humans—have a brain is for locomotion and so they can perform adaptable movement within complex environments and situations that demand displacement. Plants, on the other hand are incapable of locomotion, which is why they do not need a brain.

Not surprisingly, adaptability is a core principle of Natural Movement and its practice. With regard to movement, what do we have to adapt to? To constantly changing context, including diverse environmental variables and changing situational demands. A context is primarily a combination of an environment and a situation. Adaptability is your ability to respond, through your movement and physical effort, to contextual demands that are either chosen by you or placed upon you.

It is important to understand the difference between environmental variables and situational ones. Natural Movement inherently adapts to your direct environment and its specific parameters (muddy, sandy, icy, stony, dry, wet, cold, hot, smooth, rugged, slippery, flat, inclined, declined, narrow, wide, stable, unstable, linear, curved, and so on), as well as adapting to the situation you are dealing with (usual or unusual, safe or dangerous, predictable or unpredictable, urgent or insignificant, short or long duration, intentional or accidental). *Adaptability involves a reaction to or an interaction with something external to ourselves.* In some cases, like fighting, it is not just where the fight takes place that is the environment. The opponent's body and movement are environmental factors, with their ill intentions toward us being the situation, which makes a single individual practically a whole context to deal with. In a way, the term *contextual adaptability* is redundant because adaptability always means reacting to the context.

Imagine you're running on flat surfaces but those surfaces alternate between being soft and hard. Your gait will have to go through minute adjustments to remain as efficient as possible on both surfaces because the environmental variables are changing over distance. What about if you're running to the top of a hill and then running back down? Though the environment itself remains the same, your direction, orientation, position, and movement interaction with the environment is nonetheless modified. You are adapting to it. In fact, intentionally or not, consciously or not, you *must* adapt to it to remain as effective and efficient as possible.

Situations are also part of the context we must adapt to. A situation is not necessarily something unexpected, challenging, or even unique. For example, right now you might be casually sitting and reading. This situation implies that you'll be holding a particular position for some time, and although it doesn't seem to be anything special you have to adapt to, it actually is to a relative degree. During the day you could be working, relaxing, going through a routine, dealing with problems, having a party, doing the same old thing, or trying something new. You might be doing something you've chosen to do or something that's been forced on you and you must react to. Depending on the case, you might have to remain idle or move intensely; you might have to be physically active for only seconds or a whole day. You might have a clear and simple path in mind or have to use snap judgment and make hard decisions.

Maybe your context today is to stay in an office and sit for many hours. Maybe it is to be in the woods and hike for hours. Those are two significantly different contexts. You will have to adapt to one or the other both from a movement perspective, a physiological perspective, and a psychological perspective. Even the seemingly least physically active context demands a particular behavior and response from you, which you may not perceive because you're accustomed to it.

> **" Adaptability is being able to adjust to any situation at any given time."**
>
> —*John Wooden*

You could find yourself in a natural environment yet decide to just sit there if the situation does not demand movement from you. In this case the situation is defined by your own decision to stay idle. However, if a predator lurks nearby, or if hunger, cold, or nasty bugs start to overwhelm you, the situation will change, and you might be forced to move because of a situational demand and your self-preservation instinct. The opposite example would be that, while you are confined to a small, empty room, you nonetheless want to engage in Natural Movement practice. The range of movement you could do is still relatively broad, but because the only environmental variables you can interact with are flat, linear surfaces within a small area, it is not nearly as broad as if you were in a larger, more diverse area, such as the woods.

The *environment* is where you move, and it influences how you move. The *situation* is either what you choose to do or what happens to you. It's also how you choose to respond to what happens to you, and it influences how you should perform. Say you are going on an easy and relaxed hour-long hike on your favorite trail. The weather as you start is gorgeous, but it suddenly changes dramatically, soaking you in a cold rain and making the trail muddy, slippery, and difficult. The hike ends up lasting several hours. The sudden weather change causes a radical modification in the environmental demands, which affect your gait and overall physical effort. On a different day, the gorgeous weather might not change, but an unusual event could happen, which forces you to swiftly run, jump, crawl, and climb to the best of your ability to get back to the trailhead.

Instead of merely hiking, your physical experience turns into an intense, prolonged, and exhausting "obstacle course." In both cases, even though the trail is very familiar to you, you have a completely different experience because the context radically changes due to an environmental or a situational change. In fact, the whole context might be altered also because of you. Indeed, your ability to perform and adapt relies on your physical and mental state in the moment. Being exhausted or sleep-deprived, being cold and numb, being ill, being doubtful, afraid, or distracted are some individual parameters that can affect your ability to adapt.

You can't predict what will happen. The point is, are you ready for whatever comes? How adaptable are you?

> **❝ Life is 10% what happens to you and 90% how you react to it."**
>
> *—John Wooden*

Adapted *Versus* Adaptable

Real-life physical action occurs because of contextual demands that are sometimes predictable and sometimes unpredictable. *Context is not necessarily easy to handle just because it's predictable, and it's not necessarily challenging to handle just because it's unpredictable.* Your level of physical capability and mental control in relation to the level of difficulty of the context determines how easy or hard the context is. Regardless of whether context is predictable, context is rarely linear. If the environment or the situation changes, the context changes. When context changes, contextual demands change, and physical behavior should change.

How much difficulty can you handle before you reach the limits of your capability and how much complexity can you handle before you reach the limits of your adaptability? You will realize that levels of adaptability are the true measure of capability.

Let's use a concrete example of an individual who's fit enough by conventional standards to sprint really fast on an athletic track. This person is trained for sprinting—in short, the person is adapted to this movement and effort. Now the same person is forced to run for miles on a rocky terrain, and because she is not trained for such terrains, distance, and duration, she might get fatigued rapidly and might become injured with a twisted ankle. Despite a specific adaptation to running, the running capability of this individual is tremendously reduced by over-specialization in environment, movement pattern, and physiological effort, which means she has low adaptability when exposed to unusual types of challenges and stresses in running. *Adapted* and *adaptable* are not the same.

In the absence of contextual necessity, it's deliberate practice that is the input necessary for both adaptation and adaptability. However, adaptation and adaptability are not exactly the same. *Adaptation* is what consistent practice made you acquire, be it motor skills or physiological improvement. It's not the finality of training; it's the means to an end. *Adaptability* is what you must do and display as you move to be effective and efficient in a real context. Without practice of a wide scope of contextual demands—real or simulated—you can't develop adaptability. Just a bit of complexity may defeat you: a simple obstacle in your way as you sprint, an uneven surface where you lift or land, an unstable surface where you balance, a surface from which you hang that's much thicker than usual, and so on.

Although the environment where you move and physically perform might be random and the situation chaotic, how you physically respond is geared for a particular outcome: practical effectiveness and ideally efficient and safe performance.

Adaptability in Natural Movement is not just how you respond in the moment; it actually requires a perception and anticipation of the immediate future to enable fast responses that are both deliberate and reflexive. You only move "randomly" because you have no idea what you are doing or how to do what you need to be doing. Simply put, you do random things because you have never had to adapt to such demands before. You only feel that you must "improvise" because you've never learned techniques or consistently trained for conditions like the context you are dealing with. Your movement isn't random or improvised when you're trained and experienced to reflexively move in a way you know fits best for a given context and that you're able to instantly adapt in every way necessary, move after move; your movement is *adaptable*. There's more than one way to jump, yet how many patterns or techniques have you experimented with? On how many diverse environmental variables have you practiced those jumping moves to increase their adaptability?

 Take in every detail of your environment and adapt."

—Carlos Wallace

The biggest disservice ever done to physical training was removing natural environmental variables and demands. People doing movement patterns in isolation from environmental demands are like goldfish in a bowl—going in circles, bored, living a useless life.

Originally, or evolutionarily speaking, movement was rarely dissociated from external demands as those demands couldn't be dismissed or ignored. Environments and situations always impose changes in the way movements are performed in terms of pattern and physiology, which leaves the body no choice but to adapt at every level and to work at the level it has to.

Adaptation occurs when a specific and repetitive input and challenge is imposed to your nervous system and to your physiology; it thrives on consistency. This notion that your body adapts to demands as it experiences them consistently has been termed the Specific Adaptation to Imposed Demand (SAID) principle, and it applies to both motor skills and physiological adaptations. Simply put, with regard to motor skills and physiological adaptations, you only own what you practice.

The more diverse the contextual demands you subject yourself to, the more varied the adaptations and the more adaptable you become. The effect of linearity and predictability of most gyms and the absence of a diversity in environmental opportunities to expose and address deficiencies in physical performance leads to an "atrophy" in the movement adaptability of athletes to the benefit of a few "hypertrophied" adaptations, such as strength or metabolic conditioning. Don't get me wrong: Strength and metabolic conditioning are extremely valuable, but without adaptable movement skills to operate them, physical training is specialized, which leads to deficiencies. Although focusing on specific adaptations is understandable from a highly specialized athletic perspective, real-world capability depends on a much greater diversity of skills and adaptations.

To adapt is to move ahead."

—Byron Pulsifer

Freedom *of* Movement

From a Natural Movement perspective, freedom of movement lies in our ability to adequately respond both to a changing environment and to changing situations in the most minute, accurate, and efficient way possible. It doesn't mean being free of natural laws and efficiency principles but being free of traditional, conventional, or self-imposed limitations so you can instantly identify the most appropriate physical response to the context.

The diversity of Natural Movement techniques and movement variations doesn't stem from subjective or superfluous movement creativity that has no practical value. When you're running over uneven terrains, climbing a tree, or jumping over an obstacle, you're not being creative, really; you're just being adaptable. You're rediscovering what your ancestors collectively placed in your cellular memory, and you're making it your own. Natural Movement variety is an inherent biological necessity to physically perform and adapt to the near endless environmental complexity of the natural world.

Biologically speaking, as well as from the practical and vital perspectives of Natural Movement, it's a mistake to dismiss the context in which movement was originally shaped. Without an "in-context" assessment of your movement capability, you don't take risks, and you don't expose your potential flaws by confronting them with external demands. Your moves may be complex when they're context-free (in other words, they're performed on flat, even ground), but they aren't adaptable. Simply put, you have no skin in the game. When people train contextually they learn to adapt quickly because they aren't insulated from demands external to themselves or from the consequences of their deficiencies. Think of it this way: Meditating in a quiet place is easier than meditating in a chaotic place. By the same token, moving with control in a context-free environment is easier than moving in a complex environment.

Perfect Form

In Natural Movement, "perfect form" is seen as a highly misleading term; if I ever had to define "perfect form," I would say that it's the movement that adapts the best to context, not that conforms the best to a convention that stems from tradition, analytical interpretation of a scientific theory, or a subjective individual criteria. When movement practice is permanently absent from interaction with the environment and external variables, adaptability becomes unnecessary; in fact, we start to avoid it.

Under traditional fitness practice and theory, reaching "perfect form" starts with controlling the context by first restricting environmental variables as much as possible and then by imposing a situation where only predefined positions or movements are allowed. An example is an exercise machine that mechanically dictates the exact movement pattern

your body can follow. Another example is a tradition that conventionally dictates the exact position your body must assume. In any case, your body is either mentally or physically forced to conform to a certain behavior.

Conformism and adaptability are radically opposing notions, and a "natural" approach to physical exercise that avoids adaptable movement interaction with nature is not actually natural at all.

From a MovNat standpoint, movement is either technically efficient or inefficient, but ultimately it is the form that adapts best with your direct environment or the situation at hand that matters the most. Whereas efficient running technique normally implies, among other criteria, a straight back, you'd still better round it and lean forward to avoid running into a low-hanging branch, right? That's adaptability.

If instead you were to prioritize the dogma of perfect form over pragmatism and adaptability, you would bang your face into that low-hanging branch. There is no way you can ignore real-world conditions to fit your idea of what perfect movement should look like. This explains why taking a leg-extension machine to the woods or doing "body-weight" muscle-targeting drills in nature does not qualify as a "natural" way of exercising. Being in nature and interacting with it in a practical and adaptable way are not the same.

> ❝❝ **We should train muscles in the way we use them."**
>
> —*Gray Cook*

The naturalness of your movement behavior primarily lies in your movements' practicality and adaptability to the environment rather than in the naturalness or artificiality of the environment where you perform them. Machines and conventions do not breed adaptability; they *restrict* it.

Low Adaptability, Small Comfort Zone

We have seen how the evolutionary mismatch between the lifeways and conditions of our ancestors and modern humans is affecting us, and that includes our movement and physiological adaptability, both of which have shrunk considerably. I'm not saying that adaptability has completely disappeared from our everyday lives; we keep physically adapting, more or less passively and more or less effectively, to a variety of environmental stressors, such as the kind of seats in which we sit, how we carry children and grocery bags, the type of shoes or clothing we wear, the type of mattress where we sleep, and so on.

Yet modern culture, which promotes efficient management of pretty much everything in our lives, ends up regulating and standardizing most aspects of our day-to-day environments, and that tends to make our behaviors within such environments more homogeneous, global, and inherently predictable. Without our awareness, we tend to automatize our mental or physical behaviors to turn them into routines we can then optimize. Change becomes our enemy, and the deviation from what we've accustomed ourselves to expect becomes an unwelcome challenge that we must avoid by suppressing undesired variations and variables. This is very paradoxical of the era of abundant choice we live in.

> ❝❝ **Action and adaptability create opportunity."**
>
> —*Garrison Wynn*

The same observation applies to physical practice or training. If your environment is all square, rectangle, flat, and linear, you're in *big* trouble. Your brain and body aren't meant to live in a box. If your physical behavior is overly dictated by traditions, conventions, or programs, you also are in trouble. Your central nervous system and body are not supposed to be limited that way.

Adaptation does not take place without repetition, but adaptability does not develop out of repetitiveness in the absence of external variability. Practice wise, *repetition* is the replication of a pattern of position, movement, or effort. It is necessary for learning new skills, optimizing existing ones, or triggering particular physiological adaptations.

Repetitiveness starts when repetition stops producing improvement. It's the end of progress and the death of adaptability. Although an emphasis on the same patterns and the same measurements may be desirable from a specialized-sports perspective, from a real-world capability perspective, repetitiveness is a big issue because it causes you to lose sight of *everything* that you're not measuring, assessing, and preparing for. Your focus on particular adaptations blinds you to the big picture, which is adaptability.

Variety in physical training may imply ten or twenty different exercises, maybe more. Variety in Natural Movement implies dozens of techniques and several hundred movement variations. However, variety alone isn't enough: Natural Movement involves near constant *variability* in the way those movements are done in terms of intensity and volume, the way they are combined and transition from one to another, and environmental complexity (surfaces, shapes, angles, distances). Including variety and variability isn't a random thing; you can determine both with precision and follow a customized pattern until you've achieved the desired progress or gain. Thanks to an incredible potential for variability in movement patterns, volume, intensity, and environmental complexity, Natural Movement practice avoids ever becoming repetitive.

> 66 **Set patterns, incapable of adaptability, of pliability, only offer a better cage. Truth is outside of all patterns."**
>
> *—John Wooden*

The more you reduce exposure to variety and variability in training, the more you suppress the necessity for adaptability, which in turn shrinks your ability to become or remain adaptable. By shrinking adaptability, you narrow your comfort zone because a comfort zone that is rarely challenged does not remain at the same level; it gets smaller and smaller over time. By being overly specific, you become very comfortable with the particular movement or effort that gets all your attention and energy, but what about everything else? It doesn't matter that you may have been active while you were growing up. After decades of physically idle adult life, you tend to resist movement activity because it instantly takes you out of your comfort zone. Although your physical comfort zone was much greater when you were a kid, it has since shrunk dramatically.

> 66 **It is not balance you need but adaptability."**
>
> *—Erwin Raphael McManus*

As your adaptability and comfort zone shrink, your freedom in life also shrinks. Because you can adapt to fewer variables, you can do less and will be less daring. You become less open to imagination and opportunities because you have become unable to handle the challenges they represent. Instead, you prefer to remain confined to the safe limits of your self-imposed, controlled routines, habits, and day-to-day context. Becoming less adaptable means you become less robust and more fragile. This statement applies to movement practice, physical training, and the way you live your life. Start thinking outside of the box when you think about movement. You're not a machine. You're a human animal with an extremely versatile ability to move. You're super adaptable by nature.

Routines that cease to evolve are dead-ends, and the only way out is to go outside your comfort zone. Ancient Greek philosopher Archilochus once said, "We don't rise to the level of our expectations, we fall to the level of our training." So, the closer your training is to the kind of challenges you might encounter in the real world, the greater the chance that you'll be successful in those challenges. Knowing the incredible variety of contextual demands in the real world, you must make sure your physical practice addresses movement adaptability.

NOTE

Do you know how hard it is for robotic engineers to replicate some of the simplest movements humans do every day without noticing? We are capable of prodigious movements, starting with all our natural ones, and they all have an incredible ability to adapt to our environments. So why limit yourself to only the movements that you can do on an exercise machine?

Move in environments that encourage you to engage complex and adaptive motor skills. If you don't have a challenging situation happening to you, simulate one. Such environments and situations can even be reproduced within controlled environments to provide the necessary scalability that will ensure you safely progress to the next levels of challenge.

The increased ability to deal effectively with environmental and situational variety, complexity, and difficulty you gain through Natural Movement practice will unlock your true human fitness, and it will carry over to all areas of your life in the form of greater self-confidence, resourcefulness, and creativity. Although you might never master your environment, you can learn to master how you move through it.

You have to understand that adaptability to environmental variety involves more than movement; it also has a physiological aspect, including adapting to changing weather conditions. Introducing Natural Movement to your daily routine might at first be a big step out of your comfort zone, but you will rapidly realize that it is a huge step toward a significantly greater comfort zone in your body and life.

The more technologically comfortable and convenient our day-to-day lives become, the more we need to reclaim the value and ability of physical and physiological adaptability through strategic lifestyle practice involving progressive discomfort and efforts, which starts with Natural Movement training. Movement adaptability is both the greatest demand and the greatest reward. Adaptable movement is the "holy grail" of Natural Movement.

" The art of life lies in a constant readjustment to our surroundings."

—*Kakuzo Okakura*

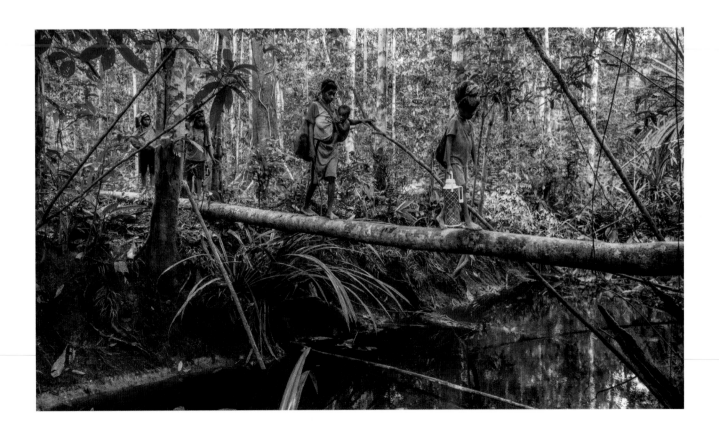

8
Environmental

"The future will belong to the nature-smart—those individuals, families, businesses, and political leaders who develop a deeper understanding of the transformative power of the natural world and who balance the virtual with the real. The more high-tech we become, the more nature we need."

—Richard Louv

As a species, we weren't designed in a lab and made from synthetic components just as we weren't meant to be physically idle most of the time or to live in artificial environments. Over millions of years of evolution, nature is the cradle where early humans organically, intuitively, and empirically experimented, tested, developed, and transmitted to the next generation their human Natural Movement aptitudes. Wild, natural environments provided the greatest number of variables in terms of terrain, surface, texture, or weather. In the previous principle, "Adaptable," I mentioned that animals have a brain for the primary purpose of solving the immense challenge that is adaptable movement to effectively and safely displace their bodies through complex natural environments. Our brains weren't designed to help us navigate linear, sterile, predictable, artificial environments.

Compound—which might also be called multi-joint or multi-planar—or full-body movement patterns might suffice to make practice functional from an anatomical and physiological standpoint, to some extent at least, but they aren't sufficient to make physical practice natural in the absence of contextual adaptability. Obviously, we must have anatomically functional bodies to effectively perform movement, but there is an enormous difference between *anatomical* function and *practical* function. Anatomical function relates to the functioning of the body and particularly to its basic movement patterns—pulling, pushing, twisting, and so on—regardless of the environmental or situational variables where such movement patterns are supposed to be performed. In short, anatomical functional exercise is "context-free."

What that means is that although some functional patterns might look complex, they are performed without interaction with complex external variables.

This is equivalent to a musician practicing without an instrument; they may move their fingers in a way that simulates how they interact with the instrument, but there isn't any external sensory feedback to assess. To become a musical virtuoso, a person must practice on an actual instrument; otherwise, the person is just playing air guitar (or air piano or air violin), right?

The beneficial aspect of functional exercise is that it trains movement patterns rather than muscles. But should you train movements in isolation from the environment where they are normally done? My answer is no.

Simplifying movement performance to its core patterns irrespective of context may be a temporary strategy, which also is used in the MovNat method; the purpose is to isolate fundamental patterns to better assess and improve them. However, systematically practicing this way is heresy. If adaptable movement within complex environments is the original reason for Natural Movement, then what is the point of systematically dissociating the two?

Whenever possible, movement patterns must be "reintroduced" within the environment where they should be done. It's vital to your central nervous system that you gradually practice motor control with exposure to diverse contextual variables, from simple to difficult. Doing so breeds adaptability, which enhances movement competency. Without exposure to realistic physical variables, the adaptability of motor control remains dormant, and low movement adaptability is not an expression of high levels of functionality.

Fortunately, this principle doesn't mean that we need to practice Natural Movement only in natural contexts; clearly one can practice or use Natural Movement also in urban or artificial environments.

Evolutionary psychology hasn't limited how we psychologically behave; it includes a natural instinct to move that's irrespective of the naturalness of the environment. This is exemplified by children who crawl, jump, hang, and climb anywhere possible, including a living room or man-made playgrounds; by climbers who train indoors on artificial climbing surfaces; or simply by any wild animal that ventures through a city. Falcons in large cities perch on top of the tallest buildings as if they were high cliffs; they prey on smaller city animals the same as they do in nature. Our Natural Movement behavior doesn't go away just because the environment becomes artificial. Even when a person's conscious motivation for running on a treadmill in a gym is that they are doing it to "stay in shape" and to maintain their "cardio," that person could very well be subconsciously expressing part of their Natural Movement instinct by running on a surface that simulates a long distance.

Because movement is contextual and the environment where movement takes place represents the primary aspect of context, the Environmental principle is strongly related to principle 7, "Adaptable." Movement should adapt to the environment where it takes place.

From the practical standpoint of readiness, adapting to the environment makes sense. Do you want to be adapted only to clean, linear, non-slippery, reliable, and predictable environmental variables, or do you want to become adaptable to a vast array of random variables? Do you want to be able to walk easily on pavement but be in trouble when you're hiking in nature? Do you want to do Pull-Ups on a pull-up bar but not be able to hang from and climb on top of a tree branch because it's thick, slippery, and unstable?

As I've said before, greater levels of adaptability are necessary for a greater level of physical capability, and such adaptability is developed only with frequent exposure to diverse, complex environmental variables. Science has proven that complex movement in complex environments stimulates and increases brain function, which encourages the development of greater body intelligence and greater mind-body connection that can carry over to other areas of life. (Read more about the mind-body connection in principle 11, "Mindful.") So, you should frequently move and practice Natural Movement in environments that encourage you to engage in complex motor skills in increasingly complex environments. Natural environments are often the most complex and least predictable environments; consequently, they're both the most challenging and rewarding.

If you live in a city or simply haven't had Natural Movement practice in a long time, you might not start in nature, but practicing your Natural Movement skills in nature should be your goal. Natural environments typically provide more variety than indoor environments—although this isn't necessarily always true—and the variety in nature greatly stimulates adaptability, alertness, and reactivity. This is because nature is not an artificially "enriched" environment": It inherently is—in most places—naturally rich. Only a dull environment, like an indoor setting, can be enriched. For example, modern zoos are now designed to replicate some of the natural variables the animals expect from their original biomes. Zoos are nothing but jails for wild animals, with each cell "enriched" enough to prevent absolute boredom, depression, and death. Wild animals need more than food and water; they need the environment that enables their natural behavior, which is a condition required to support both their physical and psychological health. Humans are no different.

" The city is not a concrete jungle, it is a human zoo."

—Desmond Morris

Urban environments are enriched with playgrounds that replicate some of the environmental diversity and complexity found in nature to provide city children with an outlet for their innate Natural Movement behavior. It is obviously beneficial to the children both physically and psychologically, even though the surfaces of playgrounds usually are made of metal, plastic, and other synthetic materials rather than wood and stone. However, we must reverse our thinking and consider whether it is a little supplemental environmental complexity (either artificial or natural) that is beneficial, or is it actually the near total absence of environmental complexity that is tremendously detrimental to us?

Do we want to regard our Natural Movement behavior within diverse and complex environments as something optional to human beings and regard the norm as being the extremely simplified modern physical behavior that we do within extremely simplified artificial environments? Or should we acknowledge that, biologically speaking, a Natural Movement behavior is a condition for optimal physical and psychological well-being and health? The Environmental principle is a reminder that a Natural Movement interaction with external variables, whether natural or artificial, is the behavioral context that our biology responds best to from a physiological perspective. In short, you need to move naturally several times a day, and you also need to interact with some degree of environmental complexity.

Environmental Stressors

The Environmental principle invites us also to consider the necessity of being more selective regarding what types of environments we interact with daily. Because we are evolutionarily shaped by nature and our interaction with it, the biological need for nature goes beyond Natural Movement. Even though modern humans are, for the most part, born and raised in artificial environments, our biological needs have not changed significantly. Exposure to nature, or lack thereof, has an effect on every aspect of our health: physical, physiological, psychological, and even spiritual. We still need the diversity and complexity of natural environments and the extremely diverse and stimulating sensory inputs only nature provides.

We all understand very common physiological adaptations—for instance, that muscle strength and size increase by lifting heavy weights but decrease by staying in bed for weeks, or that we suntan if we spend time in the sun but become pale if we never step outside and take off our clothes.

The causation—direct cause to effect—in those cases is evident, yet most people tend to be unaware that other physiological adaptations take place in our bodies because of a multitude of other influences, such as the quality (or lack thereof) of what we eat, the air we breathe, how we breathe, how we sleep, and how

we think, to name only a few. All these variables have at least a short-term—and in some cases a long-term—influence on how we feel, perform, or look simply because adaptability to environmental stressors goes beyond our movement; it takes place physiologically depending on the diverse variables of the environments that surround us. Whereas we have been taught for decades that our individual genetic code determines pretty much every aspect of who we are, we now know that other variables, called *environmental stressors*, can have a more powerful effect on how we feel, perform, or look than the genes we've inherited.

Epigenetics is a biological science that studies how the environment influences our cells and genetic expression. Epigenetics explains how consistent exposure to stressors affects us at a cellular level (including bones, muscles, brain, blood, organs, hormones, and so on), alters our physiological functions in a beneficial or detrimental fashion, and moves us toward greater or lower health, strength, vitality, well-being, resiliency, and even happiness. Again, our genes certainly play a big part in our health, but so do the environments and behaviors we consistently choose for ourselves.

Stressors induce stress, but it's a mistake to think that all stress is negative. Living and working in a city and living and working in nature both expose us to a great number of environmental stressors, but the types of stressors in the two environments are different and have different effects on our energy and health levels.

❝ Everything growing wild is a hundred times stronger than tame things."

—Forrest Carter

Imagine spending one day being exposed to stressors such as gentle natural sounds, pure air, natural light and surfaces, unprocessed food, Natural Movement, and activity that demands effort but that you enjoy doing. The next day you're exposed to loud or constant noise, "conditioned" or polluted air, artificial lights and surfaces, small and boxy spaces, windows and views with no horizon, places crowded with people or cars, heavily processed food that contains chemicals, physical idleness, and a job that makes you feel tense or anxious. Both days will have a significant effect on you physically, physiologically, and psychologically depending on how you respond to the diverse stressors. If you can feel the difference after a single day, what do you think the result would be if you spent decades of living a given lifestyle, even if you get accustomed to it? The effect of the environmental stressors that you are consistently exposed to is undeniable and unavoidable.

Epigenetics is not restricted to our direct environment. We can't look only at the influence of external environmental variables without also paying attention to our movement behaviors and how they affect our bodies. If we can understand how our food choices alone can significantly affect how we feel, perform, and look for better or worse, it shouldn't be too difficult to understand the relationship between our movement behavior or our day-to-day environments and how we feel, perform, and look.

❝ Vitality and beauty are gifts of Nature for those who live by its laws."

—Leonardo da Vinci

Our choices (both conscious and unconscious) about our movement behavior—including the kind of positions we hold and movements we do, the level of intensity, and duration and frequency—are part of those "environmental stressors" that switch our genes on or off. Clearly, the cells of your muscles don't self-modify to get stronger and potentially bigger just because your home or office is packed with barbells and weights, and you don't increase your cardio-conditioning just by looking at a vast outdoor expanse. The environment is not the only determining factor of your physiological adaptations; there must be a particular movement behavior to generate a beneficial modification of your physiology. In short, without your physical participation and engagement, the environment alone can't give you the maximum benefit. Nobody becomes an adept, strong, adaptable, and resilient "natural mover" just by sitting against a tree. Your physical behavior is an extraordinarily important pillar of your "environment."

Nature *Is* Healing

Many scientific studies support the idea that, from a human biological perspective, frequent contact with, or immersion in, nature is a requirement rather than an option for optimal physical and mental health. Nature is not a mere "jungle gym" where "zoo-humans," who live in artificial environments (which are to some extent comparable to the zoos where animals that have been displaced from nature live), can find temporary relief and reconnection to their roots.

Without exception, nature is where we all come from, but we're also made of nature. Every one of your cells is made of natural elements. This reality has a tremendous impact on who we are and on our biological needs.

Because nature contains all the environmental stressors that have contributed to the construction and evolution of our species-specific biology and the very structure of our brains, a lack of nature can lead to sensory-processing, cognitive, or mood disorders

Research has shown that simply looking at scenes of man-made urban environments produces a significant increase in activity in an area of the brain associated with fear and stress. On the other hand, exposure to natural environments has been shown to reduce anxiety, lift mood, and enhance one's ability to focus and perform other cognitive abilities. When healthy adults view nature scenes that are rich in vegetation, areas of the brain associated with emotional stability, empathy, and love become immediately more active. Nature scenes even enhance brain-wave activity in ways that have benefits like the effects of meditation.

Being in nature tranquilizes the mind—including for children who suffer from attention-deficit disorders—boosts the immune system, increases energy levels, speeds recovery from illness, and reduces mortality risks. But did we really need science to tell us this, or do we already know, at least intuitively, that nature is LIFE! The Romans had a term for this, *vis medicatrix naturae,* which means "healing power of nature." The Japanese also have a term for it—*Shinrinyoku*—which is the practice of going into nature to improve one's mental and physical health.

> ❝ **The cities may cover it up...but deep underneath is an inherent urge for naturalness."**
>
> —*Sigurd Olson*

Modern, urban, indoor, artificial environments are loaded with toxicity. It's not that they aren't stimulating; as a matter of fact, they're overly stimulating in an unhealthy way that's stressful. Air pollution, noise pollution, light pollution, food and water toxicity, electromagnetic radiation, constant flow of information that is mostly negative or superficially entertaining—not to mention some of our so-called "normal" physical and mental behaviors that are ill-adapted to our evolutionary hunter-gatherer bodies and minds—all contribute to wrecking us.

The mere absence of symptoms of illness doesn't mean that we're healthy. How many people are lacking vitality and are unhappy or depressed? Millions. Antidepressants and energy drinks are not the cure to these ailments. They provide only artificial alleviation of them; they mask the symptoms. Just because we have been led to accept artificial environments as a "normal" part of our lives and have accustomed ourselves to them doesn't mean that we have biologically adapted to them. Being optimally strong (physically, mentally, and emotionally), healthy, and happy when you live in a city is a daunting challenge.

So, consider again whether it's momentary exposure to nature that is beneficial to us, or it's constant exposure to artificiality that is detrimental to us. Removing our body from the natural world has consequences just like disconnecting our mind from our body has consequences. We can't have most people spend most of their time indoors where everything is artificial and looking at screens then expect physically and mentally healthy populations.

The value of time spent in nature and the cost of not spending time in nature are equally and vastly underrated. If you want to become a force of nature, you need to interact with the forces of nature.

Yet most people nowadays feel much safer in artificial environments than in nature, which leads them to avoid nature. You have to be disconnected from the natural world to see nature as an "environment," and you're even more disconnected if you see it as a place to systematically avoid.

Embracing Natural Movement as a normal, daily behavior and practice is the first step in reconnecting to our nature and in nurturing it, respecting it, and honoring it. Moving naturally in nature is the logical next step in remembering our interconnectedness with the natural world.

Despite a constant improvement of medical technologies, health levels in the modern world are decreasing. Maybe the solution to our most common health issues is not found in more or better pills and treatments but in "naturalizing" ourselves to natural environments and physical behaviors. Could the solution to most of our health issues be *that* simple? Even the fitness gym of the future might not have to be futuristic after all.

So, go back more often to where you truly belong, and become healthy again. Natural Movement is to exercise what organic is to food. Get out in nature and move! You might not need to move intensely. Start with remembering your true nature, your true self. It may make you feel cold, hot, dirty, or insecure; it may rough you up and give you scratches, cuts, and bruises. But it's also guaranteed to make you feel fully alive, maybe to the point of exhilaration. Natural Movement in nature is no less than a physical experience of your spirit and a spiritual experience of your body. Simply be in nature, feeling the wind in your hair, the light on your skin, seeing the colors, hearing the sounds, witnessing the movement of trees and animals around you, taking in the smell of the rain and of the Earth. The Earth! Remember the Earth!

> " Keep close to Nature's heart...and break clear away, once in a while, and climb a mountain or spend a week in the woods. Wash your spirit clean."
>
> —*John Muir*

RESPECT YOUR NATURAL ENVIRONMENT

Biophilia is the innate tendency to affiliate with other living creatures and processes. It is, simply put, the love of the natural world and life.

I've explained that the first environment that you should respect and protect is yourself. Yet you want to cultivate a sense of yourself that extends to and includes the whole natural world. If you can develop this perception, then the concern for the preservation of nature becomes as logical, natural, and important as self-preservation.

> " The environment is in us, not outside of us. The trees are our lungs, the rivers our bloodstream. We are all interconnected, and what you do to the environment, ultimately you do to yourself."
>
> —*Ian Somerhalder*

It starts with "treading lightly," or moving and practicing with as minimal an impact as possible. You are absolutely entitled to be in nature, but you can't act like a jackass just because you think that you are on top of the food chain. You must respect and care for nature as you respect and care for yourself.

We know that human activity is responsible for the worldwide alteration and destruction of nature. If we ruin all of nature, what would be the point of having a very fit, athletic, healthy body?

> " We cannot have freedom without wilderness..."
>
> —*Edward Abbey*

We need to create a culture where "humanism" is no longer the progress of mankind at the expense of the natural world but the progress of humans together with the natural world. We need to create a culture of "Nature law-abiding" earthlings.

9
Progressive

> "We are either progressing or retrograding all the while; there is no such thing as remaining stationary in this life."
>
> *—James Freeman Clarke*

Natural Movement is progressive in the sense that acquisition of movement adaptability is a relatively slow process and so is the development of physiological adaptations. Rushing the process or skipping stages only leads to issues down the road. The Progressive principle is a direct extension of principle 7, "Adaptable."

The Progressive principle is also tied to principle 1, "Evolutionary." Dinosaurs didn't turn into much smaller feathery birds in a matter of centuries, and we didn't evolve from hominids into *Homo sapiens* in just a few millennia. The evolution took place over the course of hundreds of thousands of years. Evolution is about adaptability, and adaptability relies on progressiveness.

Similarly, an individual doesn't acquire the full scope of his or her Natural Movement abilities overnight; it doesn't even happen in a matter of weeks or months. No one starts their Natural Movement journey from scratch, however; although we are born with tremendous instinct and evolutionary drive for movement, a newborn baby still has zero locomotion ability. Even days after birth, we can't crawl, let alone stand, run, or jump, because we don't have the motor skills or the strength to do so. Acquiring these skills follows progressions—known as *developmental stages*—over the course of several years. Reaching physical or locomotive autonomy and getting to the level at which adults of the species can move takes much more time for the young human animal than in most other species.

Even by the time of reaching a walking stage, a young human is still not fully physically developed. It takes years for a human body to reach a "grown-up" stage as far as both motor-skill (natural movement) aptitudes and physiological levels are concerned—as long as natural physical development is not significantly impaired or even totally stopped by social conventions or lifestyle (which is unfortunately very common in today's world).

Regressive Lifestyle

The Adaptable and Environmental principles explain that both the environmental variables that surround us and our conscious or unconscious physical behaviors shape our genetic expression at a cellular level, which affects how we feel, perform, and look. Although in some cases you can immediately notice changes, most deterioration goes unnoticed because it takes place very slowly. Except in the rare cases of an accident or a disease, nobody becomes physically weak and dysfunctional overnight. It is a process that can take place over the course of several months, years, or even several decades. How we move, sit, or stand comprises a biomechanical environment where the interaction of our body weight and gravity loads, stresses, and affects *all* our body tissues to some degree.

Kids who move a lot often have wear and tear in their socks and also in the knee and elbow areas of their clothes because they use those body parts to support themselves when they move. Biomechanically speaking, through diverse and frequent movements and the interaction of body weight with gravity and the environment, children load those areas (as well as all the body segments involved in the movements), which helps them grow and get stronger.

Conversely, if a person was to stay in bed without moving at all for days, there would be no mechanical interaction of their body weight with gravity; in the absence of loading the bones in the way needed to keep them strong, loss of both muscle and bone density would ensue. If a person sits and stands with a rounded back for years, such chronic physical behavior and biomechanical environment will literally shape that person's spine to make it permanently rounded. Of course, such structural change is not benign, and it can cause great discomfort and pain. If standing and sitting a certain way for prolonged periods of time can permanently change the shape of our spines, what other changes—most of which are not even visible—might progressively take place in our bodies and cause deleterious physical and physiological alterations without our awareness?

The point is that it's not just what we intentionally do to stay healthy or get fitter that matters; the bulk of our movement and physical behavior when we're not really paying attention to it also has a progressive physical and physiological effect.

Fortunately, we can change and improve our overall habits, behaviors, and environments, which leads to progressively restoring our functions and enhancing them.

The lack of Natural Movement is foremost a disuse issue. We become physically less strong and functional because we have ceased to use our bodies the way they are evolutionarily supposed to be used. Sitting all day and walking over short distances is nowhere near what our physiology expects. The variability of movement patterns and environmental variables is missing from our modern lifestyles; the intensity, duration, and frequency of movement has been reduced to being not biologically substantial enough for us to remain optimally functional and healthy. More movement alone might be insufficient to correct the problem because from consistent disuse ensues misuse or poor, inefficient movement patterns.

By losing a certain degree of function because of chronic physical idleness, we become less adept at movement variability and adaptability. In short, we become inefficient at movement whenever we do move. Standing, walking, and even breathing become dysfunctional. We have a body for all function, and a loss of function negatively effects everything we do physically. As a result, our avoidance and sometimes fear of movement increases as if movement is something unhealthy—something that is bad for our joints, for instance. But if crawling is supposed to be bad for our wrists, jumping bad for our knees, and throwing bad for our shoulders, then is thinking bad for our brains? Probably too much negative or stressful thinking is, but no one would ever advise you that all thinking is unhealthy. By the same token, too much movement, inefficient movement, or movement that's too intense is not good for us when we normally spend most of our time physically idle, but we shouldn't go to extremes and avoid all movement.

We have a modern cultural issue with obsessive comfort and safety. Our comfort zone is both shrinkable and expandable, depending on our lifestyle and mindset choices. The less frequently you challenge your comfort zone, the more it shrinks. The smaller it gets, the more uncomfortable you become. The more comfort we seek from external conveniences, the less comfort we create from *internal abilities*. In that sense, spending a lot of time sitting and moving as little as possible can certainly be convenient, but it progressively shrinks your body functions and movement comfort zone. The less you move, the less conditioned you get, which means you're more at risk for injury, which increases your fear of movement and leads you to move less—and the cycle continues. Constant comfort eventually becomes uncomfortable and stressful.

66 **Change is only possible through movement."**

—*Aldous Huxley*

By indulging yourself by staying physically inactive every day of your life, you basically establish a slow process of weakening yourself. Interestingly, though chronic physical idleness is a health-damaging habit, we don't see it as a "temptation" the same way we view binging on sugary foods or alcohol. However, we do "binge" on prolonged periods of physical inactivity, and we have little to no awareness that it contributes to the kind of self-transformation we do not want.

Does it matter that such inactivity is considered "normal" because it's how most people live their lives? In this case, normalcy matters less than whether the habit is healthy and beneficial. Normalcy can be a silent, invisible killer, and constant comfort is one of its most common weapons.

Deconditioning Cycle

*how inactivity or improper movement can lead to
a painful, fearful outlook on movement*

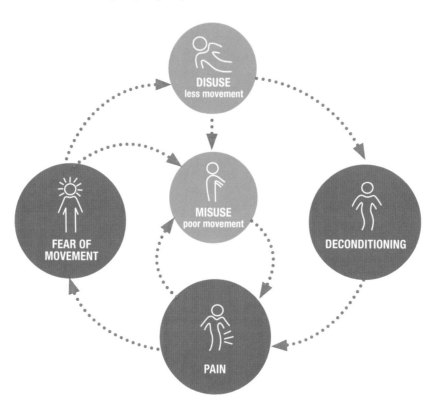

Self-Brutalizers

When many people realize they're in a state of physical neglect and weakness, they often seek body salvation through radical programs. Although it's commendable that people make the realization and follow-up resolutions, the approach they take to make improvements often is not; from a fitness perspective, long-term neglecters often become short-term brutalizers. It's funny how people, after many years of physical neglect, think they can brutalize their body back to fitness in a matter of weeks.

It is as if people subconsciously want to punish themselves for their years of physical inactivity—as if they think the adverse health effects of decades of physical abandon or idleness could be fully reversed in a matter of weeks or months. If you have neglected your body for many years, you have no choice but to embrace the idea that transitioning back into a fully functional body is going to be a slow process.

> **We either make ourselves miserable, or we make ourselves strong. The amount of work is the same."**
>
> *—Carlos Castaneda*

If you can't perform basic movements efficiently at a low level of intensity and if your most fundamental movement patterns are mediocre, what will happen when you suddenly attempt a high volume of complex movements at high levels of intensity? If your lifestyle progressively breeds a dysfunctional body and movement patterns, then the journey to reclaiming health, movement competency, and fitness should start with movement *quality and frequency* rather than movement *quantity and intensity*. People who struggle with basic moves yet push themselves to raise the bar higher are driven by either ignorance, ego, or both.

From a biological perspective of physiological transformation, there is no shortcut or quick fix; there's no instant reward. There's only a process that takes time, and that concept is easily ignored within our culture of immediacy and instant gratification.

Many people have bought into the idea of "no pain, no gain," but the reality is that when you don't carefully approach a return to good health and fitness, you can instead suffer a LOT of pain and a huge loss. When you ignore the Progressive principle, as well as a number of body signals that are telling you to slow down, and you instead inflict enormous amounts of physical stress on a body that isn't prepared to handle it, you are doing yourself a disservice. Instead of making any progress, you might get seriously injured and suffer great pain for a long time. What doesn't kill you does not necessarily make you stronger; it can also make you weaker. We see lots of "before and after" photos and success stories that promote fitness programs, but we rarely hear about the "failure stories" in which people end up with sometimes permanent injuries that can result in great financial cost and loss of quality of life.

> **Impatience never commanded success."**
>
> *—Edwin H. Chapin*

Legions of fitness and sports aficionados who have hurt themselves by doing too much too soon (and doing it inefficiently) without ever fully recovering will testify to the wisdom of progressing carefully. Strength, fitness, and health are not static conditions; they are components of a process that we must constantly and consistently pursue.

"Physical performance" isn't just for elite-level athletes or people who participate in sports. Performance is how anyone handles their day-to-day physical movements and tasks. Most of us do not need to train like elite athletes, even when the summer vacation is getting closer and we are in a rush to see quick, visible results. We simply need to move and to get back to natural movement fundamentals with variability, frequency, and consistency before we can progress toward greater levels of volume, intensity, or complexity. Nurturing health and fitness is a lifetime biological duty, and we need to approach it the smart way, which includes having humility and patience.

Progressions

The Adaptable principle explains that adaptation is specific to the type of demand. For that reason, a sprinter, a marathoner, and a long-distance trail runner don't train and perform the same way even though they all are runners. The bones and muscles of the dominant arm of a baseball pitcher are stronger than the opposite arm. Practicing complex skills, such as playing an instrument, will literally modify the structure of the brain related to that practice. The body and brain must adapt by structurally altering themselves to become better at the tasks they are consistently asked to do.

When you know that modifications take place progressively, it makes sense to make sure that the inputs necessary to trigger such adaptations also are progressive to ensure the best adaptation possible and to avoid injury. We learn early that exposing our skin to the hot summer sun for hours right after having been deprived of sun and nakedness for a whole winter will result in a severe sunburn, so we start with a few minutes of sun and stay outside a little longer every day. Moving your body at greater levels of intensity, volume, and frequency requires the same deliberate progression.

> ❝ **It might help to think of your body as more like a garden than a factory.**❞
>
> *— Matt Perryman*

The Progression principle is embedded in the Adaptable principle because you cannot brutally adapt to anything. Dosage matters a lot for the effectiveness of the process both in the short term and for the long run. The right dose, whether of sun or movement, should be incrementally increased regularly while being consistently administered. Transformation doesn't happen with a single event; it requires a succession of efforts and constant attention that rewards the dedicated. It's a process that involves countless micro-progressions, micro-gains, and even "micro-epiphanies."

Let's look at how children acquire a new skill. They go through an organic progression as they learn to move better and more skillfully through difficult movement patterns. For example, do children start doing Pull-Ups right away? Not at all. They start by hanging; they hang often, and they hang for longer and longer periods of time. They also use diverse movements, such as hanging and swinging. Eventually they start pulling themselves up as they climb so they're also using their legs. That's how they build their grip strength, upper-body strength, and coordination in climbing (or "brachiating"). Children don't rush as if Pull-Ups are the be-all and end-all of upper-body strength and fitness or because Pull-Ups are an essential "functional movement." A Pull-Up is just one of *many* climbing movement patterns. If children don't rush to do a Pull-Up, neither should adults, especially as we usually have proportionally less strength than children and have often lost a lot of our childhood physical condition.

Adults should restore the function they have lost (or maybe have never developed in the first place) before they try to enhance it. Regardless of the specific Natural Movement skill, you need to use the same progressive approach: First you address the integrity and efficiency of basic movement patterns and then you work on acquiring new or more challenging versions of the same types of movements.

> ❝ **All change is not growth, as all movement is not forward.**❞
>
> *— Ellen Glasgow*

If you respect this principle of progressiveness, you won't need "regressions," or easier versions of a movement or exercise you realize is too difficult for you, because you will start with first things first and gradually increase the challenge from there. In other words, knowing that a particular type of movement is scalable in difficulty is good, but respecting objective, adequate progressions to achieve that movement is what makes such scalability work.

Volume, Intensity, Complexity

Of course, progressive difficulty in movement complexity is not the only important aspect of progressions. Any given technique or movement pattern can be done in more challenging ways without the pattern being (significantly) modified. Typically, greater intensity and volume are the obvious variables that make the practice of a particular movement more challenging.

Volume progression is fairly evident: Either repetition (the number of times you repeat a movement in a row or within a session) increases or duration (the length of time during which you perform the movement) increases. Intensity progression relates to the speed at which you perform the movement, but it also can involve the distance, height, or depth at which you perform the movement. For instance, in the case of a jump, the weight that you are manipulating (lifting, carrying, throwing, or catching) as well as the impact you generate (in striking, punching, and kicking) affects the intensity.

Yet complexity, namely environmental complexity, is an aspect of progression that is widely overlooked. In principle 8, "Environmental," I have already shared some insights explaining why that is so. Again, there is more to your running capability than only increasing speed or duration. In this case, running on uneven terrains that gradually become more difficult is a form of progression. Increasingly contextual complexity cannot be overlooked as a progression. Increasing the number of repetitions of a given jump is a progress in volume; increasing the distance cleared is a progress in intensity; increasing the height, difficulty of take-off, and landing surfaces is an increase in complexity. An increase in environmental complexity can challenge both your body and your mind because it demands mental composure to remain in control of your movement efficiency in the presence of apprehension or even risk.

Daring to perform a movement once and succeeding is great, but developing a lasting ability is much greater. Just as you must progressively acquire physical prowess, self-confidence and self-control are capital elements of real-world physical capability you must develop gradually. Managing fear, which is an advanced aspect of the mental side of Natural Movement performance, is a matter of progression in environmental complexity. Just as consistent practice of Natural Movement will elevate your energy levels, facing fears and overcoming them frequently—yet safely—is one of the most natural and potent remedies to anxiety. Indeed, our own limitations are often found not in our bodies but in our minds.

Conversely, respecting such progressions in environmental complexity can be an exercise in practical humility for those who are reckless. You have one body and one life; one mistake can jeopardize what you are trying to achieve. By being realistic and not taking unnecessary risks unless you are really in control, you can learn to overcome misplaced confidence.

Regardless of the aspect of progression you are looking at—volume, intensity, or frequency—progressions must be well thought out. Though principle 10, "Efficient," emphasizes the crucial importance of efficient movement and principle 11, "Mindful," emphasizes how attention matters in performing efficient movement patterns, both efficiency and mindfulness are hard to ensure when levels of difficulty are overwhelming—in other words, when progressions are not respected. You should regularly make incremental increases in the level of challenge while you also ensure that you're maintaining consistency in movement efficiency.

NOTE

This chapter explains the philosophy of the Progressive principle. The "how-to" of progression is described in Part 3, "Practice Efficiency Principles." The science or knowledge behind effective progressions relies on programming. Such programming can be done either intuitively or rather meticulously and rationally.

Recovery

Recovery, which is the amount of rest your body needs to effectively achieve the physiological adaptations triggered by the input (practice), is an integral part of progression. This process does not solely take place in the body in terms of strength or energy system; it also occurs in the brain in terms of improved motor control.

> " Don't let life discourage you; everyone who got where he is had to begin where he was."
>
> —*Richard L. Evans*

You may leave a session feeling frustrated because you have not achieved the level of technique you were aiming for. What you don't realize is that even suboptimal repetitions have provided the necessary input for your central nervous system to improve your movement patterns *after* the session is over. You might be surprised to notice an immediate improvement during your next session. Progression took place while you were busy doing something else.

Depending on the type of adaptation—physiological or neural—a certain amount of rest is necessary, or even mandatory. Nutrition and overall lifestyle is also part of recovery. If you don't respect recovery, you're not respecting progression because effective adaptations are being hindered. For instance, frequency in the practice of movement patterns/technique may be very beneficial and boost progress, whereas too much frequency in training for metabolic conditioning can wreck your body. Daily high-intensity training is not sustainable because it is hormonally disruptive. Although it might look like you are "overtraining," in actuality you might simply lack enough time to recover properly.

Natural Movement practice is a process that enables the restoration of lost function, the activation of function that went dormant, the enhancement of existing function, and the development of potential function that was never developed in the first place. The word *function* could be easily replaced by *skill*, *strength*, or *conditioning*. It doesn't matter at what stage

of this process you find yourself. As I mentioned in principle 3, "Universal," there aren't natural movements for elite athletes and other movements for "common" people; there's only day-to-day movements that belong to anyone. What separates the levels of practice is not the nature of the patterns practice but the level of difficulty that you can afford in relation to your current physical state or level. Practice should never be too easy or too hard.

Just like strength, physical capability isn't a state; it's a process that is, by nature, progressive. If we quit nurturing the process, we become weak and inept; if we engage in, nurture, and maintain the process, we become and remain strong and capable. If we think of capability as a state instead of as a process, we can become disheartened. We should let go of prerequisites for worthiness and embrace the process instead, regardless of what our personal starting points are. If we can see our physical state of capability as an ongoing process, then all we have to do is to understand the necessity for consistent, continuous practice. The level of practice we can afford today might not be as high as what we could afford years ago if we went through a period of physical inactivity, but the level of practice we will be able to afford in the future is higher than what it is today if we consistently practice and continuously increase the level of difficulty.

> " It is not fair to treat people as if they are finished beings. Everyone is always becoming and unbecoming."
>
> —*Kathleen Winter*

I have seen many people regarded as "fit" by conventional standards and external appearance become clumsy beginners when starting Natural Movement practice. Similarly, the completely out-of-shape person who begins and struggles with the most fundamental moves and lowest levels of volume, intensity, or complexity may not have less merit than those who can rapidly perform more difficult movements. This is because level of difficulty and level of challenge are not the same thing. If a trained or gifted person can perform a rather difficult movement easily, that person isn't challenged. The untrained person who is struggling with a normally easy movement, on the other hand, is greatly challenged. If the latter puts their heart and effort in the movement despite the difficulty, that person has more merit than the individual who can easily perform more difficult movements but is not pushing him- or herself with an even greater level of difficulty. If simply hanging from a horizontal bar for a few seconds represents a great challenge to you and requires great courage and willpower from you, who is to say that you are not training really hard, maybe even harder than more advanced practitioners?

Two of the most important psychological aspects of practice are humility with regard to your actual physical state and ability and patience with regard to how much and how fast you should progress in terms of increasing volume, intensity, or complexity. These qualities are as important as the necessary willpower and self-discipline that are required to ensure progress. You also should have pride for the efforts that you are able to produce and the commitment that you are able to display. When you're committed to a long-term strategy, every step forward is part of a process, and with the right mindset you can feel like you're receiving instant gratification.

NOTE

I remember once having to stay several days in bed in a hospital because I was recovering from malaria. Upon coming home, I was so out of shape and my levels of strength were so low that the amount of willpower it took to achieve a Deadlift of 40 pounds was tremendous. This personal experience reminded me of something I had always believed, which is that level of effort and level of performance aren't the same, and that merit has more to do with the former than the latter.

Consistency

> ❝ **There is no failure except in no longer trying.**"
>
> —*Elbert Hubbard*

Whereas consistency does not necessarily imply progression, progression demands consistency. The path to progression—in movement efficiency or physiological adaptation—demands consistency, and the path to consistency demands commitment. There's no way around it. A lot of people become discouraged after making several short-lived attempts to remedy their issues, be it in terms of health or physical condition. They begin to think that they have literally tried everything, but they don't realize that it is their lack of commitment that prevents any improvement from progressing (or even happening in the first place). It's a product of the modern mindset to expect fast and dramatic results with little personal participation. People are not necessarily reluctant to engage in temporary change or effort; they mostly are resistant to consistency and commitment, except where their own ingrained habits and routines are concerned. Habits and routines can be both good or bad, and you must get rid of the bad ones before they harm you. Reserve your efforts toward consistency for the beneficial changes so that they become habits.

> ❝ **We are what we repeatedly do. Excellence, then, is not an act but a habit.**"
>
> —*Aristotle*

You can design yourself consciously and continuously to progressively become who you choose to be. To evolve in the direction you choose, you must be willing to step out of your comfort zone and challenge yourself. Constant comfort paradoxically becomes uncomfortable. You can only expand your comfort zone by challenging it. Habits, routines, and other lifestyle patterns that have ceased to evolve and challenge you are sterile, and they foster stagnation.

How do you know that you're out of your comfort zone? Well, if you don't know, or if you're not sure, you clearly are not out of it yet. The more comfortably numb life gets, the more stressful it is because your comfort zone becomes smaller and smaller. The strategy to expand your comfort zone is pretty simple: challenge your comfort zone frequently so you can expand it steadily. In other words, once you become comfortable with a movement, increase the volume, complexity, or intensity so that the movement becomes uncomfortable for a while. Eventually, you'll be comfortable with that new level, which means it's time to again make things uncomfortable.

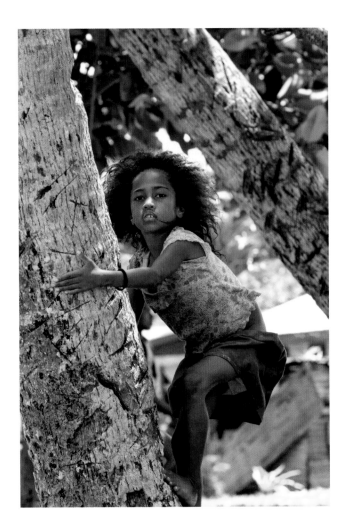

Not having the best genetics is not an excuse for having the worst lifestyle or a reason to indulge yourself with chronic physical laziness. Progress requires undertaking a lifetime pursuit of change, and the only deadline is the deadline we all have to face at the end of our lives; simply put, you are in no rush. Do you want to have short-lived New Year resolutions or a single lifetime resolution that follows a consistently progressive path?

At first, your body may not have as much skill and strength as you'd like, but with lots of strength from the heart and mind, the willingness to make achievements, consistency, commitment, and some mental effort for when things get a bit tougher, skill, body strength, and energy will eventually follow. We are shaped by anything we do, how we do it, and how often we do it, whether it shows or not—and eventually it always shows. *Any time you spend weakening your weaknesses is time you spend strengthening your strengths.* Tomorrow's physical capability and health depends on what you choose to do today.

10
Efficient

"It's not the load that breaks you down, it's the way you carry it."
—*Lou Holtz*

"Success is doing ordinary things extraordinarily well."
—*Jim Rohn*

I explain in the Evolutionary, Instinctual, and Universal principles that everyone possesses fundamental, human, innate movement aptitudes. Anyone can effectively crawl, walk, run, jump, balance, lift, and carry—to some extent at least. But can everyone perform such movements skillfully? Even if we can effectively do what is natural to us, do we always do it efficiently?

The answer is in the difference between an aptitude and a skill. An *aptitude* is a natural ability or tendency to do something. It's spontaneous and subconscious, but it can be really basic, rough, and not at all skillful. When we have movement aptitude, we perform effective movements regardless of efficiency; in other words, it's possible to be "inefficiently effective." Inefficient effectiveness isn't a failure at achieving the result we seek, but it is failure at achieving success at the highest level we could potentially achieve. A *skill*, on the other hand, is the ability to do something well; it's an advanced aptitude or expertise. Efficiency turns aptitudes into skills, whereas skills make movements efficient. Whereas effectiveness is a basic form of success, efficiency is an optimum form of success.

When we move we generate what experts call "kinetic energy"—the energy of our own motion. Obviously, producing effective Natural Movement demands some work and comes at a cost. However, we don't want to move just for the sake of moving; we move with an intention and for a practical purpose, and we expect a return on the kinetic energy we invest. Is that energy optimally employed and entirely transferred to producing that outcome we seek, or is it dispersed to some extent? The more optimal-ly it is directed and the more efficient you are, the more successful you are at safely performing a practical physical task with economy. Conversely, if your movement is mediocre—that is, less efficient—you are less successful at how you perform, which means you use more energy than needed and can potentially injure yourself. In fact, by being less efficient, attempts to perform physical actions could ultimately become totally ineffective, in which case energy is entirely wasted.

Because we are wired to move efficiently, even when we can't explain what motivates us to move that way, humans have an innate ability to notice efficient movement in others the same way they can immediately spot clumsiness. The three primary and highly desirable outcomes we can expect from efficiency are improved performance, energy conservation, and increased safety. In simple words, on top of having the ability to physically achieve more, you achieve better results by both conserving your energy and maintaining your physical integrity. Efficiency enables the minimum amount of energy to be used for a given task, which from a vital perspective of life preservation is critical.

Efficiency Outcomes

result in the highest performance, lowest metabolic cost, and greater safety

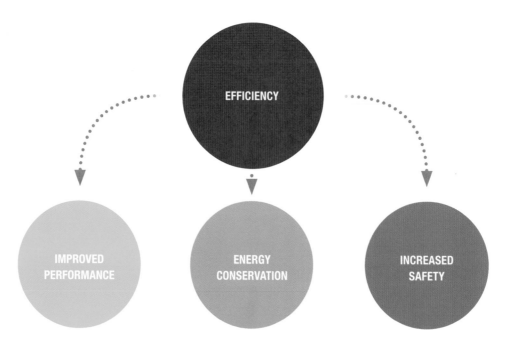

Efficiency is to the whole body in movement what dexterity is to how you use your fingers, hands, and wrists in hand manipulation, such as when you play an instrument. You can tell when you're hearing an instrumental virtuoso playing music because the efficiency is evident in how that person plays. In the same way, you can see the efficiency of a movement virtuoso. The difference between melody and cacophony or between movement control and random gesticulation is found in the difference between efficiency and inefficiency. Mastery is skillful, and skillfulness is efficient.

> ❝ **I'm pragmatic. I like efficiency. I want to read what's in front of me and not have my hands tied."**
>
> *—Susan Brooks*

The importance of efficiency cannot be taken lightly, and it helps to look at the consequences of inefficiency to understand its importance. The minor aspects of inefficiency may seem relatively benign, especially in environmentally simplified gym settings where movements are performed one repetition at a time. But in the real world, movements are always part of a continuum, and an inefficiency in performing a given movement may have consequences beyond the movement itself because it can lead to the inability to effectively transition to the next movement, lost efficiency in the next movement, or even failure of the next movement. Depending on the context, an ineffective transition could cause you a delay or a momentary loss of attention that would result in missing an important opportunity, or it could cause you to not detect a threat. Even worse, it could cause you to get injured, which can have dramatic consequences.

DEFINING EFFICIENCY

The Efficiency principle is often misunderstood as if a *minimal* amount of energy should be used, but there is a significant difference between "minimal" and "minimum."

If we want to use a minimal amount of energy then only movements that require very little strength or energy should be practiced. The reality is that efficiency implies that you should use a minimum amount of energy regardless of the level of intensity required to perform the movement.

Indeed, you can waste precious energy even when you're performing basic movements that require minimal amounts of energy; you might expend little energy but still have expended more than you should have. Conversely, you might expend significant amounts of energy while performing a high-intensity physical task yet only be using the minimum amount of energy required. Inefficient movement forces you to waste energy even when you're performing apparently easy movements, whereas efficiency enables you to preserve energy by not consuming more energy than required while performing physically intense tasks. Regardless of the intensity required, efficiency is about preserving energy by using a minimum amount of it, not necessarily a minimal amount of it; simply put, don't use more energy than you need, whether a physical action demands little energy or a lot of it.

This creates an apparent paradox when training metabolic conditioning (which is high-intensity movement aimed at improving energy systems) by the MovNat method: Expend the greatest amount of energy possible—within a given amount of time—while using the minimum amount of energy possible. While it may sound like it, this isn't a contradictory statement at all. Intensity implies that you must use high amounts of energy; efficiency implies that you must use minimum amounts of energy. "High-energy" expenditure should not imply "unnecessary waste of energy," whereas "energy-efficient" practice does not necessarily equal "minimal-energy" expenditure. Use exactly the amounts of energy needed to perform effectively—no more, no less. Seeking movement efficiency is a form of seeking comfort and finding the easiest way possible to do something even when intensity is involved; it requires some attention and effort.

Why *a* Method *Is* Necessary

Although we commonly associate the word *natural* with the word *spontaneous,* we can't assume that anything that's spontaneous is necessarily efficient. This is true for many aspects of who we are and what we do, and it certainly applies to how we move. There's a difference between an innate aptitude and an acquired skill, and even a movement that feels "natural" isn't equivalent to an efficient movement. The movement might be a bad habit you simply have gotten used to, so now it feels "intuitive" and even comfortable. We always default to our habitual patterns regardless of how efficient they are. Efficiency is not subjective, and it's more than a mere sensation. It's an outcome that can be felt by the person doing the movement, but it also can be observed, compared, verified, and, in some respects, measured by someone else.

Although Natural Movement is an innate, instinctual physical behavior, it also requires practice to make efficiency in Natural Movement second nature. We need to nurture our nature to unleash our full potential.

We are certainly all born with innate Natural Movement aptitudes and an instinct to get more efficient at any of those movements we were originally meant to do consistently. For instance, adults are able to stand seemingly effortlessly, whereas for toddlers standing is at first difficult and energy-inefficient.

But there is a problem: Years (decades even) of neglect of our physical abilities because of disuse and misuse has turned us into "zoo-humans." In the absence of physical and movement behaviors that match the behaviors of our ancestors, turning innate abilities into second-nature skills has become a real challenge. While Natural Movement originally became efficient in every individual after sufficient time of spontaneous, necessary, or even intentional practice, in modern times efficiency is not guaranteed at all. I have observed time and time again that the way untrained modern humans spontaneously perform even some of the simplest natural movements is rarely efficient, compared to the same movements performed by populations who use them daily in so-called "undeveloped" countries.

It is easy to dismiss the necessity for having a method of learning or teaching what is natural because of the romantic idea that something that's natural cannot be taught or learned. However, as I stated earlier, the reality is that what is natural is not necessarily efficient. For example, is there anything more natural than breathing? Still most modern people would tremendously benefit from relearning the proper breathing pattern they once used as children. If this is true for breathing, is it unreasonable to consider that we can also learn efficiency in every skill that is part of Natural Movement?

> " Generally speaking, if you control matter more precisely, you can get more efficiency out of any process."
>
> —*Steve Jurvetson*

Efficient movement is based on the knowledge of principles and techniques. Learning movement efficiency is a process that can be accelerated by consciously using a method. From the dawn of time, humans have developed technologies or methods for many needs and applications. To our ancestors, the purpose of developing methods of fire-making or hunting was to increase efficiency, and after they developed those methods they transmitted them through teaching and learning. A method is a systematic and effective way to learn, teach, and practice.

Natural Movement, natural processes, and phenomena are found in nature, but methods are not. There is no such thing as a "natural method." You don't stumble on a method while walking in nature. Methods are the product of a conscious, rational mind. Thanks to a method, you may realize what you never noticed in the first place and that you need to see, understand, and improve on. Methods help us make progress when instinct has been lost or reached its limits.

In an ideal world, there would be no need for a method or program for relearning what should be a universal birthright of Natural Movement mastery. Unfortunately, in today's world, the reality is that millions of people need to reclaim their birthright of competent, adept Natural Movement. In fact, the health predicament that modern humanity is facing implies that most people need an overall reform of their lifestyle. To get started, they need to begin with the most basic natural movements. There is a common belief that efficiency only matters for the more complex movements, but it can make a significant difference in some of the seemingly simplest movements, such as standing up; a lack of quality in the most basic movements will negatively impact the efficiency of the more advanced, technical movements.

Exploring your instinctive movement patterns is only the beginning of your journey to movement competence. Although you don't need a method, a coach, or scientific research to simply get outside and use your Natural Movement aptitudes, spontaneous skill is very rare. Given that most of us have been disconnected from our natural behaviors and many of our instincts have been repressed for so long, "trusting your instincts" might not give you the solutions you need.

If highly competent movers, such as wild animals that are born and raised to move naturally in nature "for a living," sometimes miss and fail their own natural movements—slipping and falling, for instance—how could the untrained, deconditioned modern human assume that he or she doesn't need to learn and practice Natural Movement efficiency? Will efficiency spontaneously happen because you've been inspired to climb a tree or have plunked yourself in nature? Maybe, but maybe not. You might make some progress, but you won't go as fast as you could with a more thoughtful approach. Fundamental efficiency and excellence in movement stems from knowledgeable, mindful, methodical, consistent practice.

The worst-case scenario is that the total absence of guidance might result in foolish movement that causes injury or in uninspired exploration that ends in total discouragement. In most cases, instinct alone will take you only so far. Fortunately, the information I share with you in this book provides a lot of support in this regard. After you read through it, it may become part of your experience, of who you are, and of what you do "naturally," and you may even forget or dismiss how much you learned from it. Nonetheless, this book contains all the information needed to turn basic aptitudes into actual Natural Movement skills.

Practice does not necessarily make perfect. Inefficient practice can make things worse, whereas efficient practice makes things better. Just as it requires consistency to develop greater levels of strength, power, or stamina, reaching higher levels of technique and efficiency demands consistency. Research has shown that in most fields, elite practitioners perform several thousand hours of "deliberate"—which means "mindful"—practice; extensive practice is a condition for acquiring expert performance in a particular skill or activity.

Clearly, in most cases efficiency isn't innate and must be nurtured enough so it can be acquired. Yet we fortunately don't need to spend thousands of hours training every skill we want to possess to become de-cently adept at them. In fact, efficient instruction and mindful practice can generate significantly greater efficiency sometimes in a matter of a few minutes. There have been many times when I have witnessed instant and impressive improvement after I have provided a student with a single verbal cue and the student has made just one attempt of the movement based on my instruction. Of course, not all progress is that fast and simple, but anyone can acquire very effective skills without having to spend even a tenth of the overall time needed to achieve an elite level of performance.

Remember: Volume practice alone is not a guarantee that you will improve if you don't also have a sound method. You could spend tons of time or energy practicing without making any gains in efficiency if you don't know what makes a given movement pattern efficient or if you aren't at least attempting to increase your efficiency every time you perform the movement. Repetition is only the key to progress if you consistently repeat with the intention to improve. You can actually get worse with a high volume of mediocre repetitions while deeply ingraining bad patterns in the process. Unexamined movement is guaranteed to repeat itself to become the default pattern whether it's an efficient movement or not; in most cases it isn't, which condemns you to perpetuate poor quality, low-efficiency motion.

Technique *Versus* Strength *and* Conditioning

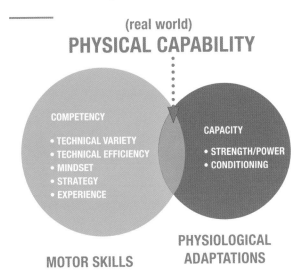

To augment your real-world physical capability, your priority is to both optimize your movement competency by making your skills as efficient as possible while also progressively increasing your work capacity (your strength and/or your endurance)*.

This is not an "either-or" proposition: Work capacity is not a substitute for movement competency, and technique does not make strength or conditioning optional. Depending on the complexity of the movement, the environment where it is performed, and the level of intensity imposed by the situation, the ratio of importance between technique and strength and conditioning may vary significantly, but neither aspect ever becomes irrelevant. Ever.

*You can read more in "Exercise-Based Performance Enhancement and Injury Prevention for Firefighters: Contrasting the Fitness-and Movement-Related Adaptations to Two Training Methodologies," at https://www.ncbi.nlm.nih.gov/pubmed/25763518

Strength and conditioning may to a degree facilitate the acquisition of movement competency, and greater movement skills dramatically improve how existing strength and conditioning are used for real-world performance. However, very few Natural Movement techniques or movements patterns require a person to have a level of strength greater than average to be performed. Anyone who is healthy can do the movements that are part of Natural Movement, such as crawling, walking, balancing, running, lifting, carrying, throwing, and catching. A person might not be able to do these movements at high intensity, but any healthy person is capable of some level of these movements. One can learn efficient lifting techniques with objects weighing no more than a few pounds. The only techniques that necessitate a certain level of strength—in the upper body—to be developed are particular climbing techniques that require hanging from the hands, and the strength required for these techniques is relatively easily gained through regressions of the techniques themselves. In other words, you don't need to be sent to the gym to be "strong" or "conditioned" enough to start improving 99 percent of the whole scope of Natural Movement; you just start Natural Movement.

Those who care more for actual work capacity than looks are a minority among fitness aficionados, and among this minority the percentage of those who value technique and movement efficiency is even smaller. To feel prepared for the demands of the real world, most people still prioritize increasing their work capacity because they think work capacity is the be-all and end-all of physical preparedness. What these people don't realize is that strength and conditioning support motor skills, but they don't *produce* any motor skills. In other words, having great power and stamina won't prevent you from drowning if you don't know how to swim, keep you from falling off a narrow surface if you don't know how to balance yourself, or help you defend yourself if you don't know how to fight.

66 **I knew I could control one thing, and that is my time and my hours and my effort and my efficiency."**

—Ryan Seacrest

People who focus exclusively on the measurable aspects of physical fitness, such as work capacity, are guaranteed significant deficiencies in their movement competency and therefore in their real-world physical capability. No extra amount of general strength and conditioning will ever compensate for a lack of motor-skill and movement adaptability. Although you also could say that knowledge of skills doesn't compensate for lack of general strength and conditioning, there is a notable difference in the sense that some specific physiological adaptations—including greater strength and conditioning—take place when you practice movement skills contextually, which makes it possible to improve technique at the same time you're getting stronger and gaining more endurance. Conversely, training for general physical preparedness generates great power and stamina, but you still need to learn all the techniques and skills that strength and stamina are supposed to support.

I'm not saying that supplemental strength and conditioning training isn't beneficial or part of the MovNat method; I only mean that it may not be mandatory when learning the majority of the techniques and skills involved in Natural Movement. As you engage in Natural Movement training, competency comes before capacity, with some capacity developing symbiotically as competency is being trained and acquired, at least until the point where movement competency is established enough that capacity might become a greater focus. For instance, you can learn lifting techniques and keep fine-tuning your skill by using objects that are quite light, until it becomes obvious that you need heavier loads to develop more strength and power. That's how it works for elite athletes, and it also makes sense for day-to-day fitness practitioners—that is, after they understand the priority value of movement competency.

Movement efficiency is not easy to quantify, but it is the primary level of performance you should be concerned about. We have been led to believe that only exercise that can be counted is productive, but so much of what really matters in movement performance can't be counted or measured. Efficiency is one of those aspects that may be challenging to measure, but it matters tremendously.

"Going strong," "training hard," and "no pain, no gain" are mindsets that emphasize the grueling side of physical training, as if you aren't doing any "real" and valuable work without sweating, grimacing, and having "the eye of the tiger." When the quest for volume, speed, or number of calories burned prevails, it is in most cases accompanied by an absence of consideration for good form or technique. Even when people have knowledge of proper form and technique, many people are willing to compromise their form if the result is better numbers—as if movement efficiency was not a fundamental part of performance or only an optional aspect of it.

Using complex movements for the sake of increasing work capacity can be very detrimental if you overlook efficient movement, and there are important issues with such an approach. First, you might develop a false sense of physical capability because you might *feel* strong and ready, but you might not *be* entirely strong and ready. But principle 7, "Adaptable," explains that adaptability stems from enough specificity in practice. Without adaptability, efficiency is immediately impaired. You may have the capacity to perform thirty Pull-Ups in a row when you're hanging from a regular pull-up bar, but you might not be able to climb on top of a thick surface because hanging from a ledge is more challenging, you lack grip strength, and you do not know what movement techniques to employ to climb on top. You might believe that the power in your lower body enables you to sprint fast, but you haven't factored in that a rugged, rocky terrain could make you significantly slow down or even stumble and fall because you are not skillful at running on such terrains at high speed.

Second, you might not detect vital body signals that indicate that an injury is imminent if you don't reduce intensity or even completely stop what you're doing. It is a mistake to think that it is okay to compromise your long-term physical integrity but not acceptable to compromise a short-term outcome.

Sadly, for most people, it is only after getting injured, dealing with the pain, going through rehabilitation, and taking time off from training that they will finally realize the mistake they made. Unfortunately, not everyone fully recovers from injuries; even some who recover and resume training are never able to reach previous levels of performance.

Last but not least, doing countless repetitions of an inefficient pattern imprints the incorrect form in your neuromuscular memory. Consequently, if you don't consciously choose the most efficient pattern, your brain will reflexively, unconsciously choose the most frequently performed pattern. What that implies is that if you do twenty repetitions of a given technique to improve its efficiency and then immediately after use this exact same technique eighty times within a high-intensity workout while badly compromising its form for the sake of greater "metabolic conditioning" or "work capacity," your brain memorizes the pattern that you have repeated the most regardless of efficiency. You thought that you got the best of both worlds with this 20/80 ratio, but you did not. You just taught your brain to make your body operate at high intensity with a poor movement. Not only are the chances of getting injured significantly greater, but you will also *automatically* revert to this mediocre pattern every time you increase the intensity at which you perform the technique. Mindless repetitions of mediocre movement lead only to long-term inefficiency.

NOTE

One thousand mindless repetitions of an inefficient movement pattern are a sign of both absolute commitment and ignorance.

There is a reason martial artists are obsessed with optimal form both at low and high intensity when they practice, and they never compromise their technique. It is because they know that in a real-world context where elements of fear or fatigue may be present, the aspects of performance that are likely to suffer are technique and efficiency. The same reasoning and martial art mindset should apply to *all* the Natural Movement skills that you practice.

It may be cliché, but our bones and muscles are our hardware, and our movement skills are our software. The most powerful hardware is useless without the right software. In other words, strength matters only if it is efficiently expressed—not brutally, mindlessly, vaguely, or inaccurately used. This applies to both the gym, the sports field, and the real world. Without a functional body and the techniques necessary to employ and develop power or energy at continuously higher levels of intensity, reaching plateaus and getting injured happen much sooner than they should. Your physiological potential is not the limit, but your efficiency is, and being inefficient can prevent you from ever reaching your full potential.

**" Become addicted to constant and
never-ending self-improvement."**

—*Anthony J. D'Angelo*

There may be functional, physiological reasons why your movement isn't efficient. In the case of a physical issue that is perceived as a threat to the body's integrity, the central nervous system (CNS) has a healthy, conservative tendency of self-limiting movement. The CNS may use diverse strategies to restrain movement, including local tension to limit range of motion in joints or lower your ability to use strength to reduce the speed or power of your movement. Because most Natural Movement involves the whole body, pretty much any body part will find itself an inherent part of most movement patterns and negatively alter otherwise normal function. In this case, we usually talk about the "weak link" in a "kinetic chain."

Learning new movements, or improving existing ones, becomes a real challenge, as the natural patterns are necessarily modified to compensate for the problem. Worse, inefficient patterns can be acquired and sometimes remain even long after the physical issues have healed or disappeared. While the issue of "nagging injury" and other functional limitations is far from being negligible in today's populations, the primary obstacle to achieving movement efficiency lies in the mind and the perception that efficiency is optional or that work capacity is a satisfying substitute for deficiencies in motor skills.

NOTE

Moving more doesn't always allow you to move better, but moving better always allows you to move more.

When movement proficiency becomes secondary or even accessory in your training, you become a mindless, inefficient fitness machine, with negative repercussion on your real-world effectiveness. Technique is absolutely not the replacement of strength or conditioning. Technique is the most efficient use of strength and conditioning. In that sense, "flow" in movement is not the elimination of resistance but the skill of optimally applying force and employing energy. The path of "least resistance" is movement efficiency. Going "strong" is easy; going smart is more challenging; going strong intelligently is obviously a greater challenge. There is no opposition between quality and quantity, between competency and capacity. "How can I do better?" is not a question that's more important than "How can I do more?"; it's simply a higher-priority one.

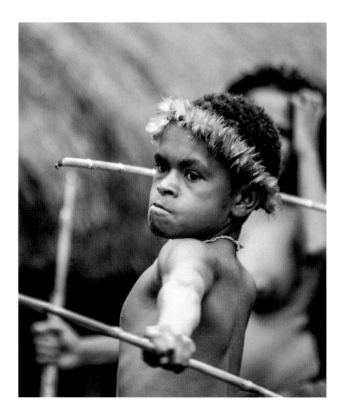

Movement Efficiency *Is Not* Enough

It's not sufficient to just have movement efficiency; you also need practice efficiency. In this book, I explain both principles of movement and practice efficiency. How efficiently you practice isn't limited to the efficiency of your movement. Similarly, how efficiently you apply your physical capability in the real world isn't limited to technical proficiency. You could be running with amazing technique and speed, but if you're running in the wrong direction or at the wrong time, you're not being effective. Efficient movement doesn't guarantee that you will be able to make the smartest decisions in real life if a situation occurs where your physical response is mandatory. You also need to have situational intelligence, which could also be called *contextual proficiency* or *tactical proficiency*.

To appraise situational efficiency and to determine the best course of action, one must consider the relationship between the contextual demands of the moment and the individual's options in relation to their level of capability when the action takes place, with the "best" course of action not always being the ideal one. Contextual parameters might require that you temporarily modify the ideal execution of a technique, which can potentially reduce efficiency to some extent.

> ❝ **When you aim for perfection, you discover it's a moving target."**
> — *George Fisher*

A suboptimal execution is a necessary trade-off; some efficiency must be lost for the sake of adaptability and ensuring effectiveness. For example, you might have the option to run around an obstacle when you know that you are not able to pass it effectively or safely, which could mean it takes longer, but you can then avoid the risk of becoming injured. In other cases, you might be forced to attempt to clear the same obstacle because you do not have the luxury of time. Your level of capability determines whether you have options, what they are, and what decisions you should make about the movements you should employ, but ultimately you must make decisions based on the conditions of a context, which is a subject that goes beyond this book. For example, first responders, such as rescue teams, firefighters, paramedics, and police officers, are taught the most relevant, effective, efficient, or safe responses to situations—yet the acquisition of experience is a never-ending process. If those professionals struggle with their movement to begin with, they're bound to struggle with the overall situation they are dealing with. Ultimately, movement efficiency, practice efficiency, and contextual efficiency are the three pillars of an overall spectrum of real-world capability.

You can never master the context where you physically and mentally operate; you can only learn to master how you will operate through it.

Flying like a bird without technology is impossible to humans other than in dreams or imagination. No technique will ever enable a human being to fly by his or her own physical means. Efficient movement and practice do not make the impossible possible, but they do enable an existing potential to become a reality. "Is there a better way?" is one of the most useful questions you can ask yourself in the pursuit of becoming more efficient.

Efficiency is indeed more than a principle; it is a mindset that makes us seek continuous improvement even when we are seemingly very adept at a given movement or physical task. This is a real paradox in the mainstream fitness industry: "Globofitness" makes basic, segmental movements—such as a biceps curl—look complex, but they're not. Efficiency makes complex, adaptable, natural movements—such as a jump over a gap—look simple, but they're not.

We have a culturally induced belief that because we start to physically decline past a certain age, it prevents us from making progress in anything new that we want to learn, but there's no truth in that belief. Continuously optimizing your movement performance doesn't depend on your age, level of health, or vitality; it depends on the strength and consistency of your intention. Does the quest for efficiency ever stop? Never, even if you simply maintain the efficiency you have previously acquired.

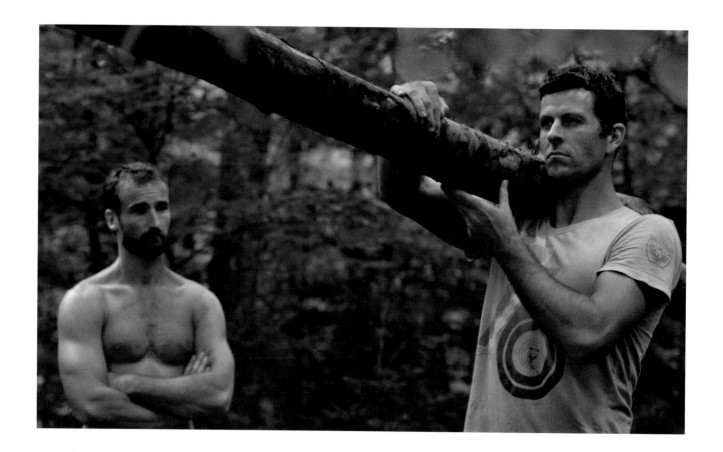

❝❝ Perfection is not attainable, but if we chase perfection we can catch excellence."

—Vince Lombardi

How much efficiency should you aim for? Do you need to reach a world-class level? Of course not. If you learn and apply the principles and techniques covered in this book, you have covered 90 percent of what you need to know to perform most movements and techniques effectively, efficiently, and safely. You will have acquired the foundation of physical competence everyone needs to perform in practical situations of the real world. Here's some other good news: It takes much longer to lose skills after you've acquired them than it takes to lose strength, and it is much faster to regain lost efficiency than it is to regain strength. If you want to become extremely adept at a skill or technique, though, you might need to seek the guidance of specialized experts—on top of spending thousands of hours practicing the skill.

Physically, experientially learning about movement efficiency helps you learn something about yourself. It is not the technique, the drill, the gym, the stopwatch, or the program that you are trying to master, right? You're trying to master *yourself*. Movement perfection might be unattainable, but self-improvement is never out of reach. Improving your movement efficiency, even in the most minute way, is a way of improving yourself. It can be as simple and easy as paying attention to how you stand and breathe. Learning efficient movement can help reduce physical discomfort or pain when you move—and when you don't move. It can add elegance to your movement. It can give you a greater sense of self-control, self-confidence, and self-worth.

11
Mindful

"That which we call thinking is the evolutionary internalization of movement."

—Rodolfo Llinás

Too often we identify our "self" almost exclusively in terms of our intellect. How does the body figure into the sense of self? How do mind and body connect with one another? Through mindful movement. But what is mindful movement? It is both practicing an intention with attention and practicing attention with intention—the two are not separate.

When you read about principle 7, "Adaptable," you learned that the reason for having a brain is to be able to physically navigate through complex environments. Trees and plants do not have a central nervous system because they're rooted and don't move. Locomotion, on the other hand, demands more than just the physical ability of displacement; it requires an ability to predict a future position in a different place, to determine the path that leads there, to anticipate the diverse and necessary steps to be made along the way, and finally to adapt every move to the terrain, the conditions, and the things that happen while traveling. This means that "purely physical" movement does not exist. You need more than muscles, joints, nerves, and fascia to move; you must have motive, or intention. Natural Movement is a physical manifestation of a drive and agenda of self-preservation, of a desire to prolong life as far as possible.

" Only organisms that move have brains."

—Rodolfo Llinás

The notion that movement or even physical exercise can be "purely" physical is absurd. Your muscles don't have neurons. They don't think. They don't get "confused." They don't know their names. They don't know how to count to ten. They have no intention of their own. Movement happens in your mind before it takes place in your body; it is an internal process before it is an external manifestation. The movements we see taking place externally are the result of the nervous system ordering the rest of the body to move. In short, movement comes from the inside out. It stems from awareness.

Rodolfo Llinás, an eminent neurophysiologist, even argues that contextually adaptable movement is at the origin of human thinking, and that self-awareness may have started with our body in motion. Although movement demands intention from the mind and awareness to have the body perform, it doesn't mean that the process relies on thinking. Rational thinking is not fast enough to keep up with the speed of most movements. In fact, thinking—as in producing thought with words and structure—is not a requirement for movement at all. We cannot move without our consciousness ordering movement from our body, but it can be done without thinking, the same way we can meditate and remain conscious without thought.

Not only can we move without thought but movement is the most efficient when it's performed without thought. Efficient awareness in movement is a wordless state of mind, a form of intelligence that is free from intellectual distraction or agitation.

Thoughtless movement is nonetheless mindful the same way thoughtless stillness can be mindful. We can even meditate while in physical motion as in physical stillness. Although the intention to move may be enough to generate effective movement, intention alone isn't sufficient to guarantee efficient and adaptable movement. Intention is the original motive for movement, but attention (or mindfulness) is what primarily enables successful movement.

However, most people have been sold the notion that exercise is something exclusively physical. As people start their practice of Natural Movement, they realize that efficiency isn't that natural. When they revert to what they are used to doing to solve most problems, which is thinking about the problem first, they also realize that it doesn't help much.

As kids, we move a lot without thinking, but as grown-ups we think too much without moving. We have been taught to experience the world almost exclusively via our intellect. Not surprisingly, adults tend to overthink the moment they try to make improvements to basic movements they "think" they "know." Developing an ability to become fully aware in movement without thinking is the antidote to overthinking movement as you learn techniques. This surrender of conscious thought is a form of active meditation that takes place through physical motion rather than physical stillness.

Mindfulness *Is the* Path *to* Efficiency

I made the case for efficiency in principle 10. I explained that a new movement that you do spontaneously is not necessarily efficient just because it came "naturally" to you; by the same token, habitual movement patterns that feel "natural" to you are not necessarily efficient. At a given moment, successfully achieving your goal might be sufficient, and you might not realize how ineptly you did it. A lot of people who are physically active still suffer from "unconscious incompetency." Although these people need a certain degree of attention to perform their movements—remember, movement is never truly mindless—their minds might not be fully engaged with their bodies as they move.

By intentionally focusing on systematically increasing the efficiency of all your movements, you might begin to recognize some deficiencies and inefficiencies in your skills. You then become "consciously incompetent." Instead of performing the same inefficient movements without a thought, you acknowledge that they need improvement and start working on making them efficient.

By first understanding what is wrong about your movement, it gives you a better sense not just of what is wrong and why, but hopefully hints about how you can start making it better. Then, by learning principles and techniques (either on your own or from someone else) and being mindful at physically applying the principles and techniques, your performance gets rapidly better. Ultimately you are able to reach a state of "conscious competency."

However, the irony of good form and efficient technique is that sometimes it doesn't feel right the first time you try it. If you have accustomed yourself to a poor movement, the modified, efficient pattern feels "unnatural" at first. In any case, at this stage, efficiency is not guaranteed and might disappear the moment you get distracted because you must consciously focus on your competency.

The last stage is when you become "unconsciously competent." At this point, you no longer need to think of what you must do to be efficient. It might even seem that you are almost not paying attention that much because your movement awareness has shifted to a subconscious level, and your conscious mind is free from the task of ensuring efficiency.

The path to unconscious efficiency relies on mindfulness and can be summarized as follows:

- **Unconscious/subconscious incompetence:** Moving naturally but poorly without knowing it. Not noticing inefficiency.

- **Conscious incompetence:** Being aware of your poor movement ability. Noticing inefficiency.

- **Conscious competence:** Having learned movement efficiency but needing to think about it. Learning, thinking, and mindful practice are required to achieve efficiency.

- **Unconscious/subconscious competence:** Having movement competency that doesn't require thinking. Thoughtless efficiency.

In the beginning, a jump is just a jump. With mindful practice, a jump is no longer just a jump because you realize that it is more complex than it looks and that it can be transformed into a much better movement. Eventually, a jump goes back to being just a jump, but it is nothing like the jump it was at first. Efficient movement has become second-nature thanks to mindfulness, but the mindfulness you have applied has helped you achieve movement competency in a wordless, thoughtless state of mind. Natural Movement demands a cognitive engagement that might require intellectual understanding at some stage but eventually becomes free of analysis. I call it *mindful movement*.

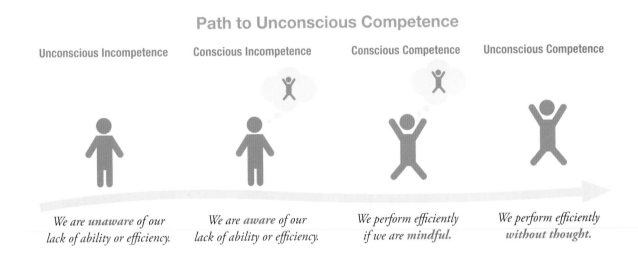

Path to Unconscious Competence

Unconscious Incompetence	Conscious Incompetence	Conscious Competence	Unconscious Competence
We are **unaware** of our lack of ability or efficiency.	We are **aware** of our lack of ability or efficiency.	We perform efficiently if we are **mindful**.	We perform efficiently **without thought**.

Mindful Practice *Is a* Feel

If the body is the "tool" necessary for movement, and technique is the tool necessary for movement efficiency, then mindfulness is the tool necessary to apply technique. Deliberate practice means mindful practice with the intention of ensuring both efficiency and continuous improvement. The central nervous system doesn't need numbers to achieve movement. "Ten" or "one hundred" might be meaningful to your intellect, but it means nothing to your central nervous system.

The purpose of mindful practice is to strive for movement efficiency rather than brute exertion. The nervous system relies on sensations of pattern, position in space, relationship to the environment, balance, timing, level of intensity, and so forth. We could talk about "internal" and "external" awareness in the sense that we could differentiate between input that stems from the internal motion of the body (proprioception) and input that stems from the environment where motion takes place (exteroception).

> **Until you make the unconscious conscious, it will direct your life and you will call it fate."**
>
> *—Carl Jung*

Mindful practice requires that you pay attention to the two primary aspects of your physical performance when you move:

- Practical effectiveness, which is the tangible goal you strive to achieve through your movement. This is a more effective way to move than thinking of the diverse muscles that you need to use to achieve the movement as you move. I'm not saying that attention to the different phases of a movement sequence and to particular body parts isn't part of mindful practice, only that it is not an intellectual exercise in kinesiology and anatomy analysis. As I previously stated, movement is too fast for the intellect to keep up with the pace.

- While your mind is attentive to the practical result, it is also attentive to your body's feedback. The practical goals are never forgotten, but the process that leads to achieving them gets special attention. Effectiveness alone is not satisfactory; efficient effectiveness is what mindfulness ultimately strives to achieve. If such effectiveness translates in part to achieving a certain quantity—say, twenty repetitions in less than sixty seconds—that is awesome. However, in the absence of mindful and efficient movement, practice is effective but inefficient, and your growth and performance ultimately are impaired. The progress that you only observe or feel is not less important than the progress that can be measured. The same goes for the "data" that you collect from practice—*the most important feedback is how movement feels.* You may use measurable data to motivate yourself, but using sensations is equally effective. The sensory feedback from your body in motion (or *kinesthetic sense*) isn't presented to your intellect in the form of numbers; it's an overall feel in both your body and brain.

Paying attention to sensations—and to thoughts or emotions that arise before, during, and immediately after movement—is essential to managing efforts and actions. "Experience-dependent" learning is a process important to brain development and related to experiences that are unique to the individual. Simply put, we must physically experience movement to learn it. The more attentive we are to these experiences, the more we can benefit from them. Attentiveness occurs through mindful Natural Movement.

It is challenging to control something that you cannot perceive well. For instance, when your hands get numb in the cold, it's hard to control your finger movement, and you have diminished dexterity as you try to use them the way you normally can. Well, moving mindlessly is equivalent to moving with a body that would be numb all over. Trusting your body sensations when you move and investing effort in better understanding and perceiving them is a healthy instinct. Feedback is only beneficial when we pay attention to it, yet it is not necessarily an intellectual pursuit. When you were a young child, each attempt you made to try to acquire or improve a new movement pattern was performed without thought. Each attempt led either to a positive or negative reinforcement (of how to move or not move) by your central nervous system (and still happened without thought).

Conscious thought can help guide your attention or objectives before movement—such as when you're studying the information in this book—or it can help you analyze visual or kinesthetic feedback after movement, which will be the case as you start practicing. We can think about our movement just before or immediately after it; it just doesn't help to think about it as we move.

Much is still unknown when it comes to how the human nervous system controls movement. Science helps us understand how diverse areas of the brain—such as the cerebellum, the basal ganglia, the brain stem, the frontal lobe, and, by extension, the spinal cord—contribute to enabling motor control. But none of this conceptual knowledge helps us move better because we can't move intellectually.

> **Can the knowledge deriving from reason even begin to compare with knowledge perceptible by sense?"**
>
> *—Louis Aragon*

In fact, you need to let go of mental tensions and mental "noise" if you want to better perceive subtle body signals with the most clarity possible while you are in motion. Practicing mindful movement sharpens your perception of the body in motion. Indeed, you can even visualize movement, how each body part moves in sequence, how the movements are timed, and the physical sensations the movement produces—without thinking...and without moving at all. This is because the central nervous system creates *somatotopic memory* of the movement, which is like a three-dimensional representation of movement patterns, except that instead of just being a visual "hologram," it also involves sensations. When you mindfully imagine yourself doing a movement, you can feel it in your body. To paraphrase Maya Angelou, you may forget the programs you once planned and the numbers you once achieved, but you will never forget how movements made you feel.

Efficient Mind

The concept of mindfulness has nothing to do with the idea of "mind over matter." You can't achieve efficient and adaptable movement and physical performance without being mindful; the key to establishing, improving, and optimizing such competency lies in consistent mindful practice. Once someone told me that they didn't need Natural Movement practice because their "mindful" practice—yoga and meditation—would enable them to overcome any challenging real-world circumstances that demanded a physical response by enabling them to tap into their innate potential to multiply their strength. I've heard stories of people who've been able to pull from a previously unrecognized source of strength in times of need, but those tales are quite rare compared to the many stories of people who have found themselves completely unprepared and helpless when life put them in situations they had never anticipated.

The only way your mind can command your body is by obeying the *rules that govern it*. Mindfulness is not a magic trick, a silver bullet, or voodoo spell; it's a straightforward, down-to-earth ability to optimally operate your body, and you can't create that efficient "mind-body" connection without practice. While practice evidently implies physical activity, the mental work needed to learn to perform new movements (or more efficient familiar movements) is much more significant than people expect. Your brain is at work as you learn and improve technique, even when you practice the simplest movements.

Contrary to what most people believe, paying attention and being mentally alert and responsive is so energy-consuming that it has a metabolic cost! It doesn't matter whether the movements are slow or fast, low or high in intensity, simple or complex; the more you need to focus to achieve efficient movement, the greater the brain activity. Greater brain activity consumes more energy.

So, to reduce metabolic cost—at any level of intensity—we need efficient metabolic conditioning and movement patterns, but to improve efficiency of movement patterns, we must be mindful. But being mindful increases metabolic cost. That sounds like a paradox, doesn't it?

I have good news, though: The metabolic cost generated by greater brain activity decreases over time, not because you will no longer need to be mindful but because your central nervous system becomes able to expend significantly less effort into making movement efficient. With each movement performed mindfully with the intention to improve efficiency, which is the very goal of practice, the nervous system remodels itself—a process called *neuroplasticity*—to optimize motor control and muscular activity. In other words, through the practice of mindful movement you can improve the efficiency of brain activity and reduce its metabolic cost.

TRAINING THE MMA FIGHTER

When I trained elite MMA fighter Carlos Condit on improving his footwork, standing stability, and speed, I used many variations of stepping, balancing, and jumping. None of the movements were very complex, and I never asked him to perform them with great intensity. (My mission was to improve quality rather than to "condition" him.)

To Carlos's surprise, he felt like taking a nap at the end of each session—a phenomenon that he had never experienced, even after some of his most grueling physical training sessions. Given his world-class athleticism and the relatively low intensity of the physical work we were doing together, there's no way Carlos was physically drained. However, his nervous system was exhausted because each session required a high level of focus to pay attention to multiple aspects of movement at once, which required great mental activity for a relatively prolonged time (two or three hours per session). After several sessions, Carlos no longer felt drained at the end of the sessions because his nervous system had adapted to become more efficient at being so intensely mindful of his movement without interruption for two or three hours straight.

So, when you feel quite tired after a session of mindful movement practice, remember that even elite athletes can become tired when they take on new challenges that require them to engage their brains as well as their bodies.

Mind-Body-Context: *Your* Brain *on* Mindful Natural Movement

Natural Movement implies a level of awareness that goes beyond the "mind-body" connection to be efficient. It demands "mind-body-context" connection, starting with "mind-body-environment" connection.

Do you remember principle 7, "Adaptable"? Natural Movement is never disconnected from the real-world context where it takes place. Although meditation is a part of Natural Movement practice, when you're in motion you cannot afford to close your eyes and isolate yourself from the world to connect to your inner world. This is a *powerful* insight: Natural Movement demands that you mindfully engage with the outer world, not retreat from it. Your senses must be sharp, your attention oriented to both internal and external input. Is this purely physical? Of course not; it's extremely mindful because the world and variables around you are real, tangible, changing, and impossible to dismiss.

If you consider the mind and the body as separate entities, a notion known as *Cartesian dualism* that's subject to intense debate, then you must connect the mind to the body, and the connected mind-body must connect with the real world you interact with through your movements. Which of the two connections requires the greatest level of awareness and mindfulness? It is often said that mind-body connection is about being in the moment—in other words, being in the "here and now"—which is indeed valuable. But it still leaves you with the possibility of becoming distracted and mentally transporting yourself to a different place and time. Adaptable movement most often does not grant you such "luxury" because the moment you get distracted is the moment movement fails. Your motion is impossible to dissociate from variables and demands external to yourself; consequently, you become naturally immersed in a mindful interaction with them. The "here and now" is the context.

Scientific studies have demonstrated that we feel better and happier when we exercise because endorphins—which have addictive properties like morphine—are generated, and they help us cope with physical discomfort during and after exercise. In some cases, endorphins also cause us to experience euphoria. Just twenty minutes of most any physical activity generates those benefits and boosts brain function, including neurogenesis (the regeneration of neurons).

If even machine-based exercise can produce benefits for your brain, what can Natural Movement—which involves mindful, adaptable, efficient movement—do for your brain? Wouldn't it make sense to assume that when we use our brains for their original biological purpose of Natural Movement that we would have a greater potential to boost brain function than when we do mechanistic exercise?

Studies also show that rich natural environments, as well as enriched artificial environments, contribute to a healthier, more functional brain and happier life. (Read more about this in principle 8, "Environmental.") This idea is implemented in zoos that are designed to replicate the wild environment where animals normally live because it helps tremendously in keeping them healthy by enabling them to physically behave the way they naturally do as much as possible. Such "enhanced environmental stimulation" is beneficial to brain function in many ways: It improves baseline chemical levels; neuron growth, size, and overall brain mass; and neural processing and connectivity between different parts of the brain, which contributes to better learning and memory. Obviously, such improvement of brain function benefits movement competency, but it also carries over to any area of life. Neuroscientists have known for a long time that brain health is linked to exercise, but they have recently started to understand that physical activity alone, such as running on a treadmill, may not be as beneficial to brain function as "cognitively engaging" with complex environments the way our ancestors used to.

NOTE

If you'd like to read more about the benefits of exercise on our brains, one source I recommend is "Brains Evolved to Need Exercise" by Alexis Blue, which you can find at https://uanews.arizona.edu/story/ua-research-brains-evolved-need-exercise.

However, plunking an animal or person in an environmentally stimulating place isn't all it takes; an apathetic or depressed person might not wake up from their mental fog or receive any benefit at all. What makes a difference in the amount of benefit derived from a stimulating environment is cognitive engagement with environmentally rich areas. In a nutshell, you cannot benefit from external stimulation without also having deliberate, mindful participation. The body won't connect to the environment if the mind doesn't connect first. The external environment must be present, the mind must be present, and you must connect the two through the body in motion.

Working memory is how efficiently you can process information, and it's been determined that working memory is even more important than IQ in determining an individual's ability to do well. In a recent study on working memory, three groups were evaluated. The first group did no physical activity at all, the second group did yoga, and the third group did a set of two Natural Movement exercises—balancing across a beam and climbing a tree. Subjects' working memories were tested before and after their activity. The first group demonstrated no difference in the two measurements. The yoga group also did not see any change, which means that form of movement did not provide any benefit. However, the Natural Movement group saw a significant boost in working memory after doing what seems to be a merely "physical" activity that seemingly did not require too much attention. Wrong. Efficiency at adapting movement to the environment demands high levels of attention, which boosts brain function. And what is attention if not mindfulness?

NOTE

You can find an article about the study about working memory and natural movement at www.medicaldaily.com/climbing-tree-can-improve-your-working-memory-capacity-50-345450.

However, not all mindful physical activity is equally beneficial to the brain. Mindfulness in the sense of "stillness" and internal "self-orientation" is not as beneficial as being dynamically mindful about something external to you that demands a cognitive interaction and an adaptable response from you both physically and mentally. Interacting adaptively with an external, complex context demands levels of awareness, alertness, and responsiveness that closing your eyes and stilling the mind can't match.

Without alertness, responsiveness is impossible. Without responsiveness, alertness is useless. It is an engagement between you and the real world through bodily motion that necessitates the most primal and ancient form of intelligence. This simple idea produces a new form of mindfulness practice, which I call the "mind-body-context connection" (and I was talking about it for years before the study on working memory was published). This is not to say that the "mind-body" level of connection and mindfulness is not challenging, rewarding, and beneficial; it's just that you can achieve higher cognitive engagement and greater mindfulness through the mind-body-context connection. Self-awareness in isolation is great, but self-awareness in relation to the real world is greater.

The importance of context is so important in Natural Movement that in the absence of contextual demands—such as when you're in an empty indoor venue with no environmental variables other than a flat floor and walls—you might want to visualize the types of obstacles or situations that you normally practice with. You can jump over and crawl under imaginary obstacles or run away from imaginary dangers. In the absence of a real context, the simulation of it gives your movement the meaning it needs and always deserves. After all, if we can anticipate our next moves before they happen, we can certainly mentally simulate the context where those moves should ideally take place. The context may be imaginary, but your movements are nonetheless real. At this point I don't need to reassert the importance of context in Natural Movement; just never lose sight of the original and fundamental reason for being able to move.

Mindfulness *and* Mindset

Mindset is the set of attitudes that we hold or the state of mind we may experience or intentionally adopt, and it's closely related to mindfulness. State of mind, mental state or behavior, psychological drive, outlook, perspective, approach, psychology, philosophy, spirit: Whatever name you want to use, mindset is something that basically stems from and takes place in the mind and has a direct influence on physical practice. Remember, movement is *never* restricted to a compartmentalized physical action that's dissociated from the mind, and we can't deny the importance of that fact. Your mindset or state of mind can be either an advantage or obstacle to your movement practice and physical performance.

" **True strength, in its broadest meaning, must be seen as the result and synthesis of physical and moral strength. It resides not only in the muscles, the breath, the agility . . . , but above all in the energy that uses it, the will that directs it, or the feeling that guides it."**

—Georges Hébert

Becoming aware of your state of mind—and even underlying emotions or beliefs about yourself or your ability—as you practice is essential to determining whether difficulty in performing is caused by a psychological reason or a physical one. Because movement stems from an intention and Natural Movement should stem from a positive one, mindfulness is not just limited to the "here and now" or the very moment when you physically practice. Mindfulness has to do with envisioning the future and anticipating in the present moment how to shape that future. This nonphysical component of your practice can be very potent. How you move *now* determines how you will be able to move in the future, and how you intentionally think about or imagine your future movement in the present can also positively influence your future abilities and experience. Your mind is more likely to limit you or incapacitate you than your body is.

"Self-talk" is an aspect of psychological practice in which we either negatively assert who we think we are or positively assert who we choose to be. By extension, that self-talk affects how we perform, experience things, handle challenges, and so on. It can be either detrimental or favorable. You don't have to wait for real events to occur to begin mentally conditioning yourself to be strong in the face of adversity. Composure, self-control, and even mettle—mental robustness and resiliency—are not just innate; they can be trained.

Some things that prevent us from achieving mindful practice include attention-deficit, distraction, lack of motivation (because the movements are too easy or too hard, because we don't like particular movements, or because we don't understand their value), mental agitation, a lack of self-confidence or self-esteem (especially when people are watching), and any kind of negative thought or emotions that are irrelevant to the practice.

Individuals with a low internal "locus of control" have learned to behave helplessly as if they have no control over the outcome of their circumstances, including their physical movement performance. It doesn't matter how much encouragement you receive; if you don't believe in yourself first, you will remain disempowered. Likewise, if you suffer from "neuroticism" (the tendency to experience negative emotions such as anger, anxiety, or depression or other expressions of emotional instability) being mindful and preventing your thoughts and emotions from interfering with your practice and performance is a challenge. Also, overthinking, or "paralysis by analysis," might occur if you stick to the theoretical details of practice rather than empirical experience. Some people do this—consciously or unconsciously—to avoid practical challenges or hard work.

Fortunately, consistent practice of Natural Movement eventually reduces, and even dissolves, most of these psychological obstacles. Positive visualization and affirmation before, during, and after practice can prove very effective and useful. Meditation and stillness are also extremely beneficial. As a matter of fact, this type of mental practice should become a habit in your life regardless of your physical practice. When you show up to practice, you bring who you are, and who you are results a lot from your day-to-day mental habits and choices. If you can mindfully improve how you operate your mind every day, your practice will be positively affected the same way physical and mental self-improvements gained through Natural Movement practice carry over to any aspect of your life and boost your self-efficacy.

  " **A pessimist sees the difficulty in every opportunity; an optimist sees the opportunity in every difficulty."**

— Winston Churchill

Not surprisingly, becoming able to intentionally adopt a certain mindset during practice supports greater performance. Different mindsets—willfulness, playfulness, a sense of collaboration, determination—fit different types of movement exercises or physical demands. For instance, before attempting a single jump that involves some risk and maybe some danger, mental determination must be composed, and

  " **They can because they think they can."**

— Virgil

you must be strong yet relaxed. A task that requires strength and speed in achieving the same efforts repetitively may demand a more aggressive state of mind (of course only for the duration of the task). The intention to physically achieve something can be motivated by the objective of being able to help others when they need physical assistance, in which case practical altruism is the goal and real-world movement capability is the means to an end.

In any case, such states of mind are used as tools, and they result from a choice and mental control; they don't randomly take place. What separates highly skilled movement practitioners from beginners is the internal level of locus of control (or how well they can control their minds) while performing physically in a variety of situations. They also have a realistic, experience-based sense of self-efficacy. Regardless of the level of practice, the mind leads and the body executes—and you're in charge of both. In the chain of command, you're at the top. You send the orders. No improvement is possible without self-discipline, and there's no self-discipline without authority on yourself.

The way we move, stand, and breathe carries much more weight than how convincingly we can discuss kinesiology, biomechanics, or exercise science. Body stances and poise are a great revealer and exposer of intention and mindset. We embody our attitudes through physical behavior. Natural Movement requires a philosophy of self-actualization and empowerment for the benefit of self and others. (This is an idea I explore in principle 12, "Cooperative.") Naturally, negative thoughts and emotions toward yourself or others have no room in the practice of Natural Movement, and they will eventually go away. If you are having fun, if your experience is mentally positive, then your love for movement will grow more. *Movement can be a more effective mood regulator than stillness.*

People who see exercise as a chore always look at the clock. People who enjoy movement lose track of time. Having a positive, rewarding, and satisfying experience depends not only on the nature of the experience but also on your ability to make it so.

As I mentioned previously, mindfulness is not limited to the specific time when you practice. You also can anticipate and visualize the progress and achievements you want to make. This process of "goal setting" is an intention for the future—a potent way to remain motivated to practice in the moment. Visualization is

mentally rehearsing your movements without physically performing them. You can imagine, sometimes very vividly, the sequence of positions the movements follow, the context where they take place, how they make us feel in our bodies and minds, and so on. In other words, my brain anticipates the feeling of the movement before I actually feel it in the rest of my body. I have visualized the movement in my mind before you see me moving. MovNat, the practice of Natural Movement, must be mentally approached the way martial artists approach their discipline: learning techniques and seeking greater efficiency through mindful practice.

Mindful, adaptable Natural Movement practice provides an immediate reward. Focus, adaptability, playfulness, and fighting spirit combined with physical motion create a potent and positive psychological experience. The instant gratification you get might not be that you acquire impressive movement skills and physical capacity in record time, but that you feel energized both physically and mentally every time you practice.

The practice of mental toughness is not a supplemental and optional aspect of Natural Movement practice, but an inherent component of it. Regardless of muscular strength and tough looks, when someone who is mentally weak is exposed to a certain level of difficulty, that person is quick at talking himself into giving up long before his body has reached its limits. It is often a surprise when unassuming individuals with no particular physical strength or skills can demonstrate impressive mental toughness. Those who have this mental quality can make faster progress than those who have natural athleticism but no willpower or self-discipline.

The "know thyself" principle isn't limited to the mind; it must include knowledge of your physical capabilities. If you don't know what your body is made of, you will never know what your mind is truly made of. Complex movements and sustained physical effort reveal the extent of your mental toughness, but context is also a factor. Mindful low-intensity movement practice cannot be the safe space where you shelter your lack of physical and mental strength. Occasionally training physically and mentally with difficult real-world Natural Movement context—which may include harsh weather or even food and sleep deprivation—forces you into a realistic space where your mental shortcomings are exposed in no time.

Shape Your Mind

People may not necessarily need scientific evidence to be motivated for movement practice; they only need to have a single movement experience that makes them feel *amazing.*

Muscle-isolation and machine-based fitness drills make most people want to mentally escape during the physical activity. Practical and adaptable Natural Movement practice, on the other hand, naturally compels your mind to engage together with your body and the outer world. A change of experience might lead to a change of perception, but a change of perception definitely leads to a change of experience.

66 **Not everything that can be counted counts, and not everything that counts can be counted."**

— *Bruce Cameron*

No single fitness drill can transform your body, but a single insight can transform your behavior, practice, and eventually your entire life. Paying attention makes anything feel like you are doing it for the first time; it keeps anything you do "fresh."

The body and how it works are immensely complex, but that doesn't mean your approach to movement should be overly sophisticated. You want to practice movement mindfully—not intellectually or analytically. When you mindfully "listen" to your body in motion, you become not only a great listener but also a better interpreter of your own mind.

In today's hectic life where the individual is being fragmented and daily life compartmentalized, mindfulness has become a rare skill and a priceless experience. Mindfulness and movement skills are an invisible and weightless kind of "gear," but they are more than a tool; they provide a whole operating system to achieve who we choose to be. Both the mind and body are trainable. The difference is that you can give the mind practice not just when the body is at rest but also when it is active.

Shaping your body is important, but shaping your mind is an even greater achievement. A strong body with an out-of-shape mind is no better than a strong mind with an out-of-shape body.

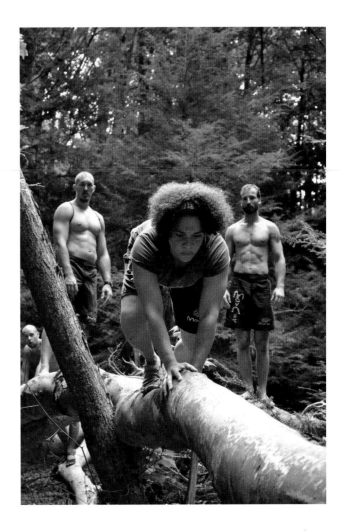

12
Cooperative

"The only thing that will redeem mankind is cooperation."
—Bertrand Russell

Cooperation between the members of the same human group, clan, or tribe was a fundamental aspect of ancestral life until very recently. All individuals of a community had to work cooperatively to ensure both group survival and individual survival. Humans, often moved in packs. This had to do with hunting, gathering, building shelter, preparing food, harvesting firewood, and transporting water (as well as pretty much everything else required to sustain the group), and it obviously necessitated Natural Movement.

Just like today, mutual help, collaboration, and good communication created strong and positive bonds between individuals, and those positive bonds greatly facilitated cooperation. Collective sustenance, safety, well-being, or success in challenges wasn't a result of internal competition within the group; primarily it resulted from collaboration within the group. Both cooperativeness and competitiveness are inherent to human nature, but cooperativeness has an equal, if not a greater, potential to make us stronger and more successful as a group than competition within a group does. Cooperativeness also makes us stronger and more successful as individuals who belong to the group which we serve. If systematic competition against each other was the rule of human existence, our lives would be miserable and short, whereas greater collaboration helps everyone who participates.

When we think of prehistoric times of mankind, we imagine outrageously selfish, typically male brutes fighting over everything, especially food. However, cultural anthropology shows that in our evolutionary past, cooperation was much more essential to survival than competition. The same thing can be observed in hunter-gatherer tribes that still survive in the world, as well as in every group that has remained faithful to its ancestral cultural heritage. Serving the group was serving oneself.

Today we are constantly bombarded with the idea of "survival of the fittest," and we approach life as if it is a constant competition in which being the strongest—and most aggressive—is the key to prevailing in any situation. The image of the superhero prevailing on all villains and single-handedly rescuing everyone or of the lone wolf overcoming harsh conditions and surviving alone in the wild are omnipresent in literature, comics, cartoons, movies, and video games. They strongly influence our perception that life is mostly a competition in which the strongest reign on top of all the rest.

66 Through the evolutionary process, those who are able to engage in social cooperation of various sorts do better in survival and reproduction."

—Robert Nozick

In our evolutionary past, surviving long term, alone, in wild environments while equipped with primitive technology was nearly impossible, and very few would have willingly chosen that lifestyle. Living alone would have resulted from someone being banished by the community, and it probably would have led to the person's death.

The importance of competition in life is undeniable, but it is overestimated, and the importance of cooperation is underestimated. We often believe that only the most competitive people are successful, and we forget that the most cooperative people also are very successful. Cooperation has nothing to do with the loss of individuality. It is not a collectivist political idea but a part of our evolutionary psychology. When the individual participates in the collective effort, the benefit is both to the self and the group.

How often do tasks you have to handle in your life or physical training necessitate cooperation with others to achieve a task? By cooperation, I don't mean only encouragement, moral support, or camaraderie—the modern equivalent of tribal bonding. By cooperation I mean performing tasks with others that you could not perform alone.

The way we live today makes it possible to completely avoid relying on any other person's physical help if we want to. Mainstream fitness has always had a tendency toward individualistic fitness training and goals. Have you ever seen an exercise machine designed so people can work out together? How many times have you had to wait in line for your turn to bench press or use the leg-extension machine? Society has become increasingly individualistic, which is a fact that pervades how we approach physical training.

As a result, new forms of community have emerged around all sorts of activities or causes that bring people together. The same sense of community has developed in the fitness world, and it counterbalances the blatant ego-centered mindset that had been prevailing. However, training *together* and training *cooperatively* are not the same: You are always training together when you are training cooperatively, but you are not necessarily training cooperatively when you train together. Again, cooperative physical training or work is based on a real, tangible interaction, communication, and synchronicity to coordinate physical action and efforts between individuals.

Training together could simply mean going through the same workout, at the same time, in the same place, but the workout itself is basically something you could do just as well on your own. Although it can be very enjoyable and motivating to work out with others, it does not teach individuals to cooperate and achieve a task that they couldn't do singly, either in the form of cooperation or mutual help.

A cooperative task could involve each person participating in carrying part of a load individually, but that could also mean lifting something collectively—something so heavy that a single person couldn't lift and carry it or something heavy enough that a single person would spend an enormous amount of energy, go very slowly, and maybe injure him- or herself by transporting it alone. Throwing and catching are also movement tasks that require impeccable coordination and cooperation—for example, to pass valuable rescue equipment or food, medicine, weapons, or anything valuable. Another extreme example is someone jumping from a height to a group of people waiting to make the catch. Mutual help is another form of cooperation, as when one person helps another clear an obstacle, reach safety, or avoid drowning.

Cooperation is mutually beneficial; you give and take, and anyone involved gets a share of the outcome that was produced regardless of how much they were able to contribute to the collective effort. Cooperation empowers everyone and leaves everyone happy—never frustrated. It makes the present more viable and the future more sustainable, both for the individuals and for the community they belong to.

This principle does not dismiss in any way the importance of individuality, nor does it discard the potential value of competition. As with principle 6, "Unspecialized," elite athletes driven by competition have achieved both personal greatness and pushed the—recorded—limits of human physical performance to new heights. Competitiveness—the desire to win or to rank the highest possible—can be a powerful drive for improvement and achievement.

However, it's essential to acknowledge that not all human prowess or achievements are born from competition. Swimming across an ocean or running across a continent are phenomenal achievements, but they might not take place within a competitive setting. Observers are quick to say that the person who achieved such feats competed against nature or against them-selves, but this is a personal view. True competition is an intention that requires at least two people. Nature is not a person; it doesn't have the intention to defeat you or prevail over you. It stays the same regardless of anyone being there, of what they're doing, and of what their intention is. You also cannot "compete against yourself." You are not two people, and you cannot win or lose over yourself. There may not be an ounce of competitiveness in the mind of those great achievers, yet they achieve something great because they have extraordinary determination and discipline. In many cases, people who achieve things individually have an impeccable support system behind them.

Similar achievements are made by pairs or groups who plan, organize, and finally realize achievements together. In this case, competitiveness between the members of the group is a very counterproductive factor that can endanger the team.

Cooperative Competition

Interestingly, when competition takes place between groups at a team level, cooperation within each of the groups is an absolute must. One of the primary concerns of all team coaches is to detect and address individualism and to maintain the greatest, most au-thentic levels of cooperativeness possible in the mind of all players. Team coaches seek great individuals who have little individualism. Although fans may be entirely focused on the aggressiveness of their team, which is necessary to secure the win, the fans often fail to realize that such aggression is totally channeled and organized into cooperative work from start to end. Individual aggressiveness alone does not win team games.

❝ **Remember that there is nothing noble in being superior to some other man. The true nobility is in being superior to your previous self."**

— *W. L. Sheldon*

Individual competition within a group can to some degree help motivate every individual to improve, and making each member of a group better contrib-utes to the success of the collective. But such compet-itiveness has more to do with the concern of giving one's best, or at least with keeping up with a baseline level of aptitude the group expects from you, rather than the desire to be on top and better than everyone else. In every group there will be always individuals who are better, stronger, tougher, smarter, kinder, wiser, more skilled, more creative, or more attrac-tive (whether they're that way naturally or as a result of some effort they make). We're all different. What matters to everyone in any group is the intention that each individual displays and the efforts each individ-ual is willing to produce. In a nutshell, authentic, gen-erous cooperativeness is what is expected from you to be recognized and accepted in the group as useful, reliable, and important. In competitive sports, most of the time preceding competition events is spent in pursuit of improving each individual's progress and preparation, and the support system provided by the coach, sensei, and other students is really what at-tracts people to the team.

Even in martial arts, training is not primarily designed to determine who prevails; it's an arrangement in which one person tries to expose the other's weaknesses and accepts that one's weaknesses might be exposed by another person; that philosophy is the key to mutual improvement. Opponents are not real opponents: They are partners within a group dedicated to everyone's betterment and continuous empowerment. They respect their partner's weaknesses as much as their fortes and enjoy seeing them evolve and make progress. They bow, hug, fist bump, and high-five, before and after sparring, and they smile and nod in appreciation during it. Cooperation, as much as competition, is omnipresent. The desire to self-improve most of the time prevails over the desire to dominate opponents. Trying to prevail is not always a finality; it is a means to the end of improving one's own capability.

Chronic competitiveness is a sign that you have no other way of being motivated. If you absolutely *need* competition to find motivation to perform at your highest, you are driven only by ego. In real life, people who always want to be better than all the rest are usually not so popular, whereas people who are always trying to support or benefit others, ensure everyone's fun and safety, or act as peacemakers when conflicts arise are most often quite popular; there is an evolutionary psychology reason for this.

> " **A person's a person, no matter how small.**"
>
> —*Dr. Seuss*

Working with others in a spirit of cooperativeness and participation to contribute to a collective effort has helped countless individuals build the self-confidence and self-esteem they were lacking. It helps engender more humility, respect, tolerance, patience, and kindness for others, and it encourages people to be more positive, constructive, open, helpful, encouraging, and friendly in life. So, I want to state again that the importance of competition in life is undeniable, but it is overestimated, whereas the importance of cooperation is underestimated.

Practical Cooperation

As you begin your Natural Movement practice, find people you can primarily cooperate with and benefit from. Learn from, share with, and train with these people, both in the sense of training next to each other and working together to achieve tasks none of you could achieve alone. Physically participate and interact with one another and with the same goal in mind. It doesn't matter who's best; what matters is how good you can become individually and as a group and how the group can improve its collective performance. Even from a situational intelligence perspective, when positive synergy occurs, the constructive interaction of two or more people often produces solutions and improved strategies superior to what each individual could have come up with if they had been working alone.

Of course, you do not have to always train cooperatively every time you practice with others. The cooperative principle neither implies the dismissal of individuality nor minimizes the importance of self-empowerment in any way. Even within a group, the real source of self-confidence is within you, and only your rigorous self-discipline and personal will can make you stronger.

Yet practicing cooperatively definitely is rewarding and beneficial. You'll learn from others as much as they might learn from you, and you might learn new things together. You'll learn to trust others and find that you can rely on them as much as they will realize they can rely on you. That mutual reliance is the goal. We could call it *reciprocal altruism*.

Nothing is more empowering than when you become inspiring to yourself—except maybe knowing that you can be useful to others. We're not more than others; we're more *with* others. "Stronger together" is not a political and gimmicky motto; it's a timeless reality that concerns us all. The pursuit of fitness without the spiritual drive to better yourself as a person and be able to help others in time of need may not be a meaningless endeavor, but it's not as meaningful and noble as the alternative.

> **True heroism is remarkably sober, very undramatic. It is not the urge to surpass all others at whatever cost, but the urge to serve others at whatever cost."**
>
> —*Arthur Ashe*

Friendly competition can be an effective additional source of motivation and fun from time to time. Competition can be the simulation of adverse circumstances that demand a physical response from you and that otherwise wouldn't exist.

However, rivalry, or competition, is not the only way—or even the most effective way—to get motivated. One of my primary motivations has been thinking of how I want to develop and maintain an ability to physically help my loved ones, friends, or even strangers in time of need. As a matter of fact, I have put such real-world physical competency and preparedness to use by rescuing near-drowning people on three occasions. My response in those situations wasn't anything special: I knew what to do, I knew what I was capable of doing, and I had trained for it with intention. Lives are saved every day by both professionals and regular people, and most often the rescues are successful thanks to the cooperation of several people who work with one another to achieve a result.

I believe everyone should be physically trained to help others. This type of training should be a mandatory part of authentic, healthy physical education programs in every school. As expressed in principle 5, "Vital," there is no guarantee that you will ever be in a situation that demands your physical capability to such an extreme, but you should still be prepared in the event that you *do* need those physical skills.

Muscle size has never impressed me, but I certainly look up to those who possess useful physical capability, a strong mind, and a big heart, regardless of muscle mass. I won't miss the opportunity to express my admiration and gratitude to all the people out there—firefighters, paramedics, rescuers, police officers, military—who at any point will put themselves in danger to save others' lives. Even if some of them may be competitive by nature, they don't behave like individualistic superheroes but as trained, cooperative team members.

> **Act as if what you do makes a difference. It does."**
>
> —*William James*

I also want to thank the mentor I have never met, Georges Hébert, whose writings inspired me to perpetuate this philosophy of cooperation. Hébert's motto was "Be strong to be useful"—both to oneself and to others. He was referring to helpfulness through cooperation and mutual assistance. Utility is for objects like tools; helpfulness is for conscious beings. Helpfulness requires your intention.

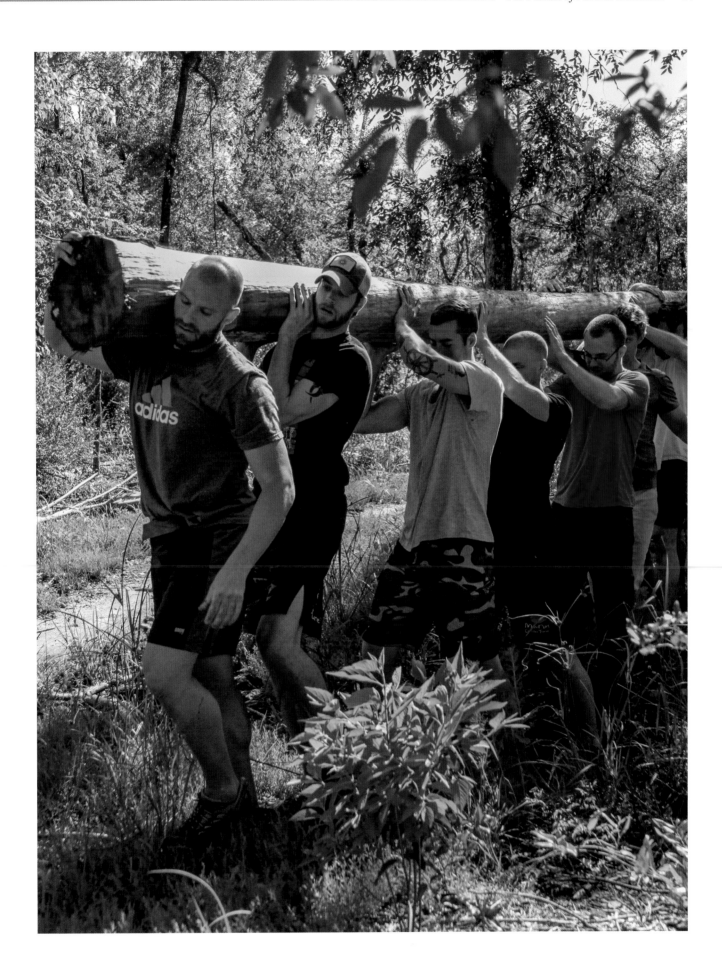

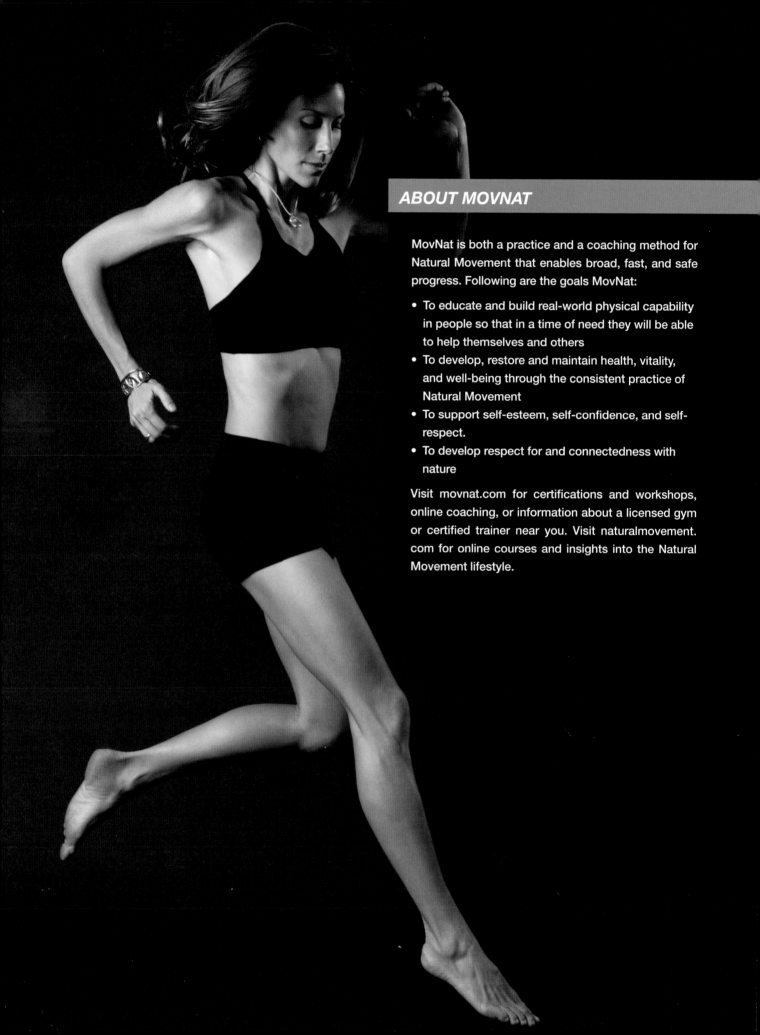

ABOUT MOVNAT

MovNat is both a practice and a coaching method for Natural Movement that enables broad, fast, and safe progress. Following are the goals MovNat:

- To educate and build real-world physical capability in people so that in a time of need they will be able to help themselves and others
- To develop, restore and maintain health, vitality, and well-being through the consistent practice of Natural Movement
- To support self-esteem, self-confidence, and self-respect.
- To develop respect for and connectedness with nature

Visit movnat.com for certifications and workshops, online coaching, or information about a licensed gym or certified trainer near you. Visit naturalmovement. com for online courses and insights into the Natural Movement lifestyle.

2

Movement Efficiency Principles

"Learning is an experience. Everything else is just information."
—*Albert Einstein*

Among the twelve Natural Movement principles, principle 10, "Efficient," gives us compelling insights on what efficiency is and why it matters so much. In this part, I want to share with you *how* movement efficiency works, which will lead us into the discussion in Part 3, practice efficiency.

It is my observation that masterful world-class movement practitioners and athletes might not have much scientific knowledge of movement, whereas world-level exercise scientists might move very poorly. My point is that experiential knowledge and conceptual knowledge of movement are two different animals, and they can exist independently. (The knowledge of teaching movement is yet another skill altogether.) However, there are universal principles that not only can be applied to human

motion but that have conditioned fundamental aspects of it. The skillful use of the body can't be achieved without the skillful application—either conscious or unconscious—of the movement efficiency principles after they have been learned spontaneously or through teaching.

I strongly believe that acquiring a basic conceptual knowledge of the fundamentals of movement efficiency should be a fast and simple endeavor rather than a long and overcomplicated intellectual pursuit. My assumption is that, even though we are cerebral and intelligent people, our main goal is to learn just enough to gain a basic, effective understanding of how and why techniques work. We want to avoid having to go through a bunch of scientific intricacies that would have little to no carryover toward a better movement practice or performance.

> ❝❝ **It is better to understand little than to misunderstand a lot."**
>
> — *Anatole France*

In short, we first need the fundamental conceptual knowledge that supports greater levels of experiential understanding—that is, knowing how to move well through our sensations. Ultimately, we need not for our brain to think of what efficient movement is but for our nervous system to remember how the efficient movement feels so we can reproduce the experience without thought. Principle 11, "Mindful," taught us that we must move mindfully, which is different than reasoning about how we move.

Therefore, some simplified notions of movement efficiency in this part work hand in hand with "perception drills," which enable a physical experience and awareness that generates a symbiotic mental and physical understanding of these principles. Mindful movement practice doesn't mean thinking of everything you know about movement or analyzing every aspect of your performance as you move; it's quietly paying close attention to what matters the most at a given moment. Simplicity in movement practice entails mastering the hidden complexity of movement without adding complication in your mind and movement. Of course, it is up to each of us to pursue advanced education related to the diverse fields—physics, biomechanics, kinematics, kinetics, kinesiology, and so on—of the conceptual side of movement study.

Keep in mind that the notions in this part don't conform to subjective conventions, dogma, or traditions that one must strictly respect. They are rational and reliable principles that you're free to apply as you wish and that you can personally verify through motion. As a result, you'll have an experiential basis for knowing that the principles work instead of being left with an assumption or mere belief.

The Formation *of* Technique

A *technique* is a movement pattern that makes movement more than effective; it makes it efficient also. Simply put, a technique is a movement strategy for a particular movement goal. By producing efficiency, the use of technique provides the three essential outcomes we're seeking: greater performance, greater energy conservation, and greater safety.

A movement pattern becomes a technique not only because it's efficient but also because the specific variables that ensure its efficiency can be strictly identified, explained, taught, learned, and—most important—applied and reproduced. Wild animals use technique without having conceptual awareness of it because intellectual understanding of it is superfluous; technique is built-in. Humans, on the other hand, can learn more efficient movements through the acquisition of technique.

Every technique involves a specific pattern of breathing, position, sequence, timing, tension, and relaxation. The first, most fundamental pillar of technique is breathing, and naturally it is the first technique I address in this part. Breathing is THE technique that supports all other techniques. Once you understand that breathing has a technique for efficiency, understanding that you can use technique to improve basically any movement becomes a no-brainer.

The end-goal of technique is optimally using the kinetic energy we produce—our physical effort—for the practical goal behind our movement. Of course, no technique—even the best one—completely conserves all the energy produced by the body; energy losses are inevitable. But the better the technique is executed, the less energy is dispersed and wasted.

It might seem that not every movement you do relies on a "technique." However, like breathing, even the simplest movement can benefit from improved technique if you're not currently doing it spontaneously with natural efficiency. Even what we call "gross" motor skills, which represent most of Natural Movement, can be improved to very fine levels of perception, accuracy, and control. This explains why untrained, out-of-shape individuals might look utterly stiff doing a basic transition from kneeling to standing with a poor movement pattern—holding their breath and having a rounded back, wobbly knees, and overall imbalance and stiffness—whereas other people could look both smooth and strong doing the exact same movement. If you belong to the first category, then learning the elements of breathing and position, sequence and timing, and tension and relaxation and physiologically adapting in the process could be considered working on technique.

When we think of movement skills, one of the first words to come to mind is *coordination*. But what exactly do we coordinate? We could naturally think of the diverse body parts (including joints and muscles) that need to integrate into full movement patterns and how these parts demand impeccable organization to work synergistically. However, joints and muscles are body tissues that function only after the central nervous system has activated and organized them. So, to achieve coordination, movement effectiveness, and—ideally—movement efficiency, the nervous system needs to ensure the coordination of position and breathing, movement sequence and timing, and tension and relaxation. (The illustration shows how these three components interact.) These principles are commonly shared by all techniques regardless of the movement skill. Now on to the efficiency principles!

Formation of Technique
by the Central Nervous System

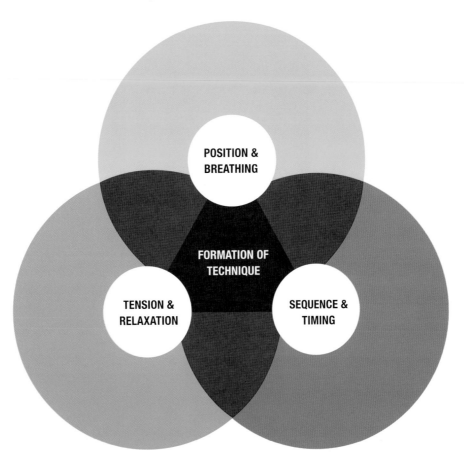

POSITION & BREATHING

FORMATION OF TECHNIQUE

TENSION & RELAXATION

SEQUENCE & TIMING

13
Breathing

"And when I breathed, my breath was lightning."

—Black Elk

Breathing is a natural movement. It doesn't involve the motion of your body through space; it's an internal movement your body needs to do from the moment you are born to the moment you die. Most of us take it for granted, but if you talk to anyone with breathing issues, they will tell you that they would give anything to be able to breathe easily.

Breathing is the control of ventilation and the set of physiological mechanisms involved in generating the physical movement of air into the lungs (inhalation) and out of them (exhalation), which is also known as *gas exchange*. Breathing is responsible for cellular respiration, which is the biochemical process that allows oxygen from outside air to be transported to the cells in the body. The cells use the oxygen and leave the carbon dioxide, which is transported back outside the body. (I describe cellular respiration in more detail later in this chapter.)

Fortunately, breathing happens unconsciously through the autonomic nervous system. However, the automatic nature of breathing makes it easy to assume that it does not have to be questioned, which makes it a component of movement efficiency that is too often overlooked. Very few people are aware that they can consciously train to develop an ability to control how they ventilate and improve the efficiency of their breathing patterns even when they are not thinking about it. However, breathing is movement skill—even though it's internal rather than external—which means that it's like other natural movements in that it can be methodically and mindfully trained.

The benefits and potency of mindful, controlled breathing has been known and practiced throughout history and throughout the world. You can reprogram, improve, and master the pattern of breathing, strengthen the respiratory system, and transform cellular respiration. Aside from supporting greater levels of health and vitality, breath control used in movement practice supports energy systems, relaxation, mental clarity, alertness or calmness, recovery, and even coordination. Needless to say, breathing well is great for your quality of life, but controlling breathing in motion supports greater levels of performance, and without it a crucial aspect of your movement competency is missing.

So, what can go wrong with the most natural movement of all—breathing? Before I tell you anything, do these two quick self-assessments while breathing exactly the way you normally do. Don't take extra big breaths because that would defeat the point of this self-assessment:

- Count how many breath cycles (one inhalation and one exhalation) you do within one minute.
- Place one hand on your chest and the other one on your abdomen just below your sternum. Just breathe as you normally do and feel what part (or parts) is moving or moving first. How much does it move? What direction does it move? Are you reflexively breathing through your nose or mouth?

For now, just remember what you have observed about your current breathing so you can compare it with the patterns I describe and/or recommend later.

Inefficient Breathing

Chest breathing is a breathing pattern that is done through the upper chest and respiratory muscles. It is what we all do when effort becomes very intense and we're breathing hard with our chests expanding to a much greater amplitude than when we're at rest. The problem is that we might chest breathe superficially (with a small amplitude) even when we're not doing any physical effort. When we chest breathe, our bellies are pulled inward and only our upper chests expand as we inhale. *Clavicular breathing*—which also normally occurs only with high intensity efforts—is even worse; in that case, only the collarbone and shoulders rise while the rest of the thorax remains motionless. With such shallow breathing, only a small amount of air flows, and it reaches only the upper lobes of our lungs, where less blood flow occurs. The result of this shallow breathing is poor oxygen absorption by the blood, and an oxygen deficit for the tissues that need it.

Consequently, over-breathing ensues. If we *over-breathe* (also known as *hyperventilating*), we continuously breathe through the upper chest with short, small, rapid breaths. It's an unconscious compensatory attempt to keep the body properly oxygenated. A person who chest breathes will always end up over-breathing.

The breathing pattern that combines chest breathing and over-breathing is deemed "normal" only because most people are accustomed to it; however, it's an inefficient way to breathe. It feels weak, it's neither relaxed nor relaxing, and it's very unsatisfying. You might not even be able to breathe deeply when you want to. If you look at a person lying down with closed eyes who is breathing shallowly in this way, it is very likely that the person is actually neither relaxed nor asleep; the person is probably anxious about something and unable to fall asleep.

A normal, healthy breathing rate should be, on average, 12 to 14 breaths (that is one inhalation and one exhalation) per minute. Although trained individuals can use less than 8 breaths a minute, most people can take up to 20 breaths or more per minute. A person who takes 10 breaths per minute breathes about 15,000 breaths a day. With 20 breaths per minute, the person is breathing 30,000 breaths each day.

With more breaths, a significantly greater volume of oxygen than is needed by the body is taken in, which paradoxically impairs proper oxygenation while accelerating oxidative damage and aging. Physical signs that accompany over-breathing are breathing through the mouth, regularly sighing, or regularly needing to take large breaths.

Movement behaviors are often unconsciously influenced, if not determined by, family, mindset, or culture. Just like the way you stand or walk, breathing is mostly learned unconsciously through mimicry, and you might have inherited the way you breathe from your parents. In addition, countless variables may negatively affect breathing, both mental (negative emotions, anxiety, mood swings) and physical (sitting too much, sitting in bad positions). Suffering from lack of movement, breathing polluted air, smoking, eating junk food, becoming sleep deprived, being overweight, inflammation, and general fatigue are some of the main variables that might factor in and lead to the pattern of over-breathing. Pregnancy also makes it harder to breath abdominally, and months of shallow breathing can result in a pattern of inefficient breathing that persists even after childbirth.

When you default to relying on superficial respiratory muscles to breathe, the otherwise primary respiratory muscles, such as the diaphragm and transverse abdominis, are weakened. The stabilization provided to the pelvic floor, spine, or sternum is also weakened, which has negative implications to your posture and to your ability to control breath through movement. Think how your performance can be impaired when you start moving, especially when you move vigorously!

Needless to say, improving your breathing patterns, starting with learning to breathe both abdominally and through the nose and to bring your breathing rate and volume to normal, helps correctly oxygenate your tissues, organs, and brain; reduces stress; and increases your levels of health and energy both when you move and don't move. If your breathing isn't optimally efficient yet, making it a real skill is the first priority and most potent way to improve your movement, physical performance, and whole life.

The importance of inhaling through the nose (nasal breathing)—except when the intensity of an effort makes it too hard—cannot be understated. Indeed, science indicates that breathing in through the nose, not the mouth, positively influences the brain and our cognitive functions, including improving the way we process emotions and memory. However, nasal breathing isn't actually a technique in the sense that all that is required to do is to keep your mouth closed.

NOTE

To read more about the positive influences of breathing through the nose, read "Nasal Respiration Entrains Human Limbic Oscillations and Modulates Cognitive Function" (www.jneurosci.org/content/36/49/12448).

Breath Control *and* Benefits

Breath competency means having optimum breathing mechanics and a highly functional respiratory system, both when you're at rest and when you're physically active. Natural, efficient breathing is centered in the abdomen—specifically in the diaphragm.

No less than ten muscles can be used for inhalation, but the diaphragm is the primary respiratory muscle we need to use. It is large and dome-shaped, and it extends across the bottom of the thoracic cavity (which contains the heart and lungs) to separate it from the abdominal cavity. When the diaphragm contracts, it pulls away from the ribs and creates an internal depression or vacuum effect that draws air into the lower part of the lungs, which are right at the base of the rib cage. The lower lobes of the lungs are where the greatest amount of blood flow occurs, which means that diaphragmatic breathing dramatically optimizes ventilation and oxygenation. This type of breathing has many obvious physical and mental benefits in both day-to-day life and in athletic and real-life physical performance.

Breath control starts with the ability to breathe slowly and quietly through the abdomen (and through the nose) when at rest. Though it is also known as *diaphragmatic breathing*, I prefer the term *abdominal breathing* because the transverse abdominal muscle (or transverse*) balances the action of the diaphragm by enabling exhalation. Another term for abdominal breathing is *deep breathing*, but that might imply that

we must take deep breaths, which is not necessarily the case when breathing abdominally. Breathing abdominally isn't exclusively about the diaphragm but about the abdominal area generally speaking. Thanks to a mechanism called "baroreflex sensitivity" that regulates blood pressure via heart rate, slow abdominal breathing lowers your heart rate and blood pressure which signals your brain that all is fine and positively influences relaxation at a hormonal level (in the parasympathetic nervous system). Reduced stress, improved mental relaxation and focus, lower inflammation (and associated discomfort or pain) in the body, more restorative sleep, and the diminution (or even disappearance of) breathing-related sleep disorders are some of the direct benefits of keeping your breath slow and relaxed when at rest.

From a movement practice and physical activity perspective, breath control is the ability to breathe at a rate with an amplitude and timing that adapts best to your current movement pattern. Some of the benefits include the following:

- Promotes improved cellular respiration, which turns into a more efficient use of existing levels of metabolic conditioning
- Supports greater postural and positional control (bracing)
- Provides greater ability to sustain high-intensity physical activity (by improving ventilation, muscular relaxation, and energy metabolism)

---

*The transverse is the deepest of all four layers of the abdominal wall (abdominal muscles). Unlike other abdominal muscles, the transverse runs horizontally. Aside from exhalation, this muscle's essential role is to stabilize the lower spine and pelvis.

- Promotes faster recovery, including in between bouts of high-intensity activity
- Helps with motivation and overcoming fear or negative emotions
- Participates in efficient thermoregulation and immunity
- Supports breath-holding whenever necessary (such as when you're under water or surrounded by smoke or toxic air)

Frequent, conscious practice of efficient breathing patterns—both when at rest and, of course, when practicing movement—reprograms the part of your brain responsible for your respiratory system to efficient breathing patterns, making it a healthier behavior both when you are and aren't paying attention. Of course, this does not shield you from involuntary, normal, and healthy reflexes that temporarily modify your breathing, such as sneezing, sighing, burping, or coughing. It also doesn't prevent alcohol, medication, weather, dust, smoke, pregnancy, occasional negative emotions, or physical activity from modifying your breathing pattern. However, breathing control helps you minimize how those things affect you, or for how long they affect you, and it enables you to return to normal, slow, relaxed breathing faster.

Before *You* Start Practicing

1 Breathing is and should stay simple and straightforward in the way it is explained and practiced.

2 Seek the purest air you can. The exercises can help you develop great ventilation, breath control, and cellular respiration, but if you breathe polluted, toxic air, your health and energy levels will be negatively affected.

3 Intentionally modifying your habitual breathing pattern can cause a minor physical or emotional response that initially might not feel good. Uncomfortable symptoms can include mild and temporary light-headedness or dizziness, which is why it is best to first practice while you're in a ground position (lying, sitting, kneeling). Don't practice breathing while standing, moving—or worst—driving until you have practiced enough to not experience any dizziness. If you feel dizzy, stop until you have regained clarity. Just don't overdo it at first.

4 Establishing the consistency of breathing efficiency when at rest—abdominally and through the nose—is your main objective. You may practice breathing exercises every morning and in the evening, or you can do it while you're sitting and doing other activities.

5 As with any exercise, you can do breathing drills in sets, and you can practice other movements in between breathing sets. Keep focusing on body sensations and quality rather than the number of sets you do.

6 You only need to practice the following drills if you encounter issues performing them correctly or easily. After you've mastered breathing efficiency while at rest, establishing breath control while in motion is your next step and the ultimate goal of breathing practice. Of course, you can always return to practicing the drills while at rest.

Maintaining breath control while performing complex movements and/or at high intensity will be the ultimate level of breath control. As a matter of fact, if you can only maintain breath control while in a resting position, but not when moving swiftly through complex environments, do you even have any breath control at all?

To the practice!

Control *of* Abdominal Breathing

Your primary goal is to make sure that you are breathing with the abdomen (or abdominal muscles) instead of the chest. You first need to locate the diaphragm by feel and make sure its movement is right.

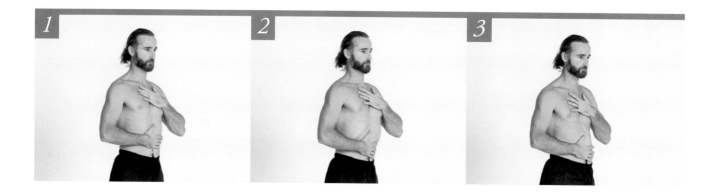

1   While in a sitting or kneeling position, place one hand on your chest and the other on your upper abdomen just below the rib cage (as in the self-assessment test you previously did). If you're lying on your back, an alternative to using your hands is to use two books for feedback: one placed on your chest and the other on your upper abdomen. You may close your eyes to enhance your perception. (Stand only if you are not subject to dizziness.)

2   Pay attention to the movement you feel as you breathe. If you perceive a little movement at chest level and most of the movement in your abdomen (with your abdomen pushing your hand away as you inhale), bravo! You're already naturally breathing abdominally. However, if you perceive the most movement at chest level with little or no movement in your lower hand (the one placed on your abdomen) as you breathe, or if your abdomen pulls in first when you breathe in, but you do feel movement and expansion in your chest, you're a chest breather. It's also likely that the number of breath cycles you counted during the self-assessment was high, which indicates over-breathing. Let's fix this.

3   Start breathing out—either through your nose or mouth—by gently contracting your abdominal muscles. As you do, the transverse contracts as the diaphragm relaxes. You should feel that your hand is drawn in as your abdomen pulls in. Don't force your exhale. Now let your diaphragm take over and expand so you can inhale through the nose, pushing your abdomen and hand out. You want to feel that your chest is completely relaxed, meaning you're not engaged in any active breathing effort. If your spontaneous reflex is to raise your chest and use your superficial, upper respiratory muscles, resist it. Visualize breathing as something taking place primarily lower and deeper in your abdomen. Your upper hand should experience only barely perceptible movement from your chest.

Only your lower ribs should slightly and passively expand sideways because of the inflation of your lower lungs due to the action of the diaphragm.

Keep breathing this way for some time, simply making sure that your chest stays relaxed and still and the in-and-out motion of your abdomen is constant. Once you start to control your abdominal breathing, you may relax your lower hand and keep only your upper hand on your chest; as long as there is no movement in your upper chest, you are breathing abdominally. You may eventually release both hands once you feel that your abdominal breathing is consistent. You may occasionally take a deep chest breath for the purpose of perceiving the sharp contrast between abdominal and chest breathing.

Now that you have identified the movement of your diaphragm contracting and pushing out as you inhale and relaxing and pulling in as you exhale, I'm going to explain how to keep expanding your understanding and control of breathing.

Perception *of* Abdominal Diaphragmatic Power

This drill is the same as the first one, except you need a partner who can give you honest feedback and help you better perceive the diaphragmatic respiratory power that lies within your abdomen.

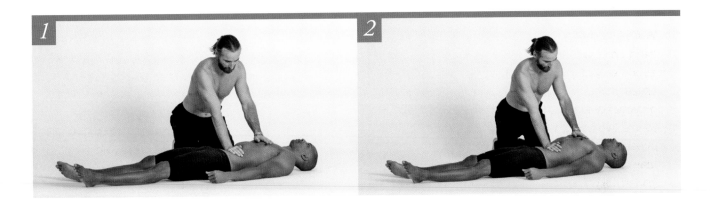

1 Place a firm hand on your partner's abdomen (below the rib cage/sternum) and a light one on the chest. Your arm should be fully extended so that you can apply downward pressure gradually and effortlessly simply by leaning forward onto your hands a little more. Your partner should relax his diaphragm to breathe out; his abdomen will pull in and lower your hand.

If your partner breathes through the chest (make sure not to forcefully prevent this), he is either unconsciously reverting to an inefficient breathing pattern or doesn't trust the strength of the diaphragm, unless you are applying too much force too soon onto his diaphragm and causing discomfort.

2 Your partner should contract the diaphragm—not the abdominal muscles—so the abdomen pushes out against your hand and elevates it. Obtain your partner's permission to shift more body weight onto your lower hand each time he inhales, which generates increased resistance to the motion of the diaphragm and helps your partner realize how powerful the diaphragm is.

Control *of* Amplitude *and* Strength

Now it's time to experience how much amplitude, or to what length, you can inhale and exhale abdominally. You do this by forcefully exhaling to the greatest extent you can so that you fully depress your lungs, and then you contract the diaphragm to the greatest extent you can (but without following up by expanding the rib cage using the upper-chest respiratory muscles).

At this point, you're not concerned with generating maximum air intake; you're only trying to reach full abdominal inhale and exhale. By increasing the amplitude of your abdominal in-breath, you naturally increase the amplitude of your diaphragmatic out-breath. To achieve this, first relax the diaphragm and exhale as you normally would, which is far from reaching the maximum exhale you could actually reach. At the moment between the end of the exhale and the beginning of the inhale, start contracting your exhalation muscles more. (With forced exhalation, a total of no less than eight muscles are involved; it's not just the transverse!) It should feel like tightening your belly in public to make your belly look smaller than it is, except that you keep pulling and pulling inward as long and as far as possible. Pull your whole waist area inward until you sense intense tightness and it feels that your lungs are absolutely empty and your rib cage is significantly reduced in size. You may voluntarily produce a sound with your throat as you exhale if it helps you emphasize and strengthen your exhale. When you feel that your lungs are completely empty—they aren't, but it will feel like it—resume inhaling normally until you reach the point between inhale and exhale where you would normally stop inhaling. At that point, keep pushing your abdomen out to the point that you cannot push it out any farther. Your belly should look as big as you can make it because your diaphragm is inflated to its fullest extent, which pushes your abdomen out as far as possible.

Through this drill of forced inhalation and exhalation, you might experience tightness, discomfort, or gentle stress in areas of your body that you might not have suspected were involved in breathing. This is because abdominal respiratory muscles play a fundamental role in stabilizing both your lower spine and pelvis through intra-abdominal pressure. (This effect is called "bracing," and I talk about it more in Part 4.) With forced inhalation and exhalation, both your diaphragm and your transverse contract to the maximum, which strongly pulls on your lower ribs, sternum, spine, and pelvic area. It also exerts pressure on your organs, which you might not be used to.

WARNING

If you experience an unpleasant sensation, either stop or reduce the strength and amplitude of your abdominal breathing. You need progressive practice to fortify your abdominal respiratory muscles as well as the diverse tissues involved in or affected by a powerful use of these muscles. In any case, bear in mind that this drill is for "perception" only; it helps you to better feel and use your abdominal breathing muscles. In reality, when in movement, you will rarely reach full abdominal inhale and exhale, which I talk a little more about at the end of this chapter.

As for the strengthening of all the muscles and tissues involved in abdominal breathing, it takes place primarily with abdominal breathing applied while in movement and during physical exertion.

Control *of* Rhythm

Now let's move on to contracting and relaxing the diaphragm and transverse alternately at diverse speeds and amplitude, which helps you generate any breathing rhythm you want. Practice the following breathing exercises, making sure to breathe in through your nose.

Slow Breathing

The primary goal is to fix over-breathing and reprogram your unconscious respiratory pattern to slow (or at least slower) breathing when at rest. Practice slowing down your breath—both the inhale and exhale—as much as you can, but do it without holding your breath. The out-breath is generally easier to slow down; therefore, the time you spend exhaling will usually be longer than the time you spend inhaling. You can measure your progress by looking at a clock and counting how many breaths you take within a minute. Make your first objective to breathe in and out no more than ten times a minute. Ultimately, you could go as low as a single breath each minute.

Though it is not actually breath-holding, this slow breathing is a potent way to improve your cellular respiration. However, it is better to aim at reaching a point where you can sustain a minimal number of breaths per minute (for at least ten minutes) rather than breathing only once per minute and then having to interrupt the exercise because you are huffing and puffing after sixty grueling seconds.

In any case, slow breathing will not just help you with cellular respiration and ingraining a slower breathing pattern; you will rapidly feel its tremendously calming benefits, which themselves can become quite addictive.

Hyperventilation

This drill is the exact opposite of the Slow Breathing Drill, and it is basically a form of voluntary, exaggerated over-breathing. The difference between this drill and unconscious hyperventilation is that you do this drill abdominally rather than superficially at chest level. The drill teaches you to become able to rapidly dissociate the tension-relaxation action of the diaphragm and transverse muscle while maintaining a quick turnover. Consequently, it becomes quite challenging to remain in perfect control of your abdominal breathing pattern without getting confused and reverting to chest breathing.

As you do this drill, it's a good idea to place your hands on your abdomen and chest so that you get instant feedback if your breathing pattern begins to elevate to the chest. Start accelerating your breathing progressively until you breathe as fast as two breath cycles per second (at least one hundred per minute), which is a very high rate that you can't sustain very long. Obviously, the faster you breathe, the more the amplitude and duration of each breath must be reduced.

You don't need to do this drill for longer than thirty seconds at a time. Once you can steadily maintain such a quick abdominal breathing pattern for about half a minute without interruption, confusion, erratic rhythm, or chest breathing, you can stop practicing.

Free Rhythm

Now that you can breathe long and slow as well as short and fast, you can imagine that you are a "breath drummer" and play with changes in breath rhythm. In this drill, you breathe and intentionally mix short, long, slow, or fast inhales and exhales, alternating them at will. You may accentuate the noise it makes through your nose or throat to make it more audible and "musical."

This drill promotes true control of abdominal breathing, and with it you can synchronize your breath with specific movement or effort at will.

Reaching Maximum Lung Capacity

After you've worked through the Slow Breathing, Hyperventilation, and Free Rhythm Drills, you can begin to learn to use the capacity of your rib cage to the fullest, which, when combined with abdominal breathing, enables greater air intake whenever you need it. Greater air intake in this case means greater air volume per inhale, which does not necessarily mean increasing your breathing rate, depending on the practical reason why you are expanding the chest. In this case, greater air intake is different than over-breathing, which is when an excessive number of small air intakes leads to an overall excessive amount of oxygen inhaled.

The ability to expand your rib cage optimally is natural and useful as you engage in bouts of high-intensity movement. It has the following benefits:

- Helps you through the effort, which increases breathing rate
- Helps you recover faster from effort, which tends to return breathing rate to normal
- Makes it possible for you to hold your breath when necessary, which decreases your breathing rate

You are not substituting abdominal breathing with chest breathing, nor are you reverting to superficial chest breathing in these situations; you're prolonging and expanding breathing thoracically, always starting with abdominal breathing (at a faster rate) and continuing with filling the lungs all the way to the top by using your upper respiratory muscles.

The objective of the following drills is to enhance your perception of the three-dimensional nature of the expansion of your rib cage and the "spaces" in which the expansion takes place, especially the sides and back of the rib cage. It's a common belief that the rib cage expands only to the front (think of a chest being puffed out), but the reality is that your rib cage expands all the way around, even though your breathing may be too weak and shallow for it to be significant and for you to notice it. The "rounded" expansion of the rib cage already happens when you take a deep abdominal breath, though it is less perceptible in

the back and front (chest) and more detectable in the sides because most inflation occurs in the lower lungs, which pushes the lower ribs out. After you have reached the limit of your diaphragmatic inhale, you should be able to expand your rib cage significantly to the side, back, and front for maximum lung capacity.

The more flexible your rib cage is—more specifically, the more flexibility you have in your thoracic spine, which involves the mobility of both the spine and thorax—the more room you have for your lungs to expand and reach full capacity. Many natural movements, including but not limited to crawling, rolling, hanging, and lifting loads overhead, contribute to making or keeping the thoracic spine supple, which consequently enables you to breathe more freely. You may also practice partial or full thoracic expansions as a separate drill to develop even greater thoracic mobility and volume.

> **WARNING**
>
> Like forcefully breathing abdominally, forcefully breathing thoracically challenges the muscles and tissues involved in the upper respiratory complex, and these drills can cause discomfort. Greater air intakes can also make you light-headed. Make sure to pay attention to warning signals and sensations, and pause or reduce the intensity of practice whenever something doesn't feel comfortable.

Start each drill with a firm, but not forced, full exhale followed by a full diaphragmatic inhale. In each area you focus on, notice the significant difference in volume between the full exhale and inhale.

Coastal Breathing *(Lower Ribs)*

1 Place your hands around your lower ribs and gently apply pressure. You may extend your thumbs toward your kidneys/back to get more feedback from all around your lower ribs. Fully deflate your lower lungs.

2 Deeply inhale through the diaphragm while constantly maintaining a bit of resistance against the ribs with your hands but allow your lower ribs to reach maximum expansion to the sides.

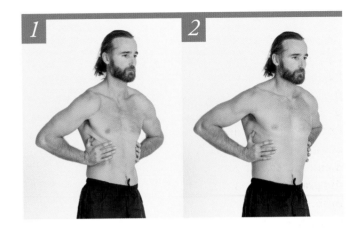

Back Breathing

The back is the space where the rib cage can expand the most and where you can potentially make the most gains in lung capacity. This explains why track cyclists can breathe quite effectively; their hunched-over position prevents their chests from expanding much but allows the back of their rib cages to expand fully.

1 From a standing position (you may also sit or kneel) and while keeping your spine straight, press your forearms tightly against each other and against your chest to prevent it from expanding. First exhale deeply (but not fully), then fully inhale (reaching full abdominal inhale, which is the point at which you cannot breathe in more through the diaphragm), which should give you a mild sensation of expansion of your rib cage in the back. Now, using your upper respiratory muscles, allow your rib cage to expand to the back as much as you can. If you have good mobility in the back of your rib cage, your back will look rounded—not because your spine is flexed but because your rib cage is fully inflated in the back.

2 Lie down in a prone position as a partner applies firm pressure on your upper back with their open hands (position may change with each inhale). Exhale deeply (but not fully), then take a full abdominal inhale that makes you feel your abdomen push against the ground. Your partner's resistance against the expansion of the back of your rib cage will be evident if you really focus on inflating that space. You will feel that your chest wants to expand as well, but it is made difficult by the ground.

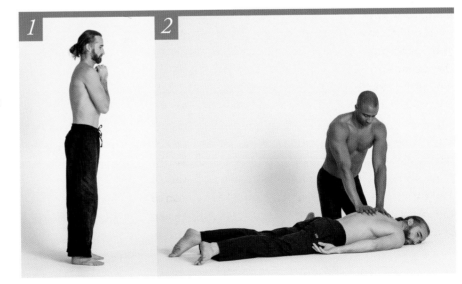

Chest Breathing

Expanding the chest is something everyone knows how to do reflexively, but that doesn't mean you can't improve your chest expansion.

1   Bend at your hips and place your hands above your knees to support your torso. Extend your upper spine as if a hand was pushing against it. Exhale, breathe abdominally, and then expand your chest as much as you can as you inhale. You should notice that your clavicles move slightly, enabling you to fill the top third of your lungs. While the movement in your collarbone area takes place whenever you are fully expanding your chest, you might feel it more this time because of the position you're holding and because you're focusing on this particular perception.

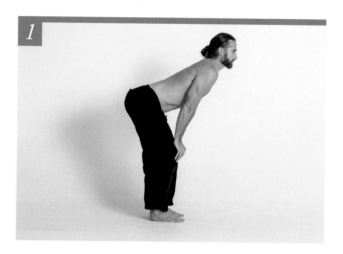

Bracing and Resistance Breathing

Resistance breathing, also known as *inspiratory muscle training (IMT),* is an effective way to increase diaphragm strength and endurance to help you maintain efficient breathing longer during effort, especially at high intensity. It also supports the improvement of cellular respiration. If you are already adept at abdominal breathing, resistance breathing occurs naturally during physical exertion when the abdominal wall is under great tension (such as when you're lifting or carrying heavy loads, power jumping, or grappling from your back). It's a reflex—and technique—called "bracing" that helps support lower spine stability. Despite the great tension, both the diaphragm and the transverse must keep functioning optimally without reverting to chest breathing. However, it's one thing to be able to breathe abdominally when you're at rest and you're paying attention, but it's a whole different animal to maintain abdominal breathing as you make swift changes in position, movement patterns, or intensity of effort, which is often the case in Natural Movement. To avoid becoming a chest breather when you're moving, you must start by developing the reflex and strength to maintain diaphragmatic breathing under abdominal tension—in other words, you develop an ability to "brace." It must become a reflex because during adaptable movement, you might need to prioritize attention to other aspects of your physical action or effort, such as anticipation, timing, precision and so forth. Bracing should reflex-ively take place at a degree of tension that's dependent on the intensity of the effort and how much support the lower spine needs to remain stable as you move.

You can already replicate this type of demand and enhance your abdominal breathing strength and endurance with the following Abdominal Resistance Drill. (Note that the Abdominal Resistance Drill doesn't improve cellular respiration unless you combine it with the Mouth Resistance Drill.) You need to keep the abdominal wall—the web of abdominal muscles and tissues—contracted to stabilize your lower spine as well as maintain the sitting balancing position regardless of whether your diaphragm is contracting or relaxing. So, whereas the diaphragm can and must relax fully upon exhalation, the transverse and other abdominal muscles must remain constantly contracted in this position—not only when you exhale. When the diaphragm contracts as you inhale, it must do so while pushing against the resistance of your abdominal muscles, which is a great way to strengthen the diaphragm.

If you can mindfully master abdominal control under very tense abdominal contraction when you're in a controlled position, you are more likely to be able to do the same as you engage in more dynamic movement that involves tense abdominal contraction. Obviously, mastering control under tense contraction also makes it even easier to breathe abdominally when tension is light or nonexistent.

Abdominal Resistance

1   Assume a balancing seated position with both legs off the ground and all your body weight on your rear, which creates great abdominal tension. While holding this position, breathe abdominally only. You may place your hands on your abdomen and chest to assess that you are able to maintain abdominal breathing without reverting to chest breathing. Given the tension, you should notice that the amplitude of the movement of your abdomen is not as big as when you aren't experiencing additional abdominal tension. You may add some front or side rocking motion while doing this, and you also may change the rhythm of your breathing. Pause when it becomes difficult to maintain the position or breathing pattern.

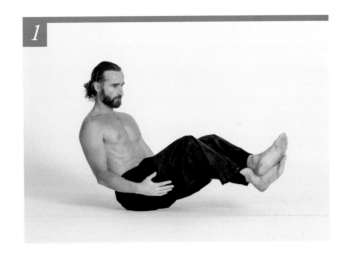

Mouth Resistance

Another way to train inspiratory muscles is to impose a resistance to air flow, either by using a device (which could be as simple as an empty pencil shaft) or by pursing your lips to make it more difficult for air to enter your lungs. The resistance happens at the entry point of the breath, which achieves two benefits:

- It strengthens your respiratory muscles because you need to forcefully, slowly, and continuously draw air until you can fill your lungs. If you emphasize the diaphragm, it will be strengthened by this exercise. If you breathe with your upper respiratory muscles, those will strengthen. You can do this training from any position or even while moving slowly, such as when walking. What matters is the amount of resistance to breathing.

- It improves cellular respiration, which is explained in the next section.

Cellular Respiration

I defined cellular respiration at the beginning of this chapter and explained that efficient ventilation mechanics are the priority way to drastically improve cellular ventilation.

Regardless of the mechanics of your ventilation, both high-intensity and endurance training improves overall metabolic conditioning, including cellular respiration. You also can improve cellular respiration through mouth resistance breathing, such as the last drill I described (or through breath-holding exercises). Because resistance breathing slows down your breathing rate significantly, you need to be patient to get the oxygen you need. If you also slow down your exhale, the impact and benefit on cellular respiration is even greater, resembling the benefit of breath holding. Whereas you aren't actually holding your breath, significantly slowing down ventilation challenges cellular respiration, forcing it to adapt.

By exhaling slowly and keeping air in your lungs over a longer period, less oxygen is available to your tissues, which significantly optimizes your use of oxygen in two ways. You will adapt to

- Extract more oxygen for a given volume of air
- Transport oxygen faster to the tissues (organs, muscles, cells) that need it

But that's not all. When you slow down breathing (or hold your breath), oxygen in your body is used and turned to carbon dioxide (CO_2), which accumulates in your body until you finally breathe out. By delaying the exhale (because you are busy struggling to inhale or because you are holding your breath), you build a higher tolerance threshold for CO_2, which is very helpful in challenging efforts, such as endurance or anaerobic efforts. This higher tolerance can really help boost performance.

Breath-holding is another type of breath training that is especially important for aquatic locomotion and competency, especially diving or swimming under water. It can also be very handy in cases of air toxicity. In my opinion, it's quite important to develop a decent ability to hold your breath for practical real-world reasons and not just for the sake of optimizing overall physical performance. A minimum of three minutes is a good goal, but breath-holding for duration requires training methods and protocols beyond the scope of this book. You may experiment on your own, and improved breathing mechanics will help you greatly.

Breathing *in* Movement

Your ability to use and synchronize breathing with any type of movement and physical effort determines how much control you have over your breathing. If you have breath control in a comfortable resting position but lose it when performing complex and intense movement, then do you actually possess breathing control?

Breathing supports mindful movement, relaxation, as well as positional control of the lower spine and pelvis, which in turn supports better position and proper timing in executing the right movement sequence of any particular technique. Breathing also helps you use your energy systems more efficiently.

To develop breathing control while in motion, paying attention is the most important factor, of course, as your attention can easily wander to other aspects of your activity—such as the detail of a specific technique you are trying to learn or improve, the changing environment you navigate, or the sheer willpower needed to achieve an intense physical effort. Because your focus can so easily stray from your breathing, it is important to start with relatively easy movements, efforts, and environments and increase those variables progressively. So, you start with only breathing and add all other variables incrementally while maintaining breathing control. For instance, a great breathing/moving practice is to do a variety of ground movements at low intensity as you maintain abdominal breathing. Whereas normally your breathing should synchronize with your movement, when starting to practice breathing control together with movement, you should place breathing at the core of the practice and align your movements to consistent abdominal breathing.

The main issues of breathing in movement are to revert to chest breathing, over-breathing, and having frequent, unwanted, and prolonged moments of unconscious apnea (breath-holding). Overall, you should focus on maintaining abdominal breathing without being preoccupied by the moment you inhale or exhale. This is true for cyclical movements such as running, where the effort is uninterruptedly shared between both legs at a high cadence, which renders irrelevant the decision of optimum timing for inhaling or exhaling.

That said, synchronicity does matter and can support movement efficiency. While the relevance of such synchronicity is very clear when swimming (when your face is intermittently immersed in water), it also matters on land when the effort is more intense and the timing more specific.

Last but not least, a very important consideration that you must take into account is that inhaling has a tensing effect, whereas exhaling has a relaxing effect, which can be used to your advantage. You can use inhaling before you "load" your body before an intense muscular contraction, and you can even briefly hold your breath to maintain the tensing effect as you produce significant levels of force, and then you relax by exhaling immediately after the contraction. You also can choose the timing of exhalation with the moment when you need the most relaxation in a movement.

However, inhaling or exhaling too hard and too deeply can turn those tensing and relaxing effects against your performance if they happen at the wrong time. As I have briefly mentioned previously, when in movement you should rarely reach full abdominal inhale and exhale unless it is necessary, just as you will rarely have to fully use your lung capacity or exhale to a maximum. In fact, efficient breathing in most movements and physical efforts implies maintaining a constant mild compression (or "bracing") of your abdominal area and avoiding prolonged inhale and exhale to the point they reach maximum abdominal amplitude. I can't show this with photos, but I invite you to experiment for yourself as you start practicing breathing control with movement.

The best way to start for this purpose is to explore a number of movement variations shown in Chapters 24 and 25, which are about ground movement.

14
Position

When you have regained efficient control over the fundamental, internal movement that is breathing, you want the same efficiency and control over the movement of your whole body, starting with the positions that you will need and use.

The world of human positions is vast. Of course, your position in the sense of location is first on planet Earth, regardless of where your current geographical location is. This generality is important because I'm going to talk about gravity and how it affects us—particularly our positions and movements.

Beyond that, position generally refers to an enormous diversity of possible physical or anatomical configurations of the human body, which also is called *human positioning*. Human positioning can be anything from the position of your fingers, toes, eyes, or tongue to the position of your whole body. The same way the scope of human movement is not limited to natural movements, the scope of human position is not limited to natural ones. Anyone can explore atypical positions or create some, such as in dance, mime, or acrobatics. Positions can also be associated with given traditions or rites (yoga, religion, spirituality). One can pose with an aesthetic, artistic, or goofy intention in mind.

Not surprisingly, this book focuses on an astounding number of natural positions, such as lying, crawling, kneeling, sitting, squatting, standing, balancing, or hanging (and more). Natural positions are all practical and can be used to wait, rest, recover, sleep, eat, defecate, meditate, work, ride, shoot, hide, protect, play, have sex, and give birth. Life is an endless succession of positions—intentional, reflexive, and unconscious.

Although our primary understanding of position is to think of it as being something exclusively static and motionless, and indeed that is part of it, we must make it evolve to dynamic positions in movement; we must view movement itself as nothing but a dynamic change of the body's position. It is illusory, though, to think of position and movement as separate. Unless you are entirely relaxed in a lying position, holding any other position demands an active participation, with some level of strength and tension to first enable a transition to a position to establish it, which is nothing less than movement, and then to maintain that position. On the other hand, movement is no less than a dynamic succession of positions you perform while following a sequence, with a particular timing, duration, and intensity. Movement is the process of transitioning positions. Strong, efficient, controlled positions provide a significant mechanical advantage in movement, optimizing balance, relaxation, coordination, and transitions to the next movement...or next position.

Understanding and mastering position means learning, improving, and ultimately mastering movement *faster*. Control position and you control movement. The better you control position, the better you move. Enter positional control.

Positional Control

Positional control is the ability to intentionally and optimally organize body segments to hold a given position or perform a given movement and physical action as effectively and efficiently as possible in a given context.

Positional control first implies *alignment*—that is, the control of how you position, or "align" each segment of your body in relation to other segments independent of the environmental complexity.* In other words, alignment is the intentional organization or relative position (orientation, angle) of bones to each other for optimum positional efficiency (in terms of maximal stability, leverage and force production, minimal energy expenditure, and minimal wear on the joints).

Because the goal of alignment is effectiveness and efficiency, perfect alignment does not necessarily imply linearity. For instance, a "straight back" is great to lift something heavy and a "rounded back" isn't, but you can't roll with a straight back; a pronounced spinal curvature is mandatory for rolling smoothly. In the former case, the straight spine is perfectly aligned, but in the latter case, a well-rounded spine is perfectly "aligned" as well.

Posture is an integral part of alignment. Conventionally, posture refers specifically to linear alignment of the spine from sacrum to neck (the infamous "straight back") when the body is in an upright/vertical position, such as when you're standing or sitting. I like to extend the notion of posture to any position that demands a straight back to be optimally efficient, such as in the Hip Hinge or the Foot-Hand Crawl, which coincidentally are among the best movements for activating the same muscles that support postural integrity and control. Postural control is the ability to maintain a stable "neutral" spine (or straight lower and upper back) and is an aspect of positional control that's of paramount importance.

When you have decent control of your positions when you're going slowly, the challenge is to be able to replicate the same level of positional integrity as you transition at a faster pace from position to position, which is what you do when you start to move.

Positions require many of the same elements necessary for movement:

- **Strength:** Except for positions where the body is fully relaxed with zero muscular tension anywhere (which is the only real "passive" position that can exist because you are either unconscious, paralyzed, or dead), assuming any position obviously starts with muscular contraction. Tension is indeed necessary to establish and then hold the position with stability at every joint involved in holding the position. I discuss more about this in Chapter 15, "Tension-Relaxation." Similarly, position influences muscle function and output.

- **Mobility:** You need to possess enough range of motion to reach positions without being limited by a lack of mobility.

- **Proprioception** (also called *kinesthetic awareness*): This is an innate ability to sense body signals relative to position, motion, and balance. In other words, when you hold a position, you are aware of the position of each of your body parts in relation to the others but also in relation to the environment and gravity, which enables you to establish and maintain balance. Balance is covered in Chapter 26, "Balancing Movement."

- **Exteroception:** This is the part of proprioception that relates specifically to positioning and the variables of environment you are directly interacting with through physical contact. Exteroception is an innate ability—although you can develop it—to sense stimuli that originate from the surfaces that support the body to enable you to determine your position and how sustainable it is. This ability enables you to balance and transition to the next movement. Therefore, a very important part of exteroception has to do with perceiving frictional resistance or "friction," which I explain in more detail on page 122 in the "Perception of Friction and Surface of Support" section.

---

*Which means that the environment is horizontal, flat, and stable, and it does not impose specific adjustments of position.

Last, but not least, positioning has to do with how you *intentionally* position each segment of your body in relation to the environment—and not the mere perception of it (exteroception). The environment can be any external variable (terrain, weather, someone else's body) that you need to adapt to so that you can ensure effectiveness and efficiency. For instance, how you position your arms on a horizontal surface to hang and rest is different than when you want to pull from it to climb on top of the surface. The environment presents demands that cannot be denied—which exteroception enables you to feel—and it dictates how you make both minor and major positional modifications. (Again, I'm talking about adaptability.)

When you have decent control of your positions when performing them at a low level of intensity, the first challenge is to maintain the same level of positional control with more intensity—for instance, going faster, jumping higher, and so on—within a simplified environment. Ultimately the challenge is to maintain such control over your positions when moving through complex ones. If you're not already able to hold fundamental positions impeccably and at will, if you're not able to make minute adjustments without overthinking (or even without thinking), or you're getting confused in the absence of intensity (speed, distance, height) or environmental complexity (uneven, slippery, moving surfaces), then what will happen when you need to replicate the positions at greater levels of intensity or within complex environments?

It's simple: You'll be in a *lot* of trouble. In Natural Movement, positioning is a fundamental skill because the more you advance your practice and as environmental complexity increases, the more intensity increases. Therefore, positional control is ultimately about anticipatory positional adjustments relative to how movement needs to be performed in a given context—environment and situation—to ensure the stability, and therefore the effectiveness and efficiency, of the next position or movement, which is the very essence of movement adaptability. When you see people moving very slowly in nature when the terrain gets rough, it is not necessarily because they need strength or cardio; it might be because it takes them a long time to figure out reliable and safe positioning with every move they make.

Like all aspects of movement training, positioning is trained by respecting progressions from simple environmental demands to complex ones and increasing the level of intensity.

Positional Variability and the "All-Purpose Position" Myth

Ever heard of the "all-purpose squat" position? Well, it is the idea that a single squat position can be used for any purpose. Any purpose? Then why are we capable of diverse variations of the squat position? That's because each variation has a purpose, a given practical context where it is best. Thank you, Evolution! Knowing what variation is most appropriate for the context in which it is being used makes you understand the actual purpose of each variation and the necessity for positional variability to exist in the first place. In fact, which position is a "variation"? Is a Narrow-Base Deep Squat with the feet pointing out a variation of a Squat in which the feet are hip-width apart and pointing forward, or is it the other way around? It reminds me of two people who speak the same language but have two different accents; which person has an accent? Both, right?

Dealing with diverse contextual variables demands varied and frequent modifications of your position. In this case, *purpose-specific* position is a more appropriate name than "all-purpose" position, even though any position variation may have more than one use.

So, forget the idea that any position is the "only," the "standard," or even the "best" and that variations of the same position should be dismissed as unimportant or less important, which is what happens when you start to believe in a so-called "all-purpose" position. "Best" means nothing without understanding a specific application. All-purpose positions simply do not exist. No single position ever fits absolutely every contextual purpose, and that's the reason why the human body is capable of many positional variations—for the sake of adaptability and efficiency. Just go and move in nature sometimes and experience this reality firsthand.

You won't need to have control over a single squatting, sitting, kneeling, or hanging position that will supposedly enable you to be comfortable and in control of all other variations. This is a myth. To develop actual positional control, you need to practice a wide variety of positions, become comfortable in and control all of them, become able to easily and smoothly transition from one to the next. Furthermore, you need to become experienced in the strengths and weaknesses of each position in different contexts so you can assume the ideal position in each situation without hesitation, without wasting time, and without losing your balance.

The notion of "power position" is contextual also. A power position in a certain context becomes a weak one the moment the context changes. In that situation, the alternative may be a position you never practice so you feel weak or incompetent with it because it's not a "power position," and you've utterly ignored it. For example, you might be able to assume a comfortable Wide-Base Deep Squat in which you feel strong, but when you must use a Narrow-Base Deep Squat, you might feel weak or off-balance even though this position should be your "power position" in the given context.

Understanding context helps you understand whether a given position is relevant or irrelevant, effective or ineffective, and efficient or inefficient. It is understanding what position has power, where, when, and what that power is. This is an important part of positional control.

Conceptual *and* Experiential Understanding

At this point there are more insights into understanding positional control and movement efficiency principles that I want to share with you, which is the "conceptual understanding" part, but I believe they are best assimilated if you can get a perceptual or "experiential" understanding of them simultaneously. Before we go through some discrete positions and patterns, I want to lead you through a series of simple "perception" drills designed to give you both a broad perceptual and experiential understanding of some of the most fundamental and universal aspects of movement. Although science can provide immensely more detailed information about such movement efficiency principles, the reality is that conceptual knowledge can take you only so far; eventually, experiential understanding rules your ability, or lack thereof, to move efficiently. Ultimately you want your "movement brain" and body to get it—not just your mind.

" All our knowledge has its origin in our perceptions."

—Leonardo da Vinci

The ten following perception drills relate to gravity. Gravity is a universal and omnipresent force that pulls every body that has mass toward the center of the Earth. Astronauts who spend time in a zero-gravity environment rapidly lose muscle mass (they suffer from sarcopenia) and bone density, but even in the presence of gravity, absence of interaction with gravity through movement has the same result, just not to the same degree and speed. You don't need to be launched into space to suffer the adverse effects of lack of gravity; all you need to do is to stop moving.

Humans have evolved in and exist in a gravitational field, and it is not just movement and life in nature but also movement in relation to gravity that has shaped the way we move. Because every movement technique is about being effective and efficient, gravity is always a factor, and you must understand how to best "negotiate" it. You can't change gravity; the only thing you can change is how efficiently you interact with it. The only way your mind can optimally command your body is by first understanding and obeying the forces that govern its movement. In that respect, gravity ranks as the number-one force.

As you work through the following drills, I suggest you keep your eyes closed so that you can better feel what's going on in your body. Let's go!

 Don't fight forces, use them."

—R. Buckminster Fuller

Perception of Gravity, Body Weight, Points of Support, and Contact Force

When you lie down and relax, why doesn't your body float off the ground and levitate? Because of the gravitational force!

Visualize Earth and the immense power of gravity. When you lie down and relax, do you have a physical perception of gravity at this moment? If yes, can you describe it? How do you feel it, or where do you sense it? You feel gravity in every body part that is supporting some of your body weight at this moment. *Body weight* is the amount of gravitational attraction between your body and the Earth. You should feel weight, or pressure, in the back of your head, shoulders, arms, legs, feet, and bottom, correct?

Take a moment to focus on the sensation of pressure on those parts. Feel all the body surface that is touching the ground: These areas are called *points of support* because they support at least some of your body weight—and sometimes all of it depending your position. Points of support can be any body part, but they are primarily our feet, hands, and bottom; secondary points of support are our knees, elbows, forearms, shoulders, belly, and so on.

Except for the occasional moments where the body is airborne, the rest of the time it is connected to the environment through points of support. The points of support are primarily responsible for your perception of both gravity and your own body weight. But we also experience gravity in the muscles, which must be contracted so you can hold active positions to resist gravity and prevent it from pulling your body weight down.

> **The foot feels the foot when it feels the ground."**
>
> —*Ernest Wood*

For every position that is not airborne, we are physically attached to the environment—the ground, a tree branch, or water. This physical connection of our body with the environment generates a *contact force* regardless of its duration. A contact force is a direct force that acts at the surface of contact between two objects but in opposite directions, such as between your points of support and the environment. For example, when you pull a heavy object off the ground, there is contact force between your hands and the object, and there is contact force between your feet and the ground. The latter force is called the *ground reaction force*. In fact, the same "ground" reaction force takes place if, for instance, you pull or push off a tree branch, which isn't technically the ground. Both contact forces last as long as you stand while holding the object. When you're running, the contact force (in this case the ground reaction force) is applied in a short burst every time one of your feet lands. Basically, the idea is that the environment provides the support for you to stand, hang, push, pull, or rebound, which you couldn't do without contact force. Points of support "anchor" the body to the physical environment, which is the reason you can't keep jumping unless you have touched the ground.

Try this drill: Lie down completely flat on your back with your arms and legs lengthened (don't cross them). Breathe in a relaxed manner and release muscular tension. Slowly raise both lengthened arms at an angle (diagonally). As the sensation of pressure due to contact force is relieved from the backs of your arms, muscular tension in your shoulders that's necessary to oppose the pull of gravity commences, which gives you both another sensation of the pull of gravity and a sense of how much your arms weigh. Now completely let go of tension in your shoulders and let gravity pull your arms back down. Gravity takes over as soon as you release tension in your shoulders.

Perception of Base of Support

Hold a regular standing position. Do you feel any pressure in the back of your body? No, you don't. You feel all the pressure of your body weight in both feet, which tells you that your feet are the two points of support that are currently supporting the totality of your body weight. The area running between and under your feet is called your *base of support*. Generally speaking, a wider base of support makes your position more stable; conversely, a narrower base of support is less stable. For example, standing on one foot is clearly not as stable as being on all fours using your knees and hands for support.

Perception of Body-Weight Shifting and Body-Weight Distribution Without Change of Base of Support

As you continue from the previous perception drill, your entire body weight is equally distributed between your feet, with each foot supporting 50 percent of your overall body weight. Shift your body weight from one foot to the other while keeping both feet grounded. This does not change your base of support or points of support, but it does change how your body weight is distributed over those two points of support. As a result, the pressure under one foot increases as it decreases on the opposite one. You can come close to putting 100 percent of your body weight onto one foot, but you can't have a full 100 percent because doing so would require that you lift one foot off the ground. A swift change of body weight distribution using the pull of gravity can generate useful momentum, which is something I cover in Chapter 16, "Sequence and Timing."

Perception of Center of Gravity

The *center of gravity* (also called *center of mass*) of your body is the point in space about which your body weight is evenly distributed. When you stand upright, your center of gravity is located around your navel. Depending on your physical makeup, your center of gravity when standing can be slightly higher or lower than another person's. The precise location of your center of gravity changes depending on your body position because the center of gravity is determined by how the weight in all your body segments is positioned in relation to each other. Changing your position changes the distribution of your body weight and consequently changes the position of your center of gravity to some degree. The center of gravity continuously shifts through movement toward the greater concentration of your body weight.

For instance, if you lift both arms, you are shifting some of your weight upward, which shifts your center of gravity upward from your navel toward your sternum. When you crawl all on all fours, your center of gravity shifts below and actually outside your body.

Perception of Line of Gravity and Balance

The center of gravity is considered a theoretical point that can be tricky to physically locate.

The perception of the line of gravity and body-weight shifting can help you get a sense of the location of your center of gravity. The line of gravity is an imaginary line that runs vertically between your center of gravity and the ground (or the center of Earth). The center of gravity, the line of gravity, and the center of Earth are always aligned. However, to be well balanced in *any* static position, which is called *static balance*, the center of gravity and line of gravity *must* be vertically aligned with your base of support. Conversely, to initiate movement, which is dynamic balance, you must shift the line of gravity outside vertical alignment with your base of support; the amplitude and speed of the shift depends on the movement you're performing.

In the standing position, feel how your body weight is evenly distributed between both feet, then visualize your line of gravity running from your center of gravity to the center of your base of support and all the way to the center of Earth as it keeps you well balanced and stable. If you shift body weight toward one of your feet, you're shifting both your center of gravity and line of gravity toward the side of your base of support, which is still sustainable but not as stable. If you keep shifting your body weight further to the side, you would end up pushing your center of gravity and line of gravity beyond and outside vertical alignment with your base of support; without the support of a base, gravity immediately pulls you off balance and toward the ground. For this reason, *vertically aligning your center of gravity with the center of your base of support is the primary condition that creates more stability in all directions.*

Following are some other ways of ensuring more stability:

- Enlarging the base of support (increasing the horizontal distance between the line of gravity and the edges of the base of support) by widening it or by adding points of support
- Shortening the distance between the center of gravity and the base of support

Perception of Linear Joint Alignment

From the same standing position, visualize and feel how centering your center of gravity and line of gravity with the center of your base of support also causes you to instinctively center all body segments and their segmental mass by stacking them from feet to head as vertically as you can, which produces the most stable position possible, while avoiding any unnecessary tension to minimize effort. It's like stacking cubes; the straighter the stack is the more stable it is, right?

Indeed, efficient static balance implies that you "center" your joints in a neutral fashion as much as possible depending on the context to obtain the most structurally stable and energy-efficient position. You do this through *joint centration,* which is organizing your joints in a linear vertical alignment to handle the downward compressive force that results from gravity and your own body weight. It's a mechanical advantage because your bones are aligned so that weight is transferred down through the centers of your joints to rely as little as possible on the support of ligaments and muscles.

We unconsciously learn this principle when we learned to stand for the first time. However, as effortless as a vertically well-centered standing position feels, it is not truly effortless for two reasons:

- A certain amount of tension, even minimal, is required to maintain the position.
- You can never take your balance for granted.

Close your eyes while assuming a standing position. Pay attention to the subtle, barely perceptible oscillations of your body moving forward, backward, or sideways and the subtle positional adjustments that accompany those oscillations. This is your *vestibular system* managing your balance for you. Holding any static position is part of movement because it is an interaction with gravity. You may try to prevent those oscillations and make them disappear by trying to relax or by trying to add tension to your body: Either way, you will fail. You cannot force your body to become perfectly still whenever you hold a static balance position. This is because you are not an inanimate object but a living being who must organize the pluri-articulated structure which is your skeletal system to find and maintain the body's point of balance.

That point of balance can be optimal, but it's never perfect; it's always temporary and never shielded from the action of gravity.

Perception of Angular (Non-Linear) Joint Alignment

Now tilt your head forward. Do you feel how the segmental mass of your head has moved outside vertical alignment with the rest of your body? Now move your head further by rounding your back. Don't you already want to reset your posture so it's straight? Your head isn't stacked on top of your body anymore, and your vertebrae aren't stacked on top of each other. The support is gone, and gravity is naturally pulling the weight of your head down, which forces you to create extra tension in the back of your neck and back and to also slightly shift your center of gravity to avoid tipping over. Unless it is contextually necessary to assume this position, this is a bad posture to hold.

Now bend at the hip and knees and feel the extra tension necessary in your body to hold this position. This is a stable position, but it would clearly be a very uneconomical way to stand, right? Absolutely, because your hip and knee joints are no longer vertically aligned with your base of support and the rest of your body. You have lost the benefit of joint centration in a number of your joints, demanding your muscles and joints to work more. However, if you had to lift something heavy off the ground, you would want to bend at the hip and knees (as well as make other positional modifications) and intentionally align your joints and body parts for maximum efficiency. (Remember: Alignment isn't always linear.) You must create angles at the joints to produce force. Could you jump upward from a standing position without first changing your alignment, bending your joints, and changing your position?

Perception of Change of Support

Changing support implies a modification of both point of support and base of support, which is the very essence of locomotion; and not just "movement." Indeed, it is possible to produce movement without producing locomotion by moving on the spot without changing your base of support or location.

From your standing position, shift all your body weight to a single foot, vertically align your center of gravity and line of gravity with it, and then pick up the opposing foot. Your base of support is now made of a single point of support and feels less stable. Extend the nonsupporting leg forward and place the foot one or two feet away from you. Voilà, you have displaced one of your two original points of support, changed the location of your base of support, and initiated not only movement but locomotion. You are not standing in the exact same place anymore!

Whenever you want to produce locomotion, you must let go of existing points of support to establish new ones some distance away. But you also must let go of your balance on the existing base of support until you can establish balance on the new one. Easy? Well, anyone can let go of their position and points of support and destroy their balance, but not everyone is confident of their ability to rebuild their balance somewhere else on new points of support. If you fail at rebuilding your balance, what happens to you? Gravity takes you down (which you've known since you were a very young kid). That's the difference between the person who moves skillfully and the one who moves clumsily, between the person who moves confidently and the person who is afraid and reluctant to.

Perception of Body-Weight Shifting with Change of Base of Support = Perception of Gravity as a Free Energy Motive

But what would happen if you were to swiftly remove one of your feet from the ground without first vertically aligning your center of gravity with the next intended base of support? By lifting a foot, you are removing a point of support and changing your base of support (from two feet to a single grounded foot). This immediately places the center of gravity outside and beyond vertical alignment with the base of support, and gravity is quickly pulling your center of gravity off-balance toward the direction where your center of gravity is already leaning.

Is having your center of gravity off-balance a bad thing? Not necessarily. If the move was unintentional

then it's undesirable because you are now off balance and must quickly react by re-establishing a new point of support that will enable you to recover a balanced position. Otherwise, you will fall hard to the ground. This type of reflex is covered in Chapter 26, "Balancing Movement." However, it can be an intentional strategy for efficient movement, which is covered in Chapter 16, "Sequence and Timing."

Perception of Friction and Surface of Support

For this next drill, you again need to lie down on your back. Bring both feet to rest on the floor close to your buttocks. Keep your back and hips on the ground and push off from your feet and legs as if you're trying to slide your body backward. Can you? Unless the surface where you lie is slippery (and maybe your clothes are synthetic), you won't slide backward. It's likely that your feet will slide forward if you try to push harder.

The reason you can't slide is because of the difference of *frictional force* (or *friction*) under the points of support, which are currently your back, rear, and feet. The frictional resistance from under your back and rear is significantly superior to that under your feet, for two reasons:

- The overall surface in contact with the ground of your back and rear is far greater than the surface of your feet in contact with the ground.
- Your back and rear are supporting much more of your body weight, increasing friction in those areas.

Because of the difference in friction level, there is only so much force from the legs you can apply to your feet before either your feet slide forward, or your hips elevate off the ground when you try to push and slide on your back. It doesn't matter how strong your legs are, if the static friction in your back exceeds the static friction in your feet, the force applied in your feet meets the resistance of your back and loses.

It would be even "worse" if the bottoms of your feet were oily, or if they were resting on a wet or icy surface. Your feet would helplessly slide forward with little effort, right? Conversely, if your feet were resting on a rugged, firm surface that provides a lot of friction, and your back and hips were on an icy surface (or if you were wearing a jersey made of synthetic fabric), sliding backward on your back would be easy.

It's frictional resistance that gives our points of support "static friction" or "segmental inertia," which is a resistance to change in its motion or position so that force can be applied in other body parts and create motion in a controlled direction. Without static friction, even for a millisecond, we can't ensure the points of support required to push or pull ourselves in any direction, and kinetic energy produced would be dispersed. Simply put, deficient static friction under a point of support reduces the amount of force we can apply to it, whereas the absence of friction renders a point of support useless. This is why it is so challenging to move on icy surfaces.

Now, from the lying position, shift your body to the left side, raise your hips off the ground, and load your left shoulder with body weight. Tense your feet and "plant" your heels in the ground with downward pressure. Push off from your heels and fully extend your legs, letting your hips move to the side and toward your shoulders. Have you now moved backward? You have, and you were able to do it not because of the absence of friction but because you made efficient use of it by changing your base of support before applying force in your legs. This is the technique called the "Hip-Thrust Crawl," which is described in Chapter 24, "Ground Movement 1: Lying, Rolling, Crawling."

What this teaches us is that we need to understand friction to move efficiently. The strength and reliability of your contact with the environment, your ability to hold a position, and your ability to produce and direct force and momentum rely on how much friction you're able to establish and maintain as you apply force and use momentum.

Friction has to do with four main variables:

- The external surface you are in contact with and that supports you, called the *surface of support.* If the rock you are landing on is wet, you will have much less friction upon landing than when it is dry—and less friction can cause you to slip. If the rock is covered with sand, you will also have less friction under your feet when landing. Different surfaces provide different levels of friction, and weather conditions may also alter friction levels.

- The external surface of the point(s) of support in contact with the surface of support: If you are landing on a dry rock barefoot and your feet are wet, you have less friction than if they are dry, which can cause you to slip.

- The total surface area for contact of your points of support: The friction from the full surface of your feet when they are flat on a surface is greater than if you stand on a smaller surface, such as your forefoot, which you might do because you are elevating your heels or because the surface of support is too small for the whole foot to be on the support surface.

- The position of your points of support in relation to gravity and the force applied to them: The more perpendicularly to the point of support that body weight or a force is applied, the greater the friction. If you place your foot on a horizontal surface of a cliff and push down, the force is perpendicular to the foot that's supported by the horizontal surface, and you can elevate your position. If you place your foot on a vertical surface and push down, your foot meets no frictional resistance, so it slides down and you go nowhere regardless of how hard you try to push on that leg. To create friction, you need to modify your position so you can push into the surface.

In other words, "friction," from a practical Natural Movement perspective of movement efficiency refers to how reliable a point of support is, which is critical when you're moving fast through unknown complex environments—natural ones in particular. The reason friction is widely overlooked or completely ignored in the fitness world is probably because neither programs nor gym environments are designed for adaptable movement and meeting the challenge of physically navigating through diverse, complex, and unpredictable environments. In a gym, unless water or sweat makes the floors slippery, accidental slippage is not really a concern.

So, is friction that important to Natural Movement? Yes, extremely. Locomotion requires constant change of support, and points of support enable you to transfer momentum and produce force. The faster you move or the more complex and unknown the environment where you move is, the more difficult it becomes to ensure friction for change of support and to avoid partial or complete slippage and a loss of energy, time, and balance that can even cause a fall and an injury. This kind of movement practice and physical performance is more demanding than moving on flat surfaces and predictable, unchanging environments. With every movement and every change of support, the perception of friction will be one of the primary reasons for success or failure, safety or injury. It is not just body weight and gravity that give us a sense of the points of support that connect us to the environment where we stand; it is also the perception of friction.

The perception of friction gives us a sense of

- How balanced and confident we can be on a given surface of support.
- What should be the optimal positioning of our points of support in relation to the supporting surface, as well as what the alignment of the rest of the body should be.
- How much force we need to produce and in what direction to ensure sufficient friction.
- How much power we can produce relative to the amount of friction we perceive we can rely on.
- How much momentum we can transfer from our base of support.
- How long we can afford to remain in a position on a given surface of support.
- Even what, where, how, and when should be our next move. An instant decision to modify the movement we were intending to transition to can be made depending on a perception of friction different than what we anticipated.

It is not unusual to witness people who otherwise have a "normal" sense of balance be challenged by their inability to manage efficient positioning (position in relation to the environment) and to trust their points of support; you may have experienced it yourself when walking in nature on rainy days. People— including athletes and fitness aficionados who aren't trained to move in nature— slow down considerably while having little ability to accelerate, especially off trails. This is because not a single surface of support is exactly the same and static friction can only be assumed. Inexperienced people don't know what to expect every time they make a move, or expect the wrong result. They experience apprehensiveness about slipping, insecurity, and even fear of falling and hurting themselves, which causes tension and stiffness in the body and increases clumsiness. Because you cannot always choose or predict the surfaces where you move, you cannot just "trust your body" in the absence of experience. To move faster, you need

to become skilled at quickly changing support while ensuring static friction, which is a task that requires lots of practice and experience when moving within a complex environment you're not familiar with and where surfaces change with every move you make.

Frictional resistance can be obtained from any body part because pretty much any body part can be used for support. However, most of the time we move while we're supported on our feet, hands, or both. Ensuring friction is probably one of the main reasons why the feet and hands are extremely sensitive to environmental stimuli for locomotion. (In the case of the hands, it has to do with both locomotion and manipulation.)

When ensuring friction is an issue, we adapt through diverse strategies to avoid slippage (changing position, positioning, gait, speed, timing, direction, intensity, and so on) to enable us to maintain the highest level of performance that is contextually possible.

In this book I show you specific positions that ensure optimal friction for each technique, *but* it is ultimately your practice with diverse real-world environmental variables that will ensure efficient, adaptable proprioception.

Here's the last drill for this chapter: Close your eyes to give yourself greater internal awareness. Slowly explore a variety of movements and positions on the spot and involve many parts of the body as points of support—for instance, the hands and the feet, knees and elbows, shoulder, buttocks, back, heels, fists, and so on. Pay attention to the interaction between the surface and the new points of support, friction, and body-weight shifting. Maintain breath control at all times.

15
Tension-Relaxation

"Maturity is achieved when a person accepts life as full of tension."

—Joshua L. Liebman

The first law of thermodynamics is that to produce work we need to expend energy. *Kinetic energy*—the energy of motion—is the outcome of the work primarily produced by the energy generated by muscular tension, which is itself the outcome of muscular strength. Muscular strength is the ability to exert tension and produce the force necessary to hold positions and perform movement. Simply standing requires some level of strength even if it's only a minimal amount. Without tension, there would be no position, sequence, and timing taking place.

Practical, Adaptable Strength

For strength to be produced in a way that fits a particular practical purpose behind movement, muscle tissues modify their length, which is called *contractility*. Strength is expressed through distinct patterns of muscle contraction, depending on the four main kinds of physical action it supports:

- Accelerating
- Decelerating
- Transitioning
- Holding

Accelerating

When you want to initiate and accelerate the movement of anything that has mass (or "weight")—a body part, the whole body, an external load or object—your muscles need to shorten to produce force, which is called *concentric contraction*. When you jump several feet away, for example, a concentric contraction occurs at the launch to accelerate your body and generate a takeoff. This acceleration is a motion in space (or displacement) at a given rate with respect to time,

which is called *velocity* (or, in simple terms, *speed*). The greater the force produced with the greatest velocity, the more *power* ensues.

Decelerating

Conversely, when you need to decelerate anything, your muscles elongate to produce force as well; this is *eccentric contraction*. After jumping, for instance, your body uses eccentric contraction to decelerate upon landing to minimize impact and bring your motion to a stop.

Transitioning

Although we could say that movement is nothing but a constant transition, it might happen that you need to transition in the sense of both decelerating and accelerating seemingly simultaneously through *plyometric contraction*, which is an extremely fast transition between eccentric and concentric contractions. That's what would happen if instead of landing to a static position, which means you only elongate the muscles in your legs to reduce velocity to zero, you have to swiftly bounce into another jump and produce great velocity by shortening the same muscles within milliseconds. This is why it is also sometimes called *elastic strength*. Indeed, the energy produced through eccentric contraction is briefly stored in the tendons and creates a recoil or "strain energy" that is transferred back to the concentric tension. I talk more about this aspect of muscular tension in Chapter 28, "Airborne Movement."

Holding

Holding a static position implies avoiding motion and therefore preventing acceleration, which necessitates *isometric contraction* with no change in muscle length. Think of holding a half squat position for several seconds before jumping and immediately after landing a jump. It is sometimes also called *yielding*. When we hold a position, "potential energy" is produced.

NOTE

Interestingly, in the examples I've just given, the same muscles handle the tasks of increasing or decreasing velocity, transitioning, and holding. Like all other aspects of physical performance, tension occurs because of our intention to move, not because of analytical thinking as we move. While moving we must feel the expression of strength rather than thinking about it.

Understanding in-depth scientific details about every aspect of strength won't turn us into amazing movers, although it helps design more effective training protocols to develop maximal strength and power and to increase capacity, which is a critical aspect of real-world physical capability. Our primary concern at this stage is to acquire simple, useful insights on how to move efficiently regardless of our current levels of strength.

Regardless of the type of muscular contraction employed for any specific movement or physical task, we know that the work produced comes at a cost called *energy cost,* which is the amount of energy used to perform such work. Naturally, we want to ensure economy so that the overall amount of energy spent for a given quantity of work remains minimal. The lower the energy cost for a given task and the more efficient we are, the more we delay lassitude and muscle fatigue. By not exerting more energy than needed, we can produce more force for a longer duration.

Tightness Mentality

Muscle strength, mass, and shape are often perceived to be the paramount fitness achievement. They are achievements without question, but not paramount from a Natural Movement perspective, as movement competency is priority.

The importance of strength for physical performance cannot be understated. However, it's always good to remember that, biologically speaking, strength in itself is not the finality; strength is the means that enables movement and locomotion for practical reasons relating to self-preservation. In

short, whereas physical movement develops and/or maintains strength, ultimately the purpose of strength is to serve movement, not the other way around.

Looking at strength as the be-all and end-all too often leads to an obsession with muscular tension and how hard muscles can be squeezed and pumped up. It's as if modern men and women want to be as hard as the marble of the ancient statues that have inspired contemporary physical culture from more than a century ago to the more modern bodybuilding movement. However, the physiques of the sculptors' models weren't achieved by muscle-isolation exercises; they were the result of diverse athletic, natural movements. We can safely assume that those ancient bodies were able to do more than pose stiffly because they were nimble and able to move adaptively. As a matter of fact, most of the original Olympian games related to the diverse physical skills necessary for warriors to fight wars. The aesthetic outcomes of such training, including hypertrophy and muscle definition, were legitimately valued the way they are today, but they weren't valued nearly as much as realistic, useful physical performance. I understand that this sounds more philosophical than practical, but you need to realize how a particular mindset turns into particular approach and expectation, which turns into particular behaviors and consequences.

If you want to achieve real-world movement efficiency, you must depart from the idea of muscle tightness and embrace the power of relaxation. Don't misunderstand my meaning: I am not implying that strength and intense muscular tension are unnecessary or that you should avoid muscular effort by relaxing and stretching all day. I'm suggesting that to achieve movement efficiency, muscular tension and relaxation must work hand in hand. You must learn selective muscular tension and muscular relaxation.

Although we obviously understand that no movement is possible without some muscular tension, we must also understand that no movement would be possible if every muscle in the body was tensed at the same time. Simply try to fully contract every muscle you can in your body while you're in a standing position and then try to run or jump. You can't do it. You have produced maximum gross tension and zero net force.

Despite the enormous amount of tension in your body, you might be able to move a small amount because, despite your intention and effort, some of your muscles are relaxed even if you don't perceive it. In any case the crazy amount of intentional tension in your body will make movement inefficient and very unpleasant, as if there is a conflict taking place in your body.

If you want to move a particular body part, you must enable the muscles responsible for movement in a given direction to tense and those responsible for movement in the opposite direction to relax, otherwise the force produced by antagonistic muscles would mutually cancel. Say you want to flex your arm (like a biceps curl) and extend it (like a triceps extension) at the same time. Could you do that? Of course not.

The *net force* is the amount of force directed in a given direction minus the force generated by the antagonist muscle at the same moment. You never need to spread tension to all muscles at the same time, and you don't need to tense muscles that have nothing to do with the task at hand. This is known as *irradiation:* intentionally spreading muscular tension to areas of the body that are not directly participating in the movement or physical task at hand. Irradiation is something that you must absolutely avoid.

The problems with inadequate tension in movement are numerous and unfortunately not limited to increasing metabolic cost by wasting precious energy. Inadequate tension throws off your coordination; decreases force production, power, and endurance; makes you less responsive and accurate; and slows down your recovery in *whatever* movement you do.

Every movement rendered inefficient by inadequate tension can also be rendered completely ineffective—again, that means that movement is failed entirely—which makes you waste time before you can recover and resume your movement or transition to the next one. The bottom line is that the whole tension and relaxation principle is a very big deal when it comes to technique and movement performance.

Selective Tension

To perform movement efficiently, muscular tension must be selective. *Selective tension is the optimal use of muscular tension to increase performance while minimizing energy expenditure.* Selective tension enables you to connect, disconnect, and reconnect body parts, sometimes extremely fast, following the sequence and timing of a given movement pattern thanks to our ability to tense or relax muscles alternately. For tension to be employed efficiently, you must consider the following things:

- **Where the tension is applied:** Body parts and muscles that do not contribute to the movement should stay relaxed.
- **When the tension is applied:** If tension is applied to soon or too late, it is wasted. Tension must synchronize with the proper sequence and timing of the movement. Before action, muscles must stay relaxed; when the job is done, muscles must return to a state of relaxation.
- **For how long the tension is applied:** If you apply tension too briefly or for too long, movement might fail or significantly decrease in efficiency.
- **How much tension is applied:** Too much tension is obviously a waste of energy, and it can also compromise the effectiveness of the movement, reduce its efficiency, or disturb the next movement.
- **What kind of tension is applied:** The kind of tension needed in the legs to jump up isn't the same as the tension needed to land after coming down (concentric contraction, eccentric contraction, plyometric contraction, isometric contraction).

To enable movement, tension takes place in the body just before actual motion occurs to ensure stability before the large muscles (or *prime movers*) that participate in overall stability generate most of the tension required for a dynamic movement. The production of power by large muscles or of momentum through the swift and wide-angle motion of body parts is bound to significantly disturb your initial positional set if it is weak from the start. Interactive disturbances are called *motion-dependent effects* and also *interaction torque,* which can modify your starting position and compromise the ensuing movement sequence you intend to perform. Whereas large, powerful muscles are responsible for generating force, smaller ones participate in directing the force efficiently—either before or after the production of force by the prime movers. A good example is the Forearm Swing-Up, where you hang on to a horizontal bar by your forearms and one leg that's hooked over the bar on one side. Your free leg must extend upward and swiftly swing downward to generate body-weight transfer and upward momentum. The motion from your leg can easily disturb your overall position, starting with the positioning of your forearms on the surface of support; if you cannot keep your upper body position stable, then you won't be able to properly transfer this momentum, and the action will fail.

In most cases, tension is not something you can think about as you move. It just happens—quickly, in many places, and with many changes as you transition from movement to movement while adjusting to the many variables of a complex environment. But not being able to think about tension doesn't mean that you can't be aware of it. Another part of your brain takes over that task so that you do it without thought. In truth, it's fortunate that you can't think about tension as you move because thinking is both too slow and too unreliable for the job.

Perception *of* Tension *and* Relaxation

It can be useful to acquire a basic perception of your ability to generate selective tension and to maintain relaxation by practicing some drills. If you find the following simple drills a challenge, what might happen when you actually move dynamically?

Perception of Selective Tension

The following selective tension partner drill is a very convincing illustration of how important the principle of selective tension is. In this drill, you must keep one arm as tense as possible, while keeping the other arm completely loose. There is complete dissociation between the two arms.

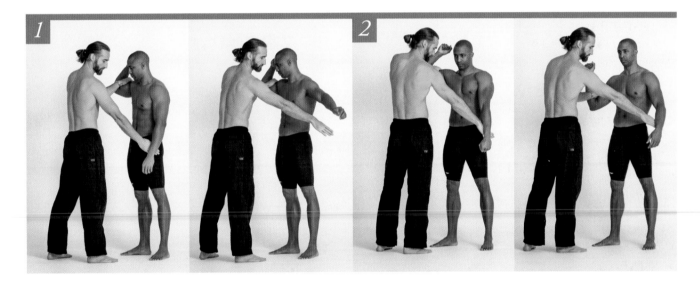

1   Stand close to your partner, facing the person. Bend one arm at a 90-degree angle and keep the other fully relaxed to the side of your body. As your partner places an open hand on the biceps of your bent arm and progressively presses down, you must resist the pressure. At the same time, your partner pushes your loose arm to the side away from your body with the top of their open hand pushing against the back of your forearm; do not resist this pressure. (Also avoid lifting your arm and pretending you are relaxed, of course.)

2   To create tension in the tense arm and resist the downward pressure of your partner's hand, you must involve other body parts to remain stable, which also tends to create tension in the arm that is supposed to be completely relaxed. You'll also tend to reduce tension in the tense arm as you're trying to keep the other arm loose.

This drill gets even more complicated when you have to repeatedly switch the positions of your arms—and thus also switch the tension and relaxation—which means you must quickly recover the same levels of tension and relaxation in the opposite arms. You will find yourself rapidly overthinking, getting confused, and probably holding your breath, looking down, and being unable to pay attention to anything else.

So, if dissociating opposite arm tension/relaxation while you're consciously paying attention to only this aspect is a challenge, can you imagine what happens when movement involves your *whole* body (as when you climb, crawl, swim, or punch) as you move on diverse terrains?

How many times will you use tension too early or too late, apply it too briefly or too long, use too much or not enough of it, and generate it in the wrong places? It's not just a matter of wasting energy; it's a matter of overall performance. Approach every new technique with concern for selective tension with proper timing, and you will shorten your learning curve and boost your progress and performance.

When you've developed great relaxation in performing a given pattern repeatedly and consistently, the first part of the job is done, but the task isn't over. Movements such as walking, running, crawling, or swimming, that tend to provide the close-to-perfect replication of a short cycle, enable you to find a "rhythm" where you can feel relaxed and in control. Any movement can feel great after enough practice, especially if you do it on predictable, smooth, linear surfaces. But the movement might become a challenge or be completely disrupted the moment the environment becomes different or more complex or when sudden, temporary transitions to completely different movement patterns become mandatory. This is what happens in the real world. You may feel relaxed as you hold a pose in a meditative stance indoors—with a sense of perfect breath control and balance—but that sense of calm is suddenly destroyed when you try to stay balanced at a height on top of

a tree branch. Where has your "self-mastery" gone? Why are you suddenly unable to relax? Will you be able to maintain the same levels of relaxation, or do you fall back into overall physical and mental tensions you thought you could keep at bay when everything—your movement and the whole context—was extremely simplified?

I'm not saying that superfluous tensions should never occur when you're dealing with more challenging environments—because the "skill" that is relaxation in movement is particularly challenging when movement is adaptable—but the tension should not exceed what is necessary to remain effective. Adaptability is not just the ability to handle more complex environments that change; it's also the ability to handle them efficiently, which means you have to remain as relaxed as possible.

NOTE

When you have a really good command of selective tension, you might enter the famous state of "flow" where you feel totally in control of your movement as if it were "effortless" (which, of course, it is not). It might almost feel as if it is happening in slow motion sometimes. Remember, when in motion, *flow*—or relaxation, for that matter—is not the absence of tension; it is the optimal use of it. Therefore, if you want to master relaxation, you first must master tension.

Perception of Relaxation

When you practice, you might sometimes find yourself overthinking and tensing, and just thinking of relaxing might not help you to actually relax. When this happens, take a short break and do the following drills with the goal of resetting your mental and physical sense of relaxation. It should take only a few seconds. Make sure that you combine these drills with ample, relaxed breathing.

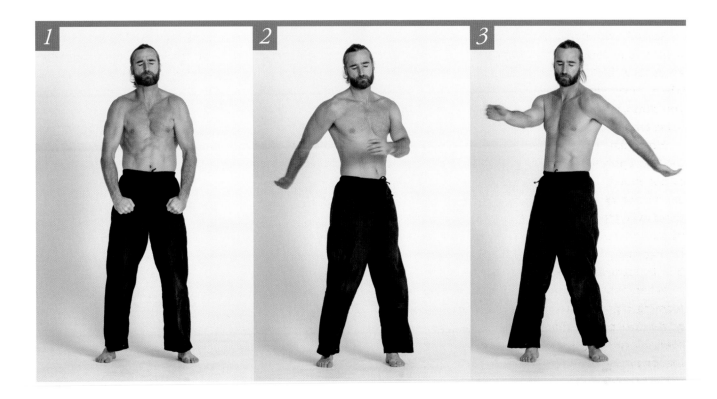

1   Assume any position you want. Hold your breath as you contract your whole body (as many body parts and muscles as you can) for five seconds. Then relax five seconds while strongly exhaling. Repeat. The goal of this drill is to paradoxically increase tension to enable the body to relax. This is a form of conscious pandiculation.

2   Swiftly rotate your hips in both directions, but let your arms be fully relaxed, so they can be moved by the motion of your hips without any active or intentional arm movement on your part. This drill reconnects you with a good sensation of tension (active hip motion/relaxation and passive arm motion).

3   In a standing position, move your hips, spine, shoulders, and neck in an undulating manner, as if you are a dancer.

NOTE

Pandiculation is what we call "stretching" as in stretching when we wake up. As a matter of fact, you could extend your arms and pretend that you are doing a morning stretch for an effect similar to what this drill is about.

16
Sequence and Timing

"All things entail rising and falling timing. You must be able to discern this."

—*Miyamoto Musashi*

Sequence and timing are tightly intertwined with breathing, position, and tension and relaxation. What is movement other than a sequence of positions and muscular tension that follow a particular timing, or in other words, a movement pattern? Coordination is nothing else but the ability to orderly recruit and activate motor units to perform a *particular* pattern. Note the importance of "particular."

We tend to see coordination as a general quality that, regardless of being innate or trained, is the answer to any movement challenge you might encounter. If you have acquired a good sense of coordination through a particular physical activity it will to some degree facilitate the acquisition of new movement patterns, but it will not spare you the time and energy required to learn to perform them efficiently. Are you as well coordinated as a karate black belt? Great. If you decide to learn judo techniques, you become a white belt again. You may or may not learn faster than someone who has zero experience in any martial art, but you still have to learn the new patterns, even if they are called "techniques." Coordination, while being a general quality, also demands lots of specificity to be efficient at particular movement tasks. The SAID principle strikes again! (See Chapter 7, "Adaptable," for a definition of the SAID principle.)

Sequence and timing are an extraordinarily important part of every movement pattern or technique. Sequence is the particular order that each body part follows as it works with other body parts to form a compound or complete movement. Timing concerns the optimal moment each part of the sequence starts and ends, its duration, and its speed.

In most cases, improper timing is what messes up movement execution. It is because of improper timing that sequence is altered (or even completely ruined), and the altered sequence disturbs your position, which can leave you confused and sometimes causes you to lose balance, waste time and energy, repeat the movement, and, in worst cases, sustain injury. The same way incorrect positions can ruin efficiency and even render the outcome of a whole movement ineffective even if the sequence and timing were properly followed, improper sequence and timing wreak havoc with even the best positional control.

Let's say you want to jump forward as far as possible from a standing position (the Power Jump), and you aren't able to swing your arms forward, which makes the normal sequence incomplete. Your jump might be effective, but it won't be efficient because of the missing segment of the sequence (swinging your arms forward). It will feel very "unnatural," and, most importantly, you will not be able to jump as far as you should. Likewise, if you do swing your arms forward but you do it too late—say you swing them just after takeoff—the sequence is complete, but its timing is off, and the result will be the same as if you had not swung your arms at all. Clearly you cannot dissociate position from sequence and timing (the same way you cannot dissociate sequence and timing from tension and relaxation).

Impeccable sequence and timing can make the difference between achieving an effective and efficient movement and failing an attempt. It makes the movement work, and it also makes it feel "natural." When the movement is cyclical, as running or swimming are, we may talk about rhythm, which is a good word that expresses smooth, repetitive sequence and timing. A movement such as the Foot-Hand Crawl can be done using the exact same particular back, leg, and arm positions, but their position relative to each other may actually follow distinct pattern variations in sequence and timing. Indeed, you can do the Foot-Hand Crawl by using an ipsilateral pattern—which means the arm and leg on the same side of the body move at the same time—or a contralateral one—where the arm and leg on opposite sides of the body move at the same time. To those who aren't paying attention or are the non-initiated, the two patterns look the same, and if you cannot differentiate those patterns when you do the Foot-Hand Crawl, then you have no option but to crawl the way you can without knowing if it's the most contextually efficient.

> **NOTE**
>
> The body has a natural tendency to "cross-educate," which means that acquired motor control in one limb or both limbs on one side of the body supports the acquisition of the same motor control on the opposite limb(s).

Also, sequence and timing may have to do with the synchronicity of breathing with movement and when an inhale, an exhale, or a brief breath-hold should take place; for instance, the timing of breathing in a heavy lift sequence is crucial. Last, the production of force or momentum, small or large, and the tension required must also take place at a particular timing of a sequence.

Force Summation

In any given movement or technique, more than one muscle plays a part. The relative contribution of each muscle to the net force exerted by a muscle group is called *force sharing*.

Force summation is the inverse perspective—the overall sum of force or momentum produced by the contribution all body parts or motor units—for example, the total amount of force produced at the moment an object is released when it is thrown. Although the notion of force summation is generally employed for throwing or kicking something, I believe it is worth applying it to any movement; there is also a force summation at the moment we take off for a jump.

When you want to generate movement, you immediately think of contracting your prime movers—those large muscle groups that are responsible for producing most of the strength or power you need, such as pushing on your legs or pulling with your arms. Inefficient movers tend to exclusively rely on the smaller body segments, such as their arms,

without considering that the rest of the body could participate to increase performance and make movement more economical. Think of a novice trying to throw hard by only extending the arm. Now think of an expert thrower who uses the whole body, starting with the feet, legs, hips, torso, and finally the arm, wrist, and even fingers. The pattern follows a particular and complex positional sequence and timing.

Involving more motor units whenever possible (and, of course, whenever necessary) in what is sometimes called *compound movement* is the bread and butter of Natural Movement. This strategy contributes to a greater overall performance if the force output is maximal, or to the reduction of overall energy cost for a given physical action compared to involving fewer body segments.

On top of involving powerful "engines" of the body such as the legs and the hips rather than peripheral limbs only, *body-weight shifting* and *body-weight transfer* are two essential strategies for increased force summation that can improve the performance of a number of movements by involving more body segments in the contribution to the overall effort and performance. In short, the two methods allow the generation of additional momentum "from scratch and on the spot."

Body-Weight Shifting

Body-weight shifting happens in one of two ways:

- When the distribution of the body weight on the existing points of support changes, which increases or decreases the load on the point(s) of support
- When a point of support is removed and the center of gravity moves outside of vertical alignment with the base of support

Body-Weight Shifting Without Change of Support

When body-weight shifting takes place from one point of support to another *very swiftly* and with enough amplitude, it generates additional momentum that increases velocity; it also can increase ground force reaction, which helps produce more force. The faster the change of distribution of body weight and with the more amplitude (wider range of motion), the more momentum is generated; it is the way body-weight shifting for the sake of efficiency must be understood.

Imagine you're in a Split Standing position and must throw a rock. Compare how far you can throw (without using hip rotation) when you start with most of your body weight on the front foot with how far you throw when you start by leaning back with most of your body weight on the back foot and then swiftly shift all your body weight to the front foot a brief moment before you extend your arm. The second option clearly makes your projectile go significantly farther because you're not relying solely on your arm to generate force. You're adding momentum to your whole body by swiftly shifting your body weight from the back of your body to the front. This additional sequence must take place with the right timing, which is just before you produce force with the upper body (pectoral, shoulder, and triceps muscles). The greater and more explosive the shift of body weight, the more additional power is generated.

The same principle could be used from the same Split Standing position as you jump forward. In this case, the forward shifting of the body weight from the back foot to the front foot not only generates momentum before force is produced by the front leg, but it also helps by "loading" it and increasing ground force reaction, which enables you to land farther than if you don't employ body-weight shifting. It is not just the force produced by the back leg to shift the body weight that is responsible for all the additional momentum; the pull of gravity, which is a free energy, also plays a part. Indeed, even if the base of support remains unchanged, gravity accelerates the center of gravity the moment it goes beyond the center of the base of support (although not as much as if it was to move completely outside of it, which is also an option available to add momentum). Through practice, you will discover a number of movements for which you will be able to use this principle.

Body-Weight Shifting with Change of Support

Swiftly removing a point of support and shifting the center and line of gravity both outside the base of support could be an intentional move for the purpose of changing direction and location, which is locomotion, in the most efficient way possible—quickly and economically. The swifter and further you displace your line of gravity and center of gravity outside your base of support, the more acceleration and momentum is generated in the direction where the center of gravity is going. The acceleration and momentum aren't generated by producing great amounts of force; it's generated by the motive (a force that produces mechanical motion) and free energy, which is the pull of gravity. While your center of gravity is falling outside your base of support, you are "off" balance yet your balance is not off; you're dynamically changing support through a controlled change of center of gravity, which is the essence of locomotion. You use this principle when you change direction while running but also in numerous other movements.

Body-Weight Transfer

Body-weight transfer happens when nonsupporting body parts or segments—and consequently their weight—is swiftly put to motion, which generates *segmental momentum* that is transferred to *whole-body momentum*. Think, for instance, of swinging your arms forward before you jump. That's body-weight transfer. The difference between body-weight transfer and body-weight shifting is that in body-weight transfer the momentum is created through a part of the body that isn't supporting any body weight. If you're standing, you can body-weight shift from one foot to the other and body-weight transfer with your arms or upper body. If you're standing on a single leg, then the free leg could contribute to additional momentum as well. If you're hanging by your hands, you can body-weight shift from one hand to the other and body-weight transfer through your legs or lower body.

A significant amount of additional kinetic energy can be produced during body-weight transfer, which results in a decrease in the amount of raw muscular strength you need to achieve a given level of performance or an increase in the level of performance you would otherwise achieve without it.

I did basic tests and rudimentary measurement to compare the Power Jump (which you might know by the name "broad jump") as I used various arm movements. The table shows the results of my tests.

No arm movement	89 inches
Forward Arm Swing starting with arms on hips' sides	97 inches
Forward Arm Swing starting with arms pulled behind the body	104 inches
Backward-Forward Arm Swing starting with arms extended to the front of the body, swiftly pulled to the back, then followed by a Forward Arm Swing, increasing the stretch reflex	111 inches

So, although these rudimentary tests and measurements show that muscular power in the prime movers represents roughly 80 percent and the most important part of the maximum distance I can reach with a Power Jump, additional momentum through body-weight transfer through the arms represents 20 percent of the distance. That's *really* significant. Now, another significant thing is that the typical partial arm swing (swinging with arms bent and starting at the hips) represents only a fraction of the overall additional distance that can be gained with really efficient body-weight transfer, a mere 9 to 10 percent extra distance compared to the no-arm distance. With a more efficient use of the arms, I got 25 percent more distance. This means that while body-weight transfer adds to efficiency for a Power Jump, efficient body-weight transfer adds even more—sometimes significantly more.

So which variables make body-weight transfer efficient?

- **Weight:** This is an aspect you have little control over, but because momentum is generated by both mass and acceleration, if the body parts you accelerate are larger and heavier, but you can move them swiftly, you generate more segmental momentum.

- **Velocity:** The faster you can accelerate a body segment, the more segmental momentum or speed you give to it and the more whole-body momentum you achieve.

- **Amplitude:** Longer segments (for instance arms extended instead of half bent) and greater range of motion (arms swinging from the back of the body to the front, and even from the front to the back and then again to the front) enables greater acceleration and therefore greater momentum.

- **Timing:** The generation of momentum must precede the production of force by the prime movers (obviously not after, but also not at the same time). Although it is commonly assumed that all movement starts with the prime movers (the larger, heavier, stronger muscles) and then ends with the smaller, lighter, less strong muscles to "refine" the movement to give it its efficiency and accuracy, when using the body-weight transfer strategy the exact opposite is true. If you were to move your arms after extending your legs and hips, they would add no momentum to your movement.

- **Direction ("vector")**: Whether momentum is produced thanks to linear or angular (rotational) motion or a combination of both, it must be impeccably directed toward where the movement goes. For instance, if you're jumping horizontally, your arms shouldn't swing at a greater angle than 45 degrees, but if you're jumping upward they should swing all the way up.

If the application of some or all of the listed variables is not adequate, it will be counterproductive to efficiency, and timing is paramount.

The Sit-Up is a good example of a combination of the use of body-weight shifting and body-weight transfer.

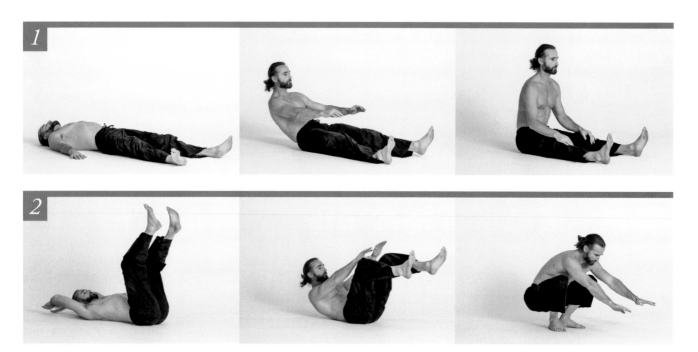

1   Lie down on the ground and perform a Sit-Up. Most people don't think of using anything but their abdominal muscles to achieve the movement, thinking "crunch" (a conventional fitness drill to strengthen the abdominal muscles) and exclusively relying on the prime movers to battle against gravity. Sitting up that way is shifting your body weight from one point of support to the other, but it is slow and strenuous. By making the same movement much swifter and constantly accelerating until you're in the sit position, transferring body weight from the back to the rear already feels much easier. That's "body-weight shifting."

2   Bring your arms behind your head and lift your legs up. You can even lift your rear off the ground. Swiftly swing your arms forward and bring your legs down: Voilà, you've achieved a

Sit-Up so quickly and effortlessly that you could even transition to a Squat! That's "body-weight transfer," and it's a much more efficient and natural sit-up movement than only using your abdominal muscles. If you want to move efficiently, you'd be a fool not to use all your limbs! This is not "cheating"; it's moving naturally with ease and efficiency.

If you aim at strengthening your abdominal muscles specifically, you certainly can do "regular" Sit-Ups instead of natural, efficient ones. Just keep this in mind: The whole-body Sit-Up strengthens the abdominals, too, but it does so while ingraining the most efficient movement pattern. There are *many* natural movements that will strengthen your abdominals in the most effective, balanced, natural way possible without you having to make it a grueling chore.

17
Local Positional Control

You now have a better understanding of the pillars of technique and how fundamental, universal laws and principles rule movement efficiency, both conceptually and experientially. Before you start learning complete movements, it's a good idea to make sure that you have *local positional control,* which is basic control over your body's simplest movement patterns, one at a time, which I'm going to tell you how to verify by standing in one spot—no locomotion yet. You're checking the alignment of your spine and the position of your head, hips, arms, shoulders, legs, or feet, as well as their basic motions. Indeed, you would be surprised by how many people have issues assuming and/or performing such simple discrete positions and movements without thinking or getting confused.

Practicing local positional control can expose basic motor-control or mobility issues or limitations, dissymmetry, and imbalances before you dive into the next chapters where you learn and practice complete movement techniques and employ whole-body positional control. You also can do the discrete movements I describe here before you engage in movement practice to check out the body's basic function, identify localized stiffness or pain, prepare for movement, or release tension. You can practice these movements when the body is otherwise almost completely idle (when you're sitting, standing, and waiting, and so on) to add movement and well-being to an otherwise movement deficient lifestyle.

To learn complex movement patterns known as "technique," you must first develop full control of other much smaller movements that participate in the complete pattern. There is a popular saying that states, "A chain is only as strong as its weakest link." Complete movement patterns—or techniques—can be considered chains. (As a matter of fact, they can be called *kinetic chains,* and each discrete movement is a "link.") A stronger link in a movement chain doesn't always strengthen the whole chain. However, a weak link in a movement chain always weakens the whole chain.

If you don't Hip Hinge efficiently, you can't lift, jump, or land efficiently. If you lack mobility in your feet and ankles, any movement on your feet is altered to an extent. Unless you pay attention to the details, you can't understand what is missing or not working correctly in the big picture. Local positional control enables you to have each part of the pattern do its job properly, which entails that particular body parts should be moving only if they're involved in the efficiency of the overall movement. Therefore, local positional control is tightly related to overall positional control and efficiency.

When I teach, I often point out small, unnecessary movements that students do without being aware of it. I always ask, "Did you notice it? Was it intentional? Did it add anything to your efficiency?" The answer is always no. With experience, you modify your positions as little as possible not out of rigidity but out of efficiency. What doesn't contribute is superfluous; what is superfluous is a waste of time and energy. Your brain must focus all its attention on the effectiveness and efficiency of movement, and if you add up constant little movements that alter your position, it is like "noise" in a symphony.

Of course, the discrete positions and movements that I describe in this chapter don't encompass the full spectrum; however, I cover the essential ones that involve all joints and all planes of motion. Eventually, the real level of function of any body part or joint is revealed by movement done in context. For instance, you may have decent and pain-free shoulder rotation when you're standing, but your shoulders get stiff and can't rotate as well when you're hanging.

The information I offer here is just a quick, partial movement screen for you to do on your own. It's not a guarantee that if all goes all right, you're ready for any movement without experiencing any issue, limitation, or discomfort. It also doesn't mean that you'll learn Natural Movement techniques without effort. In any case, the local positional control movements in this chapter may help reawaken dormant areas of your motor control. Eventually, you should be able to visualize and replicate precise positions and movements with your eyes closed.

A Few Words About Posture

One of the most crucial aspects of positional control that you need to memorize and reflexively, instantly reproduce is posture. Posture is commonly seen as holding a straight back when sitting, standing, or walking, but this is a restrictive view. Posture has to do with the linear alignment of the spine and, by extension, of the whole upper body, regardless of the particular position we hold or movement we do. For instance, posture is also present in various kneeling positions with an upright upper body, and in jumping, landing, lifting, and throwing techniques and other movements where the upper body is leaning forward at an angle.

Just like breathing, posture—good or bad—significantly affects our emotions, energy levels, hormonal balance, and so on. A "collapsed" upper body position shrinks us, compromises breathing and digestive function, and negatively acts on our cortisol levels. (High levels of cortisol are associated with many negative health effects.) We're perceived by others as smaller, weaker, less present, and less capable. Conversely a tall, erect posture expresses confidence, presence, and intention, communicating to others that we're capable, centered, in control, and self-assured; it makes us more attractive to others. There is an established interaction between posture and psychology: better posture promotes a more positive attitude, and a more positive attitude supports better posture. With good posture, things are literally looking up for you!

NOTE

To read more about the relationship between posture and psychology, I recommend the study from The Ohio State University covered in the article at www.sciencedaily.com/releases/2009/10/091005111627.htm.

For those reasons, posture is rightfully a big concern in the modern world. We are constantly told to pay attention to it. There are devices and contraptions designed to improve posture and experts specializing in fixing "dysfunctional posture" with very detailed criteria of what good posture should look like externally. To most of us, holding a "good" posture is perceived as a chore that demands constant attention and effort.

However, is there really such a thing as a standard posture? No. This would be dismissing individual variations in our anatomy, physical makeup, and measurements. My standpoint on good posture doesn't relate to arbitrary standards but to the biomechanical principle of joint centration. Whereas most animals are quadrupedal and have evolved to sustain a horizontal orientation of the spine from sacrum to neck, humans are bipedal and have evolved to stand erect. Whereas we may episodically assume positions that aren't vertical, by default we want to return to a vertically organized position, typically when we sit, kneel, stand, walk, and run. Assuming vertically "stacked" joint alignment enables us to be efficient in the way we interact with gravity, which is especially important given that such erect positions are those we assume most of the time. With rounded alignment—of the spine from top to bottom—gravity demands that we exert more tension in the body's posterior regions, such as the back, neck, and shoulders. For example, a human head weighs about 10 to 12 pounds, but looking at a smartphone with your head leaning down is equal to having a 60-pound weight pressing down on your neck. If you hold the positions for hours a day every day, such stress is very likely to cause tension and pain (and ultimately damage) in your neck. Similar issues arise with a chronically rounded spine, which used to be an issue in elderly people but is now common in much younger populations. Whereas there may not be an "ideal" posture that looks exactly the same for all, there is certainly an ideal way to interact with gravity, and individual posture is best when it is optimally aligned vertically with the base of support and gravity.

Day-to day-posture is very important, but it's only one aspect of your overall physical and movement function. It may be much more beneficial for you to look at your overall movement and physical behavior rather than trying to episodically assume good posture in the absence of the general physical behavior and even lifestyle that supports it.

The practice of the movement patterns in this chapter will help you get a better sense of your current spinal alignment. Although frequently paying attention to your posture on a day-to-day basis when you stand or sit can contribute to improving it, this isn't the most important or most effective way to address it. If you check out your posture even ten times a day and force yourself to hold a good position for a minute, your posture collapses again the moment you stop being mindful about it, and you still end up spending the overwhelming majority of your day with a rounded back, hunched shoulders, and forward-leaning neck.

Instead, you need to make posture *reflexive*. Posture needs to become something that you do not need to mentally remind your body to do; over time, it has to become a reflex of your central nervous system that unconsciously takes place in a matter of milliseconds. Without such a reflex, "postural strength" gained through specific drills becomes useless because it remains unused most of the time.

How do you reach that point? Most experts recommend that you give priority attention to how you contract such-or-such muscle (brace the abs, squeeze the glutes, and so on) in a sequence and at a certain percentage of tension so your joints and bones can "naturally" align. This might not be the best way to make good posture a systematic physical reflex as it leads people to overthinking. Instead, you need to restore the original movement behavior of your whole body as often as you can; in short, practice Natural Movement with the diversity, frequency, consistency, and, of course, efficiency it entails.

By learning to control breathing and position through many diverse movement techniques in many contexts, you synergistically learn how to organize your skeletal structure efficiently, and in most cases you will intuitively figure out, by feel, what levels of tension are required and where that tension is needed—whether it is in your abs, in your glutes, along your spine, or wherever else it is necessary—by feel. Consciously thinking of particular muscles and levels of tension may keep you mentally focused on limited areas of your posture, such as your "core," and potentially distracted to the fact that your posture is still terrible because your head and upper back may not be vertically aligned with your base of support in the first place.

You need to acquire a physical perception of what is a healthy, efficient posture both in terms of position from toes to head and with the right levels of tension needed to maintain that position, but you start with the position rather than the tension. If you start with the perception of your position being optimally aligned with gravity, then everything else falls into place.

When you're sitting at your desk, your central nervous system will remember the good feeling of aligned spine, centered joints, open chest, rib cage, and shoulder it has experienced while crawling, hanging, or lifting with efficient technique, and it will want to reproduce this good body feeling from its own initiative, reflexively.

A Few Words About *the* Core

Ever heard of the core? Of course you have. The "core" is a complex series of muscles that work together to coordinate to stabilize the midline of your body—lower spine and pelvis—in both static positions and dynamic ones (movement!). Does that relate to posture? Yes. Postural control is about the alignment of the spine from head to sacrum; in fact, it even includes the pelvis. Core stability protects the spine, especially the lower area of the spine, and protecting the spine protects the spinal cord and the ability of the central nervous system to direct motion (motor control). If you hurt the spine, you hurt your ability to move to a radical extent. So "good" posture isn't just about alignment; it's also the strength and endurance of the whole muscular system responsible for keeping the spine strong and safe, especially during dynamic and powerful movements.

The muscles involved in the core extend far beyond the abdominals. Many other muscles are involved, including the glutes and many other muscles. Trying to isolate all those muscles to strengthen them separately wouldn't be such a good idea because the core needs to be trained in concert with the rest of the body through movement. The core isn't about looking good with chiseled abs. The core has work to do—primarily to stabilize the pelvis and lower spine.

Having a strong core is significant to the big picture of efficient, practical, and adaptable movement. Doing many crunches isn't the best solution for developing the strength, endurance, and motor control that a functional core demands.

The control of abdominal breathing gives you a great head start in terms of bracing and lower spine stability, as well as supporting stability all the way to the top of your spine. It also helps your ability to relax. It is not mostly muscular strength but muscular endurance that ensures the ability to maintain posture over time. This explains why very strong individuals who can Deadlift very heavy loads may rapidly experience lower back pain when moving in nature on difficult terrains for some time; movement requires endurance and adaptability in your ability to stabilize the pelvis and spine.

The following movement patterns and techniques are very effective for teaching you postural control:

- The Foot-Hand Crawl
- The Hip Hinge, learned and practiced first separately
- The Hip Hinge applied to Stepping Under, Power Jumping, Neutral Landing, and performing manipulative techniques under load, such as the Deadlift and Front Swing Throw and Catch patterns

NOTE

Remember this: A straight posture in a living human being is not a chronic tightening of your muscles or the fossilization of your vertebrae and joints; when you're sitting or standing with good posture, allow frequent minute adjustments and movements, undulations, and oscillations of your spine and bones to conserve fluidity of motion in the spine.

Standing Positions

Photos 1 and 2 show what standing with good posture and abdominal breathing looks like.

Notice the vertical alignment from the base of support to the top of the head. The model is expressing quiet composure, confidence, awareness, and readiness, yet he is relaxed.

Intentional Practical Stances

The following standing positions are all intentional, which means not only that you are conscious of the fact you are holding them, but also that you are holding them for a practical reason. There are more variations than the few examples shown, but the point is to illustrate that standing positions, just like in any other area of Natural Movement, are practical and contextually adaptable. None of the positions shown is "faulty" or inefficient as long as it serves a temporary practical purpose.

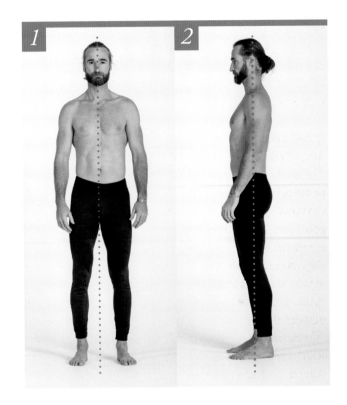

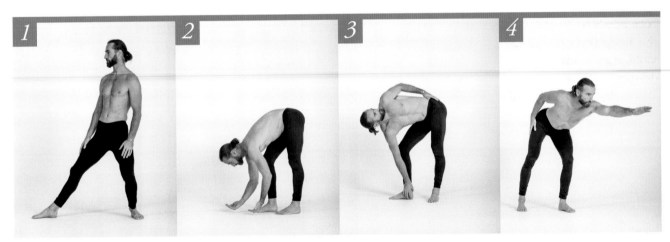

1 Split Standing with a slight backward lean: Need for stability, balance, observation

2 Split Standing, bending over: Looking for something on the ground or picking up very light objects

3 Split Standing side lean: Stepping through confined environments, looking for a passage

4 Split Standing Hip Hinge forward lean and arm reach: Reaching for something when stepping closer isn't possible

Unconscious Behavioral Stances

There are a number of standing positions we may hold that do not express the qualities I previously described. These positions might temporarily consciously or (more often) unconsciously express a particular psychological state, which we commonly refer to as "body language." Even though we see these positions as "normal" simply because they are so common, holding them by default or just too frequently is not a healthy postural habit. As you look at photos 1 through 10, you might even recognize stances that people you know often adopt. Compare the photos in this section with the photos in the first set and with how you regularly stand.

Unless they are intentional and temporary, the positions represented in photos 1 through 10 represent faulty positions because none of them displays healthy alignment or relaxation. As I mentioned earlier, the overall practice of Natural Movement, efficient movement, and positional control within context coupled with abdominal breath control and paying attention to your posture during day-to-day activities will gradually help you let go of those unconscious standing patterns and replace them with healthier ones.

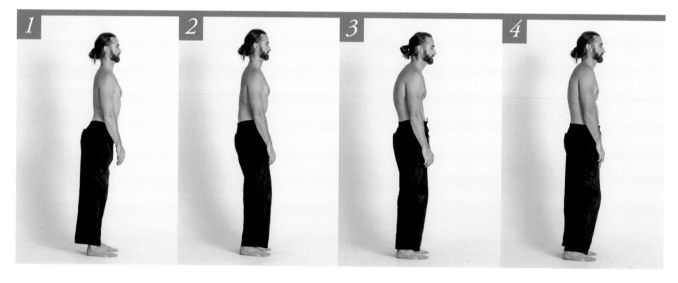

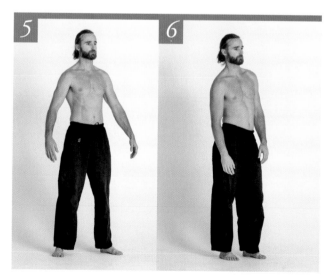

1   Lumbar hyperextension: Suggests an exaggerated self-assertion.

2   Lumbar flexion.

3   Rounded back.

4   Shrugged shoulders: Suggests insecurity, protective stance.

5   Shoulder/trapezius tension: Suggests "tough guy" attitude, showing off self-confidence (most often expressing an actual lack thereof).

6   Hip sway with most of the body weight on one foot: The *contrapposto* (Italian for *counterpose*) stance was a common pose in Antique sculptures. Suggests feeling relaxed, secure, and "cool," and but it's an imbalanced stance.

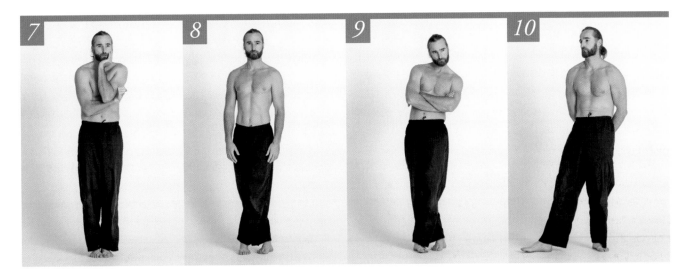

7 Crossed arm chin support: Suggests insecurity.

8 Crossed legs: Suggests insecurity, indecision.

9 Crossed legs and crossed arms with a side lean: Suggests protectiveness of self, insecurity, disagreement.

10 Rounded back with hip sway and arms crossed in the back: Suggests insecurity, disagreement, disinvolvement.

Neutral Pelvis & Lower Back

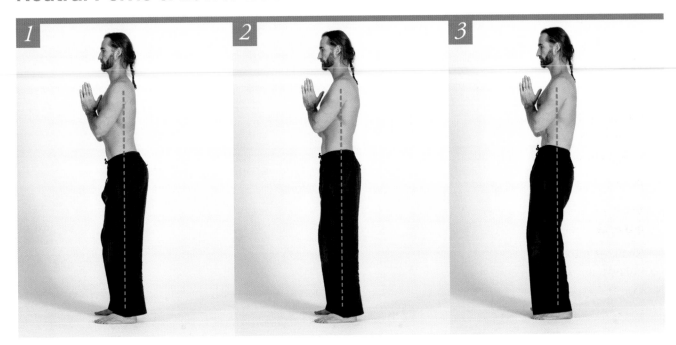

1 Anterior pelvic tilt and slight lumbar (lower back or spine) extension

2 Neutral pelvis and lower back

3 Posterior pelvis tilt and slight lumbar flexion

To help with postural control or vertically aligned standing, let's look at alignment from the base of support to the head instead of looking only at the upper back and shoulders. You're going to make sure your legs are fully extended (no knee bend) then move your attention to the lower back, pelvis, and hips (they are so closely related that the term *lumbopelvic-hip-complex* is often used) to vertically align the center of the pelvis with the center of your base of support. At this point both your pelvis and lower spine have been placed in a nice "neutral" position (the term *neutral* indicates vertical alignment with the base of support). If you can maintain a neutral pelvis and lower spine position while also maintaining a straight and upright back, neck, and head, then all the vertebrae in your spine are optimally "stacked," which takes pressure and tension off of your posterior muscles and makes you feel more stable and relaxed.

To help you center your joints and find this neutral position, try different positions for your pelvis by tilting it to the back (anterior tilt) and the front (posterior tilt) until your get a better sense of the middle or neutral position. This is something you can do in front of a mirror to get visual feedback, but you should be able to feel and "visualize" it without looking.

While you're at it, you might want to make sure that your rib cage, shoulders, neck, and head are also centered along the same vertical line, which clearly the neutral pelvis and lower back will immensely help with. A good cue is to imagine that your head is being pulled up while your tailbone is being pulled down, moving all your vertebrae apart, lengthening your spine, reducing spinal curves*, and increasing spinal stability; this is formally known as *axial extension.*

Now that you have a sense of vertical alignment from feet to head, you may start to pay attention to the tension you need to maintain the stability of your posture. When I talk about manipulation movement in Chapters 30 and 31, you learn about bracing, which combines abdominal breathing and contraction to stabilize your pelvis and lower spine under load. It is maybe the single most potent way to learn about stabilizing your core, even though significantly less tension is required in day-to-day standing compared to lifting heavy loads.

Without waiting to start learning heavy lifting techniques, you can already apply a little bracing to your standing position. Once you have set your standing pelvic and spinal position to neutral, contract your glutes (or buttocks) and abdominals about 10 to 20 percent of the hardest contraction you could generate as you maintain abdominal breathing. The level of tension you need is a little like how much you would tense if you were expecting a three-year-old to punch you "hard" in the stomach. Do you feel how this extra tension makes your midline tighter and stronger?

Assuming ground position on all fours, either in a knee-hand or foot-hand position (see Chapter 24, "Ground Movement 1: Lying, Rolling, Crawling," for some example positions), requires more tension in your core to support the neutral position. Being on all fours can help you better feel where tension happens in your body to ensure the stability of your pelvis and lower back.

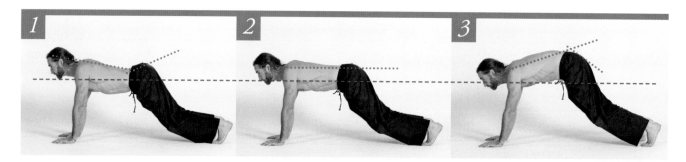

1 Lower back extension

2 Neutral lower back

3 Lower back flexion

---

*The back is never truly "flat" or straight because the spine has slight natural curves.

Hip Hinge

The Hip Hinge is a flexion at the hip joint that is performed while keeping the spine neutral and the knees slightly bent. Beyond being a position, the Hip Hinge is a movement pattern that involves both flexion and extension at the hip joint. It's by far the most important—as well as challenging—pattern among this series of local movements. It is an essential component of a number of Natural Movement techniques.

Although it's not an upright position, an efficient Hip Hinge demands postural control and benefits it greatly. The Hip Hinge teaches you to keep your spine stable and safe so the huge power of your posterior chain and hips can be harnessed. For instance, by adding an ankle extension that ends simultaneously with a knee and hip extension, you create a "triple extension" that generates most of the force in the Power Jump. While you look at the positional sequence of the pattern, you need to make sure that you are activating your core, which means performing the Hip Hinge with bracing and abdominal breathing.

People often tend to confuse the Hip Hinge with the Squat. The Squat involves an almost equal ratio of motion at the hip and knee joints, whereas the Hip Hinge is hip dominant, which means that you are moving your hips with great range of motion and your knees with slight range of motion.

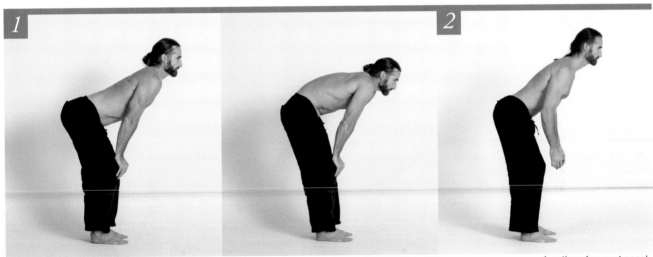

(continued on next page)

1   You can get a sense of the Hip Hinge position by bending your knees slightly and leaning forward at about a 45-degree angle as you support yourself with your arms (hands on your knees or lower thighs), then extend (photo 1a) and flex (photo 1b) your lower spine to find the neutral spine spot.

2   Hold the position for a moment without the support of your arms while maintaining abdominal breathing. You don't have to flex your hips—that is, move them backward—to the maximum at this point. But you may already play with the hip motion, coming back to standing by driving and extending your hips forward, then flexing them again to a Hip Hinge and trying to reach a greater range of motion. As you drive your hips backward and forward, your center of gravity ideally should remain vertically aligned with your base of support, which implies that the line of gravity doesn't move and ensures great stability throughout the whole hip motion.

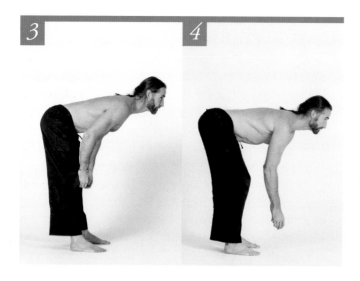

3   If you find yourself leaning at close to a 90-degree angle with your knees locked straight, you're technically in a Hip Hinge position, but it is neither an efficient nor a sustainable one (unless it is a momentary stance in a particular context and not involving the manipulation of a load). On the other hand, if you cannot reach this position intentionally, it means you lack mobility.

4   Even with a slight knee bend, if your torso gets parallel to the ground, you're pushing the hinge to an unnecessary extent that will also be unstable, weak, and unsustainable when you use the Hip Hinge as part of a more complex and challenging movement (jumping, landing, lifting, and so on).

Wall Drill

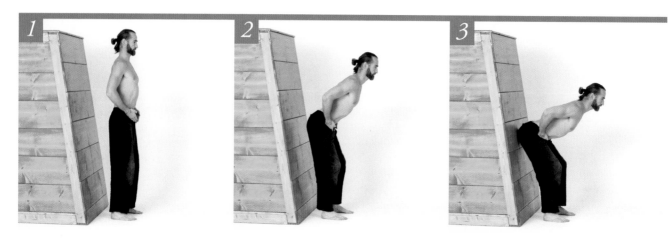

1   Stand tall facing away from a wall with your rear about a foot away from the surface it will have to reach when hinging. Place the sides of your hands on each side of the groin crease.

2   Simultaneously flex your knees slightly and initiate hip flexion while maintaining spinal alignment.

3   Keep flexion in your hips while bending your knees a little more, keeping your shins vertical and your knees aligned with your feet, and drive your rear back toward the surface of the wall until your buttocks reach the wall. Your torso should be leaning at about a 45-degree angle. As you increase the hip flexion, you should feel that your hands are firmly pinched in the creases of your hips. If you don't feel that pinch, it may indicate that you are leaning too far forward or squatting too much (flexing your knees more and your hips less). If you have reached full hip flexion but cannot touch the wall with your rear, slide your feet back a little; you probably started standing too far from the wall. If you reach the wall before achieving full hip flexion, you were standing too close. In any case, don't allow your rear to be supported by the wall; you just want to touch it lightly and briefly before you extend your hips to return to standing.

Another way to practice efficient Hip Hinge with spinal alignment is to use both hands to hold a dowel (a broomstick, PVC pipe, or something similar) behind your back; have one hand at lower-back level and the other at upper-back level. The dowel should run from your tailbone to your upper back and back of your head. Move into the Hip Hinge position without the dowel ever losing contact with any of the body parts it was in contact with when you started. If you round your back as you flex your hips, the dowel won't stay in contact with all the body parts. You can use the dowel while doing the wall drill; the dowel helps you keep spinal alignment in check while hinging, and the wall helps you with range of motion at the hip. Holding the Hip Hinge at maximum hip flexion for several seconds while maintaining abdominal breathing is also a great exercise to start building stability and endurance in the "bottom" position, which is the phase of the motion that's most susceptible to positional disruption. The next progression will be the Hip Hinge under (light) load, such as what you do in a Deadlift technique.

Neck Position *and* Cervical Motion

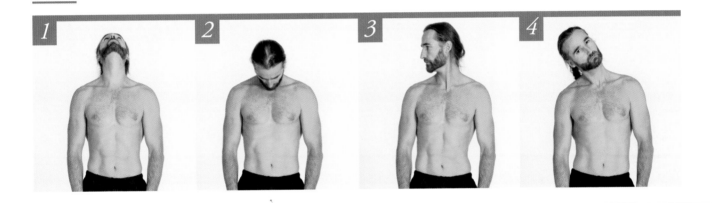

1 Neck extension

2 Neck flexion

3 Head/neck side rotation

4 Head/neck side tilt

Neck position is part of postural control, and ensuring head stability is paramount to efficient movement—due in part to the fact that most of the vestibular system responsible for balance in movement is located in the head, so minimal disturbance of the head's balance helps overall balance. The best athletes have amazing cervical and head stability in movement.

Because neck movement implies that head movement is also occurring, ensuring head stability relies on cervical stability, but it doesn't necessarily require constant linear alignment of the cervical spine. Some experts warn about the dangers of cervical hyperextension (pronounced backward head tilt), which is said to ruin spinal alignment and destroy the ability to generate power, such as when you're jumping or lifting heavy loads. This belief is not true at all except in one particular case: a hyperextended neck under the compressive forces of a heavy load, which would happen if something or someone was pushing your head back and pressing down hard on your head and neck, forcing your neck to hyperextend as it's subjected to large levels of compressive forces. In a nutshell, you would be "jamming" your cervical vertebrae and spinal cord, placing your central nervous system in a panic and protective stance called the "arthrokinetic reflex." Because of the danger of your cervical joints being at risk due to intense compression with the wrong alignment, the survival reflex of the body is to inhibit muscular activity as a protective measure because the cervical area is the most important link between the brain and the body.

The compression of the spine isn't the real issue; when lifting or carrying heavy loads, the spine can be placed under very large compressive forces, as demonstrated by Sherpas of the Himalayas or by African women who carry heavy loads on top of their heads. The real issue is a positional issue—the hyperextension of a series of joints in the neck—combined with large compressive forces. Have you ever had your hair pulled hard while you're wrestling? Has it made you feel powerless? You didn't feel powerless because of the pain in your scalp but because of the arthrokinetic reflex. This is an intuitive application of this principle in which your neck is hyperextended (in whatever direction) while a large compressive force is applied to it at the same time. So, except in some very specific circumstances, some level of extension of your neck doesn't change your level of strength.

The problem is that experts see the slightest extension in your neck as "hyperextension" and believe you should make sure that your neck and head are aligned straight with the rest of the spine no matter what. The truth is that some extension of the neck is perfectly sustainable even in the presence of some compression, as demonstrated for instance by wrestlers when they "bridge." When you're lifting or carrying a heavy load, there is the presence of intense compression, except it's exerted below the neck rather than on top of the head, which enables you to have your neck in any position you want. Therefore, a bit of neck extension, especially in the absence of any compression, doesn't cause any problem. As a matter of fact, the extension of the cervical spine is sometimes necessary to maintain an optimum line of vision. When jumping upward to grab something above you, can you not look up by extending your neck? Of course, you can, and you should.

Line *of* Vision

Even though it is not mandatory that a person can see to be able to move, vision obviously plays a crucial role in the efficiency of virtually any movement, starting with ensuring balance, because vision plays a part in your vestibular system. Vision also helps you anticipate the environment and situation where you move so you can adapt your movement rapidly and accurately. In a gym, you do not have to deal much with this type of contextual awareness, so you can maintain a neutral neck position as you work out. However, in the real world, you often have to look up, down, or sideways to have the best line of vision possible. Can you imagine being unable to move your neck and head to the best position to see properly because you were told that doing so will rob your strength? Or being unable to maintain a neutral spine the moment you tilt your head back? It wouldn't make any sense. Positional control is the ability to make minute adjustments to your position without disrupting the rest.

The influence of vision goes beyond spatial awareness, navigation, and balance; it also contributes to positional control to some extent. Turning your eyes up facilitates extension and inhibits flexion, whereas turning your eyes down facilitates flexion and inhibits extension. In a nutshell, you tend to straighten your back when you look up and round it when you look down. It's as if the line of vision precedes the behavior of the body, and looking in a given direction pushes the body in that direction; if you stand straight and move your eyes to the side, doesn't it feel natural that your body would orient itself in that same direction? This is not to say that your body and spine automatically extend if you look up and flex if you look down. Conversely, it also does not mean that you are obliged to overextend your neck to look up and to tilt your head down to look down.

True positional control means that you can establish and maintain any desired position regardless of line of vision and head and neck position, even though they are closely associated with the line of vision. However, it does imply that your line of vision may support a particular spinal alignment that is either beneficial or detrimental depending on the movement you want to perform. Therefore, you can sometimes use eye position and line of vision to your advantage. For instance, because you want to maintain a neutral spine when lifting a load, you may look up to facilitate back extension (with a little neck extension); at a minimum, you want to maintain a forward line of vision. When you land in a dive roll, you want to look toward the ground to facilitate a rounded back (without moving your head down too early).

Conversely, if you have to carefully put down a load, you must be aware that looking down at where you are placing the object tends to make you flex your spine. It doesn't mean that you can't look down, but you must be even more mindful of your postural control.

So, let me say it one more time: If you do possess postural control (the stable, linear alignment of your spine), then adjustments to your neck position—or any other body part, for that matter—should not disturb the stability of your midline or lower your ability to generate force. Neck position only disturbs postural control if you don't have it in the first place.

Trunk Side Bend

Keep your shoulders level and your hips neutral and level. Lean your trunk sideways alternately on both sides. Maintain abdominal breathing.

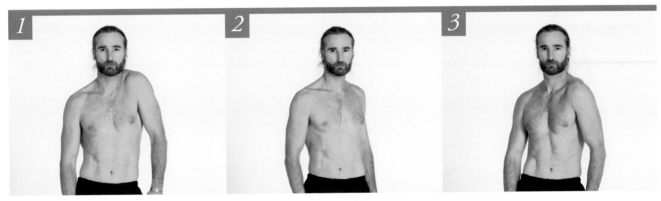

1 Shoulder elevation-shrug

2 Shoulder retraction

3 Shoulder protraction

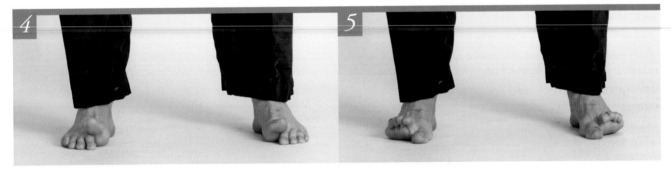

4 Big toe lift

5 Small toes lift

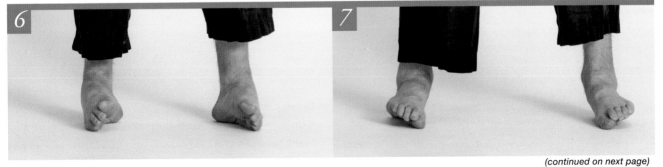

6 Foot pronation or inversion

7 Foot supination or eversion

(continued on next page)

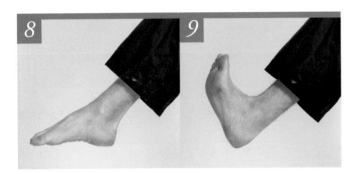

8 Ankle extension

9 Ankle flexion

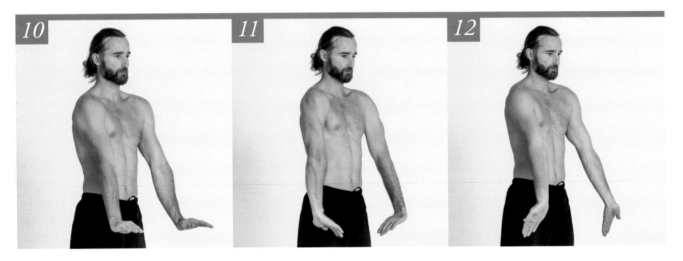

10 Shoulder neutral

11 Shoulder internal rotation

12 Shoulder external rotation

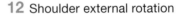

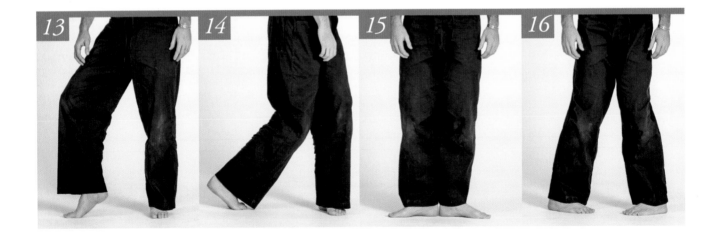

13 Single leg external rotation (with flexed foot)

14 Single leg internal rotation (with flexed foot)

15 External leg rotation (both legs)

16 Internal leg rotation (both legs)

Movement Is the Sum of Its Parts

Technique and efficient movement demand high levels of motor control. Motor control requires you to command diverse interconnected body segments to position themselves or move and apply force or relax in a given sequence and at a given time. This interaction of breath, position, tension, relaxation, sequence, and timing represents the whole spectrum of "coordination" and eventually determines efficiency.

I always start my workshops by covering the principles of movement efficiency through insights and drills, including the pillars that form technique, and I often end up demonstrating a Sliding Swing-Up, which is a climbing movement on a horizontal surface that starts with a hang and ends with your body on top of the surface. I do it with my eyes closed immediately after hanging from my hands to demonstrate that once your immediate environment has been visualized, movement happens internally before it's expressed externally. As I perform the movement slowly, I emphasize using exteroception to aid in positioning on the surface with the right base of support at different stages of the movement while ensuring friction and avoiding slippage.

Thanks to proprioception, I can internally visualize my body position—the position of my center of gravity in relation to my base of support. My positions change through a sequence and with timing I have already predicted. I apply the minimum amount of tension I need to conserve energy and stay as relaxed as I can. I also use body-weight transfer to generate momentum through my leg and make the movement much more efficient. I end up on top of the surface, well balanced and relaxed, in a smooth motion sequence that seems effortless. Every detail of the movement has been mindful and intentional, and my breathing has remained controlled throughout the movement.

This single movement encapsulates most of the principles I have covered in Part 2 that are the foundation of technique and efficient movement. *My point is that movement efficiency principles are not just about theory; they're about the effective practical application of the theory.* When you understand these principles and feel how they work when you move, you can use them to reach your full movement potential. Beyond the principles covered in this part, later in the book I cover a few additional principles of movement efficiency that are specific to particular movement skills.

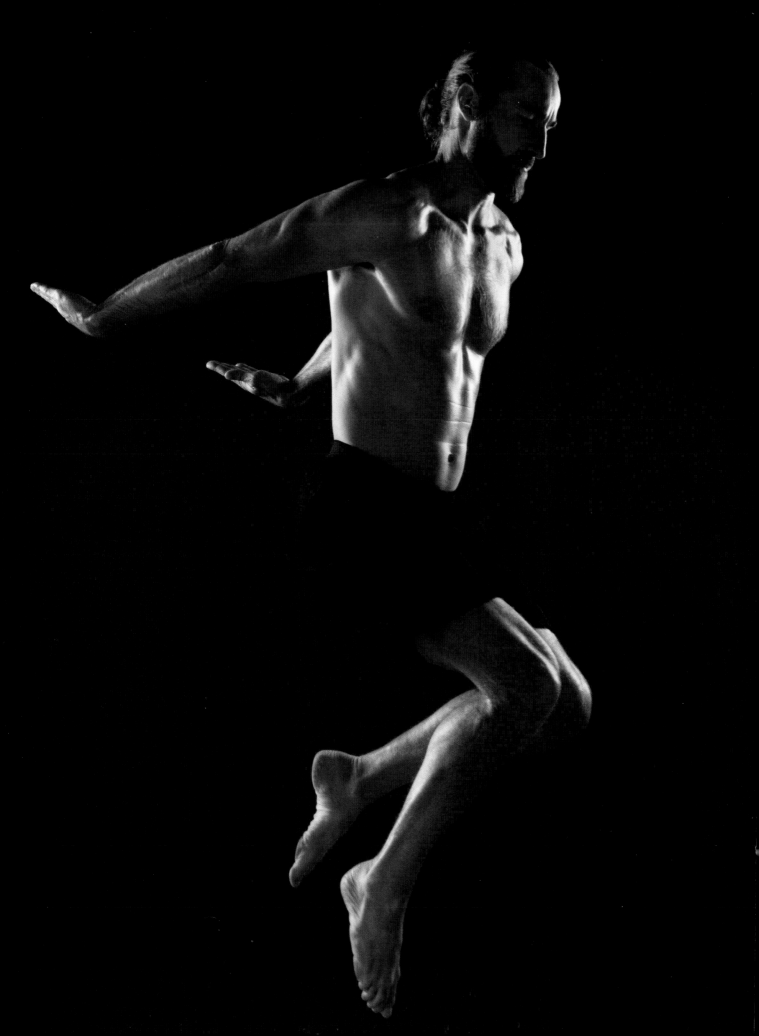

3

Practice Efficiency Principles

"I have been impressed with the urgency of doing. Knowing is not enough; we must apply. Being willing is not enough; we must do."

—*Leonardo da Vinci*

We acquire movement efficiency through practice, and that practice must be efficient. Practice efficiency requires a method to ensure that you use the energy and time you dedicate to improving your movement optimally to generate the best results.

Movement efficiency and practice efficiency naturally work hand in hand the same way movement skills and physical capacity work hand in hand. Understanding the twelve Natural

Movement principles—focusing especially on practical, unspecialized, progressive, adaptable, efficient, and mindful practice—and knowing the movement efficiency principles is obviously a great start. In this part of the book, my goal is to share practical information to help you make your self-learning practice as effective as possible to boost your progress and maximize your results.

You put practical and unspecialized principles into practice by directly starting to learn diverse techniques from several Natural Movement skills. You apply the progressive principle by starting with the simpler and easier movements before proceeding to the more complex and difficult movements. You establish quality and efficient movement before adding volume, intensity, or complexity. Thanks to the efficient and mindful principles, you engage your mind to consistently increase the quality and efficiency of every movement you make. In the process, you naturally gain mobility, stability, strength, balance, coordination, endurance, overall adaptability, and greater levels of real-world physical capability. It is *that* simple.

Yet you don't necessarily make progress just because of your intention and efforts to improve. Mindfulness by itself is not a guarantee that you will improve as fast as you would like, or even that you will improve at all. Learning whole, complex new movements or movements you've done before but haven't known how to do efficiently can be a real challenge. Even after you've learned techniques, going through the progressions to develop higher levels of efficiency, strength, and metabolic conditioning is not always intuitive.

Beyond the specifics of each technique or movement variation you learn, there are many interrelated aspects of practice you need to pay attention to, and it can be confusing and counterproductive if you don't do it right. In the absence of a teacher or trainer, you must teach and train yourself. Though the guidance and feedback of a competent person are always useful, this book is designed to help you be your own teacher. This part about practice efficiency principles is dedicated to giving you practical insights and simple, effective tips so that you can learn the art of efficient movement as well as the art of efficient practice.

66 **The greatest results in life are usually attained by simple means and the exercise of ordinary qualities.... These may for the most part be summed in these two: common sense and perseverance."**

—*Samuel Smiles*

18
Foot Freedom, Health, Function, and Strength

Studies show that populations who grow up or live mostly barefoot have significantly healthier feet. Of course, being barefoot isn't beneficial on its own; it doesn't do much for you if you sit barefoot all day. Moving frequently on diverse surfaces supports the natural health, strength, and function of our feet. Because our feet are our foundation, their health and function strongly affect the health and function of our spines.

First, let me explain the ways in which conventional footwear is detrimental to your movement practice.

Unless you are practicing the combative aspect of Natural Movement, would it make any sense to practice movement with your hands encased in boxing gloves? No, you would look silly, like a clown pretending to play the violin while wearing boxing gloves. If you were wearing gloves, you couldn't feel and grasp surfaces with your hands to efficiently ensure friction, gripping, support, and balance. Furthermore, if you were to wear boxing gloves all day, every day for decades, your hands would certainly soften and weaken. If this makes sense for your hands, doesn't it make sense for your feet as well?

Wearing conventional heavily cushioned and elevated-heel sports footwear is just like wearing boxing gloves. The thick cushioning of the socks and thick plastic and synthetic layers of the shoes disrupt the natural "biofeedback"—exteroception—that you get from your feet when they contact the ground and that enables you to adapt your gait and positional control so you can stay balanced and light on your feet. Because most movement takes place on our feet or involves them, our feet are designed to be highly adaptable in terms of position. We have no fewer than fifty-two bones, sixty-six joints, and forty muscles in our feet, but we're able to collect an enormous amount of information thanks to an extraordinary number of nerve endings* that normally need to have almost unobstructed contact with the environment to perform their job optimally.

> **NOTE**
>
> For information about a study into the value of being barefoot versus wearing footwear, read the article "Shod Versus Unshod: The Emergence of Forefoot Pathology in Modern Humans?" at www.sciencedirect.com/science/article/pii/S0958259207000533.

---

*The highest concentration of nerve endings is in our feet. We have about 200,000 nerve endings in each sole.

Natural sensory feedback from the feet is altered in two significant ways when we wear conventional types of footwear:

- Sensory feedback is significantly less intense. You may not feel as sharply as you should that a surface is unstable or stable, soft or hard, slippery or not, and so on.
- There is latency. The feedback you get from your feet about the point of support that you're establishing as you step is significantly delayed. With too little information from your feet, each step you make arrives at your brain later than it would if your feet were bare, and your central nervous system is challenged for ensuring movement efficiency because it greatly depends on the information you gain from the environment where you stand. For instance, if a surface on which you step is slippery or unstable and you can't feel it instantly and precisely, you might not adjust your position and movement with enough reactivity and speed to avoid getting off-balance. Another common issue is that, because your perception of the impact is dulled as your foot lands, your foot tends to land harder than it should. Ironically, the goal of thickly cushioned footwear is to decrease landing impact forces and minimize stress on the joints—especially the knees—but the exact opposite occurs.

Numbness in the peripheral nerves of the feet (and hands as well) is the hallmark of a disease called *neuropathy,* and it causes serious gait issues that lead to falling and injuries. To some degree, we impose a slightly milder version of this condition on ourselves every time we put on conventional sports shoes. Think of the difference between moving in socks and moving in snow boots: Which option gives you more sensitivity and reactiveness in movement?

The shoe "platform" on which your feet are resting reduces the range of motion of your feet and ankles, preventing optimal positional control during movement. The shoe also encases your foot in a plastic "cast" that prevents natural motion. This reduced range of motion, thick cushioning, and exaggerated protection of the foot for prolonged periods softens the skin and weakens the bones and muscles of the feet, which eventually reduces foot function and makes them injury-prone.

The elevated heel, which is nothing but a convention without any relevant functional purpose, forces the rest of the body to vertically align with the base of support in unnatural ways, leading to structural issues over time, such as lower-back pain. Most shoes also have an elevated toe box that keeps your toes artificially elevated unless you stand with all your body weight pressing this area down to the floor. The point of the rounded toe box design is to create an assisted rocking motion when your forefoot goes down to the ground and pushes off rather than letting the foot do the work in its natural state.

A simple way to assess whether you have grown proprioceptively dependent on footwear is to observe how you feel when you take off your shoes after having worn them for some time or immediately after physical activity. If you feel off-balance and the barefoot sensation doesn't feel "normal"—it feels awkward even on the indoor surfaces you're used to—you are already stepping outside of your comfort zone. But the true test is transitioning from shod to barefoot when you're outside in nature. The greater the change in speed and movement behavior you observe in your gait, the weaker your feet are.

It's no surprise that attempting to move barefoot in natural environments without a thoughtful, patient, progressive transition feels awkward and painful. Barefoot motion should be, by default, comfortable on most terrains, but instead we have been led to see being barefoot as uncomfortable and "unnatural," whereas we see wearing shoes as the "natural norm"—almost as if we were born wearing footwear. Your body may be strong, but if your feet are weak, then your whole foundation is weak, which has implications to your movement performance. I have seen my young children wearing winter boots—with elevated heels and rigid rubber—that caused them to start to move awkwardly and to stumble more frequently than usual. The problem was immediately solved when they returned to their usual thin and flexible footwear. The boots had an immediate effect on their proprioception, reactions, positional control, and overall gait. They made their movement unsafe. Continuing to wear the boots or similarly designed footwear during their early growth would have permanently altered their foot function over time.

Conventional footwear is ill-adapted to the natural function of the foot and promotes foot dysfunction, back issues, and even injury. Despite several decades of so-called innovation—in terms of structure or material used—from the commercial running footwear industry, injury rates among people engaged in frequent recreational or competitive running have never dropped. By protecting the foot more than necessary and modifying the foot's function and overall gait, "technical footwear" creates more issues than it solves. The best protection for the foot is efficient, natural movement and progressive strengthening and conditioning of your feet, ankles, calves, knees, and so on until you have a natural and efficient gait.

Of course, this is not to say that Natural Movement should be done exclusively barefoot. There are many reasons why you would want to wear footwear, such as for social and professional reasons or because of weather or terrain. In fact, it is a no-brainer that wearing footwear can enable you to run faster on rough terrain—such as a hot rocky desert full of cacti—and prevent deep cuts and other injuries. There is a reason why most hunter-gatherer tribes living in nature have their own form of footwear with a simple design: thin, flexible, and light. Today, there are "minimal footwear" alternatives that protect your feet from harm (cuts, puncture, burns, freezing) or help you remain socially acceptable but also enable foot function to be as close as possible to its natural, healthy form.

Aside from the times when you're engaging in Natural Movement practice, I strongly advocate barefoot movement whenever possible, although the goal is not to turn barefoot for 100 percent of your life or during 100 percent of your physical practice. Being barefoot more frequently in to your day-to-day motion, however, will start strengthening your foot structure, which in turn will support your physical practice.

Regular barefoot motion makes your feet stronger, more functional, and "sharper," which in turn benefits your functional health as well as your physical practice and performance. Walking barefoot in nature (known as *earthing*) is grounding, releases stress, and raises your energy levels. Furthermore, if you find yourself in a situation where your shoes are lost or you have no time to put them on, at least you have a basic ability to move despite the disadvantage of having no shoes.

Barefoot practice is just like other areas of physical practice: It must be progressive to preserve your tissues and allow them time to recover, get stronger, and become healthier. Too much stress in a short time can generate discomfort, pain, and even injury and can hinder the very adaptations you are looking for.

No one can tell how long it will take you to adapt to barefoot Natural Movement; it depends on the type of movement you do, at what volume and intensity, and on what surfaces. A healthy overall lifestyle also supports adaptation in this regard. A certain level of minimal discomfort is necessary to trigger adaptations in your feet as a process that should be very gradual rather than a brutal exercise in self-inflicted pain.

Pay attention to the feedback from your feet as you work on adapting. A good strategy is to consider three different "grades" of footwear, each with a progressively thinner and more flexible sole. Instead of transitioning directly from conventional footwear to barefoot, or even to minimal footwear, you could find a pair of shoes that is simply thinner and more flexible than what you are used to. When this footwear becomes comfortable enough even on uneven terrain and more challenging surfaces, switch to a slightly thinner and more flexible pair. In any case, practice barefoot whenever you feel comfortable enough and occasional discomfort is manageable.

> ❝ **I grew up barefoot, dirty, climbing trees. It made me appreciate things more.**❞
>
> —*Elle King*

19
Practice Environments

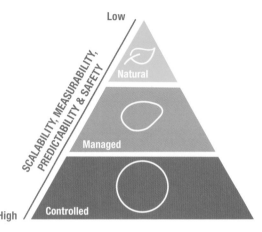

Training Environment Transition
*relationship of training factors in controlled
to natural environments*

The answer to the question "Where should I train Natural Movement?" is simple: anywhere and everywhere. Indeed, can we even talk about real-life physical capability without including a great degree of environmental adaptability? Environmental—as well as situational—complexity and variety breed movement adaptability and the motor-control and physiological adaptations it entails.

So, it might be tempting to think that for practice to be the most effective or even the purest, you must do it in the open in uncontrolled, wild environments. However, the naturalness of the movement patterns is not dependent on the naturalness of the environment in which the movement is done. There aren't Natural Movement patterns for the outdoors and others for the indoors. The minute—yet massively important—adjustments required for environmental adaptability do not depend on movements being done in natural or artificial environments but on the simplicity or complexity of such environments.

You could build very long and tall walls and an immense roof over a large patch of nature, which would limit the area and make it "indoor," but the environment would retain its naturalness and complexity. Conversely, you could take down the walls and roof of a conventional fitness gym to make it an "outdoor" location, but that wouldn't make it a more suitable environment for Natural Movement practice than the artificial fitness stations at a local park. Natural Movement practice in both controlled and natural environments can be quite similar, but it won't be exactly the same. Both present different advantages and opportunities, both have benefits, and both have downsides.

> **❝ I've always tried to seek out environments with excitement."**
> —Kenneth Chenault

Uncontrolled (Natural) Environments

By default, natural environments are uncontrolled. *Uncontrolled* simply means that the environment has not been designed, built, organized, or modified for the specific purpose of movement practice. Therefore,

urban environments, even though they have been artificially designed by people, are uncontrolled because they haven't been specifically made for the purpose of movement practice. However, urban environments are largely comprised of flat, linear, stable surfaces that are much more even and predictable than the surfaces found in nature.

Practicing Natural Movement within uncontrolled environments presents us with variables that can be advantageous and disadvantageous—sometimes simultaneously. For instance, "lack of variability" is listed both as an advantage and a disadvantage.

The advantages of uncontrolled environments include the following:

- **Variety or environmental complexity:** Natural environments can provide amazing variety in terms of height, distance, weight, angles, and surfaces—rough, smooth, uneven, angled, bumpy, holey, slippery, rugged, cold, hot. These qualities are essential to high levels of adaptability. The variety of surfaces is the aspect most difficult to re-create indoors.
- **Lack of variety:** Not all natural environments provide variety, but a lack of variety can be advantageous in that it forces you to train and adapt to particular environmental variables and become proficient with them. It can also force you to be more resourceful and patient by learning to take your time to find what you need.
- **Lack of predictability:** You can't always know what to expect or how reliable the surfaces are in an uncontrolled environment, which forces you to be mindful, alert, and responsive. As you gain experience, you will start to know how to place your foot and body weight by just looking at your immediate environment or feeling it. In that sense, the lack of predictability makes you better at predicting both the environment and how you should move next.
- **Lack of measurement or quantification:** You rely mostly on feel and observation in an uncontrolled environment. You might still count repetitions, but natural environments make it not only hard or impossible but also somewhat irrelevant to measure anything in terms of distance, height, depth, or weight. This can be beneficial to those who are addicted to the systematic quantification of performance because the inability to rely on numbers gives them an opportunity to learn to fully focus on and rely on feel, observation, and even instinct.
- **Freedom:** There are no rules in nature other than natural laws. If you respect the environment and life where you are, you can do anything you want.

- **Connection with nature:** Remembering that nature is where we all come from and what we are all made of is a powerful experience that can take place only in nature. You can't get all the benefits of nature from a pill; you must spend some time in nature.

Here are some downsides of practicing in uncontrolled environments:

- **Lack of variety or environmental complexity:** Lack of variety was listed among the advantages of uncontrolled environments, but it can also be a disadvantage. Natural environments are sometimes mono-dimensional—all ground, no trees to climb, nothing to balance on, nothing heavy to lift, and so on, which means that you might not be able to practice some skills and techniques.
- **Lack of scalability:** A lack of variety also might imply a lack of scalability. For instance, there might be a vertical surface to climb, but it is too difficult or too easy for your level of proficiency and therefore not beneficial to helping you make progress (or worse, is potentially dangerous). Uncontrolled environments are a take-it-or-leave-it/do-it-or-don't proposition.
- **Lack of predictability:** Surfaces may give way, break as you hang, or move without warning as you land. Even surfaces you believe are reliable sometimes are not. Furthermore, weather conditions can temporarily change surfaces. For example, rain makes things more slippery. A surface can be dry on top and humid underneath, which causes your feet to slide. Depending on your level of capability, the lack of predictability can be an issue, and it sometimes presents even experienced practitioners with the risk of injuring themselves.
- **Lack of progression:** Not progressing is the direct result of a lack of variety and scalability because progression is possible only when both of these variables are present. A lack of proper progression is also a major cause of injury when the increase in difficulty is too abrupt and unsustainable instead of being gradual.
- **Lack of safety:** The unpredictability of the environment is a big factor in the increase of risk of injury. The lack of scalability can also contribute to accidents because, when the setting lacks appropriate options, you might attempt to do something that's too hard for your current level of expertise.

- **Lack of measurement or quantification:** Your assessment of progressions and progress is restricted to feel and observation because it is hard or even impossible to measure or quantify distances, heights, or weights. Measurement and quantification are not only great motivators but also tools for ensuring safe progressions.

- **Lower training efficiency:** When you take all the downsides in aggregate, it makes for a less efficient practice. With lack of variety and scalability, you might find yourself spending a significant amount of time scouting the area for elements that fit the skills or techniques you would like to practice or the level of difficulty they require. Even when you know where to find settings that offer variety and scalability, they may be far from each other. If time is a concern—say you have only one hour for your practice—the distance you must travel can be a real problem. You may have to delay entire aspects of your training for another place and time. In addition, the lack of quantification and measurement may hinder your progress because you can't be sure how to compare the difficulty of your practice from one environment to another. Overall, this is not conducive to optimal practice, and it leaves you to random, instinctive training and little to no programming. While that training option works, it requires a lot of free time.

Controlled Environments (Artificial *or* Natural)

Controlled environments are custom designed for the specific purpose of scalable, progressive, and safe training because they provide predictable and adjustable environmental variables in one location. A controlled environment is always artificial in the sense that you wouldn't randomly find one in nature, but just because an environment is controlled doesn't mean that it has to be indoors or made of artificial materials. Controlled environments are most often indoor facilities filled with equipment and artificial surfaces made of rubber, plastic, metal, and other synthetic compounds, but you may temporarily arrange or permanently build outdoor controlled environments that are entirely made of natural materials, such as logs of varied length, thickness, and weight; rocks; and wood bars and boards. (*Note:* In a natural environment, you cannot, of course, control all variables, including the weather conditions and how they affect the environment.)

NOTE

Remember: *Controlled* doesn't mean *artificial. Controlled* means *predictable and adjustable.*

Practicing Natural Movement within controlled environments presents us with variables that can be both advantageous and disadvantageous—sometimes simultaneously.

A custom-made practice environment can be designed to combine variety, scalability, progressiveness, predictability, and safety in a single area to guarantee optimal practice efficiency. The following are some specific advantages of practicing in controlled environments:

- **Variety:** The controlled environment may include all the elements of environmental variety you need for practicing the full spectrum of Natural Movement skills, such as enough space to run; diverse surfaces for jumping, balancing, and climbing; and props for manipulative skills.

- **Scalability and progressions:** The equipment and props in controlled environments are adjustable in distance, height, depth, weight, and surface quality, which makes it possible to control progressions in difficulty (intensity or complexity).

- **Predictability and safety:** The predictability of the practice environment (for instance, a surface designed to provide a controlled level of instability) and the scalability of the level of difficulty greatly reduces the risk of injury and makes practice as safe as possible.

The following are some disadvantages to controlled environments:

- **Lack of variability in environmental complexity:** Unless it is specifically designed for Natural Movement/MovNat practice, practicing a wide range of natural movements in a controlled environment is a challenge and is inherently limiting. For instance, indoor gyms might have pull-up bars on which you can do only limited climbing movements. You must use your imagination to use existing elements for things they weren't designed for, and you'll also need to obtain formal authorization to do so. The natural diversity of surfaces in nature (such as bark, sand, rock, mud, tall grass, bumps, and holes) as well as weather conditions (such as rain, snow, and sun) that modify the terrain or how you interact with the terrain while in motion are also absent in controlled environments.

- **Lack of unpredictability:** When you always know what to expect, and you know that you can rely with 100 percent confidence on the surfaces and equipment you use, it's easy to become less attentive—or even to act mindlessly. Lack of attention in a gym could lead to minor injury, but in nature the consequences can be much worse.

- **Too much safety:** Knowing there is no risk of injury in attempting a difficult move because there's a crash pad or a perfectly clear and smooth area restricts your performance to being mostly a physical feat. When you have risk of failure but no actual consequence other than missing and trying again, you're not training your mental fortitude. As a result, you can get a false sense of competence that will not apply in an uncontrolled context where real danger is present.

- **Lack of freedom:** Controlled environments are often small spaces confined by walls, and there are often rules and many "don'ts" that restrict what you can do. It's easy to get a feeling of being boxed in because, as a matter of fact, you *are* in a box.

- **Air pollution:** Indoor spaces are usually filled with rubber, plastic, and chemical contaminants. They're often poorly ventilated, and they're devoid of natural materials, surfaces, and energies. Breathing bad air while training—sometimes at high intensity—is simply not healthy.

Options *for* Practice

At this point, you're probably wondering what the best solution for your practice is. The only thing you can know for sure is that you can't dissociate techniques from the specific type of environment in which they need to be executed. For example, if you want to practice balancing, at a minimum you need a narrow surface. You might have a choice between controlled complexity—a standard 2x4 on the floor—and uncontrolled complexity—a fallen tree covered with slippery moss that's elevated some distance above the ground—but the point is that to practice balancing, you have to have something to balance *on* because all Natural Movement practice is contextual. What you are going to practice really depends on where you are, what context is available or accessible, and what you intend or need to practice and at what level.

> **Do what you can, with what you have, where you are."**
> —*Theodore Roosevelt*

You want to always remain opportunistic and adaptable in finding or creating opportunities to move and practice. Don't wait to find yourself surrounded by vast natural expanses! You can't wait for the perfect environment, the perfect time, or even the perfect movement.

As a Natural Movement beginner, your priority concern is to avoid unnecessary danger and injury risk. The second concern is optimizing the (usually limited) time you have for practice by taking advantage of available variety and scalability to ensure sound progressions. Given that controlled environments are made specifically for the purpose of movement, they should provide anything a practitioner needs to ensure safe, structured, and efficient practice. A controlled environment is a perfect solution for beginners.

Unless you can find a local facility fitted for Natural Movement/MovNat practice, I suggest that, if possible, you create your own "controlled environment," which you can call a "training facility," "Natural Movement gym," or whatever term you like. You can build one with inexpensive materials. The objective is to ensure environmental variety while simplifying environmental complexity and making it adjustable for safe and effective progressions. You retain the freedom to go test your newly acquired capability in uncontrolled environments at any time!

Regardless of where you practice, eventually you are your own "controlled environment" in the sense that you are able to control your mindset, choices, and behavior. Let me explain this idea: Nothing in the modern world expects any movement from you. Your Natural Movement practice is an optional strategy for a better life. Part of this strategy is finding the time to practice. Everyone is in a hurry these days. Yet we spend an average of 33 hours a week watching TV, and that doesn't account for the additional hours spent on social media or video games through computers and smartphones. If you "lack time," search no more, because it relies entirely on how you occupy your time. It's a choice. You also should be able to control your mindset when you practice, starting with a commitment not to alter the way you train, whether there are people around or you're all alone.

> **❝ We all live every day in virtual environments, defined by our ideas."**
> —*Michael Crichton*

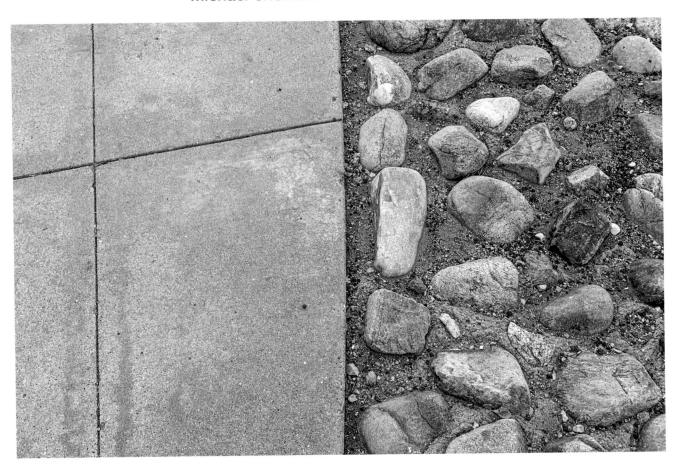

Would you choose the left or the right? Even or uneven? Flat or bumpy? Linear or nonlinear? Simple or complex? Repetitive or changing? Convenient or challenging? Dull or stimulating? Conventional or adaptable? Predictable or adventurous? Artificial or natural? Do you see landscaping on the right or do you recognize an immediate opportunity for Natural Movement?

20
Learning Techniques

Now that I have underlined the importance of natural foot function and detailed the pros and cons of controlled and uncontrolled environments, are you itching to get some Natural Movement going already? Well, I want to share a lot more information with you to help you practice as optimally as possible. However, before I get into those details, it isn't a bad idea for you to experiment with some basic Natural Movement practice. The information in this chapter will make even more sense after you've had some actual physical movement experience. I invite you to browse the pages of the book where I explain and demonstrate techniques and strongly recommend that you get started with ground movement techniques (see Chapters 24 and 25), which you might be able to do on the floor right where you are. A few minutes should suffice for now. Be curious, explorative, and willing to experiment freely and safely. At this stage, structure or programming is not a concern; there's no need to complicate anything.

Spend a certain amount of time daily—fifteen minutes, for instance. If possible, practice more than once a day. Even a few minutes devoted to short sessions throughout the day is great, and that arrangement—which for many people is most feasible on weekends—might be more beneficial than a single hour-long session in one day. Reoccupy and reawaken your body. Feel free and happy to move without judgment or a preconceived idea of how much movement you should do. Your first experience in Natural Movement is not about counting but about *feeling*.

Remember, you don't need to be fit to practice movement; the practice of movement will *make* you fit. As you explore and practice a wide repertoire of movements and focus on quality and efficiency, you will trigger many essential and beneficial adaptations—physiological and neural—that will occur without the need for supplemental drills. This functional potential has been dormant and has been awaiting the natural physical behavior required to make it become active and operational again.

Once you feel ready to start approaching practice in a more committed manner, to dig deeper into technique acquisition, and to structure your sessions more, you will need to learn and apply the information that follows.

Start Fresh

It is quite challenging to learn, assimilate, or improve movement patterns if you are already mentally and physically tired. *Get your sleep right* so you're sufficiently rested. If the goal of a practice session is to learn or improve technique, you certainly don't want to start with a grueling "workout" that physically drains you. Being tired—physically, mentally, or both—is the best way to impair the assimilation of new movement patterns. In fact, practicing technique while you're tired can not only prevent you from improving but could cause you to acquire several inefficiencies.

Movement Preparation

The term *warm-up* suggests that all you need to do before any kind of movement is to jog on the spot or do jumping jacks to get your heart pumping and stretch each body part separately. *Movement preparation* is a more accurate description in the sense that there are diverse ways to get prepared for movement. I use both terms to express the same idea; just keep in mind that whenever I use the term *warm-up*, I'm suggesting more than the conventional idea of warming up.

> ❝ **A winning effort begins with preparation."**
>
> —*Joe Gibbs*

Movement preparation isn't optional; it's an inherent part of any session because it places you in the best mental and physical conditions for your practice—which in most cases should involve more than just raising your heart rate and stretching your body. Movement preparation generally implies the mobilization of the whole body for general movement, or of specific muscle groups or body parts for a particular movement or effort. In other words, you might do a general movement preparation, a specific movement preparation, or both.

General Warm-Up

A wonderful general movement preparation includes ground movements and breath control because these two things mobilize practically all the joints and muscles in the body, which makes the muscles more active and the nervous system and mind more "alert."

However, people who have been physically inactive for a long time may also use the "Local Positional Control" movements that I describe in Chapter 17, before you do complete movements.

However, the movements available for warming up are, of course, not restricted to ground movements; your movement preparation may include movements in any Natural Movement skill. The rule of thumb is to use simple, low-intensity, low-complexity, and low-volume movements. You obviously

can't "warm up" by going full-on right off the bat. Although it seems counterintuitive to jump as part of a warm-up routine, you might perform jumps at such low-level intensity—jumping an inch high or a few inches forward at first—that it may absolutely fit the purpose of a warm-up. In fact, the only difference you may notice between warm-up and the rest of the practice does not lie mostly—if at all—in the type of movements you do, but in the intensity at which you perform them.

When you do a general warm-up, it is best to already enter a mindful state to pay attention to mental and physical relaxation, body sensations, and breath control. If you feel that areas of your body need more attention and time, movement preparation is exactly the right time to do that. Check out your sensations as if you are screening your entire body through slow motion. Soon you will feel ready to perform the movements a little more dynamically, with intermittent accelerations that will prepare you for even more dynamic movement and activate your energy systems for the more intense efforts ahead.

The younger and the more physically active you are, the faster you can warm up, and you can use a greater intensity. Conversely, if you are older or physically inactive (or both), you should take longer to complete your warm-up and keep them really gentle in intensity. Movement preparation is not a one-size-fits-all proposition, and one person's warm-up may feel like a full workout to someone else. In fact, a healthy and trained individual can start moving with intensity at almost any time with relatively little preparation.

It's true that when you're using your movement skills in the real world, movement preparation is usually a luxury; you usually need to start cold. Advanced movement practitioners occasionally practice a *cold start* by performing challenging moves or intense efforts with little or no movement preparation to get the body ready. These practitioners also have a lifestyle that enables them to stay healthy and keep themselves ready in a pinch. I strongly recommend against beginners trying a cold start because it can cause immediate injury. Advanced practitioners know their bodies and know what they're doing.

NOTE

When you need to do movements unexpectedly in the real world, even the briefest of warm-ups can be helpful. For example, if I need to jump to a depth and land without first preparing specifically for that movement, I do a quick, short series of squats on the spot to simulate the deceleration and muscular contraction specific to landing, which quickly mobilizes the joints and muscles I need for the upcoming landing. A combination of "context-free" physical and mental mobilization helps a lot when warming up properly is not possible.

As I mentioned previously, your ability to warm up quickly and effectively has a lot to do with how you live your life. If you are maintaining your body in motion frequently throughout the day on top of training regularly, you are very likely able to be ready for more intense movement practice after just a few minutes of low-intensity movement preparation.

In any case, take your time when you prepare for movement. There is no predesigned, standard warm-up routine that is appropriate for all people or situations. You can design your own warm-up, create several, or just go by feel and never do the same warm-up twice. All ground movements are wonderful for general movement preparation.

Specific Warm-Up

The specific warm-up is about ensuring that your body is specifically ready for a particular training emphasis in terms of either motor control, strength, energy systems, or all of the above. The purpose of the specific warm-up is to help you avoid injury and prime yourself for optimal performance.

In a specific warm-up, you follow simple linear progressions. For instance, your sense of balance can be relatively dormant and needs to be sharpened with a few minutes of practice before you feel that your central nervous system is fully awake and can do more complex balancing movements. If you are going to lift heavy loads and reach your maximum levels of strength, you want to start with light loads and progressively get heavier instead of trying to immediately lift the heaviest object you can. If you intend to do sprints, you want to prepare your cardiovascular and metabolic systems by doing warm-up runs and progressively accelerating. Last, if you intend to go through a "course" involving all three movements and physical efforts I've described—or more—then a specific warm-up is required for each type of movement and effort you expect to do.

A simple example of specific warm-up before heavy lifting would be to start with a light load and progressively increase the weight through single repetitions with a bit of additional weight each time until you reach close to the level of intensity where you want to train your lifting movement.

Technical Self-Learning

Feeling relaxed but alert and ready? It's time to focus on technique—one at a time of course! Pick a movement. Look at the photos of the whole movement sequence and read the descriptions. At this point, you're mentally absorbing information—conceptual knowledge—that you'll need to experience physically through movement. Reading gives you insights; experience turns these insights into a reality-based feedback and experiential knowledge. Of course, there's no guarantee that you'll immediately understand and assimilate the insights or perform immediately with efficiency; hence, the need for practice and mindful repetitions.

Assimilating technique has a lot to do with kinesthetic memory, which means that once you learn a movement pattern, you can reproduce it because you have memorized the set of positions, the timing, the sequence it follows, and the sensation it generates. The feedback of internal sensations during the movement is what makes you instantly feel that you're doing the particular pattern and lets you know how well you're doing it. Memory is about consistency and repeatability. You don't want to just "explore" new movement patterns; you want to learn and memorize the efficient patterns so you can reproduce them any time you want or need them.

There will be many obstacles on your path to technical mastery! Keep in mind that it isn't technique that fails us; we fail technique, and we do so for reasons we must become able to identify.

Are you ready to pay attention to the details of your movement, breathing and position, sequence and timing, tension and relaxation, points of support, body-weight shifting, and body sensations in diverse areas of your body? Go for it! BUT WAIT! Make sure that you first pick the simplest movements and start at a low level of intensity and complexity.

Feedback *and* Assessment

Attention to impeccable movement execution never stops—even for expert movers—but mindfulness doesn't stop the moment a movement has been physically executed; it leaves a "trace" in your central nervous system, a feedback that you want to pay attention to support continuous improvement. After you've practiced a technique a few times and you have some experience and feedback, you might have some ideas on what or how to self-correct. But that won't necessarily fix your patterns immediately or fully.

Self-correcting logically starts with assessing the issues. Do you encounter inefficiencies? What are they? Before you ask yourself what to do with your feedback, so you can modify and improve your movement, how do you know for sure that such feedback is accurate and complete? You need to make sure you have quality feedback. When you practice movement, you can use the following forms of feedback:

- **Proprioception:** This is basically a sense of the alignment and position of your body as well as the sense of how movement feels: stable or unstable, tense or relaxed, coordinated or clumsy, and so on. Everyone, regardless of the level of efficiency of their movements, receives this type of feedback. The key is to pay attention to it. Slow movement practice helps hone this sense...if you are mindful, of course.

- **Visual input:** Watching your positions and movement patterns, which is possible when you go slowly or break down a complex sequence into discrete components, provides feedback. Occasionally practicing in front of a mirror can provides very useful visual feedback, and filming your movement is even more valuable because you can watch the movement repeatedly and even see it in slow motion. This type of external visual feedback can help you notice inefficient patterns you never knew you had. You can also get feedback from another person, but that feedback is useful only if the person knows what to pay attention to and how to interpret what they see, which would imply that they are a MovNat certified trainer or at least are well-versed in Natural Movement.

As you become aware of each new aspect of your movement pattern and with every modification of your technique that you notice, you should ask yourself these three fundamental questions:

- Was it intentional?
- Was it beneficial to my performance?
- Can I replicate it at will?

Your goal is to become in control of every minute aspect of your technique. Any change you make should be intentional and should support performance (such as when you have to adapt to the environment). *Techniques are mastered only when they can be both replicated at will and also modified at will any time necessary and to the extent necessary.*

Before you rush to fix issues you have observed, felt, or seen, it is useful to ask yourself the three fundamental questions covered in the next sections.

Is It a Cause or a Symptom?

Knowing the difference between causes and symptoms is essential. Let me give you examples. You've placed a simple 2x4 board on the ground, and you're walking across it. Your arms are flailing, and your whole body is tensing in a vain effort to remain stable. You may think that you lack core stability and that you are way too tense. Indeed—good observation!

You might think you should step down to do some conventional "core strength" drills and other relaxation routines, but have you even checked the positioning of your feet? The position of your feet affects what happens "upstairs," so if your feet are misplaced on the board, your upper body is going to struggle to compensate for the unstable base of support. What your arms are doing is a mere symptom of the issue with your feet. Make sure that your feet are centered with the board, and you might immediately enjoy considerable stability and relaxation. Instead of inefficiently chasing multiple symptoms, you have tackled the single cause. *Voilà.*

Here's another example: Every time you jump forward with the aim of landing and standing on a specific area, you end up off balance and stepping forward. You notice that you tend to hold your breath and to unnecessarily tense up all over upon landing, so you manage to breathe better and relax, but you still step off balance and forward each time you land. You haven't noticed yet that you keep looking down at your landing spot, so your head is forward and down when you land, which shifts your center of gravity outside your base of support and throws you off balance. In this case, inefficiencies such as stiffness, intermittent breathing, and mental tension aren't the cause of the lack of balance; they're symptoms generated by lack of positional control. By fixing your head and neck position, which is the cause of the issue in this particular example, you will be able to perform stable landings while relaxing your breath, body, and mind.

I've explained that breathing, position, sequence, timing, tension, and relaxation are totally interconnected in movement. Bad timing can mess with a whole sequence, bad position can result in tension, bad tension messes with position and timing, and so on. Each aspect affects another and identifying what is the cause and what is the symptom and then self-correcting is part of the efficiency of your self-learning practice.

Is It Physical or Psychological?

Is the mind or the body the cause of the issue? Is the problem in the hardware or software? You might be quick to blame your body for issues that stem from a lack of attention or self-confidence. Conversely, you could be quick to blame your lack of attention because you don't realize or acknowledge that you may have a physical limitation that prevents you from performing the way you want.

Physical causes may have to do with

- A lack of mobility, stability, strength, or all of the above.
- A structural issue in your body, an injury, or a sensation of pain (explained or not). Poor technique doesn't necessarily imply dysfunction, but dysfunction or pain always leads to poor technique.
- Levels of volume, intensity, or complexity exceeding your current ability. Such mismatch ruins your efforts to learn new patterns or to

improve them and also magnifies or worsens your underlying inefficiencies; it also causes early fatigue, which only aggravates the problem.

With regard to physical causes of inefficiency, you need to be patient and progressive, and to first address the particular functional, physiological, or health issue(s) you're are dealing with that prevent you from performing the way you should. You may need to emphasize particular movements that help with a specific issue (for instance, ground movements to help with mobility restrictions), change your lifestyle (such as by making dietary adjustments to reduce inflammation in your joints), or undertake a specific therapy until the limiting issue is solved.

Mental causes may have to do with aspects of mindfulness (remember principle 11, "Mindful"):

- **Distraction or lack of concern:** Your body may do a movement correctly, and your central nervous system knows how to do it correctly. You need to invest your mind, pay attention, and genuinely value efficiency of movement to see improvement.

- **Mental tension:** Negative emotions such as agitation, frustration, impatience, and negative self-judgment disrupt your ability to focus on efficient movement execution. "Overthinking," which is a form of mental tension that causes you to think hard and even constantly self-talk as you move, can also be a problem.

- **Lack of self-confidence:** How much confidence do you have in your ability to learn? Do you believe you can learn with relative ease or with full comprehension? What is your past experience of learning something new? Self-efficacy is rapidly reduced or even completely absent when you don't trust in your ability or when you're self-conscious, such as when people watching makes you uncomfortable.

- **Fear:** Unless you are an experienced Natural Mover and you're dealing with higher level of practice that involves both risk and danger, you should not fear any movement. Ask yourself if you're trying to do something that is physically beyond what you can do effectively or safely. If that's the case, you need to lower the intensity and complexity of the challenge so you can feel secure and relax your mind. To learn more about this, study Chapter 21. If a movement involves zero danger—the risk is

that you might fail but you won't be injured—then your fear is real, but the reason for it isn't.

- **Mental rigidity:** If you refuse to try a movement in a different way, you are being mentally rigid. For instance, you might insist that you can make a given movement work a certain way even though that way is clearly not the most efficient. Another aspect of rigidity can be when you insist on performing a complete technique rather than deconstructing it to fix the one issue that's causing the problem and needs to be corrected. Either way, you aren't improving, and every inefficient repetition only reinforces the issue you have.

- **Uncontrolled enthusiasm or a desire to show off**: Feeling happy, free, and wild is great, but the body still needs to respond to and respect natural laws. A reckless movement behavior can easily turn you into a jackass and result in injury. Here's an anecdote: I was training a group by having them slowly and carefully balance on thin logs that were set at an incline running from the ground to a height of 3 feet. The logs were a bit wobbly. Immediately after I had announced that we were ready to move on to the next station, one of the students decided to attempt to literally run up one of the logs. He fell to the ground, hit his head, and lost consciousness for a few seconds. After recovering—and being checked out at a nearby hospital—he admitted that his ego had gotten the best of him and that he thought he could do better than everyone else. Everyone in the group was surprised because this person was adept at yoga and meditation and had been exhibiting very tranquil and humble behavior. The point is that this man's body didn't fail him; his mind forced his body to rush to its self-defeat.

Is It a Simple Motor-Control Issue?

Some inefficiencies relate to motor-control issues, although I consider the issues in this category to be issues that stem from the brain rather than the rest of the body. Imagine you possess the physical, functional ability to do a movement, and you are 100 percent focused each time you perform the movement. However, your body won't do the movement right until the pattern has been "written" in the brain and recorded by the central nervous system. Indeed, if your brain has not learned to operate the body in a very specific way—which has to do with motor control—the body is not the cause of the issue; the central nervous system is. Here are some examples:

- While jumping and landing, are you having trouble swinging your arms in sequence (forward, backward, and forward again) with impeccable timing? Your jumping movement looks and feels great except this arm sequence never "wants" to come out right. It's either too early, too late, too short, or too ample. You don't need upper-body strength drills; you just need to acquire the right pattern.

- Another very typical issue in learning new techniques is that as you attempt to improve a particular aspect of your movement, other inefficiencies may worsen or inefficiencies that had disappeared might return. Say you want to fix the arm-sequence issue, so you make changes. You may manage to fix it, but the fix might come at the expense of inefficiencies appearing somewhere else in the movement—one step forward, two steps backward. This kind of "trade-off" happens when your central nervous system can't pay attention to all the details at the same time, so it's forced to prioritize efficiency in some aspect of your movement while sacrificing it in others.

- A similar issue is a lack of "mind-body movement synchronicity," which typically happens when movement goes too fast for your attention to keep up. For instance, you become so focused on the takeoff step that when you land a few seconds later, you are still focusing on the takeoff. You're too late to be mindful about the landing! In other words, your mind is out of sync with the timing of the body's motion.

As you practice Natural Movement, it's likely that you *will* encounter most, if not all, of the diverse types of issues I've mentioned so far that prevent you from performing optimally.

After you have some feedback and a better sense of what goes wrong and what goes right in your movement, you need to know what strategies to use to fix the inefficiencies and effectively improve movement.

Self-Correction

While practice may help, psychological issues that impair your practice cannot be solved by practice alone. Self-reflection, honestly assessing and acknowledging negative emotions about yourself that work against you, positive self-talk, and meditation are some of the strategies you may use in addition to movement practice to help with such issues.

❝ **Brevity and conciseness are the parents of correction."**
—*Hosea Ballou*

Physical issues may be partially or totally solved by practice—something I have witnessed many times—or they might not be solved at all. The outcome really depends on what the issue is. For example, if movement causes pain, it is highly recommended that you consult a physical therapist of some sort. I am obviously not talking about minor and temporary pain as you move and is naturally linked to the particular movement or effort you are doing, such as a slight discomfort in your joint or burn in your muscles. You have to consider the magnitude of your pain, its frequency, and its duration before you decide to rush to a specialist. There are too many possible causes of physical issues and too many therapy modalities for me to be able to recommend anything more specific. For instance, a lower-back issue could have to do with a structural issue, too much sitting and not enough physical activity, too much stress and negative emotions, body inflammation, bad footwear, or all of the above. Aches and pains are common problems all people deal with in their lives, sometimes chronically, though they tend to be limited in magnitude, duration, and frequency in healthy people.

Generally speaking, therapists tend to have an immediate explanation for issues, which always happen to be exactly what they are trained to treat. Many are quick at pointing out so-called "dysfunctions"; however, physical limitations or symptoms you have may not be dysfunctions but mere deficiencies that movement practice and a better lifestyle could rapidly help with. The healthier you can make your lifestyle, the better you will feel and perform. It is all interrelated. Healthy lifestyle involving quality food and sleep, daily Natural Movement, physical therapy, the reduction of stress, meditation, and time in nature might be the most potent combination for a strong, healthy, happy life. This being said, a healthy lifestyle does not prevent all physical ailments, nor does it necessarily fix them.

Let's talk about strategies for fixing inefficient movement execution when the cause isn't psychological or physical.

Commitment, Consistency, Patience

Speaking metaphorically about movement patterns, I would say that ingrained patterns are "sticky" and new ones are "slippery." Rarely can you fix a technical issue with a single repetition. Being patient means staying calm and committing to improvement regardless of how many times you must rehearse the same movement, even if the process takes longer than you would like it to.

Spending a lot of time on anything doesn't guarantee that you become "world-class" at it; mastery is more than a matter of practice. Mastery depends on so many more variables than the amount of time you spend on practice—for example, how you do the practice, what mindset and degree of attention you have, your individual talent, your physical and mental health, and so on. While progress for beginners is often spectacular in scope and speed—because mindful practice precipitates improvement—you can't expect big revelations and breakthrough all the time. In fact, progress is often made of minute changes; they can be a series of "micro-epiphanies" that are so subtle and imperceptible that you may not even notice them. You're making progress with every mindful move or repetition without necessarily realizing it.

So, you should commit to being consistent at seeking and obtaining efficiency. A single efficient repetition is not a mark of consistency, but performing several efficient repetitions in a row is. Regardless of the strategy you use to improve your movement efficiency, it doesn't happen unless you are mindful, of course, but also committed, consistent, and patient.

Prioritization

When you first practice a technique, your attention may not be directed at anything in particular until you observe something happening or notice something that's bothering you, and it naturally draws your attention.

Most of the time, like most beginners, you'll be dealing with more than a single inefficiency. Don't try to address all the inefficiencies at once! Unless you have great mastery of your body, you won't be able to do it; you'll just waste time and energy. A step-by-step approach is much more effective than trying to address all your inefficiencies in one go. *If you try to fix all inefficiencies at once, you might end up fixing none.*

Ideally, you should tackle the most important inefficiency you have identified rather than taking on the most obvious issue. The most important inefficiencies are those that cause the problem—not the inefficiencies that are symptoms that have been generated by other issues. Fixing a "root" inefficiency always helps reduce or fix related inefficiencies. Let's say you notice that you tend to chest breathe or intermittently hold your breath and to be overly tense while doing a movement. It's very likely that you are physically tense because you are not breathing properly. You likely will fail at improving if you insist on trying to relax without first addressing your breathing. The first order of business is resetting your breathing pattern to make sure you maintain ample, relaxed abdominal breathing the next time you perform the movement. In this case you will keep focusing on your breathing until you consistently observe and feel it has been fixed as you perform several repetitions in a row. Then you may move on to another issue, making sure the one you just tackled doesn't come back, until you have taken care of them all.

Patterns of superfluous muscular tension can be some of the hardest aspects of practice to reset. Any pattern that has been rehearsed thousands of times either through day-to-day habits or through specialized training has become deeply ingrained in your neuromuscular memory, and those patterns are often the trickiest to replace.

Resetting the Body and Mind

Because we are mental creatures, we tend to think and analyze. However, *overthinking* can be a real issue. There is nothing wrong with thinking about your movement—just don't do it as you move unless you are moving very slowly and marking pauses by holding positions with the goal of learning and improving.

Too often we are conditioned to think about quantity, and we mentally count the number of repetitions we do as if the number of repetitions is the most important aspect of our practice. Focusing on the number of repetitions makes efficiency secondary. Some people tend to rush from one repetition to another without any "down time," as if movement is all about conditioning, speed, and intensity.

It's time to press the reset button. Resetting is a little like taking a break; it's a form of brief rest for the body and mind that enables you to relax and prepare for another attempt. During this time, you can assess your tensions, breathe deeply, quiet your mind, and reset your focus and intention. You can also rapidly process some of the feedback you just got from your last execution. We know that perception—how you mentally approach movement—influences physical behavior, but it's also true that your movement behavior and experience influences your perception.

By mentally directing your body to perform a specific way to modify your physical behavior, such modified physical behavior will in turn influence how you mentally approach and perceive movement, and you will be establishing a mutually beneficial mind-body interaction in the process.

Being mindful through your repetitions with the goal of constant improvement means that instead of doing ten repetitions of the same movement in a row without any time in between to process each repetition, you actually perform the movement ten times with a brief moment in between each execution. (Think of it as ten sets of one rep rather than one set of ten reps.)

Otherwise, you may mindlessly perform repetition after repetition and wonder why quantity does not naturally generate quality. Sometimes, if you feel tired of—or frustrated by—a given movement, you might decide to switch to something completely different for a moment. In fact, this is an inherent part of "combo practice," which is a form of circuit training. In that case, the variety of movements is not aiming at metabolic conditioning but at improving both movement and practice efficiency by allowing your central nervous system to reset not by pausing any physical activity but thanks to alternating movement patterns.

The "One Shot" Principle

This practice strategy is an extension of the "reset" principle, and you will indeed need to reset your body and mind to make it work. The idea is to treat each repetition (each execution) as if you have only one chance to do it right, which forces you to fully engage with and fully value your movement every single time you perform. It is about demanding complete mental and physical commitment from your practice.

In many ways this translates to some of the critical situations of the real world where you get only one "shot" at doing something because you're dealing with an actual situation rather than practicing. By embracing this mindset, you approach each repetition, every second, and each effort spent practicing as if missing means having to face real consequences.

Visualization

Visualization is the process of mentally envisioning and, to a limited and subtle degree, internally feeling your movement before you physically perform it. The goal is to prepare your mind to focus on key aspects of execution, especially when the execution time is brief because of the nature of the movement. For instance, it's difficult to slow down a jump enough that you can give attention to the diverse elements of the technique. With visualization, you can mentally break down a fast movement into a slower one in your mind as if you were observing it from the outside while at the same time you imagine your body experiencing it from the inside. You might feel your nerves trying to make your body move as you mentally re-create the intention of performing the movement even though your body remains still.

This process doesn't need to take a lot of time; a few seconds may suffice, especially if you are focusing on a single aspect of the execution, such as maintaining breath and relaxation, improving the action of your arms, or fixing the specific position of your feet. You can use visualization even with totally new movements if someone slowly demonstrates the movement or you look at a photo sequence or video of the movement.

As you observe the movement, you internally replicate the sequence and timing before you physically attempt the move for the first time.

The main use of visualization is to use it as you "reset" between each repetition of a movement or whenever you feel that you become a little confused or inefficient with a movement pattern.

Slow Movement

Slow movement is an amazing way to get started with any movement, and it helps you acquire efficiency more rapidly. Slowing down may be the simplest, most potent way to improve your form, make faster progress, and eventually perform movement faster. You can't do some movements slowly—there is no such thing as a slow-motion jump for instance—but you can do most movements at a slow pace. Slow movement also enables you to better assess your current level of efficiency and helps you better determine if you're ready for greater levels of intensity for a particular movement.

There are many benefits to slow movement. One is that you will notice many more details of the "landscape" of a movement sequence. It is akin to the difference between walking down a street rather than taking your car. Obviously, it takes more time when you walk, but you can discover so many details that you're unable to notice when you travel in a speeding car. Similarly, you can screen your movement pattern by going slowly rather than speeding. By lengthening the entire sequence of a particular movement pattern, the time it takes to execute each part of the sequence lengthens, which enables you to better understand how the sequence works in terms of position, bodyweight shifting and balance, and tension and relaxation. You're dissociating the diverse inputs, signals, and sensations that performing the sequence generates. Numbers stop mattering when your focus is entirely on sensations, observation, empirical feedback, and experiential input. Slow is truth.

You begin to consider questions like these:

- What is taking place in my foot or my hand? Are they correctly positioned?
- Am I following the right sequence with the right timing?
- Can I get rid of the tension in my neck and shoulders?
- Should I add more tension in my glutes and abdominal muscles to stabilize my hips and lower back?

- Why did I hold my breath for several seconds? Can I improve my breath control?
- Where should my attention go the most?

If you tend to tense up, if you have uncoordinated movement, or if you lack joint stability, slow movement will expose the issue while it also helps solve it.

The low intensity of slow movement enables you to improve selective tension dramatically because you can better focus on detecting and minimizing tensions you would otherwise not notice at faster speed. Moving slowly is a great opportunity to ask yourself whether you can achieve the same movement with the same efficiency but with less tension.

"Fitness cowboys" tend to have a hard time slowing down, and they don't understand that slowing down could enable them to ultimately go faster or at least avoid wasting energy if only they first could have the patience to take their time to improve movement. Slow movement requires a mindset: If you can perform a movement slowly and efficiently, you not only own the "right" to perform it at higher intensity but you will perform it much better when you do. For instance, if your mind and body are out of sync—something I have mentioned earlier—you can fix the issue by using slow movement to ensure synchronicity before you gradually increase speed and intensity while maintaining the synchronicity.

It's better to be slow and controlled than fast and inefficient. Besides, even from a real-world practical perspective, slow and controlled movements matter as much as fast and controlled ones. The physical feedback from slow movement is clearer to your brain than the feedback from same movement when you do it faster, which enables the brain to "rewrite" an improved version of the pattern in its memory. This is called *neuroplasticity*.

Switching Pace

Another useful practice efficiency principle is to alternate slow and fast execution of the movement, still with an emphasis on slow movement. The idea is to provide the central nervous system with different feedback based on the pace of execution rather than on a changing pattern. Comparing sensations when the same pattern is executed with sharply different speeds can give you valuable feedback and help you learn faster. In any case, technique is only mastered when it can be replicated with the same level of efficiency at any speed.

Deconstruction and Isolation

Breaking down a complex movement to more basic, isolated segments to improve them separately and then reintegrating them into the entire sequence they are part of can greatly help reduce your learning curve or solve a physical—or mental—block that prevents you from performing the entire sequence. Chapters later in this book that are dedicated to each movement skill start with positions that will become part of most of the techniques I cover, which is a form of breaking down the movements. Breaking down a whole movement pattern means practicing separate, smaller movement patterns that are parts of the whole sequence. Indeed, while practicing complete movement and addressing inefficiencies one at a time can be an effective way to improve, practicing first the distinct positions of a sequence a technique is made of can also facilitate improvement.

Working on separate segments helps you identify issues and solve them. For instance, you might identify an inefficiency in a complex movement sequence but have trouble fixing it through rehearsing the whole sequence, even if you do it slowly. Deconstructing the movement and practicing the troublesome part might resolve the issue more effectively. Sometimes, you may become aware of an issue without being able to identify exactly what the issue is or when it happens. Deconstructing the whole movement into parts enables you to spot at what moment of the sequence the problem occurs, and you can also tell if the issue concerns motor control, strength, mobility, or some other thing. Obviously, you need to address the issue to take care of it, which you can do quickly if it is a motor-control issue, but strength or functional issues take more time. In any case, you might not need to work on each segment of a whole movement; you might only need to focus on the problematic ones until they are improved or fixed.

However, positions are positions—not movement patterns seamlessly linking such positions. Eventually you must "reattach" movement segments one by one, link by link, until you've re-formed (and usually improved) the whole kinetic chain. You will find numerous practical examples of this strategy of breaking down movements in each chapter of Part 4.

Exaggeration of Inefficiencies

This practice efficiency principle may seem counterintuitive, but it can really help. Instead of trying to attenuate or getting rid of inefficiencies you have identified and that you may have already tried to do with limited success, you may want to intentionally—but temporarily, of course—amplify them.

> ❝ **If you want to truly understand something, try to change it."**
> —*Kurt Lewin*

It might seem strange to amplify an inefficiency, but that could be the most effective way for your central nervous system to realize how counterproductive a given pattern is, and it might lead to quicker remediation of the issue. For instance, if you tend to be too tense when you move, you could add even more tension in your whole body to help you better realize and address this pattern.

Self-Imposed Contextual Limitation

This is a strategy that has everything to do with perception as you add or simulate environmental or situational variables. Here's an example: When students jump and land, they tend to get off-balance and step forward before they can stabilize themselves on the target where they land. If pointing out the alignment issue that causes the instability doesn't work, I tell them to imagine that they are landing on a rock and would fall into a raging river if they could not achieve a stable landing. Having the student visualize an imaginary context—with the environmental part being the small landing area that doesn't offer the possibility of stepping forward and the contextual part being the dramatic consequence of falling off—sometimes solves the problem, but some people need a motivation that is more tangible than what they must imagine.

When the first method doesn't work, I stand just in front of the landing area. A student who is off balance steps forward and bumps into me, and no student wants that to happen. The result is that students look straight forward rather than looking at their feet, which helps them keep a more erect and stable position when landing. Voilà—problem solved *very* quickly every single time. There's nothing like context to make practice real and breed effectiveness and efficiency!

NOTE

So, you might be wondering why I don't use the second method from the start. Because, in the absence of the tangible context, it's important that you be able to visualize the consequence of failing the movement and taking such consequence seriously even though it is imaginary. When you practice, it's not *always* possible to have a tangible motivator that helps you stay on track. Sometimes, you have to rely on your inner eye to help you visualize risks, threats, and consequences.

Another technique involves imagining that you are at ground level as you balance at a height, which can reduce anxiety. Conversely, you can imagine being at a height when you are balancing at ground level to elevate—pun intended—your level of focus. This practice strategy resembles the "one shot" principle in the sense that you imagine facing real and adverse consequences if you miss.

Strategies like the examples I've described are designed to modify your perception to improve your performance. In these cases, the body follows the mind, not the other way around.

NOTE

Does this strategy of self-imposed contextual limitation remind you of something? It's the adult version of the childhood games of "hot lava" and "snake pit." If you fall, you burn or get bitten and die. Children intuitively use the strategy I've described to make their instinctive Natural Movement practice more realistic and engaging. Why not you? It is a brilliant and effective mindset.

Bilateral Practice

Practicing bilaterally means making sure you perform any "one-sided" technique on both sides. For instance, in get-ups, where you place a single arm on the side, or in jumps, where you step and launch from one leg, you must practice the technique on both sides equally; otherwise, you're apt to consciously or unconsciously emphasize and rely on a preferred side. In fact, you should practice more on your less-used side (or less-able side) until you can do the movement with close to equal efficiency on either side. Usually, switching sides to improve the neglected side feels awkward at first, as if one side was a "black belt" and the other a "white belt." What's good for you, though, is that what the central nervous system has learned on one side helps improving the opposite side faster than if you had no skill or experience on either side.

Knowing When to Stop

When you practice your techniques and skills, you might make many successful attempts that can be seen as partial or even complete failures, but that are the necessary path to improvement and success. Misses are inevitable and can be discouraging. They can also motivate you to keep trying until you succeed.

However, it is important to not keep pushing yourself when you reach a state of physical and mental fatigue. You will start failing in a way that becomes counterproductive because it has stopped supporting improvement, and you should avoid coming close to this type of failure when learning new movements and trying to improve your technique. Pay attention to your sensations—both physical and mental—and stop practicing when you feel and observe that the quality of your movement declines despite your attention and efforts to maintain efficiency.

21
Progressions

Progressions are the steps that take you from the basic level of practice to increasingly more challenging levels—so you can make *progress.* Progressions can refer to the learning and improvement process of a technique as well as the increase of volume, intensity, or environmental complexity of your training.

You can ensure progressions by feel, observation, and intuition without the need for detailed programming (which is a quantified, predesigned approach to training; read more in Chapter 23, "Programming"). This process is called autoregulation, and it enables you to modify the level of difficulty of your practice on the go during a session and from session to session, depending on how each specific performance and overall progress go.

The intuitive way has been working for humans since the dawn of mankind, whereas programming is a quite recent science that's based on measurements and quantification and has a goal of helping you achieve very specific results. To most modern humans who have been disconnected from nature since birth and deprived from the healthy expression and development of their full Natural Movement behavior and potential, the intuitive way may not seem and feel that intuitive any longer.

> ❝ **It is not enough to do your best; you must know what to do, and then do your best."**
>
> —*W. Edwards Deming*

The incredibly varied techniques, movements, and the diverse principles for efficient practice I'm sharing in this book should give you a solid basis for practicing on your own without an immediate need for programming. When you follow the instruction in this book, your practice of Natural Movement is not purely intuitive because it's significantly influenced by all the information I provide as well as the sequence in which I deliver it, but we could call it "intuitive" in the sense that you will adjust your practice and progressions mostly or even entirely through feel and observation rather than through programming. Practicing that way doesn't necessarily mean that what you're doing lacks structure because you could structure your practice without feeling the need to detail and quantify every aspect of it.

Going through progressions based on natural feedback doesn't mean that your practice is not effective and producing significant results. Conversely, just because your practice is entirely programmed and quantified doesn't mean that it's more effective because numbers on the paper make it look more rational or even "science based." As a matter of fact, as a beginner, you might achieve tremendous progress by feel and observation—that is, through autoregulation—and through the synergy of highly diverse and unquantifiable neural and physiological adaptations than you would if you were attempting to quantify every aspect of your movement. An autoregulated and progressive practice of Natural Movement following the MovNat method is certain to make you achieve impressively broad and fast results. All you need to do is to make sure that your practice has enough variety, frequency, volume, intensity, and complexity; similar to a programmed approach to practice, intuitive practice is structured and based on consistency.

Progression *and* Scalability

Progression is the increased difficulty in level of practice to reach the superior performance for which you are aiming, whereas scalability is the level of difficulty at which you can afford to operate as you perform in real time. Progressions might aim at improving motor control (techniques, skills, efficiency) as well as physiological adaptations (strength, energy systems) by gradually increasing the levels of stress the body is subjected to (which is also called *progressive overload*).

In MovNat, progressions have first to do with the continuity of movement patterns and technique acquisition that follow a progressive sequence independent of environmental complexity, starting with fundamental positions and movements and evolving toward related yet increasingly more challenging techniques such as Dead Hang, Front Swing (hanging), Power Traverse, Pull-Up, High Hand-Reach Pull-Up, Forearm Pull-Up, Pop-Up, Push Power-Up. Obviously, if you can't hang, you can't pull up, and if you can't Pull-Up, you can't Push Power-Up! This is more a matter of progression than scalability, even though choosing movements that you can actually perform at a given stage of your progress is part of the scalability of your practice. Scalability, or *scaling,* is specifically the aspect of progression that has to do with ensuring a sustainable level of volume, intensity, and complexity (VIC) as you perform regardless of future performance or goals; indeed, if you can't perform at a given level of difficulty today, tomorrow's intended level is irrelevant. In MovNat, the method of teaching Natural Movement, we employ the use of intelligent progressions and a wide range of scalability variables to ensure our students make efficient and satisfying progress in their practice.

When the primary goal of movement practice is efficiency, the level of difficulty as you perform should never be too easy or too hard. Therefore, you should scale up or down at any time to keep your practice optimally challenging while remaining safe.

" Achievable goals are the first step to self-improvement."

—J. K. Rowling

Let's say you are practicing several techniques mixed in a "combo" as part of a program you have designed. (You read more about combos in Chapter 23.) You have a certain number of repetitions you want to do for each movement at a certain level of intensity and complexity. However, what you have on paper and in mind is not necessarily what goes on. As you go through the combo, you might notice that the volume or intensity or complexity must be reduced if you want to be able to maintain efficiency.

You must trust what is going on in real time rather than what you programmed yourself to do. If doing fewer repetitions; reducing height, distance, speed, or weight; or simplifying surfaces is what is required for you to maintain quality movement, that's what you need to do regardless of what your training plan says. Insisting on sticking to a program when reality is proving that you can't do the plan efficiently will result in practice and memorization of inefficiencies, and it puts you at greater risk of injury.

However, scalability also means that you may increase the volume, intensity, and complexity if you feel particularly comfortable with challenging yourself more; you just must be able to preserve the same level of efficiency.

Adaptability in movement practice is not reserved only to environmental complexity; it has to do with all types of variables and how you physiologically and psychologically respond to diverse inputs. This means that a 100 percent success rate at doing a movement at a given level of intensity and complexity does not necessarily imply that your practice is too easy and that you must immediately scale it up so you start experiencing some failure. Are you being challenged despite being effective each time? Are you learning and improving in the process? If so, you might not need to immediately increase the difficulty. Although your execution externally looks right, you might be having a suboptimal experience psychologically, and you might feel that you could use more relaxation, better breathing, or greater accuracy.

Training Progression

Quality allows for three areas of difficulty to be added individually or simultaneously.

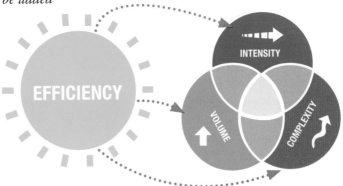

The VIC Principle: Volume, Intensity, Complexity

Volume has to do with one of two things: the number of times you are doing a movement (for instance, how many jumps you perform overall) or the duration of the movement (for instance, how long you run). Greater volume supports the development of endurance, and if you increase volume with a focus on technique, efficiency improves as well.

Intensity has to do with how fast you do the movement. Intensity also is affected by external, environmental parameters—such as height, depth, distance, weight, or force of impact—that demand a significantly greater physical effort. You can combine variables to make performance extremely challenging. For example, sprinting is more intense than jogging, and jumping ten feet forward requires more effort than jumping two feet forward. Greater intensity supports the development of strength, power, and work capacity.

Last, *complexity* relates to environmental variables (it may also relate to sophistication in movement pattern). For instance, a rounded, uneven, unstable surface is a more complex surface to land on than a flat, even, stable one. Greater environmental complexity supports the development of higher levels of movement competency and adaptability.

A typical beginner reflex, especially in young individuals, is to immediately jump as far as they can, lift as heavy as they can, run as fast as they can, try the most difficult obstacles, do as many repetitions as they can, and so on. They try to start with high-intensity, high-complexity, high-volume action. It is nearly impossible to learn a technique this way if you haven't already established a high level of efficiency.

Progressions in volume, intensity, and complexity work very well in a linear scalability, which means the consistent—yet incremental—increase of the variables involved in making your practice more difficult: higher number of repetitions; longer duration; greater speed, distance, height, depth, and weight; and more complex environmental variables. All three variables are intertwined to contribute to the development of greater capability and performance. A combination of volume and intensity supports the development of greater capacity. When intensity and complexity or complexity and volume are associated, the practice becomes representative of some of the most difficult single physical actions or prolonged physical actions that can be encountered in the real world. Depending on the level of intensity, complexity, or volume, greater frequency may support greater ability to recover or improved technique.

Great levels of any of those variables in training also fosters mental training and the increase of courage and resiliency. When you add frequency to the mix, you're developing discipline and commitment. (Frequency relates to how often you practice techniques or movement in relation to a specific level of intensity, complexity, and volume.)

Last, progressions in VIC also work wonderfully with variability, which implies that you will vary difficulty and challenge from session to session by changing any of those variables in a non-linear fashion, which "surprises" your body and breeds greater physiological adaptability.

Getting Started

So where should you start? Would you learn balancing by trying to walk along a frail log that spans a deep ravine? Of course not.

Remember the Progressive principle. As you start, your primary goal is to establish a baseline quality of movement and learn fundamental techniques to develop efficient movement, which is simply impossible to achieve in the presence of high levels of intensity or complexity. (A certain volume—that is, a number of repetitions or time spent on a given technique—is necessary.) You can equally condition through sloppy technique or through impeccable technique, with the former teaching you inefficiencies and the latter teaching you efficient movement. Either way, the amount of energy and time spent is the same. Therefore, I recommend you start with the following:

- **Simple movements that are not too hard for you to do:** The movements should be sufficiently challenging so you are not overly successful or constantly failing; you get benefit from having a mix of successes, half-successes, and failures. The movements shouldn't be so hard that you cannot perform them and become discouraged or get injured trying, but they shouldn't be so easy that you get bored. However, you also don't want to systematically skip the easy movements because they are beneficial in many ways. For example, easy movements release mental tension, might help alleviate physical discomfort, and energize your body and mind. Don't mistakenly believe that low-intensity isn't a stress on your body. Practicing even a relatively low volume of gentle movements is a form of stress, but it's stress that's sustainable and beneficial, starting with keeping you ready, or even helping you to get ready again, for more difficult movements.

" **Teachers open the door, but you must enter by yourself."**

—*Chinese proverb*

In this book, I have done my best to present you with the simpler and easier positions and movements before I progressively explain the more complex and challenging ones. It is a natural progression that you want to follow as much as possible.

- **Low to medium volume:** A certain amount of time or number of repetitions is necessary to learn technique and acquire efficiency. However, just because you *can* repeat the same movement one hundred times right from the beginning without too much effort doesn't mean that you should. You could surprisingly wake the next day and feel sore beyond belief. Instead of immediately going for high volume, first look at the quality of each movement you do while seeking constantly improved efficiency. A small number of mindful and efficient repetitions is better than many mindless and inefficient ones.

- **Relatively low intensity:** Intensity is like volume: Just because you could jump farther, run faster, or lift heavier already doesn't mean that it is the right thing to do. If you do try to push the limits of intensity, you could be in real pain the next day, which, contrary to common belief, is not productive at all. Are your movements optimally efficient? If not, then you don't deserve to work with greater intensity yet. Slow down, cowboy or cowgirl; you're still riding a green horse.

- **Relatively low complexity:** The presence of context makes practice more realistic and satisfactory, but just because it is more realistic to jump between two obstacles doesn't mean that you should start jumping a large gap between tree branches at a great elevation. Ground-level jumping surfaces will do. I talk about this more in the "Risk-to-Danger Ratio" section later in this chapter, and I explain why simplified environmental complexity within a controlled environment is where a safe and progressive path to skill acquisition and physical development should start.

You also need to manage frequency. How frequently you want to train the same skill, technique, drill, or combo depends on how you feel and respond to the movements at the level of volume, intensity, and complexity you practice them. For instance, when you practice technique at low intensity, you may use relatively high volume and great frequency; developing metabolic conditioning, on the other hand, relies on volume and intensity but not a high frequency. Your goal and how your body responds determine whether very frequent or more intermittent practice is desirable and beneficial. Everyone is somewhere on the continuum of health, fitness, movement competency, and physical capability, and each person must determine what is best based on feel, sensations, observation, and experience.

Example Progressions

Progressions in VIC can be dissociated, but it's not necessary to dissociate them. You may incrementally raise levels of all three variables simultaneously rather than separately. The following are some examples for practicing the Power Jump with a progressive increase in each of the three variables (over the course of three days or more, again depending on your body's response).

Volume Progression

- Ten repetitions, distance of 4 feet, ground level, large landing surface
- Fifteen repetitions, distance of 4 feet, ground level, large landing surface
- Twenty repetitions, distance of 4 feet, ground level, large landing surface

Intensity Progression

- Ten repetitions, distance of 5 feet, ground level, large landing surface
- Ten repetitions, distance of 5 feet 4 inches, ground level, large landing surface
- Ten repetitions, distance of 5 feet 8 inches, ground level, large landing surface

Complexity Progression

- Ten repetitions, distance of 5 feet, ground level, large/flat/stable landing surface
- Ten repetitions, distance of 5 feet, 1-inch elevation, medium/rounded/stable landing surface
- Ten repetitions, distance of 5 feet, 2-inch elevation, small/uneven/unstable landing surface

With a simultaneous progression in VIC, all three variables would obviously increase in difficulty together. However, that type of combination can be an explosive cocktail, with a significant increase in risk injury. For instance, greater volume at a low or medium level of intensity supports the improvement of technique, but greater volume with near maximum level of intensity increases and accelerates fatigue, which can suddenly destroy technique. If you also add environmental complexity, you are guaranteed to rapidly fail and are very likely to injure yourself as well.

Adjusting all three variables of progression should be approached very incrementally and wisely so that you stay effective, efficient, and safe. This being said, with very small incremental progressions, the combination of increasing volume, intensity, and complexity simultaneously can be extraordinarily valuable.

Often, a reasonable increase of complexity alone can make your practice immediately more beneficial. Let me give you an example. Say you are performing a volume of ten depth jumps with an intensity of 3 feet of depth. You have a choice between landing on the ground or landing on a 1-inch-thick, 1-square-foot board. In both scenarios, the volume and intensity are the same, but you have a choice of complexity, which challenges your attention, accuracy, and balance upon landing. You will spend the exact same time and energy going through those ten repetitions, but which of the two options is the more beneficial? You can apply this reasoning and complexity strategy to any movement you do.

How fast you should progress in terms of volume, intensity, and complexity has to do with many variables: your personal potential, your lifestyle and how it supports your practice, your commitment, how you physiologically respond, and so forth. You might have an innate ability to intuitively determine effective progressions, or you may determine progressions more analytically by monitoring such progress through methodical programming, or you may use a blend of the two. The golden rule of MovNat practice is to first establish quality of movement before you advance to higher quantity of movement, greater intensity of movement, and greater complexity of the environment where movement is performed. In other words, always respect scalability and progressions while focusing on improving or maintaining technique and movement efficiency. Never raise volume, intensity, or complexity too much or too soon. Knowing what level of volume, intensity, or complexity (or a combination of the three) you can—or rather should—handle without degrading good form is key to efficient and safe practice or effective programming. Such knowledge requires practice, experimentation, observation, experience, and humility.

You can always use this very simple yet very effective method when approaching progression in any of the three aspects of difficulty (VIC): If you can consecutively perform three to five impeccably executed attempts—and I really mean *consecutively*—then you have demonstrated enough consistency to deserve trying the same movement at a slightly higher level of difficulty. Keep in mind, though, that as with scalability, being effective at a movement at a given level of difficulty doesn't mean that you aren't challenged or improving anymore.

Risk-to-Danger Ratio

The risk-to-danger ratio is a concept that relates to practice mostly in regard to environmental complexity. Risk is the probability that you will be unsuccessful in completing a physical action and potentially be exposed to danger. Risk depends on your individual physical capability, the context, and your physical and mental state at the moment you perform the action.

For example, the risk of falling if you walk across a 2-foot-wide beam that's 4 feet long is quite low because the beam is very wide and the distance is very short. If the beam is 1 inch wide and 20 feet long, the risk becomes quite high to an untrained person, yet for a person who's well-trained in balancing, the risk remains low. However, even a well-trained person can experience risk of falling if that person is sick, strong winds are blowing, or something suddenly distracts the person as they try to balance across the beam.

Danger is the physical danger that is present if your movement fails, and it's likely that you'll experience physical harm or even death regardless of the level of risk involved. For example, the danger related to losing balance off a 2-by-4 that's on the ground is zero; if you do lose balance, you only step off the surface rather than "fall off." However, the danger related to losing balance off a 2-by-4 that's 30 feet in the air is much higher; if you fall, you'll likely hurt yourself badly—or possibly die.

Although danger has mostly to do with environmental complexity, it can also be related to your movement behavior. You don't need a high level of danger to get hurt; you can get hurt when you augment the level of risk implied with movement by doing it at a greater level of intensity or complexity. For instance, if you walk on a concrete surface, you can't really hurt yourself, but if you sprint on it and stumble, the combination of your weight, speed, gravity, and the hardness of the surface represents an obvious danger of causing you harm. If you sit on ice, you are safe, but standing and walking on it implies the danger of falling and hurting yourself.

Not all movements are dangerous, but all movements are risky. The more you move (increase volume) with more intensity in more complex environments, the more risk you deal with. Statistically, the chances that you will miss go up. If you go on a simple hike on the sidewalk, the longer you walk, the more likely it is that you'll stumble at least once. It's a risk you can't deny, even though no real danger should be associated with that risk. When you know that risk exists, being mindful means treating your movements as if none are casual as you also stay relaxed and confident.

The risk-to-danger ratio is the relationship between risk and danger. It's is generally inverse. *The higher the danger involved in a physical action, the lower the risk should be.* The higher the risk involved in a physical action, the lower the danger should be. Obviously, if the level of danger and the level of risk are both exceptionally high, you know that you are going to die. This is the extreme ratio you do not want.

> ❝ **Decision is a risk rooted in the courage of being free."**
>
> —*Paul Tillich*

If you don't know the environment where you are, or if you do but want to try something new or more difficult, you first need to assess the danger rather than the risk. It doesn't matter if the chance of missing is only one in ten; if you perform the move several times in a row, you *will* miss. What happens if you do? That is the question. What danger and what consequences will you be dealing with at that point where you miss and fall? As part of your progression in Natural Movement practice, you want to avoid unsustainable levels of danger regardless of the level of risk. Period. There is a point at which additional danger doesn't train your body; it trains only your mind. Yet if you know that missing implies great harm to your body or can result in death and that there is a risk of even one in ten, deciding whether to proceed is a choice that only you can make. Are you willing to kill yourself while trying?

Think about it: You can't manage danger; you can manage only risk. After you take the risk, you can't change the danger that exists, even if you have adjustable props that make your training environment safer, such as within controlled environments customized for practice; danger is not scalable while you're in action. You can't fix your movement once it has failed, and you can't unhurt yourself after the hurt has occurred.

To lower risk, you must gradually build up your physical capability and self-confidence. In addition, you need to become gradually experienced in realistically assessing risk level. Just as you can't expect "mind over matter" to make danger physically disappear, you can't always expect your mind to nullify the probability of failure. If an environment exceeds your physical capability, the risk is maximum, and there's nothing you can do about it. If you want to keep your practice safe, you should be able to objectively assess that there is no—or very little—danger associated with a limited risk and that you can expect to perform a movement successfully based on your experience and current sensations. Better yet, you want to scale the movement by doing it first with a lower level of difficulty, which is the most effective way to give you a realistic sense of capability versus risk.

If you are afraid of doing a movement, there could be three causes:

- You have a rational reason to fear it because of the combined presence of danger and risk.
- You have a rational fear of the movement because of the presence of danger despite very limited (but not nonexistent) risk.
- You have an irrational fear of the movement because some risk exists, yet there is no actual danger.

You will find some obstacles that you can never overcome because they are beyond your physical capability. You can only dream of clearing them. Those you *can* physically overcome are either permanent limitations or mere delays: The choice is yours. Assuming that you want to enjoy life for a long time and that you have nothing to prove, facing high danger with the risk of failing your attempt is not the best choice. So many people have died while daring to do extremely dangerous feats.

You may occasionally face limited, non-lethal danger as part of mental training. It makes you or keeps you brave, emotionally in control, and coolheaded. But, by all means, keep your practice sustainable. Reserve the highly dangerous stuff for when the real world leaves you no other option.

Not all progress and performance can be measured easily. Aspects of technique—such as positional control, ease, relaxation, alertness, responsiveness, timing, balance, and accuracy—are mostly observed or felt. But it can be useful and highly motivating to measure what is measurable. You can use basic measurements, such as how far or high you can jump, how heavy you can lift, or how fast you can run a distance.

On the other hand, you might prefer not to use any measurement because you can just feel that you move better, that you are more mobile and relaxed, faster, and stronger. You might notice that not too long ago you were unable to jump over an obstacle that you now can clear quite easily. Do you know the exact distance between two rocks that you're using in your practice? Does it really matter if you have a measurement for what you can simply observe, such as a longer distance now versus a shorter distance from before? In some cases, what you can perceive without measuring is sufficient to give you an empirical sense of your ability and also to give you the confirmation that you have made progress. It can also give you the confidence that unmeasured, nonprogrammed practice is quite effective when you are determined to get better and do better. It can make your practice simpler and save you time.

I have encountered highly fit athletes who knew exactly what their "vertical jump" height was but had no clue whether they were able to clear the distance between two rocks or walls when outdoors, let alone whether they could land accurately and in a stable way. *My point is that it's not necessarily more rational to precisely know what number or measurement you can achieve than it is to know what real-world physical performance you're capable of or what progress you've made using the simplest and most ancient method: observation.*

The important thing is to consider your mindset. Some people immediately relate to a "pure" approach of practicing Natural Movement barefoot, outside in nature, and by intuition. These people don't want their practice to include what they see as artificiality—watches or clocks, training logs, counting, measurements, quantification, planning, or programming. Other people want to integrate Natural Movement practice within a gym setting and exclusively train in a quantifiable, predesigned, and monitored fashion. In the middle ground are the people who are opportunistic and adaptable; they can practice anywhere, using diverse environments, props, gear, methods, and mindsets. You don't have to belong to a category, and you could ultimately blend both approaches. Not only is there no contradiction in approaching practice both ways, but you will learn a lot by doing so.

> " I am large, I contain multitudes."
>
> —J. K. Rowling

These two approaches serve the same purpose by using two different methods and mindsets. Neither is right or wrong, superior or inferior; they're just different.

22
Structuring Sessions

For your practice sessions, you can take the approach of not planning a particular structure; instead, you decide what you do as you go "by feel." Most of the time, even when you don't have a detailed plan of what your session should include, you will have an idea of some of the particular movements you want to practice.

Structuring sessions is optional, but it can be an effective way to organize individual sessions as well as maintain some continuity of specific aspects of your progress over several sessions. How you structure each session depends, of course, on what you intend the session to be made of and the results you expect. You can use diverse practice types in training that is part of an individually designed program or of an impromptu session. The shorter the session is, the more specific it should be. For instance, if you have only five minutes, you shouldn't be deterred from practicing, but you should avoid trying to do too much or having too much diversity unless your intention is to keep your body alert and functioning in a limited amount of time. The more time you have, the more movements you can practice and the more diverse your

practice can be. Structuring your practice sessions, even in the absence of planning, means that you know what particular improvements you're looking for and you have some basic level of organization to guide your practice and optimize the results.

Eventually, despite the diversity of movements trained, you might create your own practice patterns that you know fit you best, and some aspects of your practice will be consistent but still have a degree of variability. Sometimes, the totality of a practice session will be spontaneous. Sometimes a single session will emphasize a single technique, a single skill or physiological adaptation. In a nutshell, there are many diverse ways you can approach your practice to achieve Natural Movement capability.

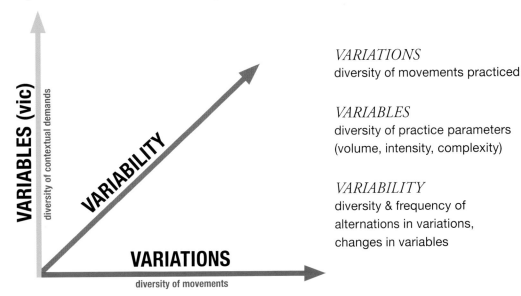

VARIATIONS
diversity of movements practiced

VARIABLES
diversity of practice parameters
(volume, intensity, complexity)

VARIABILITY
diversity & frequency of
alternations in variations,
changes in variables

Practice Types

The following suggestion is one recommendation of an effective sequence that's broken into practice types when you have sufficient time—at least twenty minutes—for training:

- **Warm-up/movement preparation:** Spend five to fifteen minutes preparing your body for movement.
- **Emphasis:** An emphasis can be either focusing on one or more specific techniques or on particular aspects of capacity (a practice session may involve several emphases).
- A technical emphasis involves selecting techniques that you want to learn or improve, with a focus on efficiency (measurable aspects of practice are secondary and counting repetitions is relevant only if it helps you evaluate a percentage of efficient repetitions). The less time you have, the more you should limit the number of techniques to be involved. You could also decide that technical practice will fill the entire time after your warm-up. Capacity emphases may involve any movement with a focus on either strength, power, and/or conditioning (as long as you don't compromise technique efficiency). Lastly, you may have an emphasis that pushes your limits in terms of both efficiency and capacity as a means to develop your ability to delay the deterioration of your technique under fatigue. In this case, it's best to limit the scope of techniques involved to at most three techniques.
- **Combo practice:** Combine at least three but no more than eight movements into a sequence, including the particular techniques you just practiced. Using a circuit of movements is a very valuable and beneficial type of technical practice. Instead of spending ten minutes each on three different techniques from different Natural Movement skills, you could spend thirty minutes alternating the same techniques, doing a single or several repetitions of the first movement, then the second, then the third, and then going back to the first movement again. The advantage is that you're not stressing the same areas of your body in the same way for too long, which is the case if all the movements belong to the same

Natural Movement skill (crawling, balancing, jumping). Also, your central nervous system gets an opportunity to "reset" every time the task changes. Another highly important aspect of combo training is that it teaches you to seamlessly transition from one technique to another. You learn to connect movements rather than practicing them in isolation, which helps your transitions to be more efficient.

Combo practice also helps you maintain motivation and avoid boredom. The same idea can be used with the goal of developing strength, improving mobility, or improving energy systems. Another way to use a combo is to mix up high-intensity movement with low-intensity movement—for instance, lifting and carrying a heavy load followed by balancing across a beam. In this case, alternating high- and low-intensity movements is a form of "interval training," and the low-intensity movements enable you to continue technical practice while under mild fatigue, which challenges your ability to maintain efficiency.

Last, a combo may exclusively contain movements performed at high intensity, which is a very effective way to develop your work capacity by improving your energy systems through metabolic conditioning.

With hundreds of techniques and thousands of movement and position variations and all the potential differences in volume, intensity, or environmental complexity variables, you can literally come up with a limitless number of combo variations.

Combo example (repeat 10 times or perform for 10 minutes):
- 100 yards fast-pace run
- 6x Forward Power Jump, distance of 5 feet, with a precision Square Landing
- 30-second Side Double-Hand Hang Front Swing
- 25-yard Inverted Crawl at a moderate pace

ONE SIZE DOES NOT FIT ALL

I could give you many examples of combos, but they're just general ideas that aren't customized to your individual ability and specific goals as they should be. Customizing practice is part of programming that you must do based on your needs. The main thing to remember is that the priority of a combo is always to maintain efficiency throughout the practice.

THE BENEFIT OF COURSE TRAINING

Course training can help you verify your capability instead of only assuming it. Therefore, part of this type of training could be to confront tough conditions that you don't normally encounter, such as cold, heat, mud, fear, darkness, slipperiness, and possibly a state of food and sleep deprivation. Undertaking these types of challenges doesn't have so much to do with testing your technique or physical ability as it does with testing your mettle. You have to be aware that the tougher you make the course, the easier it is to become injured. However, not all courses have to be turned into a physical and mental ordeal. You can keep the course safe and not overly hard, especially as you're beginning.

- **Course:** Work through a course, which is akin to an "obstacle" course. Like the combo practice, there is no standard course that applies to everyone. The course you use depends on where you are and what environmental variables you can use, such as terrain, surfaces, walls, boulders, fallen trees, and so on. The length or duration of the course will vary as well. In addition, what you include in the course obviously depends on what you are capable of.

The difference between a course and a combo is that you might not rehearse the same course several times in a row. The point of a course is not to learn and practice efficiency; it's to test capability and sometimes also willpower. On a course, if you have imperfect execution of a movement, you don't stop and do it again; you just keep going.

Another purpose of a course is to make your performance more situational than technical. There's more to working a course than the technique or what environments or obstacles you're training for; it's also about simulating a scenario. Why are you going as fast as you safely can? It's not just for metabolic conditioning; it's because you're imagining an emergency. Even though the situation is only simulated, your effort is very real. Not all obstacles are walls and ropes: speed, duration, distance, weight, weather conditions, and even fear can be tremendous obstacles, so course practice can be designed according to the type of difficulties you want to prepare for and to verify that your practice has actually prepared you for them.

- **Games:** Try incorporating games into your practice from time to time. Games are inherently playful or competitive (if you're not training solo). In fact, you don't necessarily need to make something a game to have fun. Balancing is inherently fun; so is precision throwing on a target. Games tend to imply that several players are involved, that there are rules and a goal to the game, and possibly that it's a competition with a winner. The point is this: Just like any specialized sport that's based on some specific Natural Movement skill, when you incorporate a game into your practice, you might combine several skills.

Injury Prevention

Now that I've covered aspects structuring your practice, it's a good idea to address injury prevention in more detail:

- **Environment:** Check out the environment and surfaces where you practice. If you step down or fall, is there a danger? Can you stumble on a rock hidden in the tall grass and break toes?
- **Efficiency:** The primary strategy for avoiding waste of energy where efficiency is concerned is learning technique and paying close attention to biomechanically sound, quality movement.
- **Mindfulness:** Self-preservation requires the mindset of behaving realistically, cautiously, and wisely to avoid reckless movement. Another important way to avoid injury is to anticipate fatigue—both muscular fatigue and the fatigue of your central nervous system—long enough before your form degrades too much and you can no longer perform safely. Indeed, injuries frequently occur toward the end of practice sessions or when fatigue peaks. Some issues you notice, such as significant impairments in performance or painful body signals, could turn into injury if you dismiss them, so be careful not to ignore the signs telling you to start becoming extra cautious, slow down, or even stop the activity (which are the brain's natural responses to muscular fatigue anyway). If you start practicing regularly, you will notice that you aren't always feeling "fresh" at the start of a session, but that doesn't necessarily mean that you must skip practice until your body feels perfect. You are good to practice through mild physical fatigue as long as your movement quality doesn't degrade much.
- **Progressive practice in relation to VIC:** The body in motion is subjected to the action of both external and internal forces. A single movement event at an intensity that exceeds the ability of your tissues to handle overly stressful effort may cause a trauma, such as a torn muscle or broken bone. Know your capability and limits and respect progressions in all three aspects of VIC.

- **Consistency:** How you used to perform some time ago may not be how you're able to perform today. If you haven't been consistent at practicing particular skills, techniques, or at a certain level of VIC, you can't assume that you can resume at the same level of difficulty you once could handle. The longer you have paused training, the more cautious and patient you must be before you can train at the level you used to again.
- **Variety:** We can injure ourselves when unintentionally and forcefully reaching positions past our maximum flexibility or positions that are biomechanically unsustainable. But we can also injure ourselves in positions that we are not familiar with or prepared for, in habitual positions we aren't trained to handle past a certain level of intensity or volume, or in positions unusual to us that we perform at a high level of intensity. (In this latter case the potential for injury is quite high.) This is why it's essential that our practice is comprehensive enough to have us regularly practice the full spectrum of Natural Movement and at sufficient levels of intensity.
- **Recovery:** Injury can occur from the systematic repetition of a stress-inducing physical action over time. In this case, the force is too small to cause an immediate injury, but unnoticeable microdamage can occur that will eventually lead to injury because it accumulates with every repetition. It's essential to ensure proper recovery (time, rest, hydration, nutrition) so your tissues can physiologically adapt to a greater level of stress. Otherwise, instead of your tissues getting stronger, you enable cumulative fatigue to weaken them, which leads to injury. Recovery time is highly individual and depends on diverse variables such as
  - Volume and intensity in relation to your current level of physiological adaptation
  - Type of effort or muscle involved. The eccentric component of muscular work is responsible for most muscle soreness. Large muscles recover more slowly, and large muscle groups recover slower, too.
  - Age

- **Lifestyle:** Healthy habits support health, energy, physical robustness, recovery, and resiliency, which are all necessary for sustainable Natural Movement practice.
- **Frequency:** Frequency implies that you are moving regularly and also that you are practicing a variety of movements and effort regularly enough to remain physiologically ready.
- **Therapy:** If you notice any functional issue or have a known past injury, you must give it special attention, and possibly special treatment, as it can aggravate if it remains unchecked.

With efficient Natural Movement practice—that is, if you follow my recommendations and always practice mindfully—you are taking a risk that you might occasionally injure your body in minor and temporary ways, but with chronic physical idleness you are absolutely guaranteed that your body will continuously deteriorate. Practicing Natural Movement can prevent numerous physical ailments. Physical idleness unavoidably promotes physical suffering, even when you do not link the two. The return on investment is evident, and the rewards are beyond expectations.

23
Programming

An intuitive practice will do wonders for you as a beginner. It gives you the latitude to explore many diverse movements and opens options for very diverse ways to practice without limiting yourself or having to learn the science of programming. As a beginner, programming might unnecessarily limit the overall range and speed of your progress. In short, programming is completely optional for beginners and could easily prove counterproductive. The necessity for programming mainly arises when you start to reach a plateau in a given area and need to opt for a specific approach to move beyond it. Obviously, this issue is likely to be more of a concern for more experienced or advanced practitioners who are seeking effective strategies to keep increasing their performance.

However, you might as well start programming some aspects of your training early on, as soon as you have acquired technique—for instance, to develop greater strength and performance in particular aspects of your capability, such as in lifting and carrying. From an unspecialized approach to physical training, you might want to use programming to support greater or faster progress in bringing a given skill to near equal performance with other skills. If you're a beginner, you should not drop all other aspects of your training because you want to make specific gains in a particular area; any program you decide to follow should be a *part* of your practice, not your *only* practice. More advanced practitioners may temporarily dedicate themselves entirely (or almost entirely) to improving a given aspect of their capability because they have already become proficient at the overall spectrum of Natural Movement and need a greater emphasis to achieve the gains they're looking for.

Programming is about designing your practice to achieve results over the course of days or weeks (sometimes months) by determining in advance what each training session should be made of. So if you are planning the content of a single session in detail, or even the detailed content of all your practice sessions, but you don't have any connection or continuity between sessions, that is not programming; it's just planning. Programming can address the progressive development of skills and techniques, but it can also address the development of work capacity including the strength, power, and metabolic conditioning that enables you to sustain efficient movement, effective performance, and physical action for a longer time and makes your capability more *durable*. You can design a program for progress in one skill or several, for specific physiological adaptations, or to achieve multiple gains simultaneously.

" Discipline is the bridge between goals and accomplishment."
— *Jim Rohn*

If you decide that you want to approach your training and progress systematically and determine what particular objective you want to make a priority—for instance, achieving one of the Natural Movement physical challenges or training to surpass them—you need to figure out what particular improvements you want to make in technique, strength, power, energy systems, mobility, and so on. Then you must figure out the process you will use to achieve your goals. Whereas your fundamental goal is to always increase your real-world physical capability, a program—which is by default temporary—could emphasize very specific improvements that indirectly support that fundamental goal, such as losing weight (through high-intensity Natural Movement training) or gaining in mobility. Also, specialized athletes may use a Natural Movement practice program to support performance in their particular sports.

> ## NOTE
>
> Note that I didn't say that you must approach your progress *rationally*. Using a systematic, predefined, quantifiable approach isn't the only rational approach.

Programs are only relevant if the objectives are well understood, and also if they are specific, individual, realistic, measurable, and adaptable.

- **Specific:** For a program to effectively help you achieve goals, the goals have to be limited in scope. You can't pack a program with an endless list of drills and expect specific results, and you can't expect a great variety of improvements, either. You must limit your target goals so you can better identify the strategy that will help you achieve them the most effectively. In short, keep your program(s) simple. It's well known that physiological adaptations can conflict with each other; for instance, there can be a conflict in attempting to develop high levels of power and endurance at the same time. Fortunately, this issue is not really a concern for beginners who can actually achieve very diverse improvements in gains with a general approach to their practice. The only exception is a lack of upper-body strength that prevents beginners from achieving a number of climbing movements on horizontal surfaces. The issue of needing specific emphasis and programming to break plateaus and enable further progress occurs mostly in highly specialized athletes or in MovNat practitioners who have already reached an advanced level. Natural Movement/MovNat beginners and

even intermediate level practitioners can absolutely develop greater power and endurance at the same time. In fact, by designing programs that resemble the example I give later in this chapter, you can reach your objective while simultaneously making progress in a variety of skills.

- **Individual:** Programming necessarily starts with determining what objective(s) you should reach. Your plan must be individualized and customized to enable you to reach your own goals, not someone else's. Even if you and another person share the exact same goal at a given time, it doesn't mean that you should use the exact same strategy to achieve it.

- **Realistic:** Both your objective and the strategy must be realistic. You may never be able to perform at the level of world-class athletes who have been training their entire lives—unless you specialize the way they do. You might not be able to achieve your goals in a matter of days, or maybe not even in a matter of weeks or months. Don't lose sight of the big picture, which is a relatively equalized scope of physical capability, and don't dismiss your current physical capability and health status. The process of adaptation demands time. Don't raise the bar too high too fast, but don't self-limit too much by thinking "I can do only this" because you'll end up with a very easy but boring program.

- **Quantifiable:** A systematic approach to practice implies that you will track sets, reps, weight, distance, and/or time so that you can quantify any aspect of your work and progress that is measurable. Non-measurable aspects of your progress should be validated through feel, observation, and/or someone else's feedback.

- **Adaptable:** Although you program progressions in diverse variables (numbers of sets and reps, weight, time) to be consistent, sometimes you might observe that you should modify them on the fly, either by decreasing or increasing them. The plan is the tool rather than the finality; if the plan doesn't effectively advance your goal, you must be pragmatic and flexible to modify it. Being adaptable doesn't mean that you want to extensively modify your training plan every session. Doing that would only be necessary if the program was very badly designed from the beginning. Adaptability means that you should always retain the latitude to modify your program if you believe that modifying something might make the program even more effective depending on how you physically respond to it as you progress through it. Don't force yourself to go as fast or as slowly as the plan says; make the plan follow the pace of your progress. Use common sense: Don't brutalize yourself into progress faster than you can manage or self-indulge in progressing much slower than you are capable of.

If you'd like to see an example program, visit the Beginner's Guide to MovNat page at www.movnat.com/beginners-guide-movnat/. There you can find tips for beginners as well as a four-week beginner-level program.

Remember, that a generalized program like the example is a real program, but it's not programming. If you can already perform the skills in the example program, that particular training plan is irrelevant to you (though its content still might be very beneficial to you). However, if you currently can't do he skills, this objective is relevant to you, but that doesn't mean that the way it's designed is customized to you. Maybe you'd need two weeks to achieve the same goal; maybe you'd need six months. You must look at diverse aspects of your current level of fitness and health to determine what is realistic for you. You might need to modify the quantities and measurements, which applies both to the number of sets and reps and to the duration of the plan. After you have made modifications to customize the program for your purpose, you still want to keep your plan adaptable and modify the numbers if you judge that the program will be more effective. In a nutshell, effective programming is about adapting the program to you as much as it is about you adapting to the program.

Programming is a real science, and, as in most sciences, experts often argue about the best methods and offer diverse strategies for obtaining the same results. By definition, science is never set in stone and should always evolve with new findings. The particular programming relative to Natural Movement/MovNat practice is just starting and has a highly promising future.

❝ In science consensus is irrelevant. What is relevant is reproducible results."

—Michael Crichton

❝ Success is not a matter of mastering subtle, sophisticated theory but rather of embracing common sense with uncommon levels of discipline and persistence."

—Patrick Lencioni

CONSIDERATIONS FOR MORE ADVANCED PRACTICE

This part covered the basics of the principles of efficient practice. However, it doesn't cover the full spectrum of Natural Movement/MovNat practice, which also involves developing mental toughness, physiological resiliency, and situational awareness. However, an in-depth discussion of those aspects of practice is beyond the scope of this book.

You can start developing your physical and mental toughness by progressively exposing yourself to harsh weather during movement practice. Situational awareness, though, is something that is learned through specific instruction and training but also through actual action. You can train situational awareness by simulating some of these situations as long as you do it safely—ideally in a group setting.

If you want to put your Natural Movement skills and mindset to real use and learn more about real-world contextual demands, you certainly could consider working with firefighter and rescue teams. These people always have my utmost respect and admiration.

MOVEMENT SELECTION IN THE BOOK

For the sake of keeping the volume of material in this book manageable, I decided to not include swimming/aquatic skills or combative skills. For the same reason, a number of less essential techniques and movement variations did not make it into the book. It doesn't mean in any way that they are missing from the MovNat method. It's just impossible to show absolutely everything in a single book.

POSITIONS AND MOVEMENT NAMES IN THE BOOK

When I started instructing MovNat many years ago, I quickly realized that the number of positions, techniques, and other movement variations I was teaching *far* exceeded the names that existed in sports, the fitness industry, or other movement disciplines. I also found some of the existing names to be unsatisfactory for a variety of reasons (too conventional, in a different language, associated with a particular discipline, inaccurate, confusing, or silly).

In any case, for the sake of teaching the MovNat method, each position and movement needed a name. And, of course, for this book I obviously couldn't introduce and describe so many positions and techniques without naming them. It is also my observation that we tend to unconsciously reduce the range of positions and movements we practice to those that we can name, as if they are the only ones that have value, whereas unnamed positions and movements are easily neglected and forgotten.

I made the decision to name or rename practically *all* the positions and techniques practiced in Natural Movement—which is several hundred—in a descriptive way. The names are usually longer for that reason, though some are named in a subjective way for the sake of simplicity. Ultimately, as a solo practitioner, you will not need to memorize all these names unless you find it useful to do so.

PHOTOS IN THE BOOK

My publisher and I decided that the best course of action was to shoot all the photos indoors rather than in nature, chiefly for the sake of ensuring consistency of lighting and photo quality. Another important consideration was time management, as several days of shooting were necessary to take photos of the hundreds of techniques and movement variations on the list and verify that each sequence was complete and satisfactory.

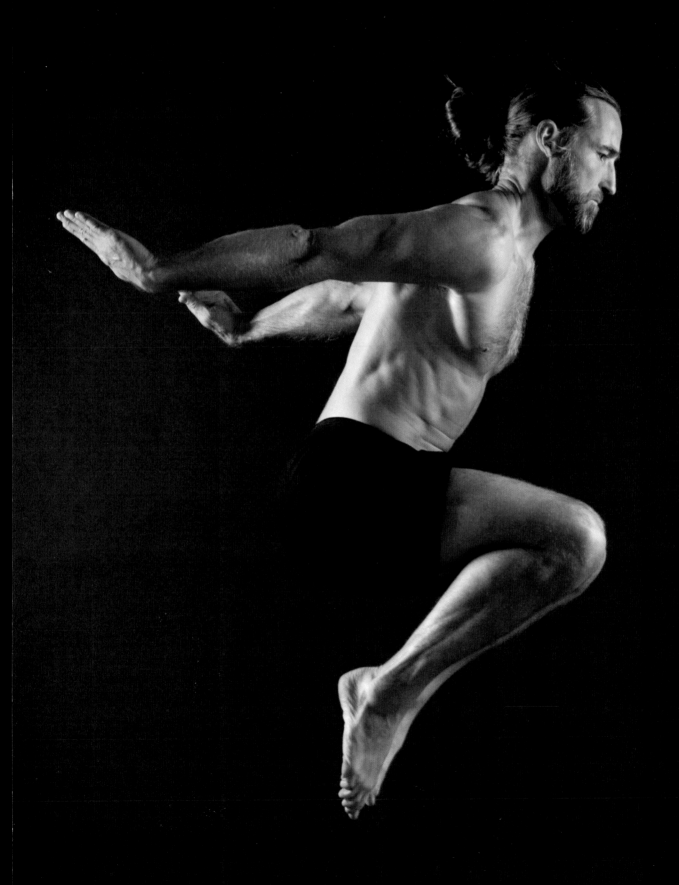

4

Techniques

24
Ground Movement 1: Lying, Rolling, Crawling

"Only by bringing peace from the ground up can problems higher in the body be understood."

—Ida Rolf

Ground movement refers to positions and movements that you do while your center of gravity is lower than your knee level when you're standing, regardless of which part of the body is the base of support. Ground movement includes lying, rolling, crawling, sitting, kneeling, squatting, and the many types of get-ups or transitions between lower and higher positions.

Place a piece of tape on the wall at your knee level, then lower yourself into any position in which your center of gravity is below that mark. You're holding a ground position or doing a ground movement.

Ground movement is where each person's movement journey begins after birth. Infants go through a Natural Movement developmental process during which they learn to elevate their center of gravity progressively until they reach bipedal standing positions. The practical value of ground movement is enormous. It's a shame that modern society has such little regard for ground movements. Most are dismissed as being "animal-like" or "child-like," or they're considered to be reserved to activities such as military training. Before you address how well you move when standing on your feet, you should verify how comfortably you move below that level.

From a practical perspective, ground movements allow infants to move around before they can stand and walk autonomously, and the movements help infants learn movement patterns that are essential to overall movement competency. Ground movements are useful for passing under or through low obstacles, handling tasks and chores on the ground, reaching something low and difficult to access, resting, lowering your field of vision, looking for something on the ground, camouflaging yourself or taking shelter under something, avoiding falling, moving when the terrain is challenging for bipedal motion, moving when standing isn't possible or is challenging (because of injury, sickness, disability, or intoxication), breathing better in smoky areas, or playing with young children.

Functionally speaking, ground positions and movements are great for the entire body: feet, ankles, knees, hips, lumbar and thoracic spine, shoulders, wrists, hands—they're all covered! No one is truly physically capable, including athletes, if they're not proficient on the ground.

If done right, ground movement can restore function in and strengthen your whole body and feel very healing, especially if you do it regularly on real, earthy ground. Even better, ground movement requires no equipment at all, except maybe a mat, and you can do it at home—either indoors or outdoors—while you visualize the potential real-life situation in which the movements might apply.

In this book, I am, of course, giving ground movement the attention it deserves. With every position and movement I present, the rule of thumb is to always maintain ample abdominal breathing. Make your ground movement practice a breathing practice for extra benefit.

Lying *and* Rolling

Lying techniques and movements are a great introduction to ground movement because they happen close to the ground, with the lowest possible center of gravity, and the movements are similar to what you learn in the first developmental stage of life. Rolling is an effective way to switch from being supine (face up) to being prone (face down) or vice versa. For some techniques, you use your limbs relatively minimally; instead, you rely primarily on the action of your core, hips, and shoulders. Those techniques are excellent for spine mobility. Other techniques require more limb action. Unlike limbless creatures that can slither, humans must use varied points of support to anchor ourselves and reduce friction to help us push, pull, or roll effectively as we perform the lowest ground movements.

In a practical sense, lying positions and movements are important in many ways. We use lying positions to rest, conceal ourselves, and protect our bodies. We also use these techniques to move when more elevated stances are too unstable or when we must creep underneath or through confined, narrow, or thick environments. Rolling enables us to rapidly switch the orientation and direction of a lying position, to transition from a landing to a lying position while dispersing high impact forces effectively, and even to quickly regain a standing position after an unexpected fall.

Positions

Unlike many other natural positions, lying positions are common in our modern lifestyles, and for a good reason: We go to bed every evening and find ourselves in diverse lying positions as we sleep. Even though you might feel like you're well-versed in lying positions, I encourage you to explore as many of the variations shown in the photos as you can with intention and mindfulness. There are more variations than what I show—for instance, the position of your legs doesn't have to be straight. You can modify the leg position to create positional variations. You do something similar for the sitting positions shown in Chapter 25. Feel your points of support and point of balance, especially in the side-lying positions, and notice how they affect your breathing.

Some positions are fully relaxed; others are "active" and require you to hold muscular tension. Also explore random transitions from any of the following positions to another position.

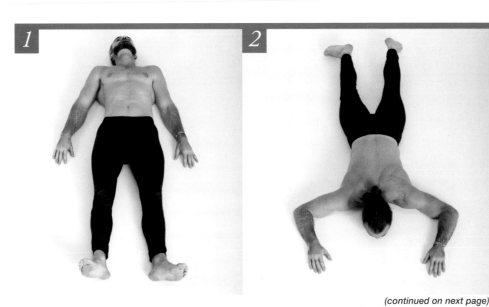

(continued on next page)

1 Supine Lying arms down to the sides (or extended to the sides, crossed over the chest, hands protecting the face, etc.).

2 Prone Lying, head up with chin on the ground, bent arms pointing forward.

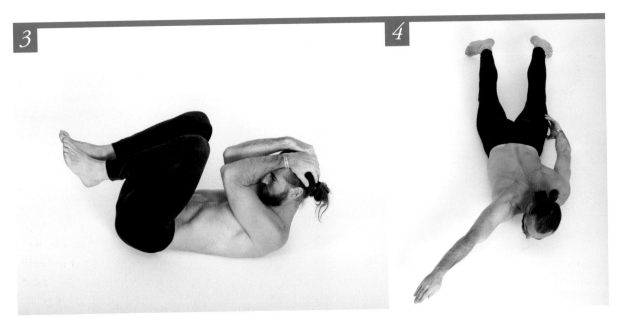

3 Protective Supine Lying, bent legs and arms, open hands on the head, forearms shielding the face.

4 Prone Lying, head off the ground, arms off the ground, one arm reaching forward at an angle.

Lying Rolls

As practice, rolling is a fun movement to do. However, the apparent simplicity of rolling movements is deceptive. For most adults, these positions and movement patterns feel very awkward at first. That's because there's a big difference between rolling randomly (and often clumsily) on soft surfaces for fun and rolling intentionally and skillfully on firm surfaces. You might lose balance. Your sense of proprioception and spatial awareness might be tricked and confused. You might realize that you lack the spine mobility and body coordination to perform efficient rolls or that you lack the abdominal strength to roll from a lying position when you haven't generated any momentum. Working on these techniques might expose physical weaknesses you didn't know you had.

I recommend that you start learning to roll on relatively soft, forgiving surfaces to avoid feeling very uncomfortable and tense. I also recommend that you start rolling from lying positions rather than standing positions. The reason is that it's easy to throw a roll using the pull of gravity, but if the roll is uncontrolled, the landing might resemble a painful crash. Starting from a lying position is the best way to ensure that you first learn a controlled, slow-motion roll. Lying rolls are both self- and gravity-powered. The first phase of the roll is self-powered, and the second phase is more gravity-powered.

If you can perform a good roll in slow motion, you can perform a good dynamic roll, but the opposite isn't necessarily true. If you want to eventually learn efficient and safe rolls from standing positions, you need to learn to perform them first from lying and in slow motion with impeccable control over your positions, sequence, timing, and relaxation.

Side Roll

Once you have become proficient at the Side Lying positions and Side-Rocking movement, rolling all the way to the other side makes sense when you need to switch your body position from supine to prone or vice versa. Possible uses for the reversal in body orientation are as a protective move or, more likely, a transitional move before you use a different crawling technique. You also might use it to get up and start moving forward immediately in the desired direction. For instance, from the Supine Lying position, if you want to move in the direction of your head, you would have to use a Shoulder Crawl, a Hip-Thrust Crawl, or an Inverted Hand-Foot Crawl (which are covered later in this chapter) without being able to look where you're going or see what's behind your back. By first reversing to a Prone Lying position, you can use a great variety of crawling techniques or even get up and immediately face the direction you're headed. You also could use the Side Roll to cover some distance on a flat terrain relatively rapidly while staying very close to the ground when there's a danger of being noticed or hit by projectiles.

You can also use the rolling move when you're going downhill, but only as a form of temporary recovery after a fall and to maintain some body position control if you can't bring yourself to an immediate stop. Although Side Rolling down a hill covered with thick grass can be fun, you never know when a stone is going to get in your way, and vital parts of your body, such as the face, back of the head, neck, and spine, are exposed to a real threat of severe injury. There are other ways to crawl or slide down a steep slope while avoiding unnecessary risks.

Supine-to-Prone Side Roll

To perform the Supine-to-Prone, Stretched-Arms Side Roll, you can roll to the side and back, then roll to the other side, alternately. When you have more space available, you can roll over a certain distance without stopping and then roll back to where you started.

Optionally, you could perform the Side Roll with your arms crossed over your chest or tight along the sides of your body. You also can include short pauses after you reach the straight Side Lying position, perform the roll very slowly, or perform the roll very dynamically. Also, nothing prevents you from using your arms to push off the ground with your hands, forearms, or elbows and facilitate rolling; however, you can learn more about the mechanics of this particular movement by learning to do it with your arms stretched (which can be necessary if you're doing the movement while holding something in your hands).

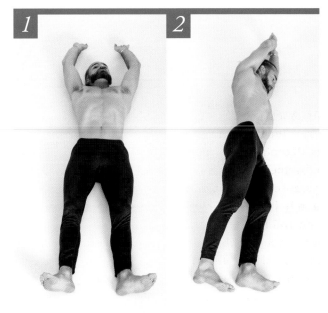

(continued on next page)

1 Assume the Supine Lying position, arms fully extended above your head.

2 Initiate the motion from a hip rotation in the direction you want to roll, shifting weight to the side of your body. You may assist the rocking motion by lightly pushing off the foot opposite to the direction in which you want to roll or by lifting your back leg (the one that's opposite the direction in which you're rolling) and swing it in the direction you want to roll.

3   As you keep driving the Side Roll through your hips, your center of gravity reaches a point beyond your base of support. At this point, you can relax and let gravity effortlessly pull you to the Prone Lying position.

4   From the Prone Lying position, you may roll back to your original Supine Lying position or roll farther in the same direction as your first roll. If you choose to keep rolling in the same direction on a flat terrain, you should use the momentum generated by each "fall" from the Side Lying position (forward when rolling from Supine-to-Prone Lying and backward when rolling from Prone-to-Supine Lying). Of course, if you use the Side Roll down a hill, gravity pulls you without extra effort on your part. If the slope is steep, you might not even be able to control your speed and will have to change your position to stop.

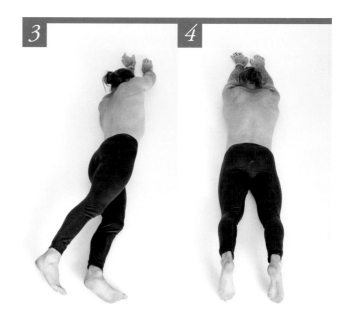

Prone-to-Supine Side Roll

The Prone-to-Supine Side Roll is slightly more difficult to execute because of the human body structure. From the Supine Lying position, our hips rest on the soft, rounded part of the body: the rear. In the Prone Lying position, our hips rest on the hard, bony part, which is a natural obstacle that makes rolling using only hip rotation quite challenging.

There are three strategies to propel your body into a Side Roll from the Prone Lying position.

- Push off from the forefoot that's on the opposite side to the direction you want to roll to assist hip rotation.

- Push off from the forefoot that's on the side that's in the direction you want to roll to shift your body weight and elevate your body slightly in the opposite direction and then use the momentum generated by gravity pulling your body weight down to roll easily in the intended direction.

- Lift your back leg (the leg opposite the direction in which you want to roll) to help lift your hip off the ground and assist your hip rotation.

Front-Rocking

You can use Front-Rocking to precede get-up techniques and make it easier to transition to a Squat or Kneel. The backward motion is also a natural part of the Backward Roll. As a drill, Front-Rocking is great for abdominal strength and spine mobility, especially if you rock back all the way to your upper back. Unlike many other movements, a supple rounded back is necessary for performing this movement efficiently.

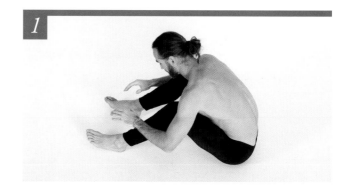

1   Position yourself in a Bent Sit, leaning forward.

SAFETY NOTE

It's important that you control the backward momentum and do not end up rolling back farther than your upper back. The back of your head may slightly and briefly touch the ground, but in no way should you shift any body weight onto it. Putting body weight on your head could potentially strain your neck. If you roll past your upper back, you're engaging in a Backward Roll, and you should shift weight to one of your shoulders. To be on the safe side, keep your rocking amplitude low at first—rolling only to your lower back before you begin rolling back forward. You can progressively increase how far back you roll.

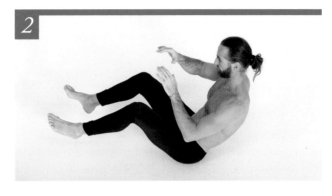

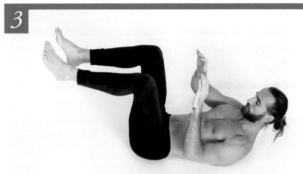

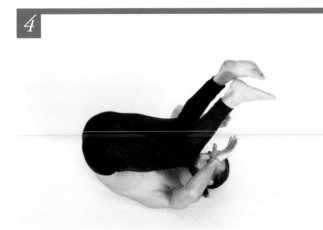

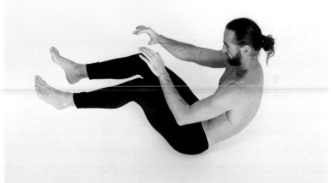

(continued on next page)

2 You may slightly push off your feet or lean backward to shift weight to the back of your rear. Your feet and legs elevate, which helps you reach a point where your center of gravity is beyond your base of support. You're pushing yourself off balance and allowing gravity to pull you back and down.

3 As gravity pulls you back and down, smoothly shift weight from your rear to your back while pulling your bent legs up and toward your chest.

4 Forcefully contract your abdominal muscles to pull your rear higher and your legs farther back so your feet are above your head or slightly beyond. You're shifting your body weight and rolling all the way to your upper back.

5 When you've rocked as far back as you're going to go, hold the position of your rounded spine and let gravity pull and rock you forward. If you rocked backward with the intention of using the forward momentum to get back on your feet, you may drive your hips and legs forward and down more swiftly to generate a stronger forward momentum that will enable you to easily transition to your feet.

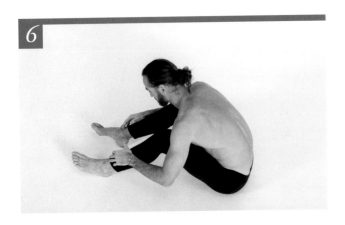

6 You reach the starting position (a Bent Sit) and are ready to rock back again if you're doing a repetitive drill. If you're using the rocking motion to transition to a position on your feet, the position of your feet and legs depends on whichever transition you're going for. (Read more about ways to get up in Chapter 25, "Ground Movement 2: Sitting, Kneeling, Getting Up.")

A progression to this drill that also increases the benefit to abdominal strength is to perform it without letting your feet touch the ground at all, which prevents you from pushing off your feet and legs to generate backward momentum. In that case, start the movement with both feet off the ground. You may bring your bent arms in front of you with your hands in front of your face or on top of your head in a protective stance.

Backward Roll from Supine Lying

The lying Backward Roll allows you to change your body orientation from supine to prone. You also can change your body direction so that your head points in the direction your feet had been pointing before the roll. The Backward Roll from Supine Lying can be quite useful in situations that require you to stay low to reduce your visibility or exposure, for switching position for observation or aiming at a target, and so on. When you start from a higher stance, such as a standing position, you can use it as a fast and smooth transition to a Prone Lying position, to disperse impact forces upon landing, or as a recovery from getting off balance and tipping backward.

As a drill, the Backward Roll from Supine Lying movement is a safe way to begin to practice for the Backward Roll; for the Backward Roll, the progression goes like so: from sitting, from a Half Squat, from standing, and finally from landing from various heights. Before you can work through that progression, you must make sure that you fully control the pattern, which you can do by practicing the roll without any momentum. The Backward Roll from Supine Lying pattern is where you begin the roll—first doing it without any rocking motion. Beginners tend to roll in random directions and end up lying at an angle; although this is acceptable, it should be the outcome only because you intend it rather than because it merely happens without your control. Your goal is to ensure a linear roll, which means that once the roll is done, your Prone Lying position is aligned with your starting Supine Lying position.

TECHNIQUE TIP

Remember to maintain ample and relaxed abdominal breathing while rolling to facilitate relaxation and T-spine mobility.

⚠ SAFETY NOTE

It's important that you control the backward momentum and do not end up rolling back farther than your upper back. The back of your head may slightly and briefly touch the ground, but in no way should you shift any body weight onto it. Putting body weight on your head could potentially strain your neck. To be on the safe side, keep your rocking amplitude low at first— only rolling to your lower back before you begin rolling back forward. You can progressively increase how far back you roll.

⚙ TECHNIQUE TIP

Some people find it helpful to start with straight legs so that they don't try to kick themselves over. Keeping your legs straight forces pure abdominal contraction that's coupled with a little momentum from your legs.

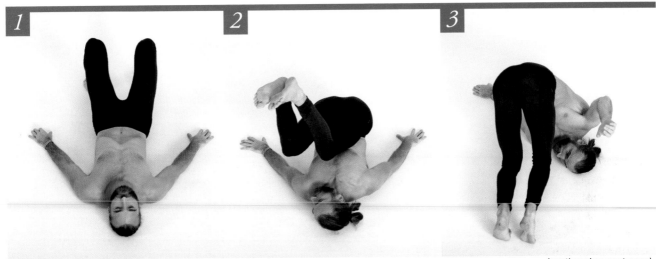

(continued on next page)

1   Start in the Supine Lying position with your legs bent. Your arms are extended to the sides of your body in a V shape, palms down.

2   Stabilize your position with your hands and arms and lift your rear and legs off the ground and toward your head using strong abdominal contraction. Your lower body is leaning slightly sideways at an angle, but not so much that you fall to the side. Start turning your head in the direction of the shoulder you will roll on, which enables you to see where you will place your feet on the ground. The more you turn your neck toward your shoulder and tuck in your chin, the more comfortable the movement feels.

3   Keep pulling your lower body up and back so that your feet are above the ground beyond your head as you shift your body weight onto the back of your shoulder. Your opposite shoulder is starting to come off the ground. Make sure to protect your neck by keeping your head clear of supporting any body weight.

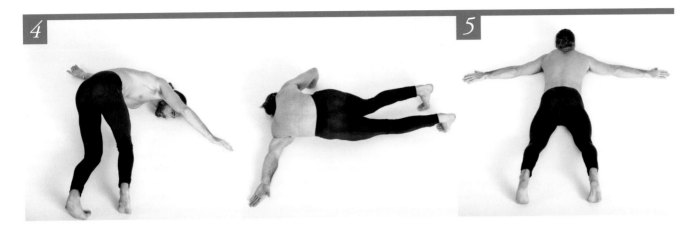

4 Your body weight is now almost fully supported by the shoulder. Use your arm on that same side to stabilize your body and prevent it from falling sideways as the balls of your feet reach the ground; using your arm also helps stabilize your position. The arm on the opposite side of your body is off the ground. If you want to roll back linearly, which means closely aligned with your original position and direction, you need to make sure that you place your feet behind your head to make an invisible straight line between the original position of your feet and head. When you reach a point of balance where your center of gravity is right over your base of support, all you need to roll is to push off your shoulder and bring your center of gravity beyond your base of support; gravity takes over at no extra energy cost. The weight of your body pushes on your legs, so you can let your feet slide on the ground at a controlled speed. As you roll back, you accompany the rolling movement of your body by rotating your shoulder and arm on the ground (see the close-up photo) to facilitate smooth repositioning into the Prone Lying position.

TECHNIQUE TIP

Remember to maintain abdominal breathing while rolling to facilitate relaxation and T-spine mobility.

5 Finish the roll with your body fully flattened against the ground and your arms fully extended to the sides of your body. Optionally, you can extend your arms overhead in front of your body.

SAFETY NOTE

With both the Backward and Forward Roll, you do not want to roll straight along the body's midline, which would involve rolling over your spine (or onto your neck) and could potentially expose it and make it vulnerable to hard objects on the ground. Instead, you roll from one shoulder to the opposing hip, with the spine contacting the ground for only a very short time on a very small area.

SAFETY NOTE

When you're doing a Forward Roll, it's essential that you not push body weight onto your neck, and it's also imperative that you turn your neck and head in the *opposite* direction of your weight-bearing shoulder and tuck in your chin. Keeping your head straight—or worse, trying to turn it in the same direction as the weight-bearing shoulder as you do in the Backward Roll—would result in straining your neck or even badly hurting it.

Drill: Half Backward Roll

The most important part of the Backward Roll is to reach the flexed-spine position while you're resting on a single shoulder with the balls of your feet touching the ground behind your body. You can reduce the movement to just that part of the movement and do it as a drill. As soon as your forefeet touch the ground, immediately push off the ground and let gravity pull your body back down into a supine flexed rocking motion. As you rock and roll back again, make sure to alternate which shoulder you're rolling to.

Forward Roll from Prone Lying

The practical applications for the Forward Roll are the same as the applications for the Backward Roll. You perform it with your arms extended along the sides of your body, extended at an angle from the body, or extended perpendicularly to the body. In any case, it doesn't make sense to try to sneak your arm underneath your torso before you roll.

As you start practicing the roll from a higher stance such as Tall Half-Kneeling or standing, one arm can be turned inward and down toward the hip before you roll. This option allows you to start dispatching the greater impact forces with a line running from the back of your hand to the shoulder instead of placing your shoulder on the ground with your arm extended.

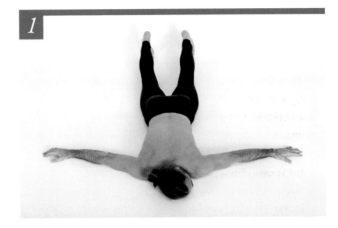

1   Assume a Prone Lying position with your arms extended perpendicularly to your body. (Optionally, you can extend your arms along the sides of your body or angle them slightly from your body). Your feet rest on the forefoot. Your head is already turned in the direction opposite of the weight-bearing shoulder.

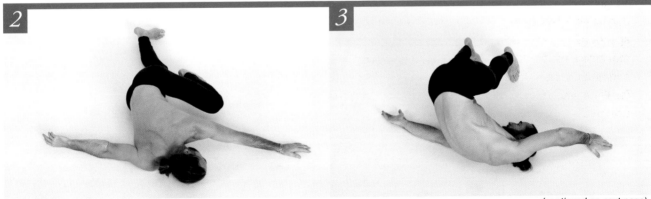

(continued on next page)

2   Push off the balls of your feet and bring the leg opposite your weight-bearing shoulder forward in a wide step, placing your foot at about hip level. This move starts positioning your body sideways in the direction of your weight-bearing shoulder. Begin protectively tucking in your chin.

3   Optionally, you can use core strength to make two or three small steps forward, elevating your hips off the ground and pushing your rear upward. Note that this option is a bit slower than the option described in step 2.

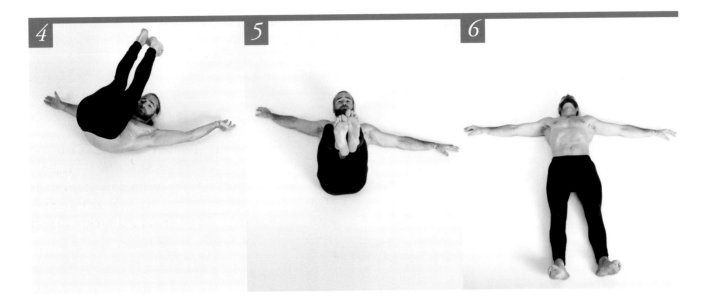

4 Push off the foot of your bent leg to drive your body forward with your rear up while you shift your weight onto your weight-bearing shoulder. Avoid pushing your body straight toward your head and neck.

5 You have pushed off your feet and fully extended your legs. The balls of your feet are still on the ground, ready for the final push that will make your center of gravity go beyond your base of support so that your body topples and unfolds to the other side. Both your arms are on the ground to stabilize your body and direct your upcoming roll. Also, you should be inwardly rotating your shoulder and arm during this phase to facilitate the smooth repositioning of your body in the Supine Lying position.

You're now rolling to the other side at no extra energy cost. Gravity is pulling your weight and lower limbs down. Immediately turn your head to verify that you're headed in the right direction.

6 As you unfold your legs, you still can adjust the direction of your body to some extent by moving your hips.

When you end, you have repositioned your body to "land" your roll in exact alignment with your starting Prone Lying position, only you're now in a Supine Lying position.

You can conveniently practice the Back and Front Rolls from a lying position because the body's orientation reverses from supine to prone as you do each roll. Make sure to practice both rolls on both shoulders, first in a straight line—reversing the orientation of your body without changing its direction—and then rolling at different angles.

Progressions for Both Rolls

- Perform a controlled roll, both slow motion and dynamically, without using momentum (such as forcefully pushing off your feet or rocking at the start).
- Perform the roll without assistance from your arms, both in slow motion and dynamically, which requires perfect core control. If you have issues not using your arms, you may bend and tuck them with your hands on your chest so that you avoid placing them on the ground.

- Roll at a controlled angle—for instance, at a 90-degree angle—so that you're oriented in a different direction upon landing.
- Roll from a higher position—such as squatting or standing—then after landing on your feet after a jump.

Lying Crawls

Lying crawls enable continuous motion over a distance as you stay as close to the ground as possible. You use a lying crawl when it's the best contextual option or simply because the context leaves you with no other option at all. Technically speaking, lying crawls are all about efficient alternation of points of support to reduce the normally large frictional surface and resistance that comes with lying positions.

Shoulder Crawl

The Shoulder Crawl is a fast way to crawl in a Supine Lying position. This crawl enables you to go under and/or through very low—and sometimes narrow and long—obstacles. If necessary, you also can hold and carry a relatively light object or load in your arms. If you tend to be stiff in your shoulders, this is a great movement for loosening them because shoulder mobility (and hip rotation) are essential for making this movement effective.

Although you might have to execute this movement in a nonlinear path in a real-life context, I recommend that you first practice this technique in a perfectly linear way to make sure you have good spatial awareness and body control.

The Shoulder Crawl is deceptively easy, especially because it is a full contralateral pattern that relies on a base of support of an opposing foot and shoulder to work efficiently. Although you rotate your hips, you must avoid hinging your hips if you want to move in a straight line as efficiently as possible. You may practice by following a line drawn on the ground (or a line of tape on the floor); try to follow the line without looking. This is a more technical movement than it appears if you want to do it efficiently.

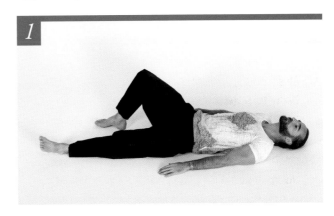

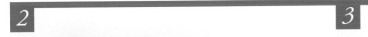

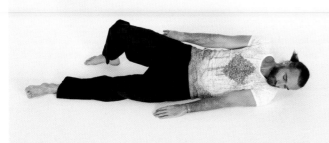

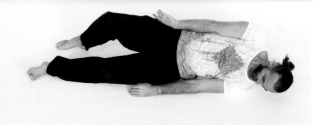

(continued on next page)

1 From the Supine Lying position, slightly flex your leg to bring one foot within a few inches of your rear and plant your heel firmly by flexing at the ankle. If the terrain is slippery, you may bring the foot a little farther toward knee level to give your heel more friction on the ground when you extend your leg. Keep the other leg extended.

2 Use your hips to shift your body weight to the side of your body that's opposite of your planted foot. This greatly reduces the surface of contact of your body with the ground. Keep your head slightly above ground the whole time.

3 Press down on your heel to maintain friction and extend the bent leg to push your body up while both your heel and weight-bearing shoulder stay anchored where they are. Extend your leg until you feel that you have reached full shoulder depression, meaning that your shoulder is as far away from your ear as it can be. As you are extending the leg, pull the opposite shoulder toward your ear.

4 While shifting your body weight to the opposite direction, slide your other foot to bring it slightly closer to your rear and plant the heel firmly to repeat the preceding steps on the other side. Keep your free shoulder pulled up toward your ear so that, as it reaches the ground, it will be placed as far forward in your path as possible, which maximizes the distance you cover per rotation.

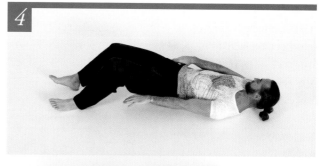

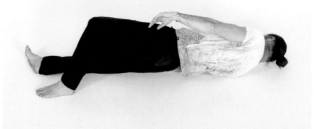

This is the exact same position that I describe in step 2, but from the opposite side. Now repeat the same sequence, keeping your body aligned on a longitudinal axis and your shoulders relaxed. Maintain ample, relaxed abdominal breathing.

There's are some faults and inefficiencies you should avoid for an efficient shoulder crawl:

- Using ipsilateral movement—in other words, trying to push with the foot and leg on the same side as the supporting shoulder, which makes you lean to a single side, makes it harder to be balanced or to press down on the heel to generate friction, and creates superfluous tensions and slows the movement.

- Bringing the foot too close to the rear and bending the leg too much. The length of leg extension should be short enough to match the limited range of motion of the supporting shoulder. When you keep pushing off the leg after you've reached maximum shoulder depression, you will force your hips to move out of line. This makes your path a zig-zag in a Hip-Thrust Crawl fashion rather than a line.

- Back pedaling if you are not pressing the heel down when you extend the leg.

- Using limited range of motion in the shoulders, which limits how much distance you cover during each cycle. If you notice this issue, sit up and rotate your shoulders backward fluidly and with maximum amplitude and then resume the crawl.

- Hip hinging or flexing the spine when the body rotates to the side orientations, which disturbs the rest of the positional sequence or could give a zigzagging motion to your trajectory.

- Breathing intermittently, which is usually related to overall stiffness, especially in the shoulders.

- Trying to stay flat on your back and slide back. If the terrain and your clothing make sliding easy and energy-efficient, sliding while flat on your back can be a good idea; otherwise, you will struggle.

Alternatively, you can practice the Shoulder Crawl in a Prone Lying position, although it's much more difficult and slower to do it this way.

Hip-Thrust Crawl

The Hip-Thrust Crawl is an effective way to move while you're lying on your side. Because you're moving in a direction opposite to your orientation, this movement enables you to put distance between yourself and a threat while you maintain eye contact with it (so you can promptly react as the situation evolves). When you use the Hip-Thrust Crawl, you also can hold and carry an object in your arm. In combat situations, you can use the same movement to bring your legs between you and an opponent who's on top of you in the mount position or side control.

In both practice and real-world situations, you can do the Hip-Thrust Crawl by pushing off both legs or a single leg and moving along one side of your body (so you move in a straight line) or alternating sides (so you move in a zig-zag). You can look at it as the human version of the lateral undulation or sidewinding that some reptiles do.

The single-leg Hip-Thrust Crawl described in the steps is more challenging than using both legs because it is a contralateral pattern that relies on opposite foot and shoulder as the base of support. Start your practice by planting both feet and pushing off both legs before you switch to the single-leg version.

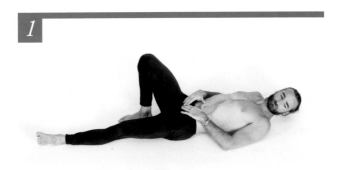

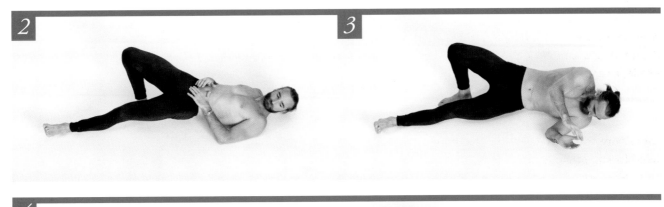

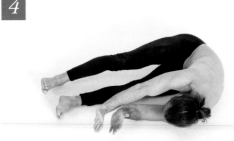

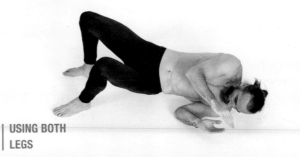

USING BOTH
LEGS

1   From the Supine Lying position, look in the direction opposite to where you intend to move and bend the leg on the side of your body that's opposite to where you're looking. Pull the foot of the bent leg as close to your rear as possible if you want to generate maximum power and distance; otherwise, you don't have to bring your foot as high.

2   Press the heel into the ground then push off it to elevate your rear and prepare for your hips to move rotationally.

3   Shift your body weight sideways toward the shoulder that's opposite your bent leg to reduce friction and allow full extension of your legs to move your hips backward. During this phase, your base of support should be located between your heels and shoulder.

4   Press down onto your heels and maintain mild ankle flexion to help maintain friction from the heels and prevent them from sliding as you forcefully push off your leg. Extend your leg fully, driving your hip as far as possible to the back, then let the side of your body come back in contact with the ground. Depending on the context in which you're doing the crawl, you may fully extend your arms during the motion as if you were pushing something away with them, flex your arms and keep them close to your chest and off ground, or bend your arms in front of your face in a protective fashion. Bring your heels close to your rear to repeat the entire sequence again on the same side. Alternatively, you can set your body to replicate the same sequence on the other side.

Half-Press & Full-Press Prone Lying Positions

With the Half-Press and Full-Press Prone Lying positions, you elevate the upper body with the support of your arms as you remain in a lying position with your legs and hips in contact with the ground. These movements are useful when you want to transition from lying to crawling or the other way around, need to crawl very low and elevate your field of vision to observe or scan your surroundings, or are trying to reach something while staying close to the ground.

The Half-Press and Full-Press Prone Lying positions start to open your hips, lumbar spine, thoracic spine, and shoulders, as well as shift body weight onto your palms, wrists, elbows, and shoulder, which is a great preparation for crawling movements. Look at the photos before following the suggested routine.

TECHNIQUE TIP

Remember to maintain abdominal breathing.

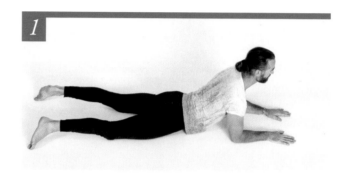

1 Half-Press Prone Lying

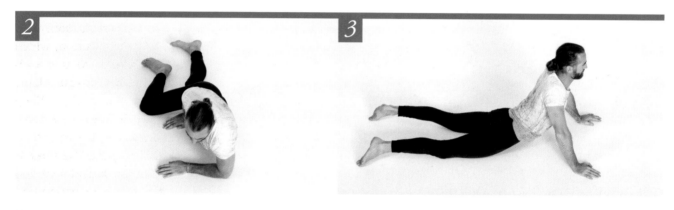

2 Half-Press Side Prone Lying Hip-Trunk Rotation

3 Full-Press Prone Lying

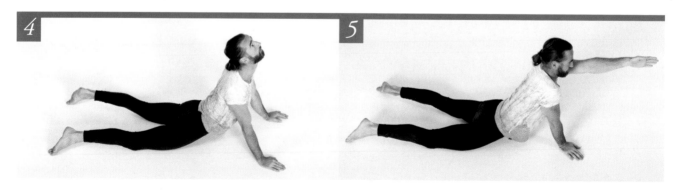

4 Full-Press Prone Lying Head Tilt

5 Full-Press Prone Lying Front-Arm Extension Off the Ground

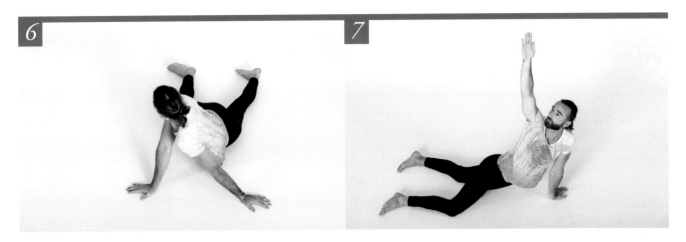

6 Full-Press Prone Lying Hip-Trunk Rotation

7 Full-Press Prone Lying Hip-Trunk Rotation with Upward Arm Extension

Half-Press Prone Lying Positions

Assume a Prone Lying position. Bend your elbows and support your upper body on your forearms with your hands open and flat on the ground. Keep your hips down, but don't force them to press all the way down onto the ground if it doesn't happen naturally. Now, change the position of your forearms to be a bit wider, narrower, farther forward, pointing inward, or pointing outward; you also could shift body weight between your arms. Maybe support your head with one hand. Stretch your arms forward or sideways. Turn your head to the side or look up.

Extend one arm forward, to the side, or up. Stretch and reach as far as you can. You could try to reach a real object or surface to make the movement completely real.

Protract one shoulder (pull it forward) and retract the opposite shoulder (pull it backward) and rotate your hips so you can look backward, on each side.

Full-Press Prone Lying Positions

Now place your open hands on the floor at about head level or just behind your head and press up. Both arms are fully lengthened, in the lockout position, which means that your arms are externally rotated with your elbow joints facing your body and your elbow creases facing forward for increased stability. Keep your hips down, but don't force them to press down onto the floor or force the lumbar spine to extend and reach a state of discomfort or pain. The same is true when you rotate your hips, trunk, and neck and extend your arms. Find and maintain a position that is comfortable or challenges you slightly. You can explore a variety of positions that are similar to the positions you did with your forearms on the ground, such as looking back or reaching with one arm to the front, side, back, or up.

Crawling *on* All Fours:
Feet, Knees, Elbows, Hands

It's time to move on to quadrupedal crawling patterns, which implies the support from all four limbs and support from the knees, elbows, and hands. With quadrupedal crawling patterns, the center of gravity is elevated above ground, which tremendously reduces friction and enables much faster motion than lying. It also gives you greater ability to clear slightly elevated obstacles in your way. From quadrupedal positions you can very quickly change your orientation or revert to lying positions, and you also can transition to standing positions much faster than from lying. You have several options in terms of the points of support you choose—feet, knees, forearms, or hands—which enables you to easily change level. Using your knees and forearms makes for a very strong and stable position but slower motion, whereas using your feet and hands enables you to move at the fastest crawling speeds possible.

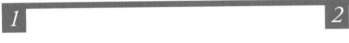

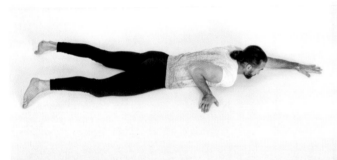

1   Start in a Prone Lying position with one arm fully bent to the back just below shoulder level; your hand is flat and externally rotated so your fingers are pointing to the side or the back. Your other arm is reaching to the front with a slight bend in your elbow; your hand is aligned with your shoulder.

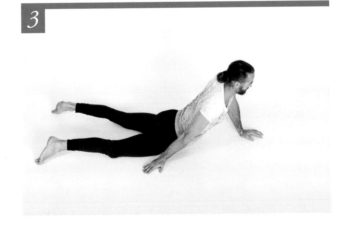

2   Push off your back hand and press down your front hand to elevate your chest slightly off the ground, then keep pushing your back arm to elevate your chest and front arm more.

3   Finish pressing off and extending both arms to fully elevate your trunk. From there you can reposition your torso and arms in their original positions, or you can switch to the same arm position using the opposite arms.

Rotational Knee-Forearm Crawl

This movement is a contralateral prone crawling technique used to move underneath obstacles that are sufficiently wide but not tall. Uses include moving into and through confined areas to stalk animals or to move to safety while avoiding being seen or reducing your visibility. This movement is also convenient for crawling uphill while staying low. The same rotational hip pattern, which is the driving motion for the movement, can be used with a knee-hand, foot-forearm, or foot-hand base of support.

Even though this crawl makes you look like you are lying, you are moving with your upper legs, hips, and trunk off the ground most of the time. Because this pattern is best known as the "army crawl," it is seen as a grueling, brutal movement based on raw conditioning. The perception is that you mainly pull yourself forward using your arms. In fact, it is a very efficient technique that mostly uses the powerful and lasting motion generated by hip rotation that pushes off the knees. Depending on the terrain and the friction you get, it is indeed sometimes necessary to pull hard from your forearms when your knees are sliding back. Otherwise, you should let your hips and core do most of the work. You should be using just the amount of tension you need in your arms to move them forward while keeping your trunk off the ground. You can do the exact same pattern in a rotational foot-forearm fashion; however, if the terrain is slippery, it won't work as well as being supported by your knees. You also can do this movement in a rotational foot-hand crawl, although a regular Foot-Hand Crawl without hip rotation is more efficient in most cases.

1. Start in a contralateral Prone Lying position. On one side of your body, your leg is fully bent and tucked forward with your foot open and flat on the ground with your heel close to your rear. Your arm on that same side of your body is tucked backward, palm down. On the other side, your leg is extended to the back, and your hip is resting gently on the ground. Your arm on that side of your body is bent and placed forward in front of your body with your hand aligned with your head. In a typical contralateral position, the arm and leg on one side of your body are close to each other, and on the other side of your body they're away from each other.

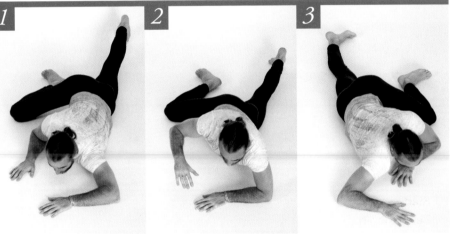

2. Contract your abdominals, then push off your back knee to drive your hips forward. As your hips and chest elevate, press down your front forearm to support your trunk off the ground and allow it to move forward. Simultaneously, pull your back arm up and forward in a relaxed fashion.

3. As your hips reach maximum elevation, your base of support runs from your back knee to your front

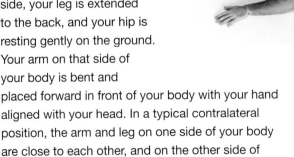

(continued on next page)

elbow. With the shoulder of your supporting arm reaching above or slightly beyond elbow level, rotate your hips to shift your body weight to the opposite side. Through this rotation and as you keep pushing off your supporting knee, pull and bend your back leg to tuck it to the front and on the ground while placing your back arm to the front of your body. The position should be like the starting stance, just on the opposite side, and you can resume forward motion.

You can move backward by reversing the sequence. Going backward is not harder or more energy-consuming than the forward motion if you keep mainly using your hips and core.

4

4   Rotational Foot-Hand Crawl

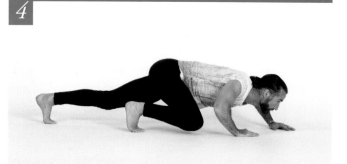

Contralateral Single-Foot, Single-Hand Drill

The Contralateral Single-Foot, Single-Hand drill could be a practical foot-hand movement if you're trying to reach something in front of you. Otherwise, this is a fantastic way to learn and develop foot-hand contralateral balance. To start, you can do this drill from a knee-hand position, especially if it is too challenging in the foot-hand position.

1   **2**

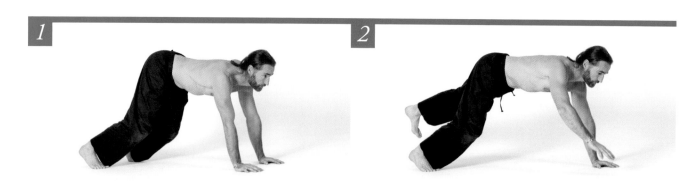

3

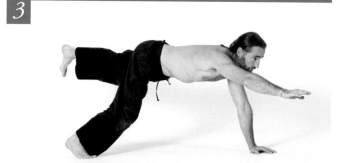

1   Start in a square foot-hand position with your feet and shoulders mostly aligned but with slightly more body weight shifted toward your feet so your shoulders are slightly behind hand level.

2   Contract your abdominal muscles and glutes. Release one hand and the foot on the opposite side to establish a stable Single-Foot, Single-Hand Contralateral position.

3   You may challenge yourself further by fully extending the off-ground leg and arm to the back and front. Regardless of how far you extend your arm and leg, hold the two-points-of-support position briefly and then get back to the square foot-hand position and replicate the same exercise using the opposite arm and leg.

Foot-Hand Crawl

The Foot-Hand Crawl is probably the most "animal-like" crawling pattern of all. As a matter of fact, it is best known as the "bear crawl" (as if bears have a monopoly on this style of crawling). Most terrestrial mammals are quadrupedal, meaning they move on all fours, as do baby humans before they learn to stand erect and walk. The Foot-Hand Crawl enables you to cover longer distances at a faster speed than any other crawling techniques. It also potentially enables you to balance on a narrow surface; pass under, over, or through obstacles; and carry a load. There are a great number of faults that can occur when you perform this deceptively straightforward and easy natural movement. Those faults don't prevent you from being effective, but they certainly lower your efficiency and fatigue your body.

Let's talk about the good form first, starting with the easier way to do it: the 4/3 points of support sequence.

4/3 Points of Support

In this pattern, regardless of forward or backward direction, the position continuously and alternately relies on four and three points of support: two feet and two hands, two feet and one hand, two feet and two hands, one foot and two hands, two feet and two hands, and so on. By alternating points of support that way, the position and movement is always well-grounded and stable. You alternate between a contralateral position and an ipsilateral position each time you regain four points of support. This sequence is a great compromise between speed and balance/stability. The position is more compact than the 4/2 points of support version. Overall, the 4/3 version doesn't demand as much joint and core stability as the 4/2 version.

TECHNIQUE TIP

Do your best to keep a neutral spine (or close to it) as you do the movement. Depending on how far you extend your hands and feet, your base of support may become a bit more compact, forcing you to round your back slightly, which isn't a big issue.

1   Start in a contralateral foot-hand position described earlier with your feet and hands staggered. Both legs are half bent, and both arms are in the lockout position. Your head is slightly tilted back; tilt it just enough to allow forward vision.

2   Shift your body weight onto the front hand while keeping your arm strong in the lockout position. Release your back hand and move it toward the front.

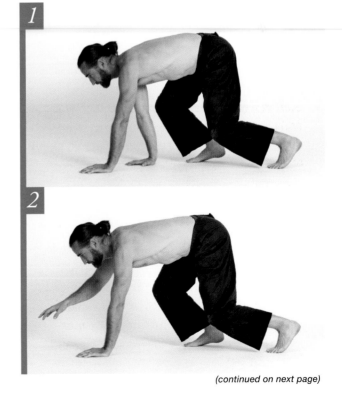

(continued on next page)

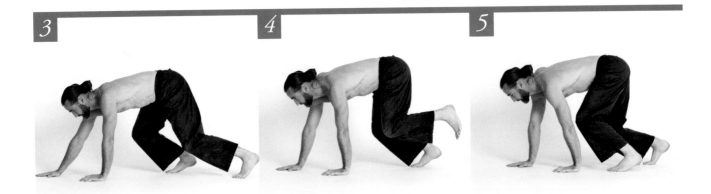

3 As the shoulder of your back arm is vertically aligned with the palm, place the hand down to the front and establish an ipsilateral foot-hand position.

4 Shift your body weight onto the front foot so you can release your back foot and pull it forward.

5 Place the foot you're moving in front of the grounded foot and re-establish the same staggered, initial contralateral position (but on the other side).

Apart from the obvious and usual positional inefficiencies, such as an overly rounded back, bent arms, hyperextended neck, intermittent breath, and overall stiffness, the following are some of the typical issues for this pattern:

- Being confused about the timing of when each limb should move, which messes with your positioning and generates even more issues. Make sure that you fully understand the difference between an ipsilateral and contralateral foot-hand stance and that you can intentionally position yourself in either position at any time if you become confused and need to reset your position.

TECHNIQUE TIP

For practice, you can reverse the sequence to go backward or move sideways either in a shuffling fashion or "weaving" with your limbs crossing the midline of your body.

4/2 Points of Support

In this pattern, the position continuously and alternately relies on four and two points of support in a contralateral fashion: two feet and two hands, opposite foot and hand, two feet and two hands, opposite foot and hand, and so on. This variation requires significantly more joint and core stability because of the contralateral phase on two points of support. Once you learn this pattern, you can more easily maintain great spinal alignment and a smooth, fluid, precise replication of position on each side, which prevents the usual inefficiencies of the 4/3 points of support pattern. This pattern also is the more reliable pattern when you're balancing on narrow surfaces.

1   Start in a longer contralateral foot-hand position than described earlier, with your feet and hands positioned farther to the front and back and your spine fully elongated. Both fully extended arms are making an inverted V shape running from your shoulder girdle down to the ground. Both your legs are half bent, and both arms are in the lockout position. Your front knee is almost touching the front elbow, whereas the back knee and front foot are aligned. Your head is tilted back just enough to allow forward vision.

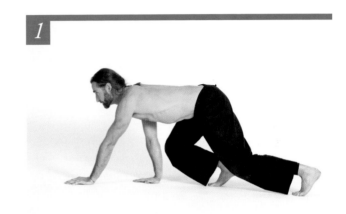

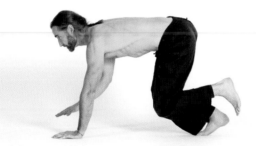

2   Shift your body weight onto your front hand and front foot so you can release both your back hand and foot at the same time. Immediately pull the back hand and foot toward the front. The moving arm and leg should pass the supporting arm and leg at the same time. You can see in the photo that the moving arm and leg are practically hidden behind the supporting arm and leg. Keep the supporting arm strong in the lockout position and the supporting foot, ankle, and knee very stable.

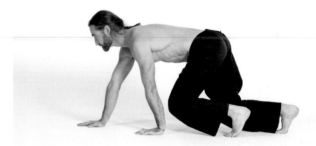

3   Keep driving your body forward until you can place the moving arm down to the front, re-establishing the exact same start position (but on the opposite side). Ideally the moving hand and foot should reach the ground at the same time, but there might often be a very brief difference of timing. You pause while you're on the four-points-of-support base; otherwise, you want to make it as brief as possible, spending most of your time on two points of support and very little time on four. Repeat the sequence.

As always, "perfect form" is that which adapts best to the context, and the Foot-Hand Crawl is no exception. You might have to lower your body to pass underneath an obstacle, which turns it into a Rotational Foot-Hand Crawl; extend your legs and elevate your hips to momentarily relieve your arms or step through an obstacle; or decide to step your feet far forward as if you were ready to explode into a sprint at any second. If you make these adjustments consciously and intentionally, they are efficient modifications. Otherwise, they are blatant faults.

NOTE

You must maintain impeccable joint stability to stay stable during this phase. Lack of joint stability alters how you land your foot and hand and your next four-points-of-support position, which itself compromises the next move. If this phase of the sequence gives you trouble, revert to practicing the contralateral Single-Foot, Single-Hand Drill described earlier.

Inverted Foot-Hand Crawl

Most people know about this movement, which is commonly called the "crab crawl" (even though I don't see the connection with crabs). However, most people struggle with the Inverted Foot-Hand Crawl because of inefficiencies, including improper breathing, position, and timing, as well as because of lack of relaxation or mobility. This technique requires great shoulder, elbow, and wrist mobility, so it's common to see people being quite uncomfortable just from assuming the Inverted Foot-Hand Crawl position.

You can't move as quickly with the Inverted Foot-Hand Crawl as with the prone Foot-Hand Crawl. The Inverted Foot-Hand Crawl is most often used when you must move down moderate to steep grade slopes with challenging surfaces (slippery, muddy, rocky, and so on). In this case the supine position on all fours, with a low center of gravity and a more erect torso, allows you to maintain greater balance and control over the orientation of the body than standing, and it prevents a backward fall from standing, which could injure your wrists, elbows, and (most importantly) spine and head. You can use this movement on flat ground to move across a slippery surface. Another use of the Inverted Foot-Hand Crawl is to go either backward or forward to create or close a distance with something while keeping an eye on what is going on. In that case, your body and head are oriented in the direction where vigilance is required, regardless of the direction your body is going.

The Inverted Foot-Hand Crawl is primarily a leg-powered movement. By default, when you have your arms locked out, they are externally rotated. It is possible to internally rotate the arm, but this tends to internally rotate the shoulders, which in turn tends to make you round your upper back, so there is zero advantage to that. An internal arm rotation uses more triceps and shoulder strength, and it's much more prone to resulting in flexion at the elbow and hunched shoulders, whereas external rotation helps stabilize both the elbow and the shoulder to stay retracted, which consequently contributes to the stability of the upper spine. The stable upper body and arm position supports pulling or pushing through your legs and enables you to pause anytime, including on a single arm, with great stability and economy; the internally rotated arm does not allow this. However, internally rotating and even flexing the arms with your elbows out can be handy if you need to press or push more from the arms and upper body, usually when there's an obstacle in the way.

There are several versions of the Inverted Foot-Hand Crawl. The 4/3 points of support variation is the most used (as with the prone Foot-Hand Crawl). In this variation, you move one point of support at a time, alternating between three and four points of support, which also alternates between ipsilateral and contralateral positions. If you don't want to think too much about your movement at first, do it this way, and in most cases, the movement comes naturally.

The 4/3 points of support method is stable but slower than the contralateral, 4/2 points of support pattern (which is also like the prone Foot-Hand Crawl). This variation is faster but more challenging because you must be more stable and have impeccable position, sequence, and timing.

Last, the ipsilateral, 4/2 points of support pattern is effective but highly inefficient. Try it for yourself. All you need to do is start in an ipsilateral position (feet and hand away from each other in staggered positions on both sides). Shift your body weight to the foot and hand on one side of your body so you can release the foot and hand on the other side and travel them forward. It's somewhat fun, but awkward and quite inefficient.

The photo sequence displays a 4/2 points of support pattern. You can use an easier, more stable 4/3 points of support pattern both for training and for real-life purpose, but in terms of skill training, it is not as beneficial as the 4/2 version, which challenges and improves your joint stability and balance much more.

Moving Backward

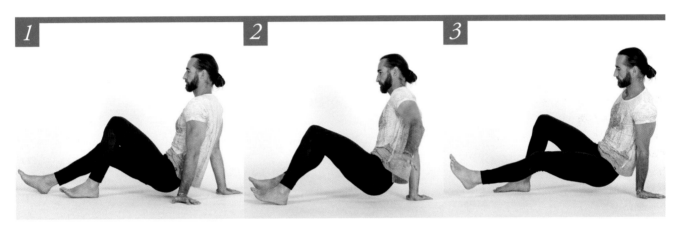

1 Start in a typical contralateral stance. On one side of your body, your foot and hand are relatively close to each other and on the other side the foot and hand are wider apart. Your ideal position should be comfortable—neither too wide nor too compact. Both arms should be in the lockout position, and your shoulders should be retracted. Lifting your foot and planting your heel firmly on the ground will get you greater friction, especially when the terrain is slippery.

2 Shift your body weight to the back foot and hand to prepare a contralateral two-points-of-support base then immediately release the front foot and hand and start pulling the arm and leg toward the back.

3 Pull the rear foot backward and place it on the ground, with your knee bent. At the same time, extend the trailing arm behind your body. Ideally, the moving foot and hand should reach the ground at the exact same time, and your body weight should shift on them so quickly that you can lift the opposite foot and hand off the ground immediately in a contralateral stance opposite to the start position.

You may mark a pause in the four-points-of-support base if needed; otherwise you want to maintain momentum and spend most of the time on two points of support and very little time on four.

Repeat the sequence entirely from the start. For optimum technique, your ideal position is replicated very closely on both sides every cycle, except when the terrain imposes modifications in changes for the sake of adaptability.

TECHNIQUE TIP

To improve your stability in the two-points-of-support contralateral stance (photo 3), hold it on the spot for a few seconds and then switch sides. You may also shift your body weight forward and backward a bit (moving your shoulder in front of or behind vertical alignment with the palm).

Moving Forward

When you're moving forward, the main technical key point is to use your heels as "anchors" and pull the body forward through the legs. This simple cue will correct the common perception that you should push yourself forward only through the arms, which is very costly from an energy standpoint. When you imagine pulling your body to the front from your feet, you use your legs much more, which distributes the load and effort more equally through the upper and lower body.

TECHNIQUE TIP

If you lack space or want to develop better technique in both directions, you may combine backward and forward motion over a short distance, moving two or three steps forward and then reversing direction.

Faults

Typical faults in the Inverted Foot-Hand Crawl (regardless of direction) include having an overly compact stance, keeping your torso too vertical with a rounded back, hunching your shoulders, bending your arms, and trying to push your body forward or backward while relying only on the arms. You want to open your position more, lock out your arms, pull your shoulders back (like you're proud), plant your heels, and pull or push from the legs to drive the hips. Remember to keep breathing abdominally.

TECHNIQUE TIP

Before I continue with other types of ground movements, I want to mention general tips about training progressions after you've learned crawling techniques. Incorporate the following progressions and variations into your practice as you gain more experience:

- Increase distance
- Increase speed
- Increase distance and speed
- Change directions
- Transition from one technique or variation of a technique to the other
- Increase environmental complexity by practicing on diverse terrains, including uneven, smooth, rugged, slippery, soft, hard, inclined, and declined surfaces
- Crawl facing the opposite direction you're going: backward going up inclined surfaces, forward going down declined surfaces, at an angle on inclined and declined surfaces
- Crawl over, under, and through obstacles, especially narrow ones
- Add a load that you carry on your back, chest, or lap
- Crawl while pushing or pulling an object

25
Ground Movement 2: Sitting, Kneeling, Getting Up

Bipedal motion is the most fundamental aspect of human movement, as well as one of the main features that make us humans. However, there is a wide range of movement patterns that we must acquire before standing is even possible. Those movement patterns are part of the foundational development that we all go through in infancy before we can stand and walk. This chapter covers ground positions that you hold, for the most part, with your torso erect as you work up to elevating the body to be standing on your feet in a Deep Squat position.

As I've mentioned in other parts of the book, our modern lifestyle has significantly narrowed the variety, frequency, and range of motion of the movements we do every day. Sitting, kneeling, and getting up suffer from the same limited range that other movements do. You might find yourself rediscovering some positions and movements that you haven't used in decades, which will lead you to realize the tremendous movement and health potential these basic movements represent.

Therefore, before we seek efficiency when standing tall on our feet, we need to recover function and movement quality with a "from-the-ground-up" approach. I teach you to progressively elevate your body from sitting to kneeling then to getting up and standing by gradually building your positions and movements toward a bipedal stance.

Unlike other natural movement skills, such as jumping and climbing, most of the movements in this chapter are inherently low-intensity. For the sake of increasing intensity, you can eventually repeat the get-ups at high speed or add a load; otherwise, the difficulty and value of these patterns resides in mobility, stability, postural integrity, breath control, relaxation, and fluidity.

Because these movements aren't flashy and are low-intensity, most fitness programs completely neglect them; people don't see these patterns as belonging to the "workout" category. At best, a small number of the movements are used as a supplemental set of "mobility" drills, but the perception is that sitting, kneeling, and getting up are not supposed to get you "results." Well, in my opinion, regaining the ability to sit on the floor, squat, kneel, and get up and down with ease is a kind of result that health-wise matters much more than losing an inch off your waistline. Do you agree?

Sitting, kneeling, and getting up are natural movements we should never abandon, and we should continue using them daily as we progress into our advanced age. As a matter of fact, the results you get from practicing all the movements in this section are vital to health and well-being. Brazilian researchers did a study that showed that the ease or difficulty middle-aged and elderly people have with sitting on the ground and getting back up without support is a predictor of longevity. Those people who needed to use both their hands and their knees to get down and back up were nearly seven times more likely to die within six years. The study also showed that this movement ability wasn't just a matter of lower-body strength; it was a matter of mobility, stability, balance, and coordination.

NOTE

If you'd like to read more about the study from the Brazilian researchers, read "Ability to Sit and Rise from the Ground as a Predictor of All-Cause Mortality" at *http://journals.sagepub.com/doi/abs/10.1177/2047487312471759.*

Consequently, a big part of this chapter is dedicated to diverse strategies for getting up and down, starting with easier movements that involve your knees and hands and progressing to the more challenging patterns that use no support other than your feet. However, getting up and down starts with being comfortable with the lower-level positions of sitting and kneeling.

The positions and movements in this section are apparently easy, but you might be surprised by how much some of them will challenge you. You need frequent practice and patience to restore great posture, balance, relaxation, and fluidity in all these movements. Remember, ease in getting down and back up is a factor in your longevity, so engaging in consistent practice every day helps conserve your freedom of movement and ensure a lengthy life.

Sitting

Is sitting worse for your health than heavy smoking? Probably not, yet scientific studies are gathering increasing evidence of the link between sedentary physical behaviors, such as prolonged sitting, and deleterious health outcomes.[1] People who sit hours a day have higher mortality rates than those who do not. The link between heart disease, diabetes, depression, and sitting is now scientifically well-established. Prolonged sitting is even linked to brain thinning, which is a precursor to cognitive decline.[2] You don't need to be launched into space to be affected by the adverse physiological effects of a zero-gravity environment, such as loss of bone density and muscle mass. All you need to do is to stay put in a chair, move very little, and have little movement interaction with gravity.

We eat meals, study, work, read, and play games while sitting still on elevated seats such as office chairs or couches; our legs are extended below our bodies with our feet resting on the floor. When we travel, we sit. When we're waiting for something, we sit. Even when we work out in big commercial gyms, we mostly sit at exercise machines! Sitting is what most of us do every day, most of the day, mostly in the same position, which is usually a bad position—and it is killing us.

[1]Stuart Biddle, Jason Bennie, Adrian Bauman, Josephine Chau, David Dunstan, Neville Owen, Emmanuel Stamatakis, & Jannique van Uffelen. "Too Much Sitting and All-Cause Mortality: Is There a Causal Link?" *BMC Public Health* 16 (2016): 635, www.ncbi.nlm.nih.gov/pmc/articles/PMC4960753/.

[2]"The More Hours You Sit per Day, the Smaller Your Medial Temporal Lobe (MTL) Seems to Become, Brain Scans Show." SharpBrains website, April 17, 2018, accessed June 18, 2018, https://sharpbrains.com/blog/2018/04/17/the-more-hours-you-sit-per-day-the-smaller-your-medial-temporal-lobe-mtl-seems-to-become-brain-scans-show/?mc_cid=9096e9c805&mc_eid=1146690848.

Throughout the history of mankind, sitting hasn't always consumed as much of our time as it does today; it's quite a recent phenomenon. There are still many countries where people do not spend most of the day sitting; when those people do sit, they do it quite differently than we do in the industrialized world. They sit directly on the floor or ground to work, rest, wait, talk, play, meditate, and pray, and they use diverse stances and usually display great posture.

Unfortunately, we cannot significantly offset the negative impact of sitting too much by exercising. Standing all day is not an effective antidote, either; the adverse effects of prolonged standing are well known. But we can look at the bright side of sitting and approach it in a healthier way whenever possible.

Let's consider the positive aspects of sitting:

- Sitting is a practical movement ability that allows you to take a break and rest, wait, observe, or work.

- Sitting can help improve or restore your mobility if your body has gotten stiff over time; sitting also helps you maintain mobility.

To become functionally beneficial, you should frequently sit by assuming diverse positions at ground level. The more comfortable you are sitting in natural, ground-level fashion, the more comfortable you will become for getting up from sitting to standing positions and getting down to sitting from standing positions.

Variety in sitting positions is important for two obvious reasons:

- From a practical standpoint, one sit position may be more appropriate for a given surface or use than other positions.

- From a functional standpoint, you should be able to hold any sit position comfortably.

Practice

Technically, sitting is a position supported by the buttocks or thighs. Your legs can be bent or unbent, parallel or crossed, and your feet level with the rear (unless you're seated in a raised sit). Your torso is mostly upright; sometimes you're leaning forward, backward, or sideways, and sometimes your arms also support you.

In this part, you're not going to learn any "sit" technique, but you will rediscover the great variety of sit positions available when sitting directly on the ground. I also give suggestions of how you can make it a mindful, beneficial, healthy practice. You might notice that the more sit positions you practice and the more frequently you practice them, the better your mobility gets.

You'll also see immediate benefits to other movement skills, including squatting.

First look at the many sitting positions I cover. To name them I have used terms that are relatively self-explanatory and describe the position of the legs such as long (extended on the ground), bent, closed (close to each other), open (apart), crossed, or side.

Start with any position and hold it a few seconds before slowly transitioning to another one. This simple practice immediately turns sitting into a movement more than a stationary stance. Unless you are meditating, are in pain, or have no other choice, you should never sit too long in one position. You may transition more dynamically as you feel more comfortable. Don't hesitate to lean forward or sideways and use some support from your hand or the tips of your fingers if a position is challenging to you. The idea is to shift some of your body weight to another body part for scalability. Over time you will gradually become able to hold more erect sit positions without support from your arms. Resist the temptation to turn sit positions that are difficult for you into a stretching workout by forcefully holding it for minutes in a row while neglecting the other positions. Instead, keep transitioning through various sit positions and go back to the more challenging positions more frequently. You also can hold the challenging position a little longer than you hold the others. For instance, you might target a challenging sit position by holding it a few seconds, switching to another position for a moment, and reverting to the challenging position. Continue alternating the positions in this way.

"Perfect" Is Meaningless

Remember that no position is "perfect" or set in stone; like any natural movement, natural sit positions are adaptable. For instance, I don't make it mandatory that all sit positions should systematically display a "perfectly" vertically aligned posture from tailbone to neck. Some do, and some don't. However, if by default your back is rounded and you cannot intentionally align it vertically, you lack mobility. Except in cases where the position is intentional, a rounded lower back when you sit on the ground shows that the pelvis is tilted in posterior position. If you are unable to tilt it to the front (anterior tilt) or at least to neutral, then this is a limitation you need to work on. Therefore, it's important to practice specifically to improve postural integrity while sitting, and the position of the pelvis is as important as the alignment of the upper back. Remember that your ability to maintain postural integrity more than a few seconds lies in muscular endurance, which requires regular practice to develop; but if you are fighting against a lack of mobility, it shortens how long you can hold erect alignment.

To make the sits even more engaging and beneficial, practice the following movements as you sit:

- Sitting with upright tall posture for a few seconds, relaxing to a rounded back position briefly, and then holding an erect posture again.
- Maintaining tall posture as you lean forward, backward, and sideways. When you lean forward, bend at hip level (anterior tilt) while maintaining a tall posture.
- Shifting body weight to each buttock alternately.
- Tilting the pelvis (anterior, posterior).
- Undulating your hips and pelvis. This means that you make your hips and pelvis move in a wavelike motion.
- Undulating your spine all the way to the neck (it can be done together with the hips and pelvis).
- Reaching your arms in many different directions. This is a fantastic way to open up the upper body (shoulders, scapula, and thoracic-spine) because reaching isn't achieved through the arms alone. You can reach in many positions beyond ground positions, and it helps with skills such as catching, climbing, grappling, or striking. When you practice arm reaches, always imagine that you are trying to grab something that is almost out of reach because that thought pushes you to extend as much as you can and immerse yourself in a practical mindset. Make sure that you reach with both arms alternately and do not hold your breath.

Just explore, explore, explore! It's even more fun, practical, collaborative, and engaging to combine sitting with throwing and catching a light object (ball, stick) with a partner while both of you constantly switch your sit positions. Whichever way you choose to practice your sits, always maintain breath control.

Surfaces

You can practice your sits anywhere that is flat and allows you to switch freely from position to position. If you need a bit of cushioning, a mat, thick rug, folded blanket, bolster, grass, or sand will give you the comfort you need. Avoid surfaces that are too soft because they give you a false assessment of your mobility and ease and prevent your joints from truly benefiting. Avoid surfaces that are too hard—unless you feel sufficiently comfortable on them—because they might hurt your bones and discourage you.

When to Practice

The best way to practice is to substitute conventional and functionally detrimental sitting with natural, healthy sitting as often as you can. Try sitting on the floor or ground whenever possible to eat, read a book, work on a laptop, watch TV, and so on because these are times that you would normally be sitting anyway. When you're practicing a series of diverse natural movements, you may use sit variations as part of a routine that emphasizes mobility, or you can add sits between high-intensity movements that you're doing in intervals (you spend the low-intensity intervals practicing sit positions). Once you have acquired ease and comfort in most or all sit positions, keep practicing your sits regularly as an integral part of your Natural Movement lifestyle.

Sit Positions

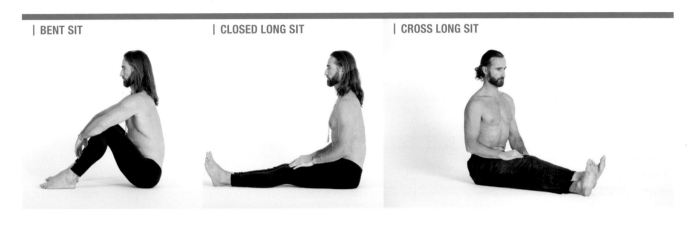

| BENT SIT | CLOSED LONG SIT | CROSS LONG SIT |

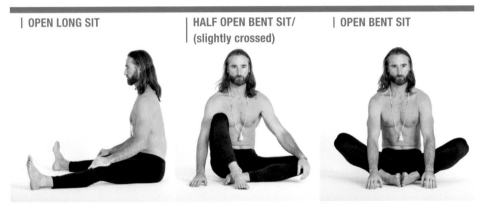

| OPEN LONG SIT | HALF OPEN BENT SIT/ (slightly crossed) | OPEN BENT SIT |

In the Open Bent Sit, both feet are placed in front of your pelvis; your soles are against each other.

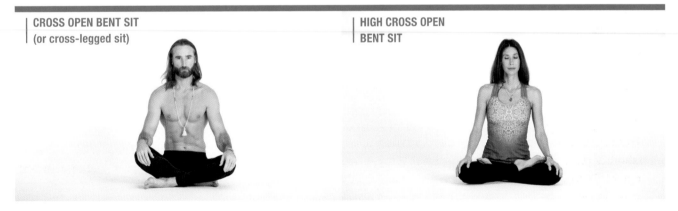

| CROSS OPEN BENT SIT (or cross-legged sit) | HIGH CROSS OPEN BENT SIT |

The Cross Open Bent Sit position might be the most common sit position across all cultures; it's also known as "tailor" or "Turkish" style. In Japan it's called *agura,* and it's considered to be a position that's exclusively for males. Each foot is placed underneath the thigh of the opposite leg.

In the High-Cross Open Bent Sit, rest each foot on the opposite upper thigh so that the soles of your feet face up. A variation involves having only one foot resting on the opposite thigh while the other rests on the ground. This position is best known as the Lotus.

| BENT LONG SIT | OPEN BENT LONG SIT

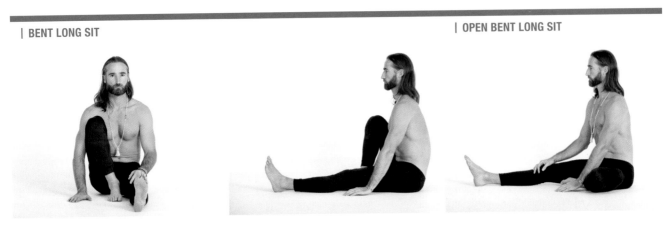

| SIDE BENT SIT | OVER CROSS OPEN BENT | CROSS HALF OPEN
                                   | LONG SIT | BENT SIT

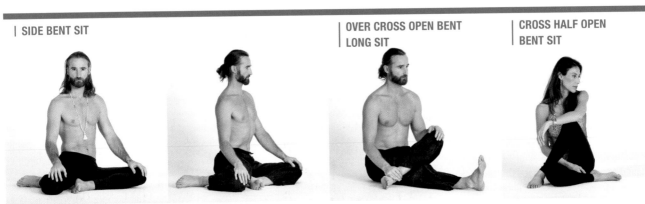

In the Side Bent Sit, your base can be wider with your
front foot and back knee apart, or the base can be
narrower with your back knee resting on your front
foot.

Below are examples of sit positions that have been more or less modified for practical
or practice purposes or for the sake of comfort.

| CLOSED LONG SIT WITH ARM | BENT LONG SIT WITH SLIGHT | CROSS LONG BENT SIT WITH
| REACH | SIDE LEAN AND ARM SUPPORT | SIDE LEAN, ONE-HAND
                                                               | SUPPORT

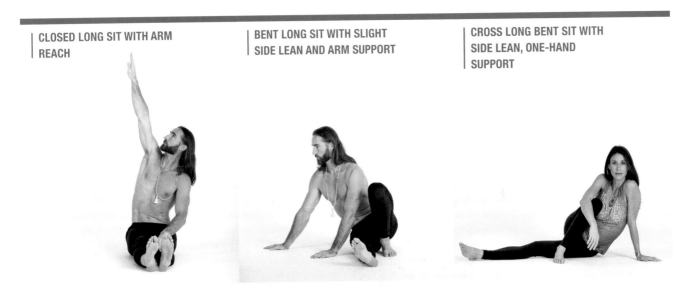

OPEN BENT SIT LEANING BACKWARD,
TWO-HAND SUPPORT

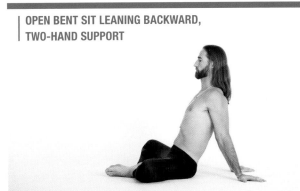

CROSS BENT SIT SIDE LEAN WITH THIGH AND
FOREARM SUPPORT

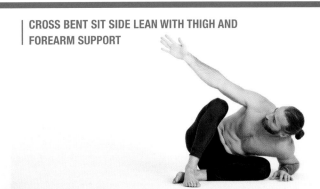

HIGH CROSS BENT SIT, PRONOUNCED FORWARD
LEAN, ARMS EXTENDED AND RESTING

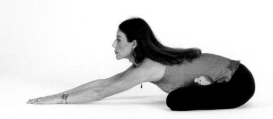

SIDE LONG BENT SIT, PRONOUNCED
FORWARD LEAN, ARM REACH

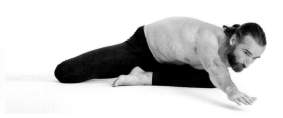

Raised Sit

Most elevated surfaces can be used as seats for humans, whether they are man-made specifically for sitting, such as chairs, stools, and benches, or natural items like dead trees and rocks. An elevated surface by itself doesn't make a raised sit; indeed, you can sit on an elevated surface while keeping your feet at the same level as your rear as if you're on the ground.

In most cases, what constitutes a "raised" sit is the fact that your legs are extended down away from your rear and below your body, usually with your feet resting on the ground. (Of course, there are differences in how you can hold your legs—for instance closed, open, crossed, forward, backward, feet at ground level, feet elevated on a footrest, or feet dangling.) This form of sitting isn't "unnatural" per se, and it's not bad in any way if you do it for relatively short periods of time with good posture.

NOTE

An alternative form of raised sitting is straddle sitting on a low-elevation surface with your legs bent and your knees and feet above the ground or very lightly resting on it.

Remember, it is the way we sit—raised and with a rounded posture and poor breathing for extensive durations—that is harmful. The problem with the raised sit is that mobility is in no way necessary in the same way it is when we sit directly on the floor or ground with our feet level with our rears. For instance, prolonged raised sitting causes overall muscle tightness, including shortening the hamstrings. The result is that over time it becomes difficult to sit with comfort on the ground, and we experience mobility and function issues that decrease overall movement performance. Also, most people end up rounding the whole back and having slouched shoulders, which in turn impairs breathing and has numerous physiological consequences. If you are going to be in a raised sit position for long periods, you won't be able to avoid the negative physiological consequences of almost complete physical idleness, but you can at least reduce the negative consequences of prolonged rounded back and poor breathing by ensuring the best position you can.

NOTE

If you spend hours sitting and could use a way to mitigate some of the negative impact of it, you can regularly press down on your flat feet as if you intend to stand up. You naturally start pressing down on your feet to ground yourself and start contracting your legs and rear, which also lengthens your spine. You can go as far as tensing your muscles enough to actually lift your rear for a brief moment. This would be some very beneficial movement if you could do it every few minutes. A "hidden" benefit of doing this is that it makes you physically want to stand up and move, as that's the reflex grounding your feet triggers.

Side Bent Sit Reverse

The Side Bent Sit Reverse is a good example of one of those sit transitions I have encouraged you to do to turn sitting into a movement practice (in this case though, the position itself is the same, just held on the opposite side). Switching the Side Bent Sit directly from one side to the other is a fantastic hip opener movement.

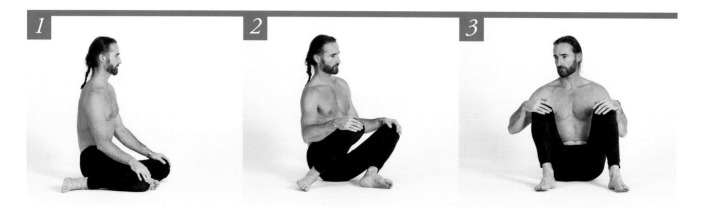

1   Start in Side Bent Sit (or, if you start in the Bent Sit, you need to move your legs sideways to the side stance). Rest your hands on your knees. Let your knees naturally reach the lowest position without forcing them down with your arms.

2   Lift your legs off the ground. You initiate the motion from your hips, or "core," not the legs.

3   As soon as you reach the neutral Bent Sit position, look to the other side and keep focusing on driving the motion through your hips, not your legs.

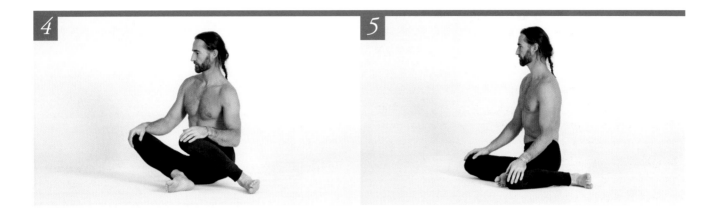

4 Depending on your mobility, this is maybe the lowest point you will be able to reach without discomfort and without trying to force your legs down by pushing them with your arms. Accept whatever range of motion you can reach. Just try to relax tension that you feel. Exhale longer to help release muscular tensions. Another way to help progress is to post one arm for support and to lean back on it to allow your hips more space to move until you gain the mobility you need to do the movement without arm support.

5 If possible, reach the full range of motion with both legs touching the ground while keeping an erect posture as much as possible. Maintain abdominal breathing always, spending more time on the exhale.

Kneeling

Kneeling is most often held with the whole body resting on both legs, which are bent under the body, and the rear sitting on the heels; it's primarily used as a rest stance. (See the photos on the opposite page.) But kneeling in Natural Movement involves many more variations—used to wait, work, listen and/or observe, meditate or pray, and even hunt or fight—beyond the neutral "kneeling" stance everyone is familiar with.

With Natural Movement variations, kneeling means any position where most of the body weight is supported by both knees, or even a single knee, while the rear is or isn't resting on the heels; the position may involve diverse leg positions (especially with half-kneeling positions). Clearly, this makes kneeling more than a rest position; it's a varied set of highly adaptable positions with many practical uses, such as staying low and close to the ground to stalk, wait,

observe, work, paddle a canoe or raft, and transition to crawling, squatting, or standing.

To name the positions and describe their distinctiveness, I have used simple terms:

- **Tall:** The position is elevated with the rear away from the heels.
- **Half:** One leg is being supported by the knee, and the other is supported by the foot.
- **Split:** One knee is in front and the other is behind.
- **Open:** The knees are wide apart.
- **Open-Foot:** The foot is externally rotated and resting flat on its inside.
- **Flexed-Foot:** The ball of the foot is resting on the ground.
- **Single:** Standing on one foot or one knee only.

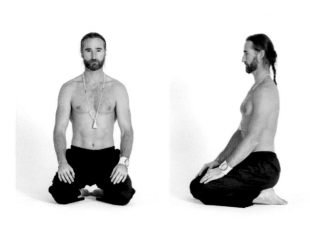

- **Extended:** You're in a half-kneeling position with your hips driven all the way forward toward the front foot.
- **Long and side:** The leg is positioned or oriented in a certain direction in half-kneeling positions.

As I've previously mentioned, none of these positions is a "pose" to be exactly replicated with "perfect form"; they're natural, adaptable positions that are subject to endless modifications for the sake of practicality, comfort, or specific mobility benefit.

To start practicing kneeling positions, review the "When to Practice" and "Surfaces" sections for the sit positions (see page 223).

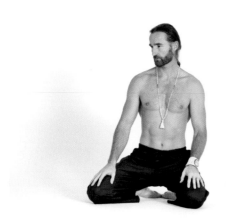

In kneeling, which is known as *senza* in Japanese tradition, your knees can be closed or wide open, feet crossed or apart, neutral or internally/externally rotated. Your body weight is evenly distributed between your knees, shins, and the tops of your feet (although the distribution of body weight can vary).

| KNEELING WITH ARMS EXTENDED UPWARD | KNEELING WITH BACKWARD LEAN | KNEELING WITH PRONOUNCED FORWARD LEAN AND HEAD TILT |

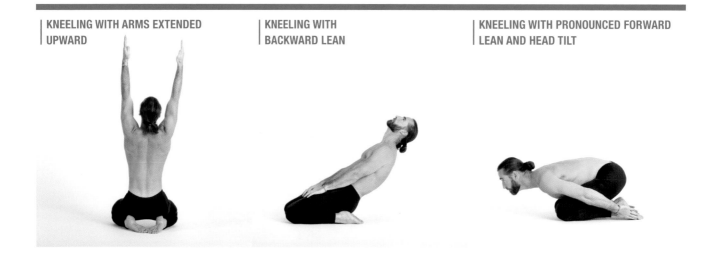

KNEELING WITH SIDE LEAN AND SIDE ARM EXTENSION

SINGLE OPEN-FOOT KNEELING

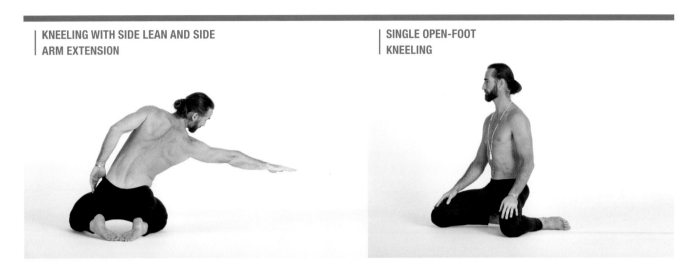

TALL KNEELING
(base can be neutral, closed, or wide)

FLEXED-FOOT TALL KNEELING

SINGLE-KNEE TALL KNEELING

TALL KNEELING WITH SIDE LEAN AND UPWARD ARM EXTENSION

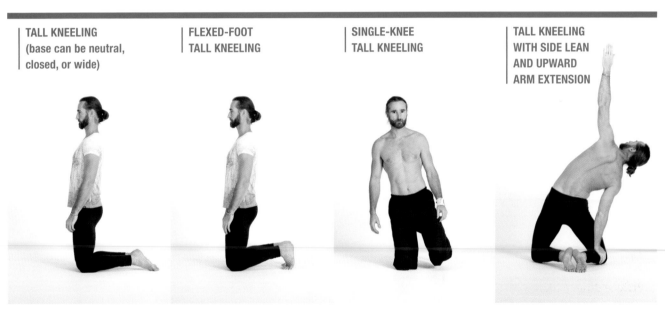

TALL KNEELING WITH TRUNK ROTATION

FLEXED-FOOT TALL SPLIT KNEELING

SPLIT KNEELING

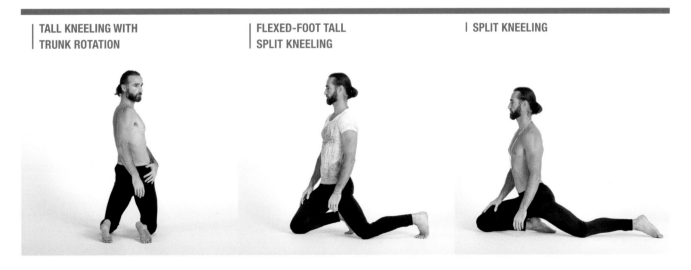

TALL SPLIT KNEELING

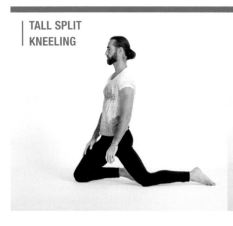

SINGLE OPEN-FOOT SPLIT KNEELING

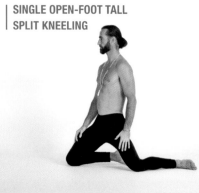

FLEXED-FOOT OPEN-FOOT SPLIT KNEELING

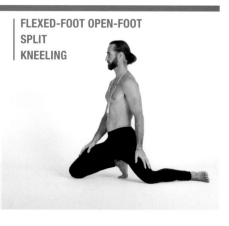

HALF-KNEELING

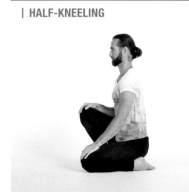

FLEXED-FOOT HALF-KNEELING

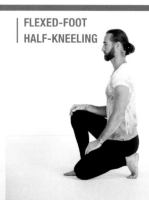

OPEN-FOOT HALF-KNEELING

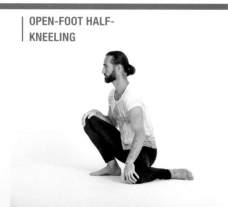

LONG HALF-KNEELING
(leg extended to the front)

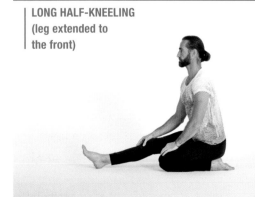

LONG FLEXED-FOOT HALF-KNEELING
(leg extended to the side)

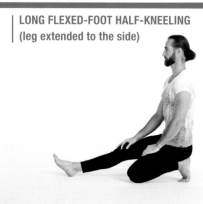

SIDE LONG FLEXED-FOOT HALF-KNEELING

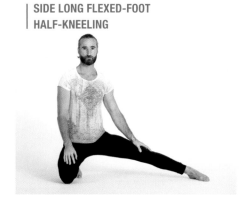

OPEN HALF-KNEELING

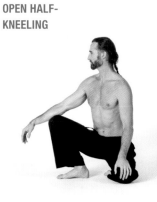

OPEN FLEXED-FOOT HALF-KNEELING

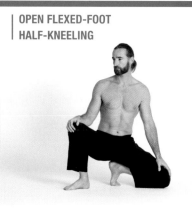

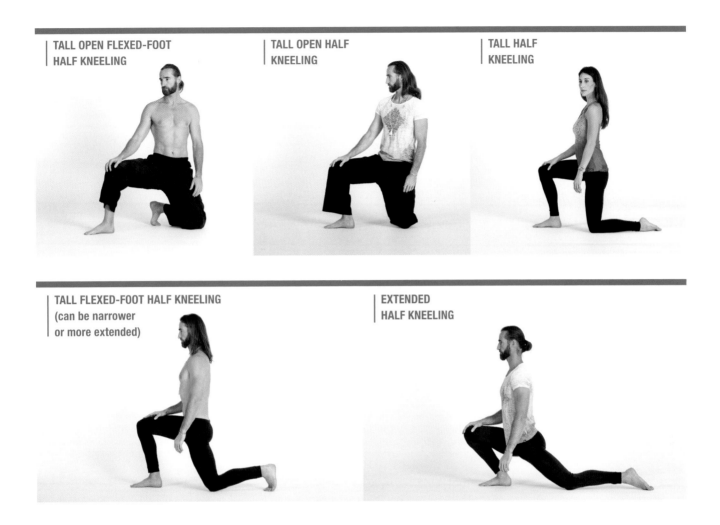

TALL OPEN FLEXED-FOOT HALF KNEELING

TALL OPEN HALF KNEELING

TALL HALF KNEELING

TALL FLEXED-FOOT HALF KNEELING (can be narrower or more extended)

EXTENDED HALF KNEELING

Kneeling Movements

If you've practiced several of the kneeling positions I've described, you have already been practicing kneeling movements, which implies entering and exiting kneeling positions. Movements don't have to be of great magnitude to be movements; a simple shifting of body weight from one knee to the other or elevation of the rear off the heels turns kneeling from a position to a movement. These small adjustments are extremely important and valuable. You can turn any of these types of movements into an endless list of drills to practice several times in a row. For example:

- Kneeling, shift body weight from side to side
- Kneeling to Tall Kneeling

- Kneeling to Flexed-Foot Tall Kneeling
- Half-Kneeling to Flexed-Foot Half-Kneeling
- Flexed-Foot Half-Kneeling to Side Long Flexed-Foot Half-Kneeling
- Half-Kneeling to Tall Half-Kneeling to Extended Half-Kneeling

Any of the kneeling transition movements you can create on your own can be turned into short routines with wonderful benefit to lower-body mobility. One of these transitions, the Open Half-Kneeling Reverse, has *enormous* benefit to foot, ankle, knee, and hip mobility.

Open Half-Kneeling Reverse

You could be resting in the Open Half-Kneeling stance while observing something or conversing with someone and need to reverse your orientation. Instead of elevating your body to a taller position before switching orientation, which is slow or could draw un- wanted attention, why not smoothly reverse your position while keeping your body level?

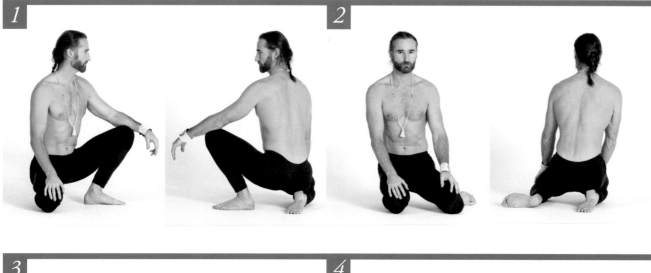

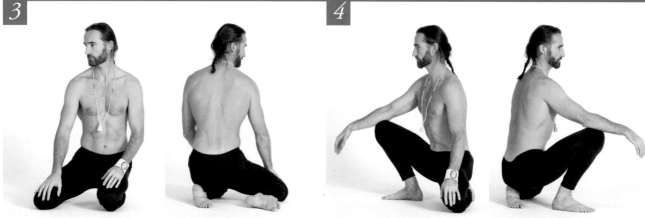

1 Start in the Open Half-Kneeling position.

2 Shift all your body weight to the leg that's bent under you, which removes all body weight from the side leg. Bring the side leg and knee all the way down, keeping an open foot flat on the ground.

3 Now shift all your body weight onto the opposite leg while making sure that the open foot internally rotates underneath your rear. Make sure the other foot externally rotates to an open-foot position that points toward the side you are turning to. The rotation of both feet happens simultaneously.

4 Lift the opposite, non-supportive knee while turning your torso to the side. As the foot naturally repositions itself flat on the ground, drive your hips slightly forward to re-establish a balanced base of support over both legs. You may rest your arms on your knees or wherever you need them to be.

Unless you do it intentionally, moving to the Tall Open Half-Kneeling position or leaning the upper body forward before reversing—or both—is a sign of deficient mobility, a sign of inefficiency (you possess the mobility to do the same movement better), or both.

Squatting: *The* Position

Entering the bipedal, on-feet positions and movements is a huge step (pun intended)!

The squat is one of the most natural, fundamental human positions. (Standing is another one.) As a matter of fact, squatting precedes standing and walking in movement development. There would be no human, bipedal motion like walking, running, or jumping—or such ability would be significantly impaired—if we didn't first acquire the ability to squat.

In healthy humans, the squat is a rest position, a work position, a wait position, a stalk position, a play position, and a defecation position. All toddlers can do the squat masterfully before they even stand up and walk. For not-so-healthy humans, squatting has become an "exercise"—a punishing mobility drill we must force ourselves to do to regain basic function that we've lost through years of "normal life" that involves hours of elevated sitting every day and poor movement the rest of the time.

Squatting is more than just the ability to hold the squat position itself for its practical value; it's also the ability to transition down from the standing to the squat position or to transition up to squatting from a lower position.

Here I'm addressing the fundamental squat position (the Deep Squat) first. Later I explain squatting as a get-up movement, which is a complex transitional sequence; performing it well requires great amounts of mobility and stability in the most essential joints and muscles. Therefore, if you've already made progress with the Deep Squat position, you'll have more success with improving your squatting skill as a movement pattern.

Improving your squat—both the stance and the movement pattern—and honing optimally functional squat mechanics have tremendous benefits to many Natural Movement skills, to your overall natural athletic potential, and to your physiological health. This is the reason we study both in detail. First you need to be comfortable in the "bottom" position—the Deep Squat; otherwise you will be quite challenged squatting up or down, and you'll need to choose other movement strategies to get up from low positions to standing (or the other way around).

Why Practicing Squatting Is Important

Daily practice of holding the Deep Squat and other squat variations is fundamental to your freedom of movement, movement performance, and health. It assists with offsetting some of the damage done by hours of sitting or other forms of physical idleness. It helps improve other Natural Movement skills and enhances performance in these skills. It helps with bowel movement and improves your physiology and health. Unlike some other natural movements that may not need to be practiced every day, you should include squatting in your daily practice, and you should ideally do it more than once a day.

From a movement practice standpoint, squatting is a phenomenal exercise that provides easy progressions, regressions, and almost endless variations in positions and transitions. Squatting targets diverse gains in mobility, lower-body strength, and power, resulting in greater performance in many other areas of Natural Movement such as running, jumping, lifting, or striking.

Why You Can and Should Squat Practically Anytime, Anywhere

Here are practical examples for creating squatting opportunities in your day-to-day life: squat while watching TV, while reading a book, while working on your laptop, while brushing your teeth, while drinking your coffee or tea, while waiting for the bus, train, or plane. Squat to pick something up from the ground instead of bending over.

Why Improving the Squat Isn't Achieved by Practicing Only the Squat

Don't overemphasize passively holding one single squat stance for long periods of time at the expense of other squat variations, both in positions and transitions. Variability is key to making greater and faster progress. Similarly, don't obsess on only squatting to improve your squat while neglecting other ground movements. If you practice many natural movements, your overall mobility will profoundly benefit.

Is There Anything Like "THE" Squat Pattern?

When I teach squatting in one of my Natural Movement events, I like to show what looks like a horrendous squat form, with a fully rounded back and my knees caving in and touching each other. I ask my students if I'm using proper form. Almost unanimously everyone shakes their heads in disapprobation. However, my answer is different. If this is someone's squat form by default, and they can't hold any other squat position, then it is a horrible position. However, if someone uses this squat form intentionally and temporarily—for instance young kids often rest or play in that position—and the person could seamlessly transition to other squat variations, then that position is fine. I have said before that there is no such thing as an "all-purpose" position. Just like any other position or movement, the squat is not a one-dimensional position.

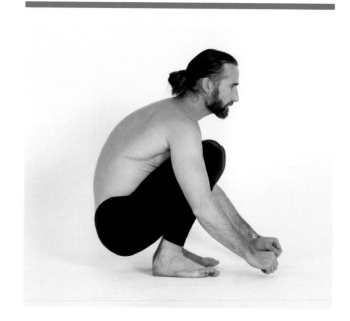

The squat is adaptable and should be easily adjusted for practical purposes (activity, terrain) whenever necessary.

There is a "neutral" squat position that should look approximately like what is shown in the photos. Here are the characteristics of that position:

- Your center of gravity is vertically aligned mid-foot (or center of the foot).
- Your feet are shoulder width or slightly narrower.
- Your toes point straight ahead or slightly outward (no more than 10 to 15 degrees).
- Your feet are flat, and your heels are fully connected to the ground. You don't have any tension in the feet and toes.
- Your thighs are relaxed; your hamstrings are resting on your calves/ankles.
- Your rear is horizontally slightly above, level with, or below your ankles. (The wider your base, the higher your rear.)
- Your knees are vertically aligned with your toes or are slightly forward and outward.
- Your lower back is slightly (but not overly) rounded.
- Your back is slightly leaning forward, but it remains straight or slightly rounded.

- Your head and neck are erect.
- Your arms can be relaxed in any position that doesn't throw your body off balance.
- Your breathing is ample and relaxed.
- Overall, your body feels well balanced, comfortable, and relaxed.

Neutral Base Deep Squat

This "ideal" squat might not look exactly like your own ideal, most comfortable squat form because you may naturally make some minor variations to suit your own individual body type. If we examine a line-up of several people with no mobility limitations who are holding the Deep Squat position, we might notice minor variations.

Keeping your feet pointing forward in the Deep Squat position challenges hip and ankle mobility more, but is it a good thing to forcefully stick with that detail when you're dealing with significant external loads (such as in a heavy loaded Squat Get-Up or Clean technique), the dissipation of force (such as in landing or catching), or intensive volume over a short period of time, when it already doesn't feel the most comfortable when holding the Deep Squat? Probably not.

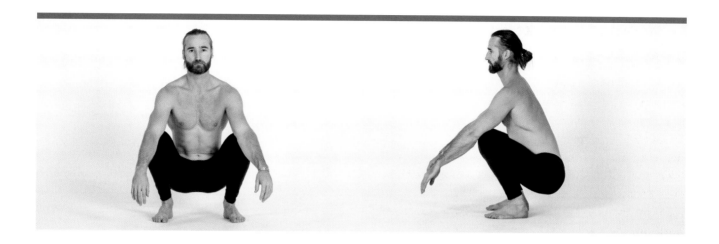

For instance, the inability to squat very deep may have to do with your body type (congenital skeletal structure) or physical history (accident, disease, specialized sports training) that is not reversible. So, it could be that nothing is wrong with "your" squat. Explore diverse squat variations, and you might find the ideal squat position for you. However, always ask yourself if other squat variations are not easy because of your physical makeup or because of mobility restrictions. In most cases, the reason is the latter. Be honest with yourself. If you are not too far off from the form shown in the previous photo and detailed in the checklist, you're good.

To assess your own Deep Squat position, you can do it in front of a mirror, have someone film you, or take a photo of it so you can have a more objective visual feedback of your position.

Lower yourself in a squat as deep as you can and adjust until you're in the most comfortable position. If you can't squat without falling back or assisting yourself with your arms to maintain balance, you have important mobility issues that this book will tremendously help you with. Once you have established your ideal bottom position in the squat, use the previous checklist to do a self-screen to compare your position with what I've described.

Following are the four main faults when you hold the Deep Squat position:

- Lack of depth (the rear cannot reach lower or much lower than knee level)
- Overly rounded back (upper or lower spine)
- Heels not connecting with the ground
- Knees collapsing inward

It's important to realize that positional issues with the squat such as those listed might be the symptoms of other underlying issues. (This is true of other movement techniques, too.) For instance, your rounded spine may be caused by deficient hip or ankle mobility that force you to round your back to shift your center of gravity forward above your base of support as much as possible. However, even in the absence of these four main issues, other issues can make your Deep Squat position suboptimal. Unless the squat is already easy for you (which is rare nowadays), you could try to force your body into replicating every single aspect from the checklist and manage it for a few seconds while you stiffen your muscles all over and hold your breath. But that will not make you skillful at the Deep Squat, will it? Other clear signs that indicate you haven't mastered the whole spectrum of squatting include the following:

- By default, the so-called "ideal" neutral squat position has become your only comfortable squat position.
- Transitions to other variations of the squat position aren't easy. It is fine that you can hold a so-called "ideal" neutral squat position, but you should be able to fluidly switch from one squat position to another.
- It's difficult to enter or exit the neutral Deep Squat to move from and to sitting, kneeling, or standing.

If your squat positions suffer from some or all of these issues, you are still far from being proficient at squatting. More practice is required!

Squat Position Variations & Drills

In this section, I describe diverse practical squat positions for you to discover, rediscover, and explore. Find out which positions feel easy or challenging, strong or unstable, and adaptable and imagine what practical purpose you could assign to each of them.

If you are comfortable in a Squat position you may try the following adjustments:

- Slide your feet to slightly widen or narrow your base.
- Point your feet and/or knees in and out.
- Rotate your legs internally and externally.
- Shift your body weight from one foot to the other.

- Slowly elevate and lower you rear (you may hold the position at different heights) or use a slight and light bounce.
- Elevate your heels and then lower them.
- Lean your torso and reach with your arms in different directions.

If you are comfortable in several positions, you may start practicing slow and controlled transitions from one position to another. Try transitioning from a Deep Squat to a Half Squat, a Deep Squat to a Deep Split Squat, a Neutral Deep Squat to the Narrow-Base Squat, a Deep Split Squat to a Half Split Squat, and so on.

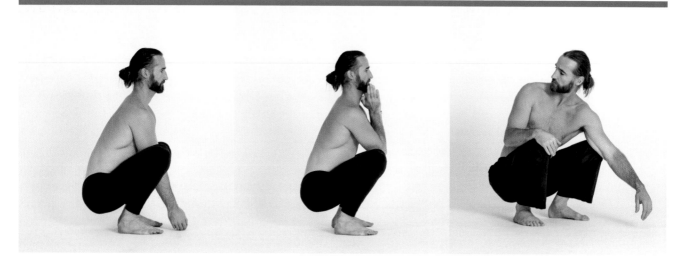

Neutral Base Squat, arms down, arms bent, arms resting on knees with trunk rotation

Narrow-Base Deep Squat

A Narrow-Base Deep Squat is handy when you're in a confined area with no space on the side of your body or when you're squatting on a narrow surface, such as a small rock in the middle of a stream. You can use this position when you're trying to keep a very low profile or to save body heat by keeping your body compact (in this case, wrap your arms tight around your legs and knees, rest your forehead on your knees with your arms covering your head).

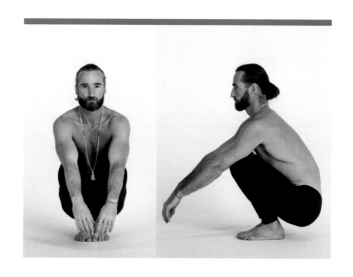

The Narrow-Base Deep Squat requires optimal joint mobility, which makes it challenging to a great number of people. To prevent being pulled back and off balance while staying as relaxed as possible, you need great ankle mobility to drive your knees and body forward as much as possible. When the stance is challenging for you, you can intentionally keep your lower back rounded, your arms to the front of the body, and drive your head forward to shift your center of gravity forward more.

Wide-Base Squat

A wide base is useful when you're trying to be more balanced when you're on unstable surfaces or between the edges of a gap. It's also helpful when you're wrestling or lifting something. Even when you let your rear go down as much as possible, it can't go as deep as the Neutral or Narrow Base Squat, and your rear can't rest on your calves. The wider your base, the higher your rear. There is a general limit to how wide the base can be, as well as an individual limit to how wide the base can be as you hold the squat while resting in the position.

The Wide-Base Squat is not considered a "half" squat in the sense that you are resting at the bottom of the position, even though the bottom position is naturally higher than when you use a narrower base.

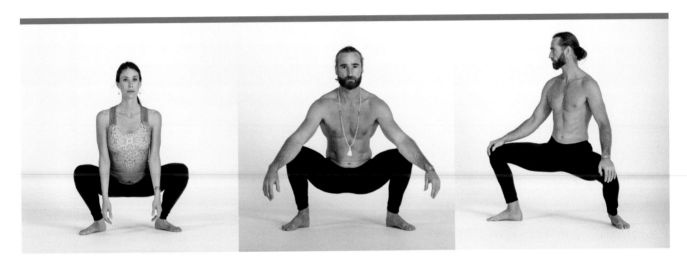

Half Squat

When you're in a Half Squat, there is tension in your leg and glutes that prevents you from resting in the deepest, bottom position. For this reason, the Half Squat is more an active position than a rest position; it's at the junction between squatting and standing. You can briefly hold a Half Squat when you're lifting or carrying or to prepare for fast transitioning to a standing movement. You can hold the Half Squat with a neutral, wide, or narrow base. You're exiting the squat and entering standing when your hips and rear are higher than knee level.

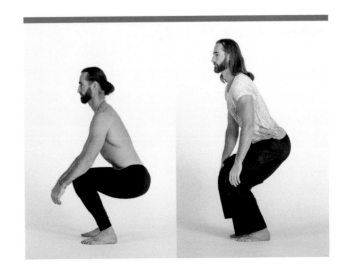

Deep Split Squat

The Deep Split Squat provides a base of support with one foot in front of the other instead of your feet being aligned. This stance forces one heel to go up in a flexed-foot position. For that reason, the Deep Split Squat technically is a mix of a Deep Squat and a Deep Knee Bend stance. If more body weight is shifted on the front, flat foot, the position is more of a squat. If more body weight is on the back, flexed-foot, the position is more a Deep Knee Bend. The base can be of various widths.

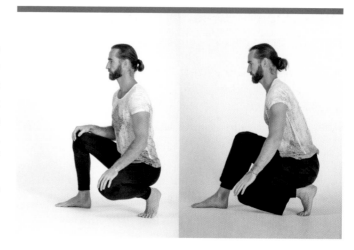

Extended Split Squat

The Extended Split Squat is commonly called a "lunge." The base is very wide. The position of the back leg could be more or less perpendicular to the front leg.

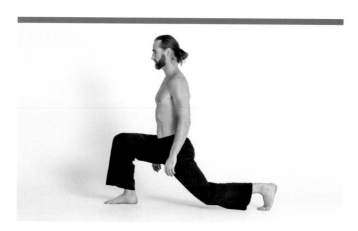

Single-Leg Deep Squat and Half Single-Leg Deep Squat

The difference between the Deep Split Squat and these positions is that your body weight is entirely or primarily supported by a single foot; the other leg is extended to the front. Even when the opposite heel rests on the ground, the body weight it supports is not significant. This position is not a rest position; it's a transitional position used in some get-up strategies that are addressed later in this chapter.

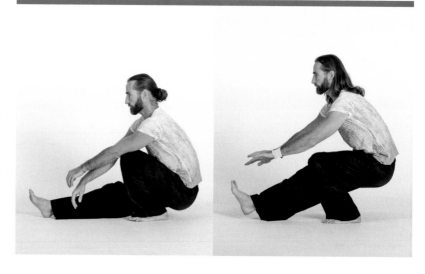

Improving the Deep Squat Position with Supported Movements

If you're not comfortable enough in the Deep Squat to hold the positions or do the drills I've described, you may use some assistance to support your position and facilitate your practice and progress.

If you're at this stage of reclaiming your squat function, don't make form a big deal, and don't stay static and stiff. Instead, while constantly maintaining breath control to help you relax, play with small motions that allow you to release tensions and let your body explore ranges of motion it has lost. You may round the spine, shift weight from side to side, rotate both legs externally, extend back to a brief sit and pull yourself back up to the squat, bounce slightly, and so on. Basically, do all the movements I recommended; just do them with some support. Depending on how comfortable you are, you may start with 30 seconds, stand and do some other movements, then return to a squat; soon you'll be able to do it significantly longer than thirty seconds. It's better do something five times for two minutes at a time throughout the day rather than do a ten-minute "workout," which can turn into an ordeal that leaves you sore and stiff.

The idea is to progressively loosen up, allow more motion in your hips, ankles, and knees, and reduce the amount of external help you need. You support yourself less and less until you finally feel ready for a Deep Squat without support. More strategies and drills will be provided as I address the Squat Get-Up further.

| HANG SUPPORT

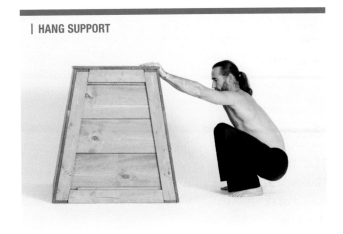

You can hang from pretty much anything. Hanging allows you to reach the lowest squat position you can, and it helps you explore great positional variety.

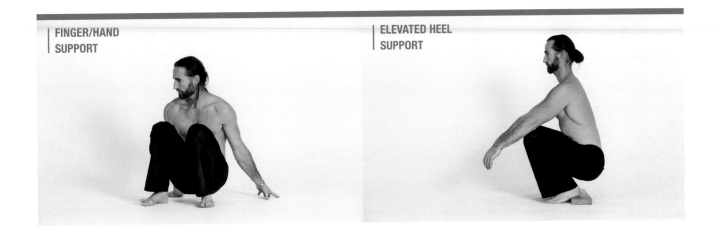

| FINGER/HAND SUPPORT

| ELEVATED HEEL SUPPORT

You may use a board, a book, or any declined surface.

The **Deep Knee Bend:** *The* **Position**

With the Deep Knee Bend, we are moving on to raised positions that are slightly higher than the Deep Squat. The Deep Squat and Deep Knee Bend are often confused as they look similar; they are also frequently linked while in movement.

From a practical standpoint, the Deep Knee Bend position is a very common and convenient position for resting briefly, getting close to the ground to pick up something light, looking for animal tracks, becoming less visible, and so on. Because your feet aren't positioned flat on the ground, the Deep Knee Bend isn't as stable as the Deep Squat, and you can't hold it as long.

The Deep Knee Bend is a good starting point as well as a convenient substitute for those who are unable to hold the Deep Squat. The Deep Knee Bend is excellent at improving foot strength, foot and ankle mobility, and stability, and it is much more challenging than the Deep Squat in this regard. Because the body is fully supported by tiny points of support (the balls of the feet), Deep Knee Bend positions can easily be turned into balancing movements without requiring that you stand on a narrow surface.

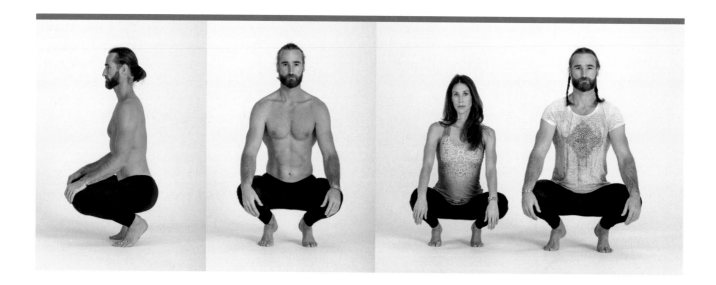

The Deep Knee Bend is like the Deep Squat in that the back of the thighs rest on the calves. Following are the main ways the Deep Knee Bend differs from the Deep Squat:

- Your base of support is on the balls of your feet with your heels off the ground, which requires much more foot strength and ankle stability.
- Your knees are lower and away from the body, horizontally aligned with your hips and rear.
- Your joints are aligned vertically from top to bottom.
- A much greater range of motion is possible in the hips.

Transitioning Between the Deep Squat and the Deep Knee Bend

This is a quite short yet very useful transition that is also deceptively challenging to perform seamlessly with balance.

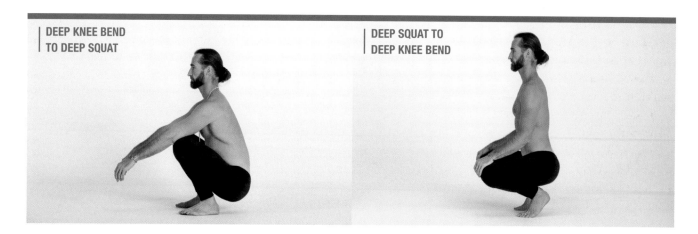

Lean your torso forward as you lower your heels and rear to counterbalance and ensure a smooth and stable transition to a Deep Squat.

Initiate a limited rocking motion by leaning your torso and shifting your body weight forward onto the balls of your feet. As soon as your heels elevate, drive your hips forward and your torso up to realign in an erect position vertically above the balls of your feet, which helps you avoid falling off balance.

Holding the Deep Knee Bend

If you are not yet used to the Deep Knee Bend, you very quickly feel the "burn" in your feet and your calves, and your balance and ability to relax in the position will be quickly challenged! Here are a few tips to help you:

- Focus on maintaining stability of your ankles at a comfortable angle. The strength of your big toes and your ability to maintain tension in this part of your foot is essential for stability.
- Control your posture, alignment, and balance mainly through your hips. If you feel unstable or get off balance, use hip drive to stabilize yourself rather than going for compensatory patterns such as leaning forward, rounding your back, extending your neck, pushing up on your legs, or using your arms to counterbalance.
- Keep your arms relaxed and resting on your knees and breathe abdominally.

Variations of the Deep Knee Bend

Variations of the Neutral Deep Knee Bend position include the following:

- Narrow or wide base of support.
- Knees closed.
- Knees wide open with feet either pointing straight or out.
- High Heel Deep Knee Bend (heel raised as high as possible and vertically aligned with the toes). This variation demands and develops phenomenal foot strength and ankle stability.
- Half Knee Bend, which is an active, more elevated position in which the heels are still off the ground but the legs and glutes are contracted to prevent the back of the thighs from resting on the calves. Usually your torso leans forward, but you can keep it vertical by driving your knees forward.
- Split feet (Split Deep Knee Bend position).
- Single-Foot Deep Knee Bend.

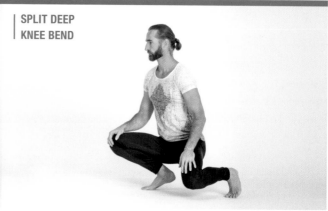

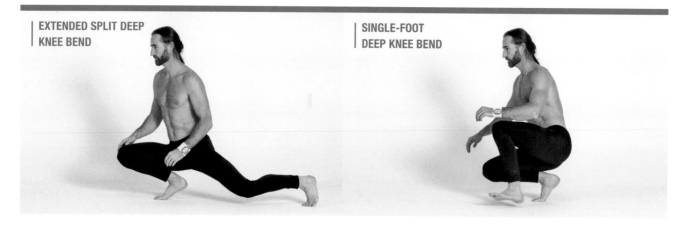

These different positions allow you to practice transitions from one Deep Knee Bend variation to another. Following are some other valuable drills:

- Tilting the pelvis forward and backward
- Driving the hips and knees forward while maintaining posture
- Driving the hips and knees forward while leaning the torso backward
- Elevating your rear to an active Half Knee Bend
- Shifting your body weight from one foot to the other
- Shifting your body weight to one foot to briefly lift the other one an inch above ground, on both sides
- Externally and internally rotating the legs (knees pointing out and in)
- Hip rotations (body pivoting to the side on the ball of the feet to a Split Deep Knee Bend position on each side)
- Narrowing and widening the base
- Raising to the Half Knee Bend
- Raising to the High Deep Knee Bend and getting down to the Neutral Deep Knee Bend
- Holding the High Heel Deep Knee Bend
- Trunk rotations and arm extensions

Deep Knee Bend Hip Drive Exercise

The idea here is to use hip motion to modify the Deep Knee Bend to reach two opposite directions in a very controlled fashion. First lower your heels very slowly until they are as close as possible to touching the ground, then maintain great foot and ankle stability as you slowly drive your hips forward until your knees are really close to touching the ground. You should control the motion and balance through your hips, keeping your arms lengthened and relaxed. Counterbalance by slightly leaning your torso backward as you drive your knees to almost reaching the ground.

Becoming adept at all these variations, transitions, and drills will be a great help when you start balancing training!

Getting Up & Getting Down

Now that you have learned to lie down, crawl, roll, sit, kneel, squat, and deep knee bend, it is time to learn diverse strategies to elevate yourself to an erect, upright standing position and get down from standing to grounded, low-center-of-gravity positions. Aside from a few exceptions, all get-up techniques are reversible sequences, which means you can both get up and get down by following the exact same pattern. It doesn't matter which of the two comes first; just keep in mind that when you read "get-ups," it also implies that you can use the movement for a downward transition to the ground (and vice versa). In practice, the difference between an upward get-up sequence and a downward sequence is in the type of muscular contractions required. (Eccentric contractions on the way down, concentric contractions on the way up, and isometric contractions both ways when certain positions need to be held until they're stable.) When particular aspects of positional control need special attention to facilitate efficiency—usually with a get-up movement—additional details are provided.

I first address the Squat and Deep Knee Bend Get-Ups. These two get-ups are restricted to the limited transition from and to standing without involving lower ground positions such as kneeling or sitting. After those, the following get-up strategies involve transitioning to and from kneeling and/or sitting positions, with the most approachable methods being those that use one or two hands for additional support. (However, virtually any get-up can be done with some assistance from the arms.) The next level of difficulty is the no-hand support get-ups that transition through support on the knees, and the most difficult get-ups transition through the Deep Squat position.

By learning all these different get-up strategies and techniques, you will also learn diverse strategies for transitioning from one position to another, such as from sitting to kneeling, half-kneeling, and split kneeling (as well as many others). To learn, practice, and improve any of these diverse transitions, you may remove the standing-up phase to simplify the techniques to the most critical part of their entire sequence; it is also true that in the real-world you may not necessarily always transition from or to a standing stance anyway. Following are some examples of transitions and drills:

- Side Bent Sit to Split Kneeling
- Open Bent Sit to Deep Squat
- Long Bent Sit to Deep Squat
- Split Kneeling to Deep Squat
- Deep Knee Bend to Deep Squat
- Deep Knee Bend to Tall Flexed-Foot Kneeling
- Deep Squat to Tall Split Kneeling

By looking at the photos and names of the diverse sitting, kneeling, and squatting positions, you may attempt many other short sequences that combine no more than two or three positions.

In any case, all the transitions I just listed and more will be naturally involved as they are "built in" to one or the other of the diverse get-ups that I am about to describe. You should learn to perform all the get-ups both dynamically and slowly with equal balance and fluidity.

Squatting: The Get-Up Movement

Squatting as a movement is most commonly understood as restricted to the downward transition from standing to the bottom squat, rest position. However, getting out of the Deep Squat to standing is as important; both sequences are closely related and should be performed with equal ease and quality of form.

The Deep Squat and Deep Knee Bend Get-Ups are not bad for your knees unless

- Your knees are bad already (because of past or current injury, degenerative disease, dysfunction, inflammation, and so on), in which case you should avoid these movements.
- You insist on doing 1,000 repetitions a day with terrible form.

SAFETY NOTE

No matter whether it's acute or mild, persistent or intermittent, pain is important feedback that signals an issue. It's always a good idea to consult a physiotherapist to discuss the issue.

Otherwise, these get-ups help restore healthy knee, ankle, and hip joints, and they also help promote a healthy lower back and spine.

It doesn't matter if you start in the standing or squatting position; you must practice both alternately: squat down, stand up from squat, repeat. That's the complete Deep Squat Get-Up. You can use it in many ways, including for lifting a heavy load. I've seen countless people taking this movement for granted— squatting down by just bending at the knees, awkwardly swaying forward and backward with a horribly rounded back as they were lowering themselves, arms extended as they were looking for something to hold on to, and painstakingly managing a not-so-deep Deep Squat position for only a few seconds.

Furthermore, as you read more about the various transitions, you will realize that squatting is a much more diverse skill than you might ever have thought before. When you do it with great emphasis on breath, position, sequence, pattern, tension, and relaxation, then a full Deep Squat Get-Up helps counteract many musculoskeletal issues such as weak glutes, tight hips, and a lack of trunk stability.

I share with you some technical aspects that make the squatting movement from and to the Neutral Deep Squat position not just effective but efficient. Remember that small children (including you, once upon a time) can hold a Deep Squat before they can stand up and ultimately walk. At some point early in your life, you owned it fully. You have lost it, but the pattern you once owned can be recovered. Also keep in mind that there is not a single, perfect form to the squatting movement with a Neutral Deep Squat position, although there is a position that's most biomechanically efficient for you because it accommodates the uniqueness of your body. Squatting as a get-up movement is adaptable to the context, and your form will vary according to the diverse squatting positions you use to enter or exit the movement.

Warming Up for the Squat Get-Up

In Part 2, I explain the Hip Hinge pattern. That pattern is going to be highly useful in learning efficient squatting form. When you squat, you won't need to drive your hips backward as much as you do in the Hip Hinge, and your knees must be bent all the way down. But the Hip Hinge teaches you essential characteristics of efficient squatting form: the flexion and extension movement of the hip joint as you maintain a neutral spine. You may conveniently use the hinge movement to warm up for the Squat Get-Up.

TECHNIQUE TIP

Make sure to practice ground movements that will help your joints loosen up, especially squat position variations.

One "Layer" at a Time

Improving a complex movement pattern that is deeply ingrained in your neuromuscular memory can be quite challenging, especially when you are trying to pay attention to and modify many details at once. Choose one aspect at a time to address, starting with the most important one; practice until that aspect has been improved enough that you can switch to the next.

The four main faults when getting up or down are like the main issues of holding the squat position: knees collapsing, lack of depth, rounded back (upper or lower spine), and heels up (Deep Knee Bend).

Getting Down

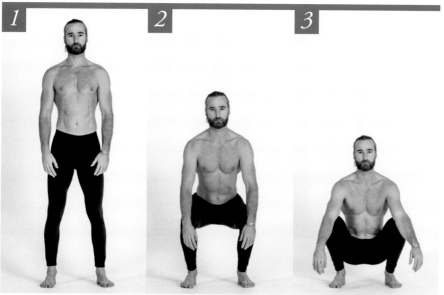

2 Hinge slightly with a neutral spine; while keeping your hips stable, flex your knees in a controlled and relatively slow fashion to lower your rear to a Half Squat. As you lower yourself, maintain a neutral spine, vertically align your knees with your feet and toes, and make your heels flat to the ground.

3 Finish lowering yourself into the Neutral Deep Squat. The details of a quality Deep Squat position have been described earlier.

1 Start in an erect, aligned standing position with your feet shoulder width apart or slightly narrower. Your toes are pointing straight ahead or slightly outward (no more than 10 to 15 degrees).

As I said previously, it's pretty simple. Here's an even simpler breakdown of the movement:

1 Start standing (that's a no-brainer).

2 Push your butt back and bend your knees a little, then lower your butt as if you want to sit down on a very low chair. You have a superhero stance with a big, proud chest and strong flat back all the way. Your heels are screwed down tight into the ground, and your knees are so strong they won't move an inch toward each other.

3 Quietly "sit" in a Deep Squat with the indestructible confidence of a supreme warrior.

But, seriously, squatting is simple. Before you squat, remember that you Hip Hinge a bit, then bend your legs while keeping your back as straight as you can. Push your knees out all the way down, and never let your heels go up.

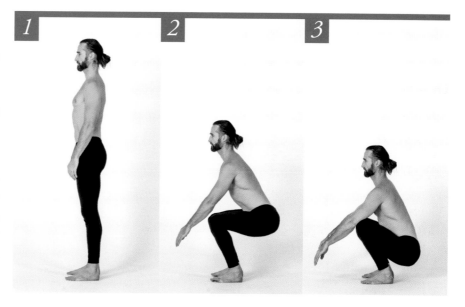

Getting Up

1   Start by turning a relaxed, resting bottom position into an active position by generating tension in the muscles of your abdomen, lower back, glutes, hips, pelvic floor and quadriceps. The tension should be enough to slightly move your hamstrings away from your calves, which will also slightly elevate your rear.

2   Elevate your position to the Half Squat by pushing off your legs and maintaining a neutral spine. Extend your legs a bit more to allow your hips to elevate a little higher than knee level, and then squeeze your glutes to initiate hip extension to drive them forward.

3   Let your torso naturally regain an erect, vertical position as you finish and extend your hips fully into a standing position.

Keep Your Body Weight in the Center of Your Feet

The body-weight pressure you perceive under your feet should feel equally distributed. If you shift all the body weight to your heels, you're at a greater risk of being pulled off-balance backward. As you're lowering yourself all the way down from standing to the bottom squat and elevating your position all the way up from the bottom to standing, your center of gravity should be aligned with the center of your foot all the way down and up rather than being aligned with your heels. Similarly, the moment your body weight shifts to the balls of your feet, your heels might elevate and make your movement unstable (if your heels elevate just a little). Elevating your heels relates to a lack of mobility—not necessarily at the ankle but maybe at the hips—which causes you to reflexively extend your ankles to help shift your body weight forward to maintain balance over your base of support and avoid toppling backward. Likewise, there should be no foot pronation—the outside of your feet elevating and your ankles caving in—which would cause your knees to collapse inwardly.

Keep Your Knees Aligned with Your Ankles and Feet

Your knees should remain vertically aligned with your ankles and feet; they shouldn't internally or externally rotate. The most common issue is to let the knees cave in, which is an internal rotation. When that happens, remind yourself (or have someone remind you) to "push your knees out." That cue is good as long as it helps you maintain vertical alignment of your knees without pushing them to the point that they rotate externally with your knee joints beyond vertical alignment with your ankles and feet. In fact, when you assume a Half Squat stance with your knees vertically aligned with your feet, look at your knees; from that perspective, it should look like your knees are slightly outside a vertical line with your feet (even though they truly are vertically aligned with them). If they look like they are significantly away from a vertical line with your feet to the side, it means you are pushing your knees out too much. If it looks like your knees are aligned with your feet, your knees are caving in, and you need to push them out over your feet.

Keeping your knees over your feet and ankles is about maintaining the most stable stance when you get up or down. The moment your knees cave in, your position becomes weak and highly unstable. Your position is also unstable if your knees move forward beyond vertical alignment with the center of the foot. However, your knees will naturally and slightly move forward and beyond a vertical line with your toes when you reach the bottom of the position.

Hinge Enough but Not Too Much

If you don't let your hips move backward and your torso lean forward enough, either your knees will compensate by moving forward beyond vertical alignment with your toes as you bend your legs deeper, which puts a lot of stress on them, or as you lower your rear you will start to fall back. A relatively pronounced hinge and forward lean angle of your torso with the hips leading and flexing before the knees (known as a "deep hinge"), on the other hand, are not issues if you know how to be stable. So first find the angle of your torso in relation to your hip that feels right for you as you hinge; then maintain this angle relatively constantly until you reach a squat deeper than knee level, at which point you start regaining a more erect torso at a less pronounced forward angle.

The Bottom Flexion

Some people's hips display posterior tilt, and those people have a mild flexion in the lumbar spine as they are reaching very close to the bottom position. This particularity may have to do with a lack of mobility, with the skeletal structure of the person (hip socket depth), or a combination of both. If you experience this problem and improved mobility doesn't fix the issue, then you have a structural issue that you can't fix. You're one of these people whose physical makeup does not allow them to reach the Deep Squat. Not to worry; you can keep squatting naturally. It only becomes an issue if you're using the Squat Get-Up for heavy lifting or strength training. Unless you reduce the depth of your squat before the bottom lower spine flexion, adding intensity (load) and volume (repetitions) would put a great mechanical stress on your lower spine with a serious risk of disc injury.

TECHNIQUE TIP

The strategies to improve your Deep Squat Get-Up are no different from those involved in improving the Deep Squat position itself; if you're comfortable with the Deep Squat position, it's unlikely that you'll have trouble with the get-up.

As a matter of fact, you don't necessarily need to achieve the Deep Squat position before starting to improve your Deep Squat Get-Up; by holding onto something as you try to squat down as low as possible each time, you could improve both the Deep Squat position and Deep Squat Get-Up simultaneously.

Be consistent: Practice every day—ideally several times a day, even if you can practice for only a minute. Ultimately, you should be able to extend your arms in front of you or hold them over your head while you maintain upper spine alignment and stability. Once you are proficient at the unloaded squatting pattern (with no additional weight), you may start squatting with a load as an exercise for gaining lower-body strength and power.

Deep Knee Bend: The Get-Up Movement

As a movement, the Deep Knee Bend allows an easy and quicker transition (to standing or to a low position) than squatting, but it's also potentially less stable. As a matter of fact, you can use the Deep Knee Bend movement both for getting up and down before and after holding the Deep Squat position, which is not technically the squatting movement any longer (because of the additional transition to the Deep Knee Bend). All you must do is to switch from the Deep Squat to the Deep Knee Bend position before standing up or the other way around before reaching the bottom Squat stance.

Unlike the Squat Get-Up, the Deep Knee Bend Get-Up is very straightforward: You stand up or lower yourself with your heels elevated above ground the whole time (except when you're actually standing) with your joints following a rather straight vertical line and without having to lean forward or hinge. The Deep Knee Bend Get-Up is "knee dominant," whereas the Squat Get-Up is "hip dominant." You may occasionally use this get-up in a manipulative way, such as when you're holding a light load, but it's not suited for heavy loads because it's way too unstable and would put an enormous stress on your knees.

Before practicing the movement, you must be able to comfortably hold the Deep Knee Bend stance with vertical alignment as you keep your arms relaxed. When standing or lowering yourself to the Deep Knee Bend, visualize and ensure a controlled, stable transition with great posture, relaxed arms, and moving along a straight vertical line. From standing, all you need to do is to start raising your heels; then you bend your knees and start lowering yourself. Voilà!

Hand Support Get-Ups

As you start to move on to get-up methods that involve kneeling or sitting, I want to start you with the easier ones that are done with some assistance from the arms. As I stated before, virtually any get-up technique can be assisted this way. There may be practical reasons for using your arms, such as when you need to get up or down faster, move more slowly and safely, assist the lower body when it's injured or painful, enable the movement when you feel weak, or carry a load on your back.

Tripod Get-Up

The Tripod Get-Up is a staple of MovNat, especially when you practice it while balancing on a narrow surface. But you primarily do it on the ground to ease sitting down or getting up from sitting; sometimes you can use it to kneel. You can do it very swiftly in case of emergency, and it has notable value in combative situations. The Tripod Get-Up enables you to lift a load up or put it down securely as you use one arm for holding the object and the other for ground support, although you can use it to lift heavy objects.

Getting Down

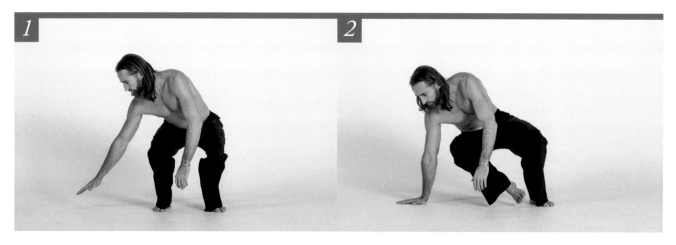

1   From standing, lower your center of gravity to a Half or Deep Squat. Simultaneously, lean sideways and reach out to either side with your arm on that side.

2   Place the palm of your reaching hand on the ground. The space between the hand on the ground and your opposite foot is ideally 1 foot wider than shoulder width. (You can make this space narrower if you don't have adequate room, but if you make the space too wide, the movement becomes unstable.) Extend your arm fully with your palm, wrist, elbow, and shoulder aligned, then externally rotate your arm to create even greater stability before shifting body weight to it. You now have a three-pointed base of support; shift your body weight between your outside hand and the opposite foot, so you can free the inside foot from supporting your body weight and drive the leg forward through the rotation action of the hips.

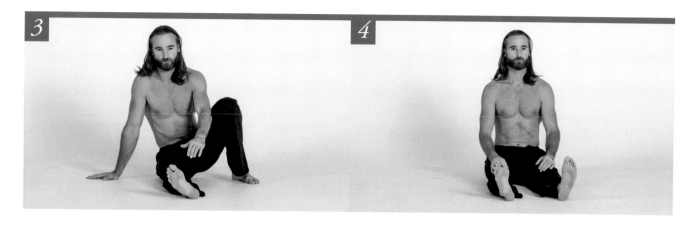

3 Supporting your weight on your planted arm and the outside leg, extend your inside leg in front of you, and then lower that hip to the ground. Keep your arm fully extended until your rear is seated on the ground.

4 Extend the other leg and release your hand; bring your torso to center over your hips so that you're in a Long Sit position.

Getting Up

1 From the Long Sit, bring the heel of one foot (or both) toward your rear while you extend your arm on the opposite side to place your hand on the ground.

2 Shift more body weight to your palm and, while keeping your arm fully locked out and externally rotated, push off your heel and begin to lift your rear off the ground and elevate your hips; meanwhile, bend your inside leg and start driving your hips and leg backward.

3 Bring the foot on the ground to the Tripod stance in a Deep Squat or a square Half Squat stance and push off your palm to immediately start standing up.

No-Hand-Support Get-Ups

The get-up techniques in this section are normally done without the help of the arms. However, for the sake of practice (and occasionally for a practical reason), these movements can be assisted at any time by one or two hands on the ground. While the ratio of lower-body muscle strength to overall body weight is an important factor in your ability (or lack thereof) to get up and down unassisted by your arms, lower-body mobility, stability, balance, and coordination are very relevant aspects to it.

Getting up from and getting down to sitting on an elevated surface may not seem to be a "ground movement," but it actually is no different than other get-up strategies that involve transitioning from a base of support on the rear to the feet. The difference lies in the fact that the sitting surface is raised, which significantly reduces the range of motion involved. Because this is a movement pattern that most of us do several times daily, it's a good thing to look at ways to do it better. Instead of only looking at our posture while sitting, we're also going to be mindful of how we get into and out of the sitting position. If we can learn to mindfully enter and exit raised sitting systematically with efficient movement, we help ingrain a better sit position as well.

Sitting Down

Start standing very close to (but not against) the seat. Approach sitting down with the intention to maintain good posture all the way down and while sitting.

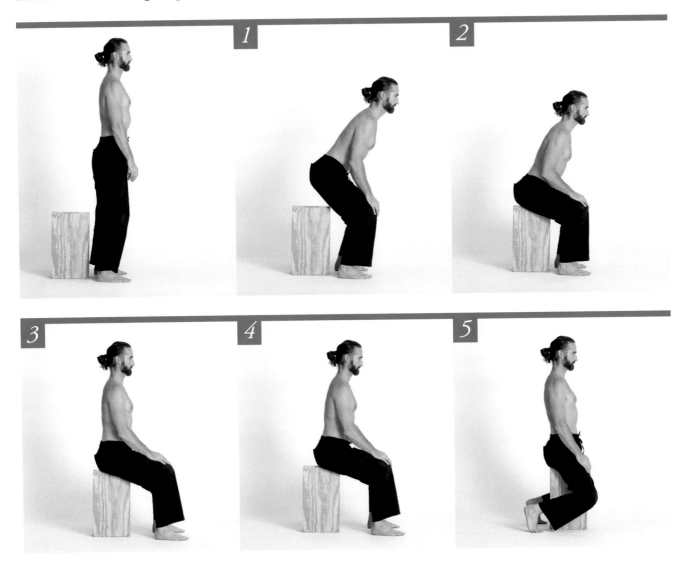

1   Hinge from your hips and start bending your legs as if you were going to squat. Keep your knees vertically aligned with your toes. Maintain posture.

2   Maintain tension in your lower body so you can control your descent until your rear smoothly reaches the seat. Don't rush to lean back.

3   Once your rear is positioned, lean back until your torso is upright.

4   Alternatively, you could lean slightly forward (or lean back if there's a backrest).

5   You also can change the position of your legs to a straddle position or other positions.

Standing Up from Raised Sitting

1   Look at the Sitting Down photos in reverse.

2   Start slowly leaning forward, hinging from your hips.

3   Generate tension in your legs and drive your hips up and out of the seated position.

4   Re-establish the upright standing position.

If your intention is to spring out swiftly from the raised sit so that you're running forward, you want to quickly lean forward and drive your knees vertically beyond your toes to shift your body weight onto the balls of your feet and load your legs faster so you can keep leaning forward as you stand up. The lower the raised surface you sit on and the more movement there is to the pattern to enter and exit the sit position, the more the sit becomes a squatting motion rather than a hinging one.

Kneeling Transitions

This subset of no-hand-support get-ups transition through Kneeling or Half-Kneeling. Some start and terminate in a kneeling position; others start or end in a sitting position.

Kneeling Get-Up

The Kneeling Get-Up is a simple transition from standing to kneeling (or the other way around), which can be limited to the transition between the Deep Knee Bend and Kneeling positions. It is a highly practical movement sequence that also has fantastic value for mobility and stability in the knees, ankles, and feet. When you assist the movement with your arms, you can reach forward with your arms and swiftly get down in a forward sliding motion until you're kneeling.

1 Lower yourself from standing or start directly in a strong, stable Deep Knee Bend position. You may optionally start squatting before transitioning to the Deep Knee Bend.

2 While maintaining great stability in your feet and ankles, start driving your hips forward to lower your knees while leaning your upper body backward. Shifting your body weight in the opposite direction (shifting your lower body forward and upper body slightly backward) allows you to stay balanced with equal distribution of body weight over your base of support through the whole motion, which brings your knees smoothly to the ground and helps you avoid counterbalancing with your arms. Establish the Flexed-Foot Kneeling position.

3 Lean forward slightly to shift some body weight onto your knees so that you can slide and extend your feet horizontally below your rear, then lean back and sink into the Kneeling position with a tall posture, relaxed arms, and your hands resting on your thighs. Alternatively, the final position could be the Flexed-Foot Kneeling position.

Getting Down

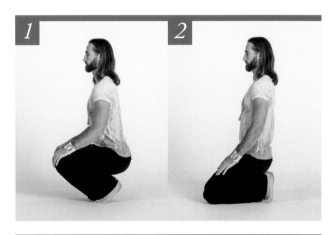

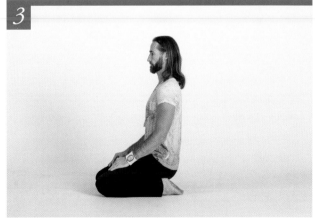

Getting Up

Getting up to standing is pretty straightforward; simply reverse the sequence. From the Flexed-Foot Kneeling position, there are two options to facilitate a smooth transition to the Deep Knee Bend. The first is to simply lean your torso backward enough to start elevating your knees off the ground. The second is to elevate your rear to a tall(er) kneeling position and then sit back on your ankles, which elevates your knees off the ground as well.

Tall Half-Kneeling Get-Up

This get-up involves a single forward or backward step to a Tall Half-Kneeling position before you kneel or stand.

Choose this option if you intend to create a bit of distance from where you stand before kneeling or to immediately keep walking forward after getting up.

Getting Down

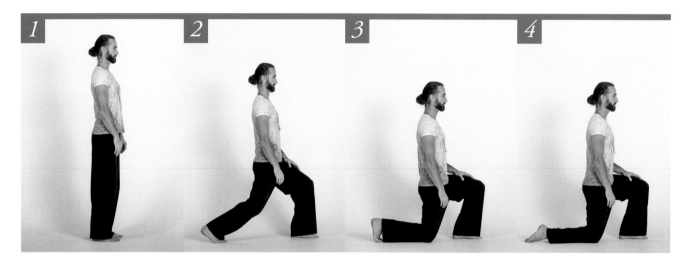

1 Begin in a standing position.

2 Step forward or backward into a relatively wide Split Stand; the distance between your feet should be about the same as the width between your shoulders so your base of support is stable. Keep your body weight evenly distributed over both feet, your spine straight, and your hips and back foot facing forward.

3 Lower your back knee to the ground into a stable Flexed-Foot Tall Half-Kneeling position.

4 Extend the ankle of your rear leg to point your toes. (Optionally, you could skip the Flexed-Foot Tall Half-Kneeling position and immediately step down with an extended foot in a Tall Half-Kneeling position.)

5 Briefly shift your body weight to a Single-Knee Tall Kneeling position and pull your front leg to the back; bring your front knee down next to the back knee to establish a Tall Kneeling position.

6 Lower your hips to sit on your heels in a kneeling position.

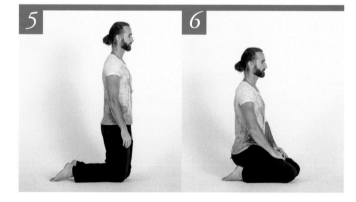

Kneel-Squat Get-Up

A very dynamic, no-hand movement involves leaning backward, elevating the knees, and then pushing off the top part of the forefoot to propel the body into a very brief airborne phase at a level sufficient for you to land on your feet in a squat position.

Getting Up

To get up from a Tall Half-Kneeling position, simply reverse the sequence. As when you get down, you must ensure great stability of the knee joint between the Tall Half-Kneeling and the Split Standing positions. You may optionally use the Flexed-Foot Tall Half-Kneeling position if you want to strongly push yourself up to get up and even transition to running quickly.

Split Kneeling Get-Up

This get-up exists in two variations and allows you to start or end the movement from diverse sit positions, transitioning through both the Side Bent Sit and the Split Kneeling positions. Because of this particularity, you end up moving your orientation slightly to the side, unless you initiated it directly from the Side Bent Sit. This get-up can start from and end in the Deep Knee Bend or standing.

The first variation transitions through the Deep Knee Bend before the ending in the Split Kneeling position.

Getting Down

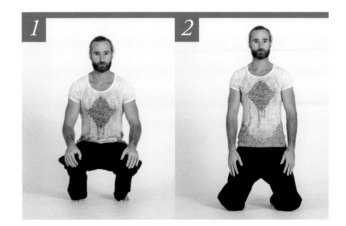

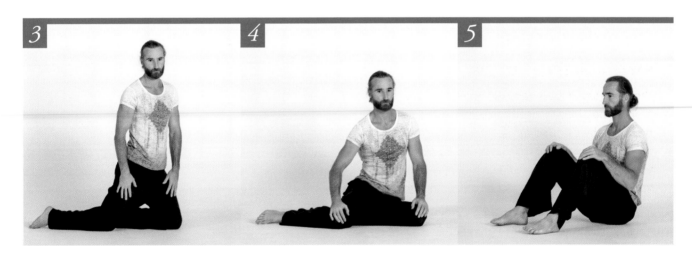

1   Lower yourself from standing or start directly in a strong, stable Deep Knee Bend.

2   Lower your knees to the ground with control, entering a Tall Kneeling position.

3   Rotate your hips to rotate both legs to either side to establish a Split Kneeling position with your torso facing perpendicularly to your legs.

4   Shift your body weight back and lower your seat to the ground behind your feet to enter a Side Bent Sit.

5   You may keep the Side Bent Sit or rotate your hips and pull both legs up to a Bent Sit.

Getting Up

Reverse the sequence to turn it into getting up. The key difference lies in the transition from a Side Bent Sit to a Split Kneeling position; you want to slightly lean the torso forward (you may slightly round your back), then drive and extend your hips forward and up to elevate your rear off the ground until you reach the Split Kneeling position. You may add a little rocking motion from the Bent Sit to facilitate the transition.

Squatting Transitions

The second type of No-Hand-Support Get-Up is a direct transition from sitting to standing through a Squat or Half-Kneeling position. Some of these get-ups start and terminate in a Kneeling position; others go to and from a sit position. The transition through the squat is quite challenging to most people, however it is a quicker way to get up or down than through kneeling, especially when you add Front-Rocking, which is not always possible with kneeling.

NOTE

The Side Bent Sit to Split Kneeling transition is the most challenging part of the whole sequence. You can isolate it to make it a drill. Otherwise, it can be useful when you're sitting and need to briefly scout your surroundings from a more elevated position.

From a functional practice, these squat get-ups push your mobility to a higher level. Basically, if you can't do these get-ups slowly without using rocking momentum or hand support, your squatting skill is not as good as you think. However, practicing the squat get-ups first with some help from your hands by rocking and then progressively starting to do them without those aids is a good strategy to improve your skill.

Cross Squat Get-Up

This is a very common way to get up and down with no arm support. It's also the movement that's most accessible to people of all levels of skill.

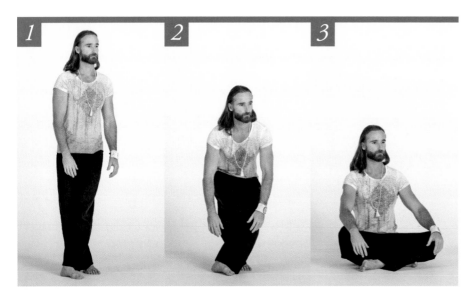

1 Begin in a Cross Standing position.

2 Move your hips back and lower your center of gravity, keeping your chest facing forward. Allow one foot to stay flat on the ground while the other rests on its external edge, which shifts more weight onto one foot, with your torso slightly leaning to the side; alternatively, you could tilt both feet so that your weight is supported on the outsides of your feet, keeping your body weight evenly distributed.

3 Lower your rear to the ground and enter a Cross Open Bent Sit.

Narrow-Base Squat Get-Up

One squat get-up that is easily done by all young children—but is a feat of high-level mobility to grown-ups, including some of the fittest ones—is the Narrow-Base Squat Get-Up. Everyone who can Deep Squat will be able to get down this way, but not everyone who can Deep Squat has enough mobility to get up this way. If you can do this movement without rocking from the sit position, your mobility and Deep Squat are great.

SAFETY NOTE

Don't attempt this movement on a slippery surface and/or while wearing slippery pants, or you will slide back when you start to push off your rear to transition to the Deep Squat.

Getting Up

1 Reverse the movement by pulling your heels as close to your rear as you can to create a base of support as narrow as possible; the effect of this movement is reducing the distance your center of gravity must travel to become vertically aligned with your feet. Keep your heels against each other and press them firmly down to the ground. Open your legs to allow your torso and arms to reach forward, then immediately and swiftly shift your body weight forward to elevate your rear. Optionally, you may rock backward on your back and then rock forward to generate momentum and get up faster. In any case, you need friction under your rear to push off it; if the ground, your clothing, or both are slippery, the movement might become completely ineffective. Make sure to keep your heels close to your rear and keep pressing down through your heels to maintain friction so you can pull forward with your legs as you rock forward. During the pulling motion, your knees are outside a vertical line over your feet, not for stability but to ensure that your torso can lean forward enough to shift your center of gravity to the front. You should bring your knees over your feet as soon as you are in the Squat position.

2 Finish shifting your body weight onto your feet in a Narrow-Base Deep Squat. Stand up if needed.

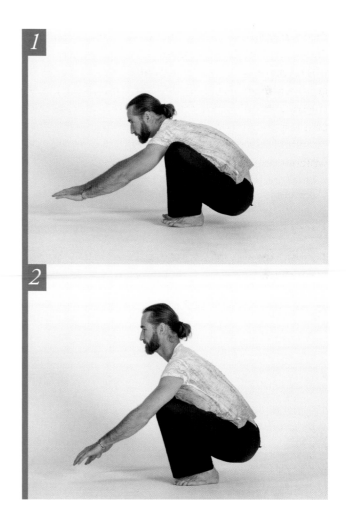

TECHNIQUE TIP

Apart from using Front-Rocking to facilitate the transition to the Deep Squat, you may also find a slightly inclined area outside and start the movement facing downhill. You also may assist yourself by holding and pulling on something, or you can push off with your hands or fingers. You can make it a collaborative practice with a partner by facing each other and helping each other up and down by holding each other's hands. In the latter case, the idea is to try to slow the movement as much as possible while also relying less and less on your partner's help.

Single-Leg Squat Get-Up

This is a squat get-up that transitions to a Single-Leg Squat position. For this reason, make sure to practice it on each side, left leg then right leg, and if one side is more challenging than the other, practice more on that side.

TECHNIQUE TIP

The Single-Leg Squat Get-Up is a perfect example of how apparently "simple" movements can be deceptively complex and technical. Even though you may add assistance or momentum to achieve the movement at first, work on your ability to perform it slowly. It's always tempting to hide stability issues by speeding the execution of the movement.

Getting Down

1 From standing, lower your center of gravity by squatting, or start in a Deep Squat.

2 Shift your body weight to one foot with your center of gravity vertically aligned with it.

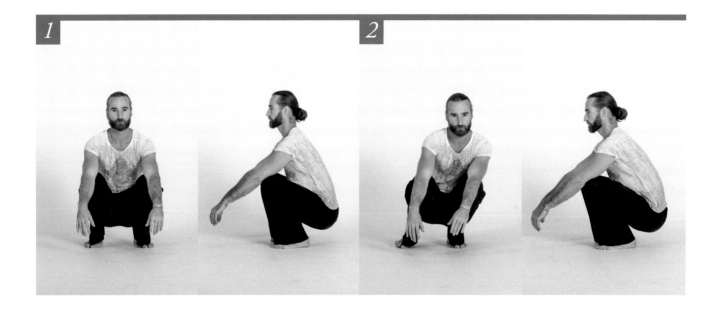

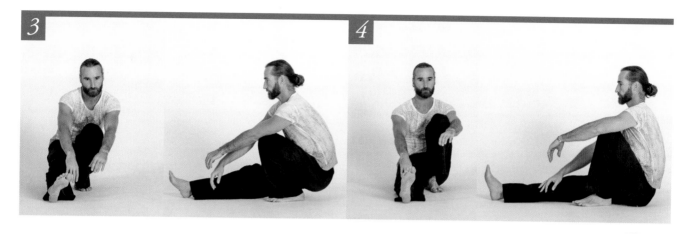

3 With the opposite foot free to move, release it by extending the leg forward, entering a Single-Leg Deep Squat.

4 Lower your seat to the ground and extend your legs so you're in a Long Bent Sit. From there you may choose any sit variation you like.

Getting Up

Getting up follows the exact same sequence in the reverse order. The key moment, which also is the most challenging, is the transition from the Long Bent Sit to the Single-Leg Deep Squat. If the main cause of your ineffectiveness is a lack of mobility, especially in your ankle and pelvis, you first need to first improve that area because no technique will compensate for such a deficiency. Unless you are already aware of such limitations and have first checked that your technique is right on, don't start blaming a supposed lack of mobility right off the bat.

Sprawls

A "sprawl" isn't just a clumsy way to fall on the ground. A sprawl can be used intentionally and be done in a controlled manner forward or backward.

The main function of the sprawl is to get down and reach the ground as quickly as possible by using the pull of gravity so that you end up lying flat against the ground. You can use it in a case of an imminent threat that demands you quickly lie down to a prone position, quickly hide, reduce your visibility, take shelter, transition quickly to crawling, safely recover from getting badly off balance, or avoid a takedown by an attacker (in this case you'd used a Back Sprawl).

The most explosive way to perform sprawls involves an airborne phase where your whole body is briefly off ground, which could be associated to a form of jumping, especially when you're moving and covering some distance horizontally in addition to go-ing down. Sprawling down to the ground is a highly dynamic movement that is physically demanding and intimidating at first.

In sprawling practice, you may start performing sprawls from a lower position rather than from standing—in this case, with your hands already on the ground and your body extending backward (Back Sprawl) or your feet down on the ground and your body extending forward (Front Sprawl). You may also start training on a soft, forgiving surface such as a mat, grass, or sand.

By definition, sprawling implies a downward motion only. However, a sprawl sequence may be done in reverse, when physically possible (which makes it a get-up). However, you can't always exactly get up the same way you get down—either as fast or as economically.

Back Sprawl

Getting Down

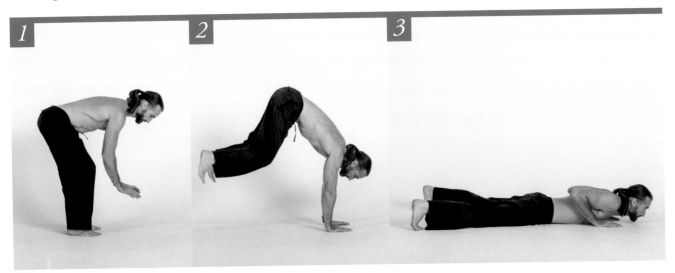

1   Start from a standing position. Hip Hinge and reach both hands toward the ground in front of you and directly underneath your shoulders.

2   As your hands approach the ground, push off both legs to elevate your hips so that your feet come off the ground as you shift all your weight onto your palms. Immediately allow your hips to start dropping. With your feet still airborne, extend both legs so that they are fully extended when your feet reach the ground behind you. Flex your feet so you land on the balls of your feet, and spread your legs slightly to widen your base and disperse the force of landing.

3   Lower your hips and chest to the ground with control, entering a Prone Lying position.

Depending on practical variables, you may modify your body position when sprawling, such as by doing the following:

- Start the sprawl from a Tall Kneeling position. This is a good option for beginners.
- Jump backward before sprawling.
- Leave your feet on the ground and let your whole body slide backward with four points of support during the whole motion.
- Use a single arm for support before sprawling.
- Deep hinge, bend your legs more to place your forearms down on the ground, and sprawl from this lower starting position.

- Push off your arms strongly to move your body backward some distance as you sprawl down.
- Push off your legs and drive your hips backward before your hands reach the ground, creating a brief airborne phase.
- Keep your legs close together.
- Let your feet reach the ground before they are fully extended and finish by fully extending them as your feet slide backward on the ground.
- Press on your arms to keep your chest and head up.
- Extend your arms fully to the front or the side.
- Turn your head to the side or even flip your entire body to one side before landing.

Getting Up

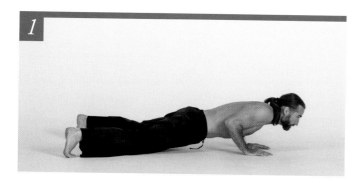

1 To reverse the movement, make sure the balls of your feet are planted on the ground in a flexed-foot manner; press on your arms to bring your hips and torso off the ground. You can either press up all the way to a plank position then push off your arms to drive your body weight back onto your feet with your legs bent before jumping your legs toward your hands, or from the plank you can pull your lower body forward with your feet sliding toward your hands.

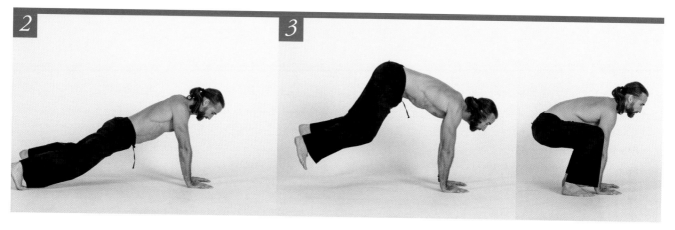

2 Once your hips are back, your legs are bent, and the balls of your feet are loaded, push off your legs to elevate your hips and bring your feet off the ground as you shift all your weight onto your hands. Keep your arms locked out so your support stays strong.

3 Bring your knees forward and land with your feet just behind your hands, so you're in a Half Squat. Shift your weight onto your feet and straighten your spine before standing up.

Front Sprawl

Getting Down

From standing there are two ways to initiate the front sprawl.

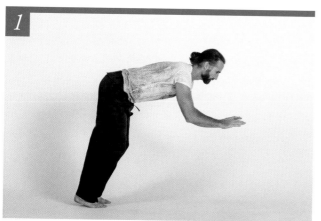

1 Reach both hands in front of you with your palms down. Lean forward to shift your center of gravity beyond your base of support; you're intentionally losing balance and initiating a forward fall. The body may stay fully extended or only slightly bend at hip level. (Think of a tree falling.) This movement starts slowly but quickly accelerates as you get closer to the ground.

(continued on next page)

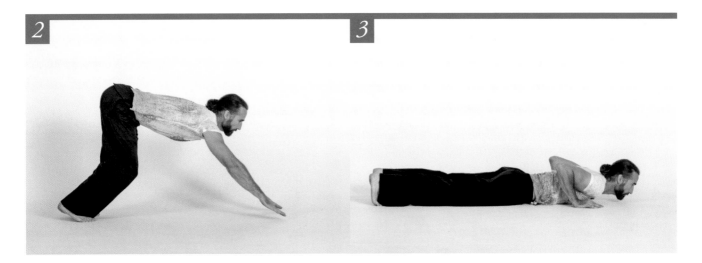

2   Reach both hands out in front of you with your palms down. Bend your legs in a Hip Hinge to lower your center of gravity as much as possible, which shortens the distance your hands must cover before landing and reduces impact forces upon landing. This is how beginners should start.

3   Land on your palms, bend your arms to decelerate as you lower yourself fully but smoothly in the Prone Lying position.

Getting Up

To manage getting up the same way, you need to powerfully push yourself backward, fully extending your arms as you hinge your hips to drive them backward, then bend your legs to load your feet as your hands take off. It makes the complete movement, of both the get-down and get-up, a quite challenging alternative to regular push-ups. Otherwise, you can get up the same way that was described in the getting-up description for the Back Sprawl.

Rolls

Rolls, like sprawls, are fast ways to smoothly and quickly transition to the ground from standing, or even after jumping from a height. They also can be done intentionally or unexpectedly upon losing balance and to dissipate impact forces while avoiding bruising or injuring oneself. Rolls are reversible sequences: The Front Roll used to get down becomes a Back Roll when you get back up, and vice versa. The advantage of rolls is that they allow you to enter or exit the get-up from a variety of positions: standing, Half-Kneeling, sitting, Prone or Supine Lying. For instance, you may roll forward or backward from standing to standing.

It may seem strange to roll forward to a sit from standing instead of using a different get-up strategy that goes straight down on the spot, or to roll back-ward from standing to standing, but it could have a practical purpose, such as putting distance between yourself and a threat or to disperse impact forces. You shouldn't see rolls as flashy moves with little practical purpose; learning to roll smoothly and skillfully from and to diverse positions and at diverse speeds really matters to your real-life physical competency.

I previously covered the Front Roll and Back Roll from lying positions in Chapter 24, and those movements are where learning rolls should start. As you start practicing rolls from more elevated positions, you might want to train on softer surfaces. However, efficiency should become your best cushioning, even when you're rolling on hard surfaces.

Front Roll

TECHNIQUE TIP

Here are some pointers before you get started:

- Though it is called a "Front Roll," the body rolls over a single shoulder in a diagonal line between the supporting shoulder and the opposite hip.

- The neck and head should never become a point of support and bear any body weight during the roll.

- Start on a compliant, soft surface!

1   From a Split Standing position, do a Hip Hinge. Reach the arm that's on the same side as your lead leg to the ground just in front of and inside your lead foot.

2   Lean down and shift your weight forward so that you begin to come off your feet. Lower the forearm of your lead arm to the ground and bring both shoulders down. Place the palm of your other hand on the ground below and just outside your head to assist with lowering under control. This assisting arm will become unnecessary as you become proficient at the Front Roll, but you can use it whenever you need it. Optionally, the arm on the side of your supporting shoulder could be extended outwardly instead of tucked inwardly. In this case you need to bend down to contact the shoulder directly on the ground, or very close to it, before rolling forward.

3   Lower the back of your lead shoulder to the ground, maintaining contact with the ground along the entire length of that arm. To avoid landing on your head, tilt your head to the opposite shoulder. This phase and position are like the lying Front Roll except that it happens much faster.

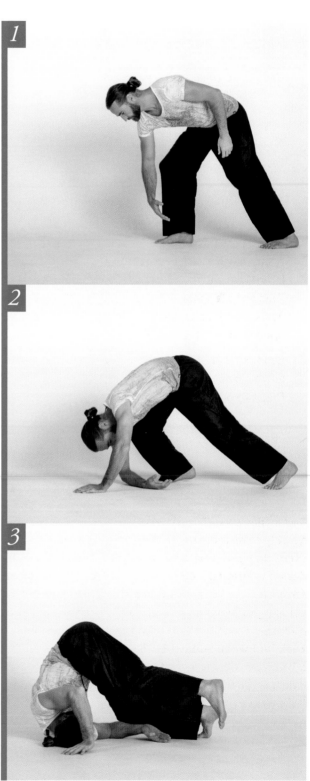

(continued on next page)

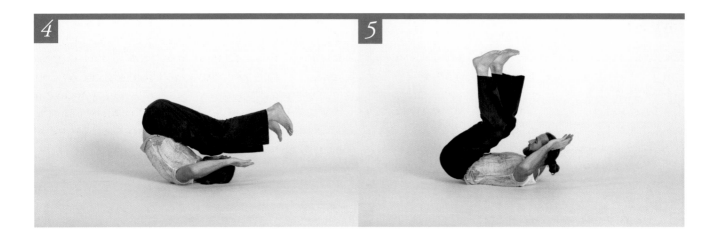

4   Allow your feet to come off the ground as you roll onto your back.

5   Maintain a rounded spine by contracting your abdominals as you swing your legs over and let your body roll all the way in a diagonal path from your shoulder to the opposite hip.

6   Unless you decide to end the roll lying down, you want to keep dissipating the momentum by transitioning to kneeling or even standing. Roll across your back, from your lead shoulder to the hip on the opposite side, as you start bending the leg on the exit side.

7   Allow your momentum to carry you up as you tuck the lead leg, so your shin is perpendicular to your direction of travel and extend the other leg slightly to place the heel of that foot on the ground. As your rear elevates with the momentum, push off your grounded thigh. Optionally, you could flex the foot of your tucked, grounded leg so it can assist in pushing your body up.

8   As you roll over your shin, pull yourself up with a pulling motion of your extended leg's heel and enter a side Half-Kneel.

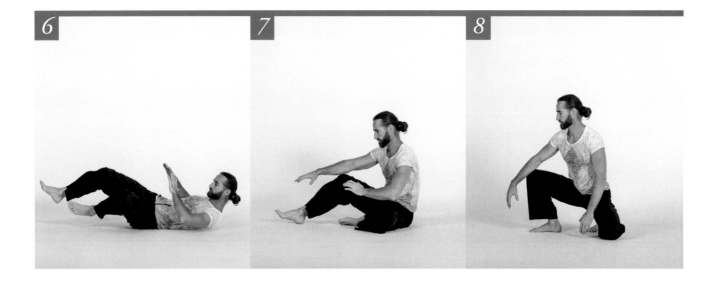

Dive Roll

The Dive Roll is a highly technical landing strategy. You use it when the peak level of impact forces will be greater than what other forms of landing can disperse. The Dive Roll is useful when the height from which you launch the jump, the forward distance you'll cover before landing, and your speed and forward momentum while jumping are significant. Without rolling, your legs would bear the brunt of dispersing impact forces, which would easily exceed the power of the eccentric contraction and could potentially damage your joints or break bones. The Dive Roll is an extremely dynamic transition primarily aimed at adding distance between where your feet contact the ground upon landing and where the supporting shoulder enters the roll. By immediately bouncing forward to cover distance in an airborne fashion before rolling, you ensure maximum distribution and dissipation of impact forces.

Less frequently, you can use the Dive Roll at ground level to clear an elevated obstacle, such as a fence, with your whole body extending above it and exiting through a roll on the other side.

The two key aspects of the technique happen while you're standing on the ground, and the most substantial part of the technique is the roll. This is the reason why I consider it a ground movement. From a practical perspective, the Dive Roll is mostly a one-way, forward movement. You can reverse it to some extent; for instance, you could roll backward and push yourself up and move back to create backward distance. However, there is no way to reverse this movement to the point where you return to the spot from which you initially jumped.

Increasing the displacement of your center of gravity upon landing, by leaning or rolling forward, reduces the peak force by dispersing kinetic force along a greater distance. You want to choose this landing option when you expect the forward momentum or impact forces upon landing to exceed your muscular ability to dissipate them in a standing position, to conserve energy, or to advantageously use the momentum to continue your course of action without slowing down. This is especially the case in rolling where kinetic energy upon landing is dissipated through a maximum number of body segments contacting the ground in a sequence.

In the photos illustrating the technique, I'm standing on a surface that's elevated 8 feet. A target is marked on the ground about 8 feet along a vertical line extending from my feet. The distance between the target and the surface where I stand replicates a real-life gap or distance that I would cover by jumping after running (although such distance could be greater with more momentum or height).

SAFETY NOTE

Although I am showing the technique from jumping from a height to make the movement realistic, for obvious safety reasons this technique is best practiced first from a Tall Half-Kneeling or standing stance on a soft surface.

Being too aggressive when you try this movement for the first time by starting too high with a run and then landing on a hard surface is very likely to leave you injured. If your roll goes wrong, you could experience a variety of injuries, including displacing a shoulder, smashing your face, breaking your wrist or arm, landing very hard on your back, and so on. A healthy respect for progression is more important than ever when learning this move and practicing it at a greater level of difficulty. Start by developing good technique at ground level.

TECHNIQUE TIP

I enter the movement with a Broad Jump, but how you enter it may vary. You can initiate it from a Depth Jump, Split Jump with or without a run up, a Vault, or even a Front Swing from Hanging.

Take Off & Airborne Phase

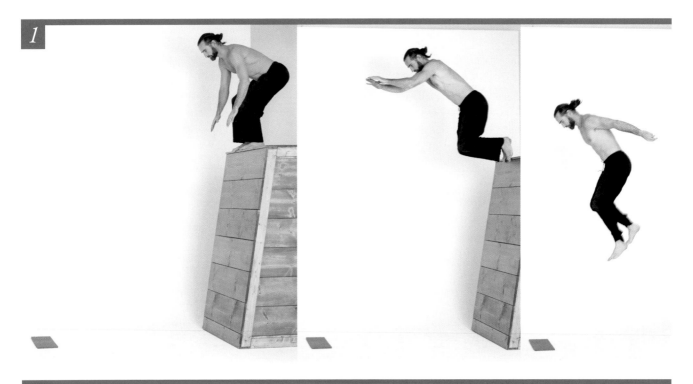

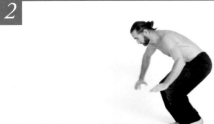

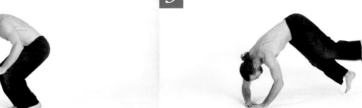

1 From the top of the surface, highly focus and look down at the area where you intend to land, including the exact area where you want your feet to contact the ground. Knowing the ratio of height to depth and the distance you need to cover tells you how much power you need to cover the distance. You need to lean forward at an approximate 30- to 40-degree angle upon landing. You can't calculate any of it in your head or on paper; only incremental progressions in training and experience will inform you.

2 The moment your feet contact the ground, bend and load your legs to start decelerating. This immediately converts some of the elastic energy stored in your legs and posterior chain into a powerful push and forward dive. Your arms and hands are ready to extend forward.

3 You are diving forward. As your whole body becomes airborne again for a moment, slightly orient your upper body and head sideways toward the side on which you'll be rolling. This is important as you want to be able to roll from one side of your body to the other in a diagonal line between the entry arm and shoulder and the opposite hip. Place your hands in a V shape pointing inward in front of your body as soon as your hands contact the ground. As your body moves forward (pushed down by momentum as well as pulled by gravity), your arms start bending to absorb pressure and to guide the controlled fall.

4 Generate some tension from your arm to start dispersing some of the impact forces as you start rolling in a sequence starting from your forearm to the back of your upper arm to your shoulder.

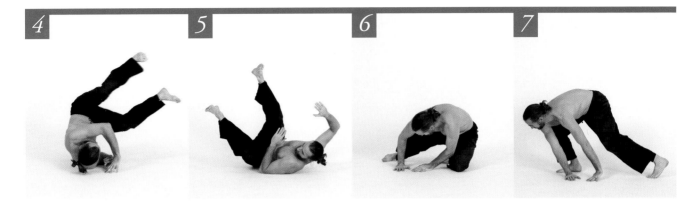

5   Keep rolling, following a line that runs diagonally along your back from your shoulder to the opposite hip.

6   As you're pushed by momentum, you briefly transition to a sit with your upper body upright. Bend one leg to use it as a point of support to keep pushing yourself forward and upward. Optionally, flex your foot so you can push off rapidly as you stand up.

Place your hands on the ground for support if the momentum is still strong enough to push you off balance and to help push yourself back up to standing.

7   Push off your arms to stand back up.

TECHNIQUE TIP

If you have managed an efficient dive, your body's position during the roll is the most crucial part in making the movement efficient and safe. It's best to acquire the specific pattern of this roll by slowly and mindfully training it at ground level as shown in the next six photos.

It's natural to prefer rolling on one side rather than the other, but you should practice it on both sides, as you do with every unilateral movement. Progressions toward a more challenging dive roll involve rolling from standing, rolling following a Broad Jump, rolling following a low Depth Jump, rolling following a jump with a depth and distance ratio, and of course adding a run-up to increase forward momentum before you jump.

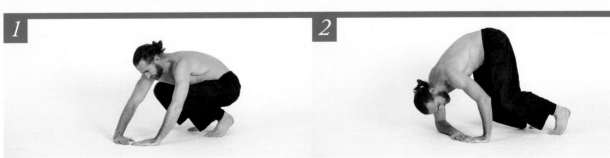

(continued on next page)

1   Start in a Deep Knee Bend, leaning forward with both hands in an inverted V shape. Slightly rotate your trunk toward the side where you'll be rolling.

2   Push off your feet to lean forward and down as you bend and lower your front forearm to the ground. Keep turning your body toward the side to which you're rolling by using a rotational hip motion. Your head starts turning in the opposite direction.

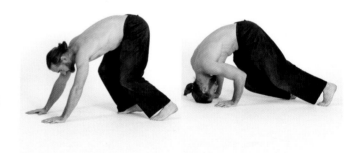

3 While tucking your shoulder and head in, keep lowering your shoulder to the ground as your hips keep moving forward above your shoulder. Your feet are now off the ground.

4 Roll diagonally across your back, starting to look in the direction where you'll exit the roll.

5 Roll on your back all the way toward the hip opposite the shoulder on which you entered the roll.

6 This phase is like the sequence I explained before.

Faults

The main faults happening with the dive have to do with the following two things:

- Rolling immediately upon landing without diving or without diving far enough. Entering the roll too violently can cause you to wreck your shoulder, elbows, head, neck, or back.

- Miscalculating the angle at which you lean upon landing. If you lean even slightly backward, you fall on your rear and ruin your knees. If you stand vertically or barely lean forward, you might go down quickly and land hard on your knees. If you lean too much you might fall flat.

Here are four of the main faults of the roll after the dive:

1 Your hands are level rather than in a V shape, which directs your body straight forward. Your head could knock the ground, or you could push up and over the head to roll directly along the spine. You might even land heavily on the back.

2 Both your hands are pointing outward, which prevents the rolling arm from bending properly and guiding the body in the right position.

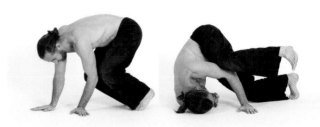

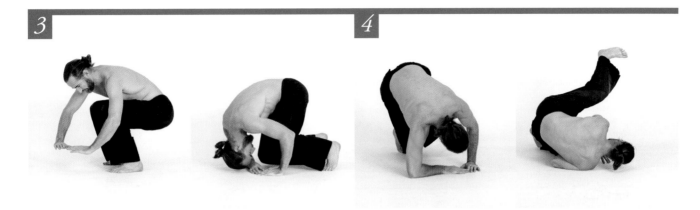

3 The position of your body is too compact and vertical (the result of not leaning forward or not diving/bouncing forward), which puts all the impact on your legs, hips, and lower back and prevents you from rolling at all or pushes your head directly to the ground.

4 Your body is leaning too much to the side and falling sideways instead of rolling diagonally across the back.

Like any other area of Natural Movement, ground movements may involve some form of external load and manipulation, such as carrying, lifting, throwing, catching, pushing, pulling, or dragging a load or object. All the get-up strategies—except the sprawls and rolls—can be turned into manipulative movements that enable you to lift or put down an object or a person (usually of a relatively light weight). More effective techniques for lifting or putting down heavy loads are covered in Chapters 30 and 31.

26
Balancing Movement

Balance is primarily an ability to maintain your center of gravity in vertical alignment with the center of your base of support with minimal sway in any direction; secondarily, it's the ability to control movement when your center of gravity is intentionally out of vertical alignment with your base of support. So, really movement is just a constant act of balancing yourself, or, in other words, movement is your controlled interaction with gravity.

Balance is required in any of our activities of daily living, even when you don't notice that you are balancing, such as when you get to your feet to stand. For example, sitting on a chair requires a certain level of balance. Balancing starts the moment that you begin elevating your center of gravity above your base of support, even though balance also occurs while your base of support is entirely above your center of gravity or when you're airborne.

However, there is a significant difference between the basic balance necessary for day-to-day movement, or even in broad Natural Movement practice on wide, stable surfaces and the advanced balance that we need to negotiate narrow or unstable surfaces. We take the former type of balance for granted, but the latter requires us to be highly attentive.

When we talk about natural balancing specifically, we aren't talking exclusively about balancing on two feet as we stand and walk in a vertical position, which is commonly referred to as postural balance. There is so much more to practical and adaptable balancing. We also aren't talking about creative ways to balance in improbable positions that have zero practical relevance, even though that type of balancing can be lots of fun and potentially functionally beneficial (so we shouldn't dismiss it completely).

Balancing from a Natural Movement perspective implies diverse positions and patterns such as lying, crawling, sitting, getting up, standing, walking, and even climbing, but all movements are done on surfac-

es that are either narrow, elevated, rounded, uneven, inclined, declined, slippery, unstable, or a combination of these variables. Such variables create complex environments in which we become mindfully absorbed in the highest priority, which is conserving balance to prevent falling and is a much greater risk than when we do movements on wide, stable surfaces. Therefore, it's the type and level of complexity of the environmental variables that force us to use the skill of balancing.

To practice balancing, we must hold positions that are normally rather easy to hold and do movements that are normally easy to do, but we must do it on surfaces that can easily destabilize us. In that sense, walking on small, unstable surfaces starts to become balancing even in the absence of elevation. Ultimately, practice is done at a certain elevation, which means we must mentally deal with the risk of falling and the possibility of injuring ourselves.

Depending on skill, environment, and mental state, balancing can be play and great fun, but in the real world it can also be a struggle, and you might have to deal with fear as you engage in life-or-death situations.

Benefits *of* Balancing Practice

On top of expanding your real-life physical competency to surfaces where movement effectiveness, efficiency, speed, and safety are immediately challenged, balancing practice provides other benefits. First, the extra sense of balance developed by training on narrow or unstable surfaces might give you increased balance when you do the same movement patterns on wide, stable surfaces. Practicing also dramatically develops greater joint stability, which contributes to greater motor control as well as injury-prevention and rehabilitation. And the benefits aren't restricted to just the lower limbs, as balance is also controlled through the rest of the body.

These benefits of increased balance to overall movement ability might serve the specialized athlete very well, not only in terms of skill and performance but also for preventing common injuries such as ankle sprain; the growing teenager trying to master his or her new body; or an elderly person who's trying to avoid the deadly threat of a fall and a hip fracture. Indeed, one out of three people aged 65 and older fall each year; one out of four people older than 50 who break their hip as they fall die within a year after injury because of the extended recovery period and complications related to the injury. This is a very serious risk to all of us. General Natural Movement training, and balancing in particular, decreases the risk that you will lose balance and fall. If you do fall, the risk of fracture also will be decreased because you might fall in a softer way and because regular movement practice keeps your bone density higher than in individuals who are physically inactive. So, don't wait until you are in your old age and a physiotherapist or occupational therapist introduces balance training in your treatment plan because you've lost motor control or suffer from osteoporosis or a neurological condition. You can't avoid aging, but you can reduce and slow the damage it does to your body, your movement ability and autonomy, and your day-to-day quality of life.

Balancing training can generate instant frustration because it can be quite challenging to do, but you also will get instant gratification because it is always so fun to do. So, get your balancing ON!

How Balance Works

Unless it is a deliberate action, avoiding toppling is what moving is all about. We all understand that toppling means losing balance, but what it implies is that the normally vertical line that passes through your center of gravity and the middle of your base of support shifts to an angle. The shifting of the center of gravity outside a vertical line with your base of support—if not remedied rapidly—produces an acceleration that becomes rapidly uncontrollable and results in complete loss of balance, which precipitates a fall.

Sensory Inputs

Three sensory systems work in concert to achieve and maintain the body's balance both statically and dynamically in relation to the environment and gravity: the vestibular, somatosensory, and visual systems. Will it help your balance to learn in-depth scientific knowledge behind each of them? Not at all. You feel your balance, not think it, and that's what these systems do: provide diverse sensory inputs to regulate your balance through sensation or "feel," without any intellectual analysis on your part.

However, here is a basic overview of each of the systems:

- The vestibular system is the input from what's called your "inner ear"; it detects gravity and both linear and rotational movement.
- The somatosensory system receives input from your joints, muscles, and skin that tells you their position relative to each other and to the surface where you balance. This system reads feedback about pressure and friction in your points of support relative to the surface of support. For instance, if you stand on your feet and more body weight shifts forward, you feel more pressure in the balls of your feet; if the shift wasn't intentional, the somatosensory system informs you that you need to readjust your body weight distribution; otherwise, gravity will pull you off balance.
- The visual system receives the input from your eyes, which has a lot to do with perceiving how vertical your body and head position is in relation to your base of support and the surface supporting you. In a world ruled by gravity, verticality really matters. When a person balances with their eyes closed, postural sway dramatically increases. Even reduced peripheral vision can challenge balance and increase postural sway, which clearly shows how important visual input is for balancing. For instance, it can be useful to focus on a fixed object, especially a vertical line. But if your feet are positioned in a crooked way on the supporting surface, if they're numb and you can't feel them, or if your inner ear is impaired and you feel dizzy, you will feel very off.

No sensory system really prevails. All three systems are equally important and must work together in harmony to interpret all three inputs, generate coordinated reflexes, and avoid unintentional toppling. This process obviously takes place when performing any movement, but it is especially critical when balancing, which again is the skill of maintaining balance while moving on surfaces that greatly challenge our balance.

Righting and Tilting Reflexes

The brain uses two ways of controlling the body's balance that have been called the righting reflex and the tilting reflex. Both reflexes have to do with deciding what positional adjustments must be made—in terms of direction, magnitude, and timing of body-weight shifting—to stabilize the body. This process can last less than a second or much longer.

The righting reflex helps you correct your position when your center of gravity is taken out of vertical alignment with its base of support while you're on a stable surface. When you balance on stable surfaces, your body should "right" its position by ensuring balance through optimum joint stability. The fact that the supporting surface doesn't move should enable "static equilibrium," which simply means holding a still position. As I describe in Part 2 of this book, even a stable balancing position never goes unchallenged and requires attention and energy to be maintained; we may experience a sensation of stillness, yet almost imperceptible oscillations occur because of the segmental structure of our bodies.

While you balance on unstable surfaces, your base of support, say your feet, moves in space together with the surface that supports it, forcing your brain to do much more complex calculations to keep the center of gravity dynamically aligned with both a moving base of support and moving surface of support. That's what the tilting reflex handles—anticipating optimum alignment in relation to a constantly shifting support surface. It is a significantly more challenging task than static equilibrium, as holding the exact same position is virtually impossible because of the instability of the support surface.

In a nutshell, the righting reflex enables you to balance in a stable manner on a stable surface of support, and the tilting reflex enables you to balance in an unstable fashion on unstable surfaces of support.

The SAID Principle Applies to Balancing

The righting and tilting reflexes often act together as stable surfaces are not always totally stable, and unstable surfaces are not always highly unstable. The bad news is that the two reflexes aren't interchangeable or transferable. A gymnast who's an expert at balancing on a beam, which is stable, does not become an expert surfer who can balance on highly unstable surfaces (or the other way around).

From a general physical competency standpoint, you must possess both reflexes, and the SAID principle informs us that if we want to be good at balancing both on stable and unstable surfaces, we must train on both types of surfaces. The SAID principle also tells us that your proficiency at balancing depends on more than the relative stability or instability of the surface; balance is also affected by factors such as how narrow, flat, rounded, and slippery it is, your experience with specific positions and movement patterns, your ability to maintain breath control, your joint stability and muscular relaxation, and your mental freshness and ability to focus with great intensity. Don't forget that environmental factors—such as visibility, wind, and rain—can play a significant role. At some point in your balancing practice, you must confront all these variables.

NOTE

You can read more about the Specific Adaptation to Imposed Demand (SAID) principle in Chapter 7.

Needless to say, fitness methods that claim to improve balance without having you actually practice balancing on diverse surfaces or that limit your practice to a few drills are not fully delivering in the balance area. Unless you frequently expose yourself to various balancing motion patterns on various surfaces, you know little about your actual balance. You want great balance? Then practice all sorts of balancing.

Learning to Not Use Your Arms to Counterbalance

Even on stable surfaces, a certain amount of sway is inevitable. There will always be small disruptions along the kinetic chain, some of which are barely perceptible. The goal of mindful practice is to train your body's automatic responses to "right" these disturbances quickly before they become out of control. Flailing your arms around is a natural reflex in untrained individuals for maintaining or recovering balance. It is usually a sign that shows that the disturbances are getting out of control or that you lack stability in control where it's needed to prevent the disturbances or adjust to them rapidly.

From a practical effectiveness perspective, it's essential that you learn to not rely on your arms to adjust your balance (or that you rely on them minimally). There is both a functional and a very practical reason for this.

The practical (and most important) reason is that you might need to use your arms for something other than helping your balance—for instance, gesturing, throwing or catching a light object, aiming at a target with a weapon, holding or stabilizing a load, or swinging your arms to transition to jumping off the surface. If you haven't learned to balance without using your arms for counterbalancing, either you will be unable to perform any additional task while your arms are busy balancing your body, or your balance will be threatened as soon as you stop using your arms for that purpose.

The competency aspect of learning to not use your arms for counterbalancing is obvious: Keeping your arms down and loose places a higher demand on the rest of your body in terms of ensuring stability. You may first learn to better counterbalance through your legs by balancing on a single leg while the other is counterbalancing. Indeed, single-leg balance is a great indicator of standing balance. Ultimately, you may become able to primarily adjust your balance through minor hip and spine motions.

NOTE

Later I give examples of single-leg positions and movements that are extremely helpful in developing standing balancing.

Learning to not rely on your arms might significantly increase sway in your hips and knees in the beginning, but over time you will learn to adjust and will develop much greater lower-body and core stability, and you'll be able to use your arms independently. The musculature surrounding your ankles, knees, and hips also will strengthen, delaying fatigue in these areas and making your ability to ensure balance more durable.

Obviously, this is a practice perspective, not a real-life one. If you are balancing in the real world and suddenly find yourself off balance, then counterbalancing with your arms immediately to avoid a fall is a no-brainer—especially if the surface is significantly unstable, in which case you need to do all you can to counterbalance your whole body.

Cause or Symptom?

Imagine that you're practicing balance on a 2x4 board at ground level, standing and walking forward. Seems straightforward and easy, right? However, you might find yourself flailing your arms (or trying to prevent yourself from doing so), stiffening your arms, and holding your breath. Your hips might be badly swaying, and your knees might badly shake. You have no choice but to go off balance, step off the board, and try again. You may try to focus more and do your best to prevent your knee and ankle joints from being so wobbly, yet your balance isn't improving at all. Have you mistaken the symptom as a cause? Maybe your feet are not centered and aligned; they're crook-

ed on the board, and from there a whole inefficient kinetic chain is formed. It originates in your lack of positional control, affects your ankles, knees, and hips, and everything else that can go wrong along the line. You won't fix what happens "up the chain"—that is, the symptom—before you fix the cause (your ill-positioned points of support). This is true for any natural movement, but it's especially important in balancing. Rather than checking your positional control from "head to toe," check it from "toe to head" (or from whichever body part is your base of support)!

Breath Control, Tension, Relaxation

Maintaining impeccable breath control is one of the main keys to skillful balancing. Joint stability is not created by overall tension but by selective tension in the muscles required for some joints to be stable in a position. Without breath control, you're nearly guaranteed to be tense all over and prevent relaxation. A lack of relaxation in balancing doesn't just cost you extra energy; it also prevents both the righting and tilting reflexes from doing their jobs and adjusting your position. You may "instinctively" think that tensing your whole body will reduce sway. It might do that, but it also can make you fall like a marble statue that topples off its pedestal. Keep breathing abdominally, so both tension and relaxation can do their part properly and harmoniously.

Losing Balance *or* Falling? Crashing *or* Landing?

Despite consistent skill training and mindfulness in movement, no one is ever unfailing. Whereas physical action may most of the time be effective despite being inefficient, sometimes it's neither efficient nor effective. Your training is not an absolute guarantee against ineffectiveness. Losing balance may happen because you're not paying attention, because the supporting surface is unpredictable and causes slippage,

because you're pushed, or because you want to fall for a reason. When you get slightly off balance momentarily, you often can recover by counterbalancing to get back to the same original position or by changing position without falling—for instance, by promptly lowering your center of gravity or by using some of the vertical transition techniques that I cover in this chapter.

Falling off the supporting surface is clearly the worst scenario. The danger you face when you fall off an elevated surface without an ability to land on your feet depends on the height, but your position upon impact and the impact surface also play an enormous role in the likelihood of injury and its severity. In short, you may crash or land. Crashing implies a complete lack of control over your landing position or movement, whereas landing implies total or partial control over it. The aim of landing is to avoid collision and crashing by intentionally positioning your body, or moving it, in a way that optimizes the dissipation of impact forces and turns the fall into a controlled landing (or a landing that's as controlled as possible). This is a self-protective reflex similar to a sprawl when you run and stumble rather than face-planting.

While no amount of technique or training will prevent you from severe body damage if you fall from a great height, sometimes a shorter fall is more dangerous than a longer one because there is too little time for positional control before impact. A longer fall increases the velocity of the trajectory and potentially the force of the impact, but it might enable you to position yourself in a way that enables optimum dissipation of the greater downward kinetic energy—through a front roll, for instance. The distance gives your brain enough time to become aware of the nature of the fall (speed, body position, angle/trajectory, duration, landing surface) and come up with a reflexive movement strategy to attempt landing and reduce the chance of trauma as much as possible. If you fall while balancing at a short height in a bad position, you might crash badly on your back or hit your head. If you fall the same way from a greater height, you might have enough time to land on your feet—if you know how to change your position while you're airborne and probably scared.

Practice *and* Progressions

The more challenging the surface, the more the risk of falling increases, which, in most cases, forces us to significantly reduce our speed to ensure control and safety. Falling is an inherent part of balancing practice. Consequently, it's recommended that you start at a low level of complexity and danger, just as you do with all other skills.

I advise to work through the following general progressions tips:

- Start on flat, stable, wide surfaces at ground level then slowly transition to rounded, elevated, and slightly unstable ones. If you aren't stable on non-moving, flat surfaces at ground level, why would you try to be stable on unstable, rounded surfaces that are elevated?
- You need to know what happens if you do fall. What is your ability to recover safely? One of the simplest answers is to step down if you're balancing close to the ground or to jump down if you practice at a greater elevation. But can you land safely and repeatedly from the height where you're practicing?

You must have satisfying answers to these questions before you engage in balancing.

Hold Your Position (or "Slow Down Cowboy")

From a technical standpoint, the ability to effortlessly or comfortably hold balancing positions is essential to your ability to move in balance efficiently. Indeed, balancing movements are nothing but the step-by-step establishment of balanced positions in a sequence. Positions that are flawed, uneasy, unstable, or inefficient will become apparent as you try to move dynamically through a sequence. For instance, beginners asked to walk across a balance beam will do it too rapidly, not just for fun but because they try to use speed to help them get across before they lose balance entirely. In this case, speed is a conscious or unconscious strategy to hide and compensate for a lack of stability. Instead of speeding the movement, you need to slow it down to expose your inefficiencies so you can start addressing them. Knowing that your ability to hold static stances is essential to your ability to perform dynamic balancing movements efficiently, the practice of static positions and slow-motion movements is the best way to expose flaws and improve balancing when you begin.

This is the reason I start with the positions that first need to be held with control; the goal is more dynamic, coordinated movements based on positional control and solid fundamental positions. From a practical standpoint, holding stable positions, even briefly, goes beyond supporting efficient movement; we often start and finish balancing with static equilibrium, before we transition to balanced movement. We also need to be able to stop and hold standing positions anytime, to reset our balance and resume moving or to rest, observe, listen, or ensure a smooth transition to a different movement, such as climbing or jumping down.

What, Where, When

To build up your skills and increase your options, you need to practice every position and movement separately and mindfully, and then practice skillful transitions from one to another. You can pick one balancing movement a day and practice a new one every day or every new practice session. Alternatively, you can work on two or three movements within the same session or pick one movement to practice for a whole week or until you feel that you've mastered it. The goal in the beginning is to enjoy practice, and changing movements makes the practice more fun by keeping it fresh and satisfying each time. Plus, there is a chance that the gains you make in a certain balancing pattern may transfer to others, at least to some extent. However, some people prefer to establish specific patterns and routines and make sure that they make progress with one thing before they change to something new. If that is your preference, just do that.

For most of these techniques, you can start on a simple 2x4 board on the floor, which is a flat, stable, not-too-narrow surface. It's also a cheap prop and great for warming up. Warming up in balancing is physiological, of course, but it also has a lot to do with awakening the central nervous system, which is best done at a low level of environmental complexity.

With techniques that involve sitting or transitions to and from balancing (stepping up or down, for instance), you need an elevated surface, but you can keep it at the minimum height necessary for basic practice. As your skills and confidence improve, switch to more challenging surfaces, such as a narrower beam or a surface that's rounded, smoother, more slippery, slightly unstable, inclined, declined, or uneven, then add elevation or a load (such as a backpack or weighted vest) very gradually.

Adding elevation has a lot to do with the following:

- Training your mental coolness more than your balancing reflexes (even though the difference of visual input can be disturbing at first), especially if you stand above a hard surface.
- Knowing what happens if you do lose balance and assessing with honesty your ability to recover safely from it. You need to find out if you can jump down with control or if you can swiftly sit or hang.

Past a certain level, additional environmental complexity becomes either unsustainable and/or unrealistic. Slacklining is a great example because it presents an approach to movement that is unrealistic. If you had to traverse across a canyon, or above a river on a thin, unstable surface, maybe while carrying a backpack, what would be the fastest and safest way to do it? You wouldn't balance; you'd hang underneath by your arms and legs. The point is that you shouldn't minimize in any way the benefits of highly challenging and specialized balancing modes, such as slacklining, surfing, or skiing, nor the immense gratification that stems from them. Instead, you should emphasize that Natural Movement prioritizes the most basic, realistic, useful, natural, and safe applications of human movement potential. For instance, humans may learn to balance on their hands in an inverted position, but fundamental aptitudes of balancing on your feet prevail over the accessory ability of balancing in a handstand. Both balancing on your feet and balancing on your hands have physiological benefit, but the former holds much greater practical value. Without dismissing creative ways of balancing your body, the most useful and frequent techniques should prevail in terms of time and effort dedicated to practice.

Mixing movement skills—for instance, carrying, throwing, or catching something while balancing—is another important step in training. Finally, you learn to integrate your balancing movements with other natural movements within "combos" that you change up frequently. You will soon realize that balancing in isolation and balancing after lifting heavy or sprinting hard is not the same at all. Practicing such transitions will help you develop greater, more realistic experience and a greater sense of your real-life physical competency.

Remember, there is no single "best" balancing position or movement you should confine your balancing practice to. Like other natural movements, the best balancing position or movement is that which adapts best to a given context at a given time. That means you should develop ability with any of the positions and movements listed in this chapter. In the real world, what is otherwise seen in practice as something to avoid, such as counterbalancing with your arms, rounding your back, and even using your knee for support, can be the best thing to do at a given time. The question is, do you intentionally place yourself in a position out of adaptability, effectiveness, and efficiency? Or do you helplessly find yourself in a position or doing a movement because you lack positional control and technique, which forces you into inefficient, risky position and movement options?

Balancing *on* Feet: Standing

Think of making your way across a fallen tree that links the two banks of a river. From a practical standpoint, walking across might not be the only physical action involved. Indeed, you might need to stop and hold a standing, two-footed position at any time to reset your balance, rest, wait, or observe. Learning to maintain joint stability from head to toe, first on two feet and then on one foot, is essential to your ability to hold steady, controlled balancing standing stances and ultimately to walk in balance skillfully. For now, let's start with the fundamental standing positions and then we'll progress to movements.

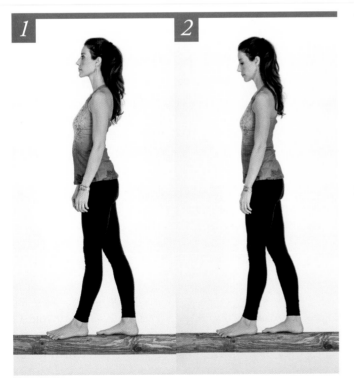

1   Step on the beam with one foot in front of the other in a Two-Footed Standing position. Keep your feet aligned with the beam from heel to toes. You should feel that the pressure of your body weight is equally distributed toward the center of your feet. Assume a tall, vertical posture with your arms down and relaxed, your head up, your eyes looking forward. Breathe calmly and minimize postural sway.

2   If you need to look down, do so without tilting your head down (or just barely tilting it).

Don't fret if things don't work exactly this way right off the bat. Even if you manage to effectively stay on the beam, inefficiencies might occur: Your feet might move out of alignment with the support surface, your back might be rounded, your torso might lean forward, your head might tilt down too much, your hips might sway, your ankles and knees might shake, your shoulders might shrug, you might be tense all over, or you might hold your breath. All are issues that are likely to lead you sooner or later to lose balance completely.

At this stage, if your immediate reflex is to use your arms to counterbalance and minimize sway in your knees, hips, and torso, try to do it minimally, and with your arms in a set position. Controlling your arms might feel counterintuitive at first, but before you know it, reverting to using your arms because the rest of your body isn't doing its stabilization job is what will not feel right.

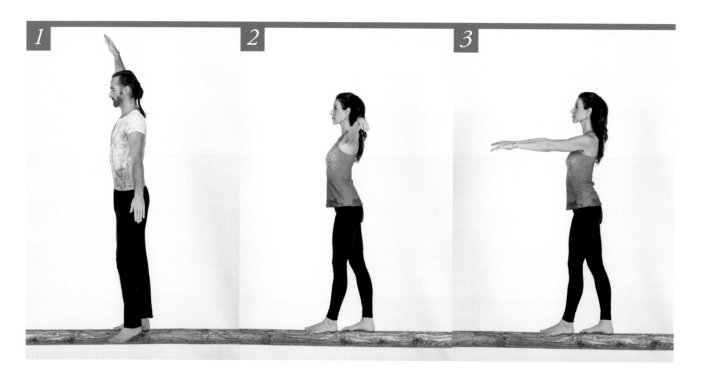

1   Practice the same standing position as before with your arms counterbalancing in uneven positions to your sides.

2   Bring your arms level with little sway.

3   Bring your arms straight out in front of you. This position is a little more challenging than keeping them to the sides. It is one step closer to not needing your arms.

Trying to let your arms down too early may result in compensatory issues:

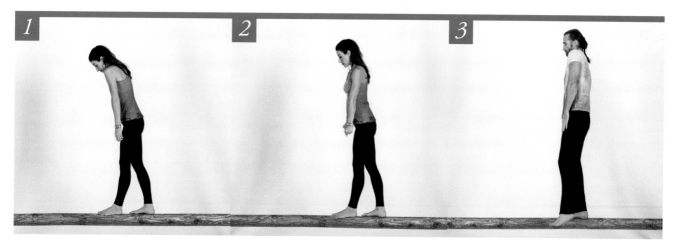

1. Your head and torso lean forward to look down at the beam.

2. You look down, clench your fists, and tense your arms.

3. You have a tall posture and look straight, but you shrug your shoulders and press your arms hard against your body.

Once you have mastered a neutral Two-Footed Standing stance with minimal sway and without arm counterbalancing, you can try more challenging variations. Always keep in mind that variations have practical value when balancing is done in context.

First while keeping the same base of support:

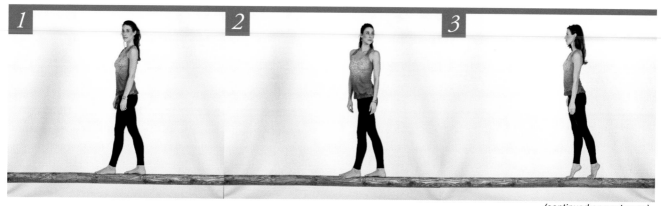

(continued on next page)

1. Turn your head to the side. You could also tilt it up and down or sideways. Head movements are an easy way to put your vestibular and visual systems in a higher state of alert or confusion and disturb your balance, yet they are very useful for observation and orientation even when balancing. Turn your head very slowly in the beginning without generating instability. Then do swifter head movements as if something required your instant attention in another direction.

2. Rotate your head and trunk. This variation has the same practical purpose as the variation in step 1. Practice it the same way.

3. Tiptoe. This is an essential transitional position that elevates your field of vision or allows you to reach something above you. This drill develops great foot strength and ankle stability. Additionally, once your heels are elevated, you could pivot sideways on the balls of your feet using hip rotation.

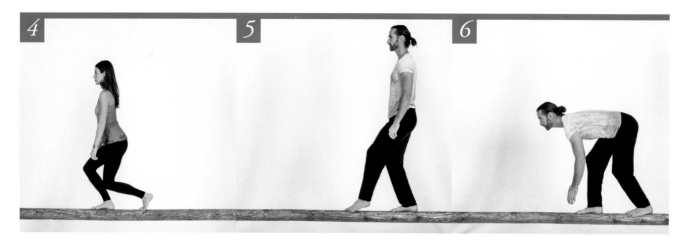

4 Shift body weight to the front foot in a Half Split Squat. Use this variation to lower your center of gravity to adjust balance, transition to a lower position, or duck under something. It demands more strength and joint stability from the leg and hip that supports most of your weight.

5 Shift your body weight to the back foot with the front heel up. You use this variation to wait or correct balance when stepping forward is challenged or when you're stepping backward. It demands more strength and joint stability from the leg and hip that supports most of your weight.

6 Assume a deep Hip Hinge while still looking forward. This is useful to duck under an obstacle or to prepare for crawling or sitting down.

Once you've mastered, or at least greatly improved, each of these individual stances and movements, start practicing slow transitions from stance to stance and movement to movement in any order you want. Over time, start to do faster transitions. Because you're in a split stance, make sure to switch your front and back feet regularly. Additional movements could include extending one arm or both arms in various directions or turning or tilting your head to change your line of vision; all are positional changes that could quite easily affect your balance and even make you lose it, but that can easily happen in real-world situations. Really, you can do any variation of position you can think of that you can assume intentionally and with control. An additional, useful, and fun drill, which I like to call "the noodle," involves making yourself very loose and intentionally creating as much sway as possible while you stay balanced on the beam.

Balancing on the Balls of the Feet

Holding your balance on the balls of your feet is a practical necessity when the support surface is very narrow. Balancing this way improves foot and calf strength, ankle mobility, stability, and postural alignment. The functional benefits of this movement transfer to a better ability in establishing or adjusting your balance when you're entering balancing by stepping or landing. Beyond that, it transfers greater stability in any movement on your feet, including walking, running, lifting, and landing.

An innate instinct is to try to center your feet on the surface of support to increase the surface of foot that's supporting your body weight and reduce ankle instability to make yourself more stable. Although this may occasionally help, it's a strategy that usually works against you. The reason is that it reduces range of motion at foot and ankle level, but range of motion is essential to letting your righting reflex adjust position. By "locking" your feet and ankles in a set, near-immobile position, all adjustments become the responsibility of the joints above the ankles, which increases postural sway and might throw you off-balance. Although learning to tiptoe makes you much more unstable at first, it also supports the development of much greater ankle mobility and stability, and ultimately much greater ability to balance on your feet. You can start tiptoeing on a 2x4 board with your feet aligned it, but this position will not let you lower your heels below the level of your forefeet. When in a side position with your body parallel to the supporting surface, and you're on the edge of it with your heels in the void, your heels can move lower than the balls of your feet.

All you need to start practice is a stable low box, a flat stone, a stair, a curb—any surface that is flat, stable, and about 3 inches tall.

Step up to a level stance, heels off the surface and horizontally aligned with your toes. You may start with half your foot on the surface and half off the surface, then progressively slide your feet backward to reduce the surface area of your feet in contact with the surface to make it more challenging. Make sure to maintain a tall posture, have your arms down and relaxed, and your head up. Always control your breathing.

Single-Leg Standing Balancing

Imagine a surface so small that it can hold only one foot, such as a rock that barely breaks the surface of a river. You must jump and land on it on one foot, balance there on one leg for a moment, then do a Leg Swing Jump to reach the next rock that is otherwise too far to step to.

Supporting all your body weight on the small surface of a single foot is not a small feat at all! But if you learn to balance on one foot skillfully, then all movement balancing on two feet becomes much easier.

Single-Leg Balancing is arguably the best indicator of bipedal, standing balance (or lack thereof). Indeed, the balancing version of walking is the same step-by-step replication of a sequence alternating single-footed and two-footed standing positions, only this

time it's on a narrow, rounded, or unstable surface. This makes the single-leg phase of the movement, which is the longer one, significantly more challenging. If your single-leg balance is troublesome, it is guaranteed to directly translate to an ugly struggle when you attempt to walk in balance.

Another practical advantage of the ability to balance on one foot is that you can always counterbalance using your free leg rather than your arms if they are unable to assist (maybe because you are holding something), which is very helpful. Whenever you are practicing single-leg positions and movements, make sure to switch feet regularly!

First, practice following progressions as you did with the Two-Footed Standing position.

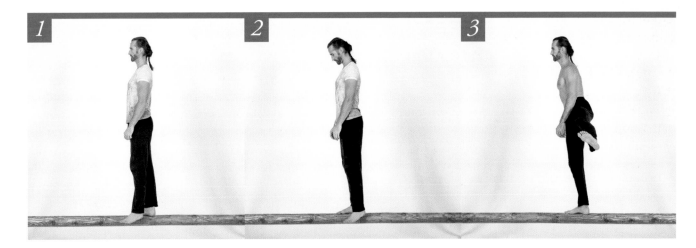

1 Establish the Single-Leg Balancing position with a tall posture, arms down and relaxed, minimal postural sway, and controlled abdominal breath.

2 Look down if it helps at first.

3 Learn to use your free leg for counterbalancing instead of your arms so you can keep your arms down and your head up. Extend your free leg to the side, ideally as low as possible.

Backward Standing Balancing Walk

Walking in balance is a common way to traverse narrow obstacles such as a fallen tree, a beam, or the ledge of a wall. Moving back to where you came from is sometimes necessary when your forward progression is stopped by an obstacle or danger that you may not have foreseen when you were standing some distance back. Reversing your orientation could be difficult or time-consuming, or it may be necessary to keep an eye on the situation in front of you as you move backward away from it.

You might think it's counterintuitive to start with Backward Standing Balancing Walk, it is actually very beneficial from a practice perspective. Going backward immediately forces you to place the ball of your foot on the surface of support rather than leading with the heel before you shift body weight backward to the rest of your foot, which is also the safest way to walk in balance when you're moving forward (except when the surface is wide and stable enough to walk with the usual heel-ball sequence). You're also hard-pressed to look at your feet while going backward, which forces you to use proprioception and exteroception—in essence, feeling your way rather than using visual input to ensure positional control. Go slow at first and work on minimal postural sway and counterbalancing before you increase speed.

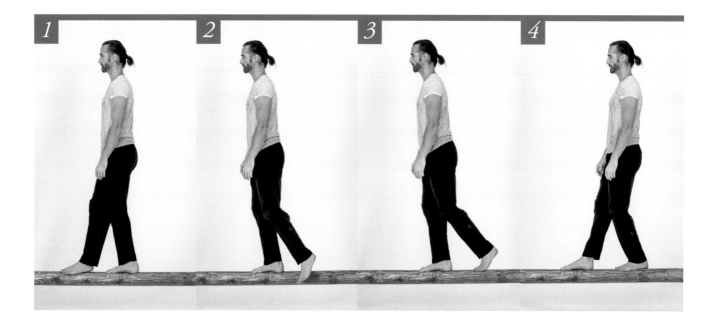

1 Start in a neutral Standing Split Stance, with tall posture, arms down and relaxed, head up and looking forward.

2 Shift your weight to your back foot, with your knee slightly bent, then release your front foot and pull your front leg toward the back while maintaining joint stability from feet to head.

3 Shift body weight to the back foot and move the front leg backward as in a regular forward step to place the ball of your foot on the surface behind you. At this point, almost 100 percent of your body weight is still on your front foot. Horizontally align the ball of your back foot and your ankle with the beam so that when you shift your weight to your back foot, your whole foot comes flat in a stable manner and is well-aligned with the supporting surface.

4 Push off your front foot and shift all your weight to your back foot, pressing down so your entire foot comes flat and is well-aligned with the surface. You will find yourself in a Split Standing stance with your back leg slightly bent and more body weight on the back foot, ready to repeat the same sequence.

Here are some progressions or variations that are just as beneficial and practical as only trying to walk faster across the beam:

- Bend your legs more, while keeping your upper body upright.
- Bend your legs more with a slight Hip Hinge (straight back).
- Bend your legs more while crouching (with a rounded back, see the next movement).
- Take wider steps.
- Slow your walk and lengthen the time you spend on a single leg.

- Walk across while changing your head position and field of vision.
- Practice walking with your feet at an angle with the beam. Although this is not recommended as a default pattern, it is beneficial to train this way as an option.
- Walk on slightly inclined and declined beams.
- Add light transverse bars perpendicular to the beam, which forces you to either step over or under as if branches or obstacles are in your way. If you don't have such props, simulate them.

Standing Side Shuffle

The Standing Side Shuffle with your body parallel to the surface of support and your heels off the support is not as convenient or safe as walking forward because you cannot counterbalance through your legs and must mostly rely on shifting the hips and center of gravity forward and backward—but you can use it when you must keep looking straight ahead at something or when you anticipate stepping or jumping off the surface in a forward direction. How far you step to the side depends on how comfortable you are with the movement or how much friction you get on the surface. If the surface is slippery, it's safer to take short steps. When practicing, start with small steps and then progressively increase the distance per step.

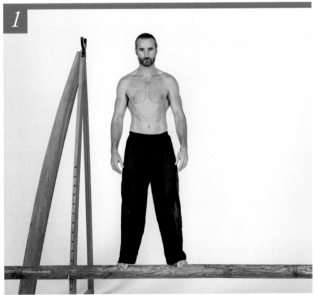

(continued on next page)

1 Assume a stable standing side stance, then shift your weight to your foot that's in the direction you are headed (the front foot) so you can pull your other leg forward. Once your weight is on your front foot, you can pull your back leg (the one opposite the direction you're going) forward close to your front foot. You may slightly lift your foot off the surface or slide it if the surface is sufficiently smooth and even. You may look straight forward, in the direction where you are headed, or in the opposite direction.

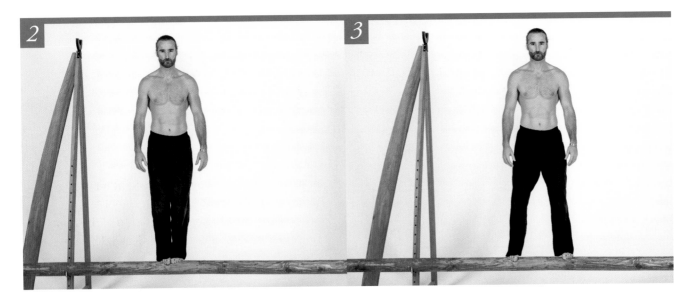

2   Place your back foot against your front foot. Alternatively, it can be safer to place it some distance forward, but not all the way against your front foot. Immediately shift your weight to your back foot so you can extend your front leg forward.

3   Pull your front leg forward and place your front foot on the surface, ready to repeat the sequence.

Reverses/Reversing

Reversing while balancing is an important skill. Reversing means changing body orientation but not necessarily changing travel direction. This simple concept can be confusing, as direction and orientation are often understood as being the same thing. Direction is where you go regardless of where you face. Orientation is where you face regardless of where you go. If you are facing and walking forward and then decide to step backward, you would be changing direction while maintaining the same body orientation. Conversely, if you are facing and walking forward then turn your body 180 degrees to face the opposite direction and resume stepping in a backward direction, you have reversed your body orientation while maintaining your original direction. In most cases, a reverse of orientation implies a change of direction as well because it's always easier and safer to face the direction where you're going.

Unless you're already in a low position, standing reverses are not the most stable options, but they are faster because you don't need to lower your body then stand back up. For greater safety, you may decide to Straddle Sit to reverse your body orientation, and then stand back up (as in the Straddle Sit Reverse).

Cross Reverse

The Cross Reverse is a step-by-step approach to reversing that is more stable and therefore safer than other standing reverse options, but it's a little slower. It is a good compromise when you must reverse relatively quickly but safely. The Cross Reverse can be easily modified and used to reverse from a standing side stance to the same stance facing the opposite direction.

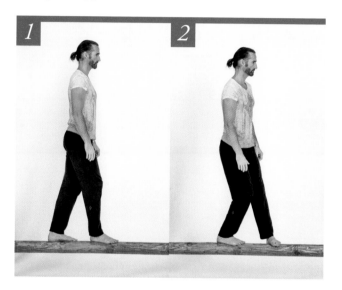

1. Walk forward.

2. While keeping all your body weight on your back foot, bring the ball of your front foot perpendicularly across the surface of the beam. Another option is to start the Cross Reverse from a Split Standing position, shift your body weight to your back foot, and then rotate your front foot perpendicularly to the beam.

3. Once your front foot is in position, you can safely shift your body weight onto it. Bending at the knee helps you balance in this position because it allows more range of motion, such as to rotate your back leg externally.

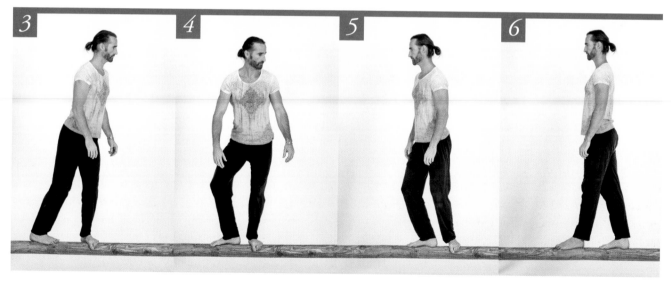

4. With all your weight on your front foot, you can easily rotate your back leg externally so your back foot pivots on its ball and reverses orientation by 180 degrees. If your stance is too narrow, though, you either are forced to pivot on your heel instead of the ball of your foot or to let the ball of your foot slide forward after it pivots. Your back foot must be well aligned with the beam. You may turn your head in the same direction before, simultaneously, or after the rest of your body moves.

5. You now can shift your body weight to your back foot and rotate your hips. At this point, your back foot has become your front foot because you have fully reversed your body orientation.

6. Bring your back leg to the front and resume walking either in the same direction while oriented in the opposite direction, or in the direction opposite to your original direction (but in the same direction as your body orientation).

Pivot Reverse

The Pivot Reverse is the swiftest of the three standing reverse techniques, and it's also the riskiest. It doesn't work well for narrow or slippery surfaces because the risk of losing your balance is too great, including the risk that one of your feet will slide off the surface, which makes you fall instantly. Although it is possible to pivot relatively slowly, doing so might increase friction and cause instability, which defeats the purpose of choosing this technique over others for the sake of speed. If you can't Pivot Reverse quickly, a safer option is to use the Cross Reverse. You can use the Pivot Reverse to change your orientation 90 degrees rather than 180 degrees; in that case it is not a reverse but a change of orientation from a front to side standing balancing stance (or the other way around).

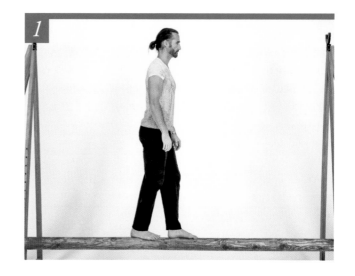

1   Start in a Standing Split Stance.

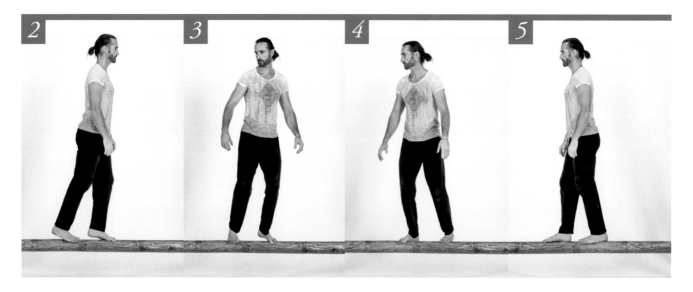

2   Keeping your body weight evenly distributed between each foot, slightly lift both heels at the same time to shift your weight onto the balls of your feet.
Lift them just enough to reduce friction. Elevating too high makes balancing more challenging.

3   Start turning your head then swiftly rotate your hips, which makes you pivot. Turning your head first helps your vestibular system get a sense of direction and position in space more quickly and helps you know where to stop your motion when your head and vision are aligned with the direction of the balancing surface. Your body weight must remain evenly distributed between both feet during

the turn. Keep your arms relaxed and allow them to swing naturally and follow the rest of the body.

4   Your head should fully face the opposite direction before the rest of your body does.

5   You can now bring the rest of your body to align with your head. Once your whole body is lined up facing the direction opposite the one in which you started, lower your heels to the surface of the beam and resume moving either in the same direction you were moving (although your orientation is opposite what it was originally) or move in the direction opposite your original direction (which is the same as your new body orientation).

Deep Split Squat Reverse

The Deep Split Squat Reverse is a safer way to reverse than standing because your center of gravity is low. In case you go off balance, it's easy and quick to lean forward to support yourself with your arms or lower yourself to a Straddle Sit position. You can do a Deep Split Squat Reverse in a slow and safe step-by-step fashion or in a swift pivot motion like the standing Pivot Reverse. I recommend starting with the slower version because it exposes potential stability issues and teaches you the pivot sequence better. Increase the speed of the movement progressively until you are ready to switch to the swifter Deep Split Squat Pivot Reverse.

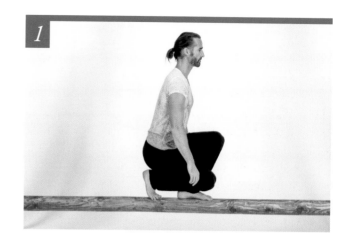

1   Assume a stable Deep Split Squat Stance with tall posture and your arms down.

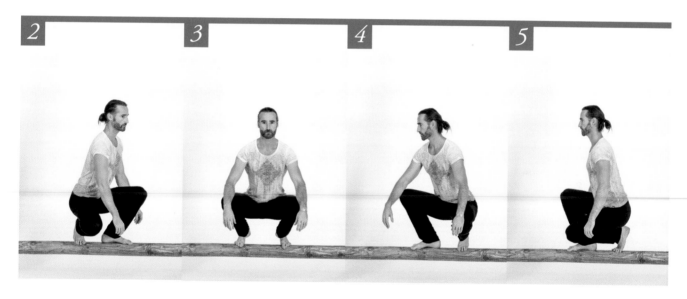

2   Shift a bit of weight to your front foot so you can externally rotate your back leg easily.

3   Rotate your front leg internally to position yourself in a Deep Knee Bend. You may pause here to stabilize if needed.

4   Turn your head and trunk in the direction you're headed while externally rotating the leg on that side.

5   Complete the reverse by internally rotating your back leg, which puts you in the Deep Split Squat position facing the opposite direction.

To perform the faster Pivot Reverse from a squat, lift both heels simultaneously and use a swift rotational motion from your hips to reverse all the way to the opposite direction, which is like the standing Pivot Reverse but is in a Deep Split Squat position. It is essential to constantly keep the balls of your feet centered on the beam during the pivoting motion to maintain foot and ankle stability. With both options, let your arms naturally follow the motion of your body, or you can rest them on your knees.

Balancing *on* **Feet** *and* **Hands**

Going on all fours to lower your center of gravity can be a safer approach to balancing because you are balancing on three or four points of support instead of two. Also, you might be able to transition quickly to the more stable balancing positions of sitting and lying, which is helpful if the surface is slippery, unstable, or both, or if you're loaded with a backpack. (However, the safest approach of all is to traverse while sitting, which I cover later in this section.) Together with the squatting, lying, and sitting balancing positions, balancing on all fours is the balancing version of ground movement, with a very low center of gravity.

Foot and hand positions also can be transitional stances when you are getting up onto a narrow surface from climbing or sitting or when you're moving from standing to lower positions, including hanging underneath the surface of support.

I cover positions that start on all fours, two feet and one hand, one foot and two hands, and even one foot and one hand. I cover these plank positions when I talk about ground movement, but practicing them while balancing is a whole different story. Not all of them have the same importance in balancing because some are less likely to be used than others. All the positions require great levels of core and joint stability, and for that reason are excellent ways to develop stability—especially in the case of the positions that have a base of support of fewer than four points. The effort required to elongate your spine and keep it level with your hips as you maintain abdominal breathing also holds phenomenal benefits for postural rehabilitation that can carry over to a whole spectrum of movement.

Positions *and* **Movements** *on* **Feet** *and* **Hands**

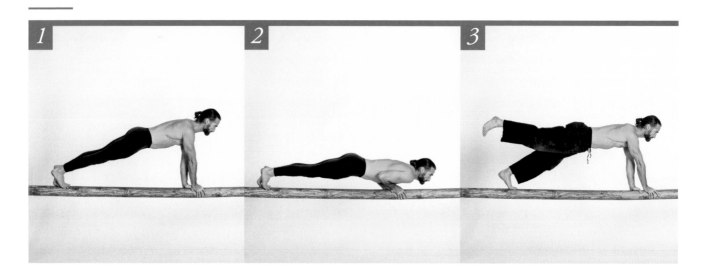

1   Long base with extended legs, level feet and hands for the foot-hand position. Joints are aligned from ankles to neck, and your arms are in the lockout position.

2   Same as position 1 with your arms fully flexed.

3   Long base with extended legs, slightly staggered hands, and a single-foot support. Joints are aligned from ankles to neck, and your arms are in the lockout position.

Foot-Hand Crawl

The pattern, sequence, and timing of this balancing movement is like the Foot-Hand Crawl movements described in Chapter 24, "Ground Movement 1." The difference is in the position of the points of support; in the balancing variation, all four points of support are aligned with the body's midline, which narrows the base of support. If you were to take a photo from the front, all you would see would be a head and two arms, with most of the rest of the body hidden behind. The narrow base of support makes stability quite challenging.

My advice and reminders for efficiency are the same here as they were for the ground movement variation except that I want to stress the importance of all aspects of efficiency in this technique even more than I did before. Any mistake will cause you a moment of imbalance from which you may not able to recover, and that will make you fall off the surface where you're balancing. Focus on keeping your back level, locking out your arms (especially during the phase where you hold the position on one arm), and breathing abdominally to avoid unnecessary tensions.

This is especially the case when you practice the balancing variation of the 4-2 points of support technique, where you must hold a contralateral stance on one foot and one hand only every cycle. From a practical standpoint, the 4-2 points-of-support sequence is less stable and riskier than the 4-3 sequence, so I don't recommend using it in a real-life situation unless you are in perfect control. However, from a practice standpoint, it is a formidable way to develop optimal stability in the Foot-Hand Crawl.

One of the most common reflexes when performing the balancing Foot-Hand Crawl is to try to use your hands for stabilization by strongly grasping the narrow surface that's supporting you. Although this occasionally can be useful, you want to train to rely on positional control rather than grip strength. If you lose balance while on all fours, no amount of grip strength will save you from falling into a hanging position. A better training strategy is to refrain from superfluous tension in the hands and forearms, and a better recovery strategy is to push your body weight away from your hands and toward your feet, which have a much greater ability to support body weight and provide stability.

Before I finish this section about foot-hand balancing, I want to address a few more positions that use feet and hands and can be held and used for a variety of practical reasons but also prove particularly useful in various get-up strategies and techniques. As usual, it's a good idea to practice these positions so they become stable and efficient before you integrate them within complex movement sequences.

Balancing Sitting *on* Your Rear

Sitting allows you to rest, observe, communicate, look for something in your bag, throw or catch something light from a steady position, and recover your balance or sense of safety.

You may sit on your rear, with both legs on one side or straddling, with or without the support of your hands and feet. You could even traverse in such Straddle Sit positions by using your arms. It creates many possible position variations.

The following sit positions also represent important stances that are essential to getting up and down.

These positions are ideally practiced separately. Once you have mastered them and become comfortable, they naturally integrate with more complex sequences.

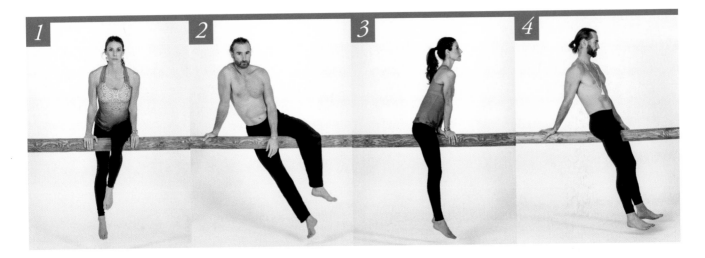

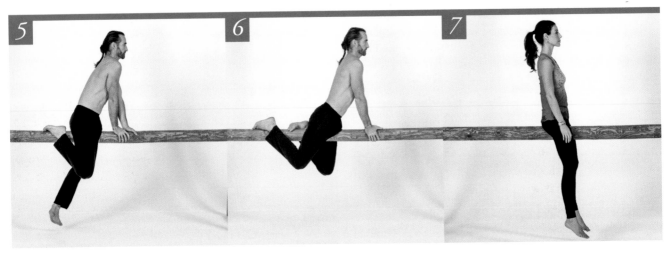

1   Side Straddle Two-Hand position. Your rear and back of the upper part of the supporting leg bear most of the weight (which is different than the Double-Hand, Single-Leg Hook climbing position).

2   Side Straddle Single Opposite Hand position, leaning sideways. The weight is equally distributed between the leg and the arm.

3   Front Straddle, Two-Handed Sit. Slightly lean forward to shift your weight to your hands and use them for greater stability.

4   Front Straddle, Rear-Hand Sit. Lean backward and shift some weight to your rear hand to help with overall stability. Keep a hand to the front to secure your position.

5   Single-Foot Hook, Two-Handed Front Straddle Sit.

6   Double-Foot Hook, Two-Handed Front Straddle Sit.

7   Front Straddle Sit, no hands. Be ready to lean forward and place your hands on the surface in case you get off balance.

Straddle Sit Movements

Sitting while moving in balance across a surface is a slow but secure way to move. People afraid of heights often manage to overcome their fear by moving in a sit. Though it does make traversing or reversing movement slower than other movements, it also significantly increases stability and therefore safety, especially if you are carrying a load on your back. I would choose this approach if the risk and danger I am exposed to are significant.

If the surface is too wide to Straddle Sit comfortably, then crawling would be probably a better option; on the other hand, if the surface is too narrow and unstable, I would probably hang traverse it from underneath. Movement choice is always a matter of context.

Balancing Lying *on* Thighs, Belly, Chest, Hands

The diverse prone or side-lying positions are great positions for rest, observation, hiding, or trying to reach something. They offer a wide, reliable, and safe base of support, and they even allow you to entirely let go of your legs and arms if necessary. It is always possible to be thrown off balance of even the most stable positions, but the great advantage of the lying position is that you can spin around on the surface and end up hanging from beneath it (if the surface of support is narrow enough for your body to hang from it).

You might notice that there is no photo that shows me balancing on my back in a Supine Lying position, and that's for a good reason. Although it's not impossible to use that position when balancing, it's very unstable. If you lose balance, which is bound to happen, you're unable to recover by hanging, and a fall is guaranteed. So, a Supine Lying balancing position has very little practical value. However, you may attempt it at a low height—let's say for movement feedback, experience, or fun. If you ever happen to rest on your back—for example, on a tree branch—make sure it is wide enough. You've been warned!

By using your legs and arms, you will be able to traverse forward and even climb in balance if the surface is inclined. As always, you want to practice these positions separately before you train transitions or actual movements.

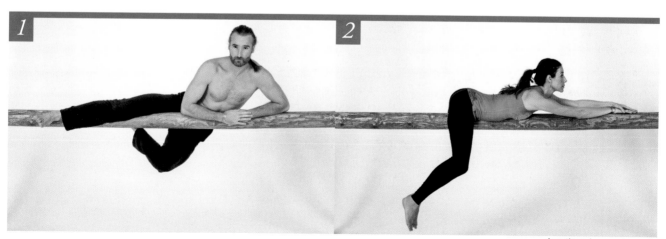

(continued on next page)

1 Forearms Side Straddle Lying

2 Front Straddle Lying, overhand extended arms

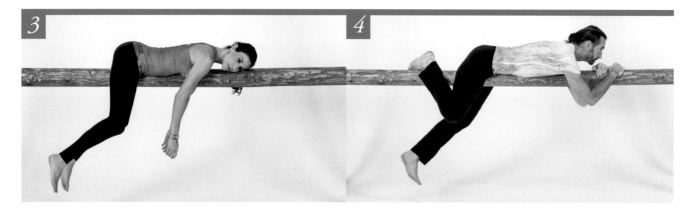

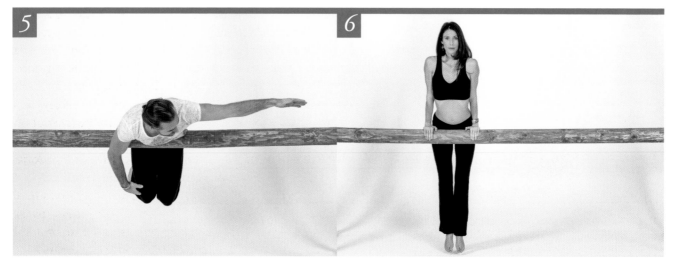

3   Front Straddle Lying, relaxed/loose arms

4   Single-Foot Hook Front Straddle Lying, overhand bent arms

5   Side Belly Lying, arm reaching

6   Vertical Hand Press

Getting Up *and* Down/Vertical Transitions

There are many reasons why you might need to elevate or lower your position and center of gravity in relation to the surface of support where you're balancing. You may do it after entering or before exiting balancing, to move faster, to be more stable and secure, to reverse your orientation, or to prepare a transition to another movement skill or surface (such as climbing down, jumping off, or climbing up).

The purpose of all the techniques I'm presenting is precisely to enable such vertical transitions both upward and downward (except for the fall recovery technique that only works going down). In some way, all these vertical transitions are climbing—up or down—movements as well. However, the nature of the environment (narrow and/or unstable) and the level of balance and stability they require categorizes them primarily as balancing techniques. No doubt movement improvements made to balancing may benefit some areas of climbing. Even though there are fewer balancing get-up options than in ground movement, if you have already become proficient at ground positions and movements, these balancing patterns and sequences will feel familiar, and you will become adept more quickly.

Techniques are shown starting from low and going upward. Like the get-up techniques in ground movement, you simply need to reverse the sequence to learn the downward movement.

I call the lowest balancing position the Vertical Hand Press and explain various strategies for you to move your position up from it, either by sitting first or directly placing your feet on the surface of the support in a foot-hand manner, then moving to either a Deep Knee Bend or a Deep Split Squat. Your initial and final positions when getting up and down depend on your training objectives in practice and on context in the real world, but I cover all your options in this section.

As for which get-up technique you should preferably use in the real world, it depends on a lot of factors:

- Who is doing the movement, in what environment and situation, with what level of efficiency for each of these techniques?
- Which movement is the fastest, or rather which one can you do the fastest?
- Which movement is the safest, or rather which one can you do most safely?
- Which movement is the most adapted to your environment or weather conditions?
- Which movement is the most adapted to the situation you're facing?
- Which movement places you in the best position for the next move?
- Are you carrying something? If so, is it heavy, and does it impair your freedom of movement or create instability?
- Are you insecure or afraid?
- Are you physically tired? What is the level of danger and the level of risk in relation to the danger?

Given that you can't predict anything, you'd better train as many techniques as you can for optimum competency and preparedness. That way, if you ever find yourself in a real-life situation, you can choose the most appropriate option without even thinking of it. That's unconscious competency.

Vertical Hand Press Drills

The Vertical Hand Press is the single most important transitional position between climbing and balancing. It is, in most cases, where balancing starts after you've been hanging and you're climbing up, and sometimes where balancing ends when you're climbing down to hanging. The Vertical Hand Press is the lowest balancing position; your center of gravity is slightly above the surface of support. You hold your position with your body in a side position, oriented perpendicularly to the surface of support and fully supported by both hands (with some contact and support from the belly); your arms are in the lockout position. Once this stance is established, you can transition to a Straddle Sit and then to the Deep Split Squat, or you can go directly to a Deep Knee Bend.

Your ability to hold the Vertical Hand Press in an efficient and comfortable way has paramount importance. You will find diverse techniques leading to this movement in Chapter 29, "Climbing Movement."

The following drills are designed to help you develop the essential upper-body strength, joint stability, and short-range motions you need to get up efficiently from the Vertical Hand Press. These drills also tremendously help you with vaulting techniques (in Chapter 28, "Airborne Movement").

Vertical Hand Press Forward-Leaning Drill

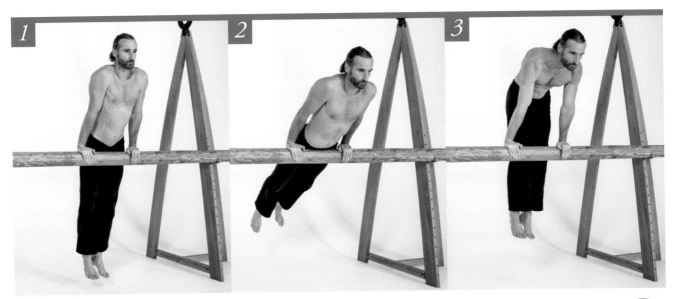

1. Assume the neutral Vertical Hand Press position. Your hands are placed just outside your hips, your palms support your body weight, and your arms are in the lockout position with your elbows fully rotated externally for optimum stability. Your shoulders are down and away from your ears.

2. Without bending at the hip or elbow or compromising your straight posture, lean forward until you feel that you can't lean forward more. Do this drill slowly at first and then do it dynamically.

3. Maintain your arms in the lockout position and keep pulling your body up by leaning slightly forward. Use abdominal strength and elevate your hips above the bar (or to the highest point you can reach). When you perform a transition from the Vertical Hand Press to the Tripod Transition, you might not need to pull your hips as high as shown in the photo, but for the purposes of training strength and positional control, it is useful to reach the maximum elevation you can.

SAFETY NOTE

You may use a crash pad or spotter, unless you are physically ready to roll into a Down Hanging position.

Vertical Hand Press Body-Weight Shifting Drill

To practice this drill, start in the neutral Vertical Hand Press position and then shift your body weight from side to side, always keeping the supporting arm in the lockout position. You may hold the position on each side for several seconds or switch sides quickly.

Single-Hand Press

Learning to balance in a Vertical Hand Press on a single hand obviously takes more strength and joint stability than using two hands. It can be a practical position if you need to temporarily use one hand for something other than balancing. To stay balanced, you need to vertically center your hand and arm with your body, aligning your base of support and your center of gravity. Hold it for 3 to 10 seconds in the lockout. This drill will greatly help with the Vertical Hand Press Traverse.

Vertical Hand Press Traverse

After you've learned to shift your body weight from side to side and hold the Single-Hand Press, it becomes easy to traverse to the other side of the bar. First shift your weight to your front hand (closer to the direction you're going), which allows you to bring your trail hand closer to your front hand. Then shift your weight to your trail hand so you can bring your front hand farther up the bar. If you want to cover more distance per cycle, try to reach farther with your front hand, but also bring your trail hand right next to the front one.

High Vertical Hand Press

This movement is essential for allowing you to elevate your hips and legs before a balancing Tripod Transition. You can practice this movement separately, but it's also part of the balancing Tripod Transition techniques and associated drills shown later in this section.

Side Tripod Get-Up

The pattern of this technique is quite similar to the Tripod Get-Up I discussed in Chapter 25, but it's adapted to the height and narrowness of the surface upon which it is performed. When done while balancing, the Side Tripod Get-Up becomes a highly technical move. It starts or ends either in the Vertical Hand Press position or in an angled Straddle Sit, and it transitions to either a Deep Knee Bend with the body's orientation perpendicular to the surface of support, or a Deep Split Squat with the body's orientation parallel to the surface. If the support surface is inclined, make sure to place the supporting hand at a level above the supporting foot.

Vertical Hand Press to Deep Knee Bend

1 Assume the neutral Vertical Hand Press.

2 Aim to place one foot on the bar next to the outside of your hand. Start pressing on your hands to lower your shoulders while elevating your hips above the bar. Shift more body weight to the hand opposite the side where your foot will be, then pull your leg up to the other side. Depending on your mobility, you might need to elevate your waist to manage placing your foot right next to the outside of your hand. Accurately and firmly position the ball of your foot on the bar with your leg fully bent, your knee vertically aligned with your foot, and your body leaning slightly forward and very slightly toward your supporting hand.

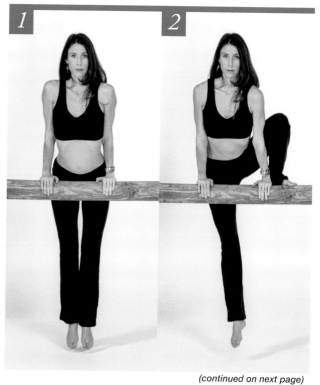

(continued on next page)

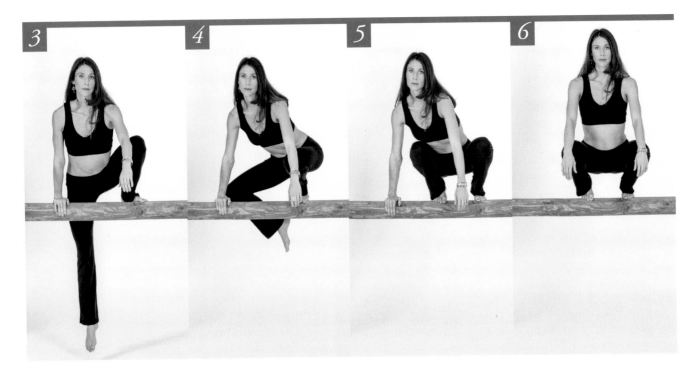

3 Shift your body weight to your supporting foot to create a two-point support base between your foot and the hand on the opposite side; this enables you to release your inside hand. Your supporting arm remains in a strong lockout position. Your center of gravity is well adjusted over your base of support to keep you as stable as possible. Optionally, you could rotate your supporting hand externally if it adds comfort (depending on the surface).

4 Using both your supporting leg and arm for stability, push strongly off your foot to elevate your hips as they move backward and more or less sideways, with your foot supporting most of your body weight (which shifts your center of gravity horizontally closer above your foot than your hand). You want to create sufficient vertical space that you can bend and pull your lower leg up high enough for your foot to smoothly reach the top of the bar. However, limit hip motion, the distance traveled by your rear foot, and the time spent during this transition to as little as possible. You may use your free arm for counterbalancing, if needed.

5 Place the ball of your trail foot right between your supporting hand and foot, shifting most of your body weight to your feet.

6 Push off your supporting hand to fully shift all your weight to your feet, releasing your hand and establishing a stable Deep Knee Bend, with your arms relaxed and resting on your knees.

Faults

Even if you've mastered the ground version of the Tripod Get-Up, the balancing version can easily generate mistakes that, at best, will make you lose energy and time; at worst, these faults will make you fall. Let's review the main issues.

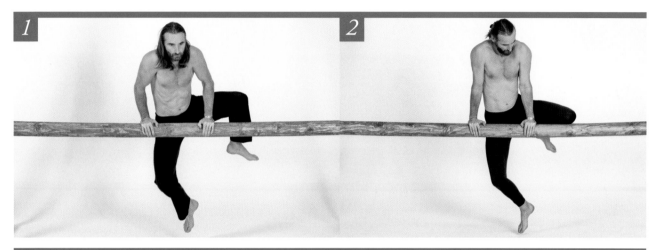

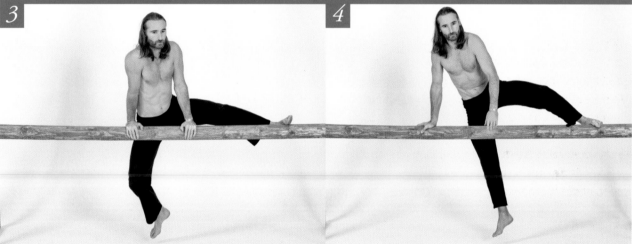

(continued on next page)

1 Having bent arms prevents you from elevating your waist, which in turn prevents you from lifting your leg high enough for your foot to reach the top of the supporting surface.

2 Having your arms in the lockout position, but instead of elevating your waist you sink low in your position with your shoulders higher than they should be and your head lower, which prevents you from raising your leg and foot high enough.

3 Trying to bring your foot on the bar with your leg extended straight out to the side because you haven't elevated your waist high enough. Even if you manage to put your foot on the bar, your leg won't be positioned so you can push off it, and you will stay stuck in that position.

4 Placing your foot on the bar way too far to the side. This position creates a base of support that is very wide and unstable. With your leg barely bent, your knee and foot are not vertically aligned, and you're forced to exaggeratedly lean sideways. You might manage to push off your foot a little, but you'll have insufficient hip motion range and might not be able to create enough vertical space for your inside foot to reach the top of the bar. Even if you succeed at placing your foot on the bar, you'll find yourself in a very difficult, unsustainable position. There is also a good chance that the supporting foot will simply slide away as you attempt to push off it, making you fall back to a hanging position.

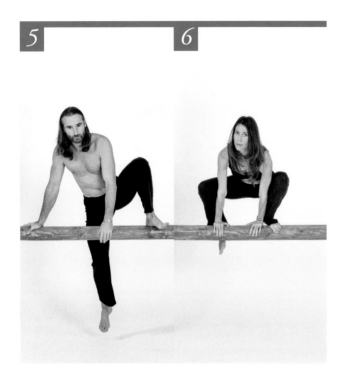

5

6

Other inefficiencies include the following:

- Your supporting arm comes out of the lockout position as you try to elevate your waist and pull your lower leg up, which immediately generates instability and makes it impossible to create the space needed to pass your leg through.

- Having a very narrow base of support in the Vertical Hand Press with your hands close to each other and bringing your foot right next to your hand with a very narrow base of support during the get-up. It can be effective if you have great lower-body joint mobility and upper-body joint stability, but unless the context is such that you must use this narrow base of support, it is not the most convenient and efficient way to do it.

- Having an overly wide base of support in the Vertical Hand Press with your hands apart significantly more than shoulder width. If you place your trail foot outside your hand, your base of support is way too wide and unstable.

5 This position is almost correct, but the heel is at high risk of abruptly sliding forward as you start pushing off it and release the hand next to the foot. If this happens, you might lose balance backward and fall back to a hanging position or fall all the way off the bar.

6 If you don't trust your balance in the position using a single supporting arm, you might keep both hands on the support, waiting until the last moment to release your inside hand. You might manage to lift your hips and leg higher, but a lack of mobility may prevent you from shifting your weight to your outside foot and releasing your inside hand. Therefore, you might not be able to create the space necessary to place your trailing foot on the bar, and you'll be stuck in a very precarious and unsustainable position. This option is manageable only by experienced practitioners who have great mobility.

Side Tripod Get-Up Beginner Drills

Drill 1

From the neutral Vertical Hand Press stance, elevate your body to the High Vertical Hand Press position, then lift one leg up and to the side. Bring the ball of your foot just outside your hand and just above the bar without touching the surface. You may look at your foot or learn to position it accurately using proprioception only. Get back to the neutral position and lift the opposite leg. (See photos 1 and 2 for Drill 4 on the next page.)

Drill 2

Same as Drill 1, but this time you place the ball of your foot on the support and shift weight on it to enable you to release your inside hand and establish the Side Opposite Single-Foot, Single-Hand vertical position. Stabilize and maintain the position a few seconds, then get back to the neutral position and do the same on the other side. (See photo 3 for Drill 4 on the next page.)

Drill 3

Establish the Side Opposite Single-Foot, Single-Hand Vertical position then push off your foot strongly. Use both your supporting leg and arm for stability, pull your trail leg up and elevate your waist. You need to push your body back (or to the side) toward your foot with your arm to shift your center of gravity close to above your foot. Keep your trail leg straight, instead focusing on elevating your waist as high as you can to create vertical space while maintaining optimum stability. You may use your free arm for counterbalancing, if needed. Once you have reached the highest waist elevation you can, you get back to the Side Opposite Single-Foot, Single-Hand Vertical position, then repeat again. After a few repetitions on one side, switch to the other side. (See photos 4 and 5 for Drill 4.)

Drill 4

Practice the entire sequence from the neutral Vertical Hand Press to the high Side Opposite Single-Foot, Single-Hand Vertical position (photos 1 through 5).

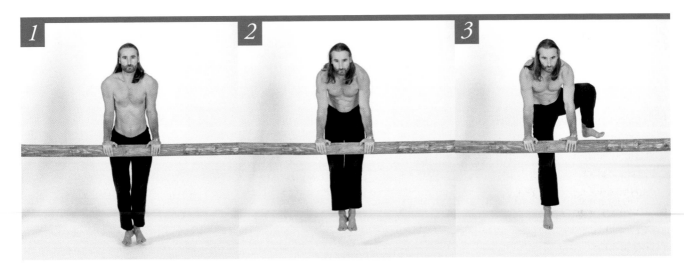

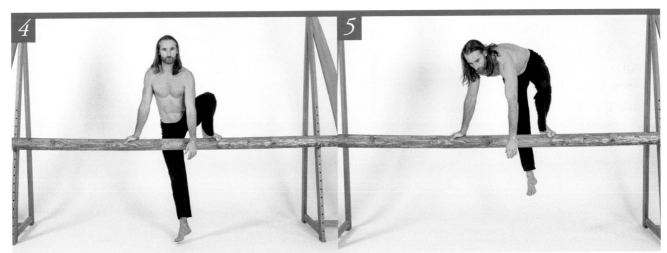

Sit *to* Deep Split Squat Get-Ups

The following get-up lets you transition from the Front Straddle Sit to the Deep Split Squat while maintaining the same orientation. It's more secure and relatively easier to do than a tripod get-up because you are using both hands for support (although you also can do it with single-hand support), and you do the movements without hip rotation.

Single-Foot Hook Get-Up

1   Start in the Straddle Sit, with your hands close together in front of you and your upper body leaning forward.

2   Pull one foot up behind your rear and hook it on the surface of the bar. It's easier to pull your foot onto the supporting surface if you extend your leg behind you with your foot away from your rear, but this widens your stance and limits your ability to elevate your hip. If you lack the flexibility to pull your foot close to your rear, you can elevate your waist by pushing off your arms. You need enough foot surface to be on the support to feel that you will be able to pull from that foot and support body weight on it; just the tip of your toes is not sufficient. However, do not position the upper, harder part of your foot near the ankle on the surface, as it will be uncomfortable, provide little range of motion, and be much more prone to slippage.

3   Having positioned your foot adequately to create friction, you now can pull from it and elevate your waist, while leaning and shifting weight a little more toward the front.

4   Having created the vertical space you need, you can pull your free foot up onto the top surface of the bar and place it flat on the bar.

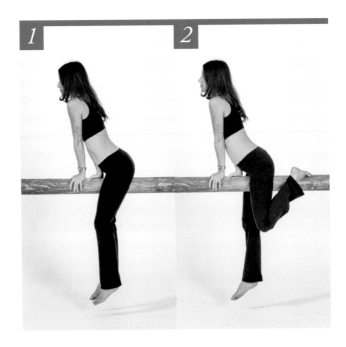

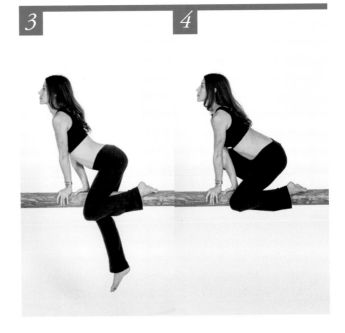

5 Modify the position of your back foot from hooked to bent (dorsiflexion) on the ball of your foot. From there you can push backward off your hands and front foot in a Deep Split Squat.

6 Establish a stable Deep Split Squat with good posture and relaxed arms.

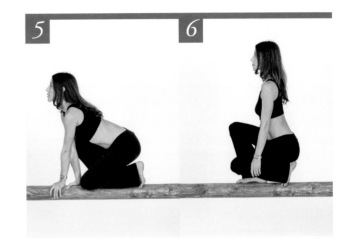

Deep Split Squat Get-Up and Deep Knee Bend Get-Up

On both the way up and down, the Deep Split Squat and Deep Knee Bend Get-Ups are either natural extensions of all the get-up strategies you've seen so far, or they're short, stand-alone get-ups if you remain on your feet from start to finish. It's essential to realize the importance of being able to swiftly lower your body from standing to the Deep Split Squat or Deep Knee Bend when your balance is challenged, rather than struggling in a standing position too long and compromising any chance of recovery. When the righting reflex fails when you're standing, or before it does, the "right" thing to do is recover balance by swiftly lowering the center of gravity and even immediately supporting yourself with your hands.

The balancing version of the Deep Split Squat Get-Up is like the same pattern on the ground, but you need to ensure positional control and impeccable joint stability to minimize postural sway. It starts with the ability to hold a stable balancing Deep Split Squat and Deep Knee Bend, of course.

Once you are comfortable enough in these low-center-of-gravity positions, you can start practicing the transition to and from standing.

TECHNIQUE TIP

Although you want to start slowly and focus on joint stability, ultimately you want to develop the ability to lower or raise your center of gravity at any speed. However, keep in mind that the ability to swiftly get down is paramount.

For practice, try using the following speeds:

- Down slow and up slow
- Down fast and up fast
- Down fast and up slow
- Down slow and up fast
- Combine any of the above

Variations *on* Balancing

So, before reading this section did you think that balancing was restricted to standing and walking on your feet and a list of three or four "functional fitness" drills on a BOSU or slackline? Those activities are great, but they represent a tiny fraction of what balancing has to offer.

Even though balancing from a Natural Movement perspective emphasizes the most realistic and practical ways to balance, overall balancing is open to many more creative and fun ways. There are more ways you can make balancing more adaptable to more environmental variables as shown in the next set of photos. If you want to get creative with non-practical ideas, the list becomes endless!

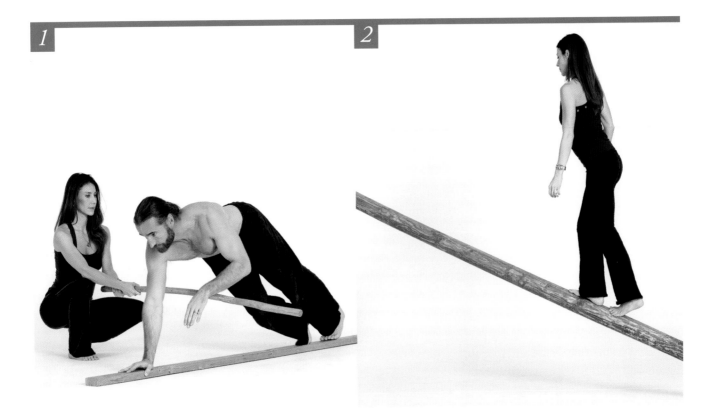

1   Stepping over in a Foot-Hand Crawl position. The obstacle can be attached to something and held in a fixed position, or a training partner can hold it. It should be at a level that is challenging for the person practicing without being impossible.

2   Inclined or declined surface, depending on your direction. The surface can be fixed at a given angle or held by a training partner and adjusted by changing position. For instance, the person holding the bar could be squatting, tall kneeling, kneeling, and so on. It's essential that the person holding the bar prevents it from rolling sideways.

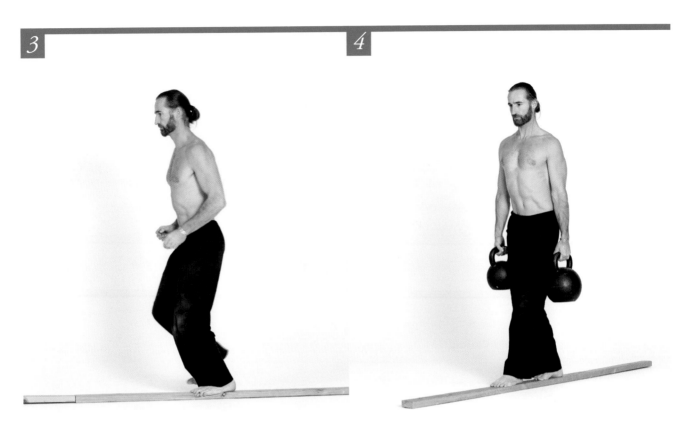

3 Skill-mix balancing and running (or running in balance, if you prefer). This is best practiced safely at ground level. This practice is great for developing accuracy.

4 Skill-mix walking balancing and hand carrying. You could hold a single object with a single hand, or Waist Carry, Chest Carry, or Shoulder Carry a variety of objects with different shapes and weights, on different surfaces, at different speeds, for varied distances. The possibilities are almost endless. Balancing carries on inclined surfaces notably help dorsiflexion, which is one of the main reasons for struggling in the Deep Squat.

So, is that all? Of course not! There is even more potential for skill-mix drills. Also remember all the possibilities I have already mentioned—going fast or very slow; accelerating and decelerating; holding positions; going in various directions (forward, backward, sideways) with different body orientation; looking up, down, or to the side; closing your eyes; reaching with your arms or legs; switching from and to different balancing positions and movements; or alternating balancing moves with other movement skills. Also, you can make volume, intensity, and complexity progressions, such as doing more repetitions;

practicing for a longer duration; increasing the elevation or narrowness of the surfaces; making them inclined or declined at a greater angle; making them more rounded, unstable, slippery; or a combination of all the above.

You can turn balancing practice into games, such as trying to destabilize and push an "opponent" off a beam where both "opponents" stand. It's up to you to always be creative and surprise your body and challenge yourself at a higher level. If you do so, you will never reach a plateau.

27
Gait Movement

> "Our grandfathers had to run, run, run. My generation's out of breath. We ain't running no more."
>
> —*Stokely Carmichael*

In human beings, *gait* is technically and scientifically defined as bipedal, biphasic, forward locomotion achieved solely through the movement of the lower limbs, with continuous or temporary contact with the ground. In simple words and from a Natural Movement perspective, gait is a particular manner of walking, stepping, or running that generally involves a certain rhythm and cadence while also being adaptable to contextual variables. Such adaptations might include intermittent shuffling, skipping, hopping, changes in pace (slow walking, brisk walking, jogging, and sprinting), and directional changes.

Early humans evolved and specialized for long-distance movement through both walking and running, as is still observed in many contemporary hunter-gatherer groups. Today, we all hold the same potential for such long-distance movement on our feet, even if it remains dormant in those of us who walk little and never run or who cover only very short distances when we walk or run.

Walking is by far the Natural Movement skill most frequently used by humans, and it's also a pattern that we've evolved to become highly efficient at. A regular heel-first walking gait, though slower compared to running, has been proven to expend about 70 percent less energy than running for the same distance. A difference of such magnitude proves that humans are primarily walkers by evolutionary design. Walking is the most economical and efficient gait when it comes to covering significant distances. This is universally true across all human cultures, minus slight gender differences in gait patterns; women generally tend to walk with a relatively narrower step width and more pronounced pelvic movement than men because of their particular skeletal structure.

NOTE

Gait is bipedal because we exclusively use the feet to support the body, and it's biphasic because, in most cases, the body is supported alternately by each foot in a cyclical manner.

The fact that we are fundamentally bipedal and primarily move on our two feet makes the foot the very foundation of human motion and the most important, valuable, and amazing piece of organic equipment we possess. When you walk or run, the human foot will support 100 percent of your body weight on an area of the body that is tiny in proportion to the size of your whole body. In fact, a single foot can support up to three times your normal body weight as it lands when you're running at fast speeds.

The human foot is a complex structure, with no less than twenty-six bones, thirty-three joints, and more than one hundred muscles, tendons, and ligaments within a small part of the body. Thousands of cutaneous sensors on the sole of the foot support finely tuned exteroception and sensitivity to ground parameters. The under-surface of the foot even shows a tough pad of fat underneath the heel bone that cushions the rear of the foot and reduces the loads on the skeletal system when we walk on hard surfaces or when we run and occasionally land on the rear of the foot. In any case, a strong, healthy foot can handle very large forces.

Like the hands, the sole of the foot can wrinkle ("get pruney") when water enters the sweat glands, which is a physiological adaptation that enables the foot to change its surface to generate greater friction in wet environments. The human foot is a masterpiece of biomechanical structure and sensory input that is both sensitive and tough as well as highly stable and mobile; it's designed to adapt to great variations in terrain.

Nonetheless, a common perception of human gait reduces it to the idea that walking and running are only done with a tall posture, linearly in a forward direction, mostly on smooth, flat, predictable surfaces. The reality of gait in Natural Movement is much richer, challenging, and more rewarding. Like any other natural movement, gait is influenced by many factors, including habit or specialized training, terrain, footwear (or lack thereof), weather, physical makeup, gender, age, mindset, pain, dysfunction, disease or other disorder, or a combination of any of these things. In the absence of dysfunction or pain, modulations in gait might have to do with temporary adjustments required for effective contextual adaptability. Those practical adjustments generate many diverse manners of walking, stepping, or running. Such variability may involve not just the pace or speed of the gait, but also the foot and overall body position that is most practical or efficient based on the terrain and surface where you're walking.

Based on the context in which you're walking, you might need to vary your position in sequences to clear obstacles—for instance when stepping over or under something. Instead of standing with a tall posture, you might alter your gait to have a center of gravity so low that the movement might be perceived as "ground movement." The direction of gait when stepping is not necessarily forward; it can be backward, upward, downward, or sideways, regardless of pace. These reasons alone make for a broad approach to gait in both comprehension and practice.

I also could argue that although humans are mainly bipedal, they aren't exclusively so, as shown by the hunter-gatherers who live in the wilderness and regularly use a variety of "on-all-fours" crawling patterns. Therefore, quadrupedal movements that I previously covered in the Ground Movement chapters could be equally considered to be "gait." As a matter of fact, humans who suffer from gait abnormality or *astasia-abasia* (the inability to either stand or walk in a normal manner) due to a degenerative disease, a stroke, brain damage, or phobia may in some cases revert to quadrupedal motion temporarily or permanently.

NOTE

The permanent fear of standing or walking is a phobia that bears diverse names such as ambulophobia, stasiphobia, stasibasiphobia, basiphobia, and stasophobia.

In addition, gait may take place on narrow or unstable surfaces and become a balancing pattern in Natural Movement even though they are also technically "gait" movements either in a bipedal or quadrupedal fashion.

In this chapter, I specifically address the fundamental human standing, bipedal, and biphasic gaits of our species.

Walking

One of the simplest ways to feel good when you're stressed out or anxious is to step outside for a simple walk in nature or a nearby park. Health benefits of *ambulation* (a more formal term for walking) are numerous.

On average, children begin to walk on their own when they're about eleven months old, which probably means you've been walking for a very long time already. But does that mean that there is nothing else for you to learn or rediscover about walking?

Using a Natural Movement approach to walking and practice obviously departs from both the obvious few steps we do to get in our cars, go to the bathroom, or take the occasional short promenade around the block on flat, even, predictable, artificial surfaces. It also differs from the highly specialized racewalking sports. However, any of these types of walking can be part of your practice, and they're certainly better than sitting all day.

Walking from a broad, natural perspective includes more than changes in speed, distance, or duration, and it isn't just about hiking outdoors. I'm talking about walking as an adaptable Natural Movement skill that involves great diversity in gait, speed, and duration but also includes stepping in diverse directions on varied surfaces in various weather conditions. It also includes the ability to walk skillfully for long distances on a variety of terrains while handling simple obstacles and potentially carrying a load. This kind of walking is incredibly more challenging and rewarding, but it requires a healthy body with great lower-body mechanics; foot, ankle, knee, and hip mobility; and stability. Fortunately for you, all the sits, kneeling positions, and transitions to standing help to recondition your foot, ankle, knee, and hip joint mobility and stability, as well as promote your core strength, in the most progressive, functionally natural and potent way with a direct benefit to your walking and running.

Technically speaking, walking in a standing fashion implies that you are moving using a simple "double pendulum" cycle where you are supporting your body weight on a single leg (called the *stance phase*) alternately while the other leg is traveling from the back to the front (called the *swing phase*), with a brief phase in between where you support yourself on both legs. It simply means that when you walk you are always in contact with the ground. In contrast, when you run, you become airborne with both feet off the ground between each step.

The main difference between walking and running is gait, rather than speed because speed can obviously greatly vary in both types of gait depending on factors such as height, weight, age, terrain, surface, weather, load, health, physical conditioning, fatigue, mindset or situation. Human walking speed averages 3 miles per hour (5 kilometers per hour), and people might walk much slower or faster than that when you take all the variables into consideration.

I'll start with the most common type of walking: standing and moving forward on relatively flat surfaces. Though it is a complex movement, it is pretty straightforward (no pun intended).

Standing Walk

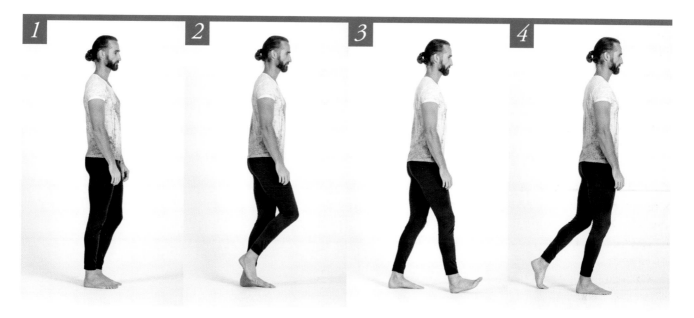

1 Start standing, shifting more body weight onto the foot you intend to support you. You may slightly bend the knee of the intended supporting leg.

2 Slightly move your center of gravity forward beyond your base of support, so gravity starts gently pulling you off balance. To begin the "first pendulum," slightly rotate the hip and bend the leg you intend to move forward to release the foot. As you slowly lean farther forward, the ankle of the supporting leg flexes. It's a whole-body lean with the foot, hips, spine, and head aligned without a Hip Hinge.

3 Extend your free leg forward without pushing off your back leg until your heel lands softly on the ground, and you establish a base of support with both feet. At this point most of your body weight is still supported on the back foot.

4 Shift your body weight onto your front foot by "rolling" it down all the way to the toes, while the heel of your back foot elevates so that only the ball of your back foot is on the ground, and your foot is in an extended position. The heel-toe motion of your foot (or "inverted pendulum") transfers more energy from step to step compared to directly placing your foot flat on the ground. From this position, keep driving your center of gravity forward to initiate the "second pendulum" and replicate the exact same sequence, this time supported on your opposite side and leg.

During the walk cycle, the center of gravity reaches its highest point as the moving leg passes the supporting one, and its lowest point when the legs spread apart, however the change in level is slight and shouldn't translate to a visible up and down motion of the head and body (unless you were to step out significantly). Except in special circumstances, it's natural to land on the heel when walking. People who have issues with this are people who have issues with their health, such as being significantly overweight or having bad knees or back issues, and they can't handle their own natural motion without discomfort or pain. In this case, gait issues are a symptom, and health is the cause of it.

Common Standing Walk Faults

Unless you are suffering from motor-control issues, such as swaying with such a magnitude that you are nearly falling (the *marche à petits pas*, which is an abnormally short-stepped gait) or you are intentionally modifying your gait for an experimental or adaptable purpose, the following are inefficiencies:

- Pronated or supinated feet
- Feet pointing out or splayed in a "duck" style
- Heavy stepping
- Dragging feet (when they rub against the ground)
- Little to no flexion at the knee
- Hip "collapsing" sideways upon shifting body weight onto the stepping foot
- Excessive movement in the lower back (lack of stability)

In addition, as you would expect, any postural issue you have while standing in one spot carries over to each step of your walking pattern. The better alignment you have from feet to head, the more balance and relaxation you have in walking. You can address some of the walking faults you have through practicing mindful walking—for instance, fixing splayed-foot stepping by leading each step through the knee with it pointed straight forward and avoiding external rotation of the leg. Some faults will indirectly and gradually improve or even ultimately disappear through consistent Natural Movement practice.

Fast Walking

To walk faster, you increase the traction from the front foot to thrust the swing leg faster and extend it farther forward, which is helped by an accentuated hip rotational motion. As the foot of the swinging leg lands, the center of gravity is almost immediately above it with greater forward momentum, which makes the double-support phase much briefer. Friction at the foot will be maximized to provide greater traction from the foot, which allows the hip to act upon the rear leg with greater force. Once the rear leg starts to swing, the leg is flexed at the knee; however, unlike running, the heel is not kicked toward the rear. Upon forward extension the swinging leg must land with minimal flexion at the knee (on flat terrain). The accentuated rotation of the hip must be counterbalanced by the motion of the arms. Your arms are bent, but your shoulders should stay low and relaxed with no exaggerated upward/backward arm swing motion. Your arm motion is a natural counter motion and counterbalancing motion rather than an active propulsive motion. Despite the rotary motion of the hips, it's essential that your feet point forward upon landing. Your hips are more forward and downward; they don't sway with lateral rotation. There is no up-and-down wave motion as you move forward along a horizontal plane.

Adaptability in Walking

Because walking is an adaptable skill, minor or major positional adjustments may occur anytime because of contextual demands, especially when you're walking in nature on uneven terrains. You may walk forward, sideways, backward, or, if you're scanning your environment as you move, by rotating 360 degrees as you change your orientation circularly with every step. You may use small or wide steps, have a wide stance, or walk with your feet in line. Walking gait variations may also include (but are not limited to) the following:

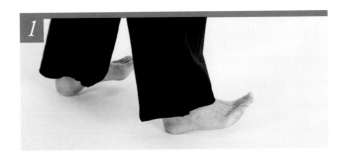

1 **Heel-only stepping:** In this variation, you walk on your heels with the rest of the foot off the ground. You usually use this style when walking barefoot on a terrain covered with sharp or pointy elements such as puncturevine (goatheads), shards of broken material, or thorns because the heel area is tougher than the rest of the foot.

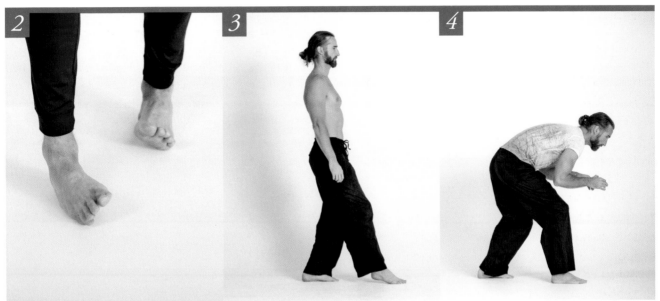

(continued on next page)

2 **Walking on the sides of the feet:** You can use this variation to minimize the area of contact or soften your steps to be quieter.

3 **Forefoot-heel stepping:** You can do this to soften your stepping and make it lighter on your body, for stalking, or when the ground is unsure, especially when you're walking barefoot without visibility on the terrain (tall grass, darkness, shallow waters, when situationally having to focus somewhere else than the ground), and you're concerned about hurting your feet.

   The idea is to keep your body weight on your rear foot, often with a slight backward lean of your torso, and feel the ground with your front foot to avoid any threat to the foot (puncture, cut, instability) before you shift all your body weight onto it.

   The lead foot comes flat to the ground, and, in the absence of an issue, you push off the rear foot to shift all your body weight to the front.

4 **Crouching walk:** With this lower center-of-gravity walk, you usually use wider steps for greater stability. Use this to handle low obstacles or ceilings or to make yourself less visible. It's also a combative stance. Alternatively, you can do this walk in a Hip Hinge fashion with a straight spine.

TECHNIQUE TIP

A lot of people who are trying barefoot movement want to use the forefoot-heel stepping variation because their feet are unprepared to handle rough terrains. They unconsciously stiffen their feet, with tension in their face and body, as they anticipate the upcoming pain. I recommend you do the opposite to accustom yourself to let your feet totally loose so they can better absorb protruding surfaces as you shift your body weight onto the foot. You can sometimes even voluntarily stomp the ground (not too hard) as you walk. The point is to relax your feet to keep your muscles loose and to spread your bones to better distribute body weight over a greater surface of your feet.

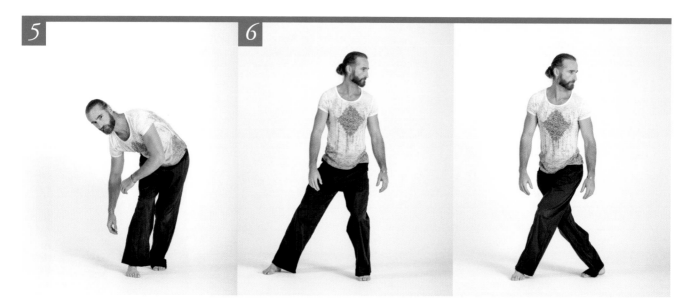

5 **Stepping through or under obstacles** may require several positional adjustments, such as leaning both forward and sideways at the same time.

6 **Shuffling:** This style can be done with varied body orientation (front, side, back). You can shuffle while keeping the same lead foot or alternating your feet.

Stepping Under

The way you should step under an obstacle depends on how high or low the space underneath it is, how wide and long the obstacle is, and how fast you want to pass it. Clearly, below a certain height, you have no option but to crawl. However, with enough vertical space you might decide to stay on your feet—for instance, if your hands are busy, or if the ground is un- safe or unclean. Although stepping under a low obsta- cle can be done in a Half Squat or Half Deep Knee Bend manner as described in Chapter 24, which allows the torso to remain relatively vertical, those methods are much more energy-consuming and often slower than the following two options.

Forward

Stepping under an obstacle with a forward orientation is effective, but it's not the most efficient movement, although it may be the only option you have if the space underneath the obstacle is too narrow or too long to approach it sideways.

1 A common approach is to lean forward with your back rounded and head down, which allows you to not bend your legs too much, which saves energy. The main issues with this approach is that you are likely to bump your back and potentially hurt your spine when you step, and you also must look down, which is a problem if you need to go fast while staying visually alert. It also holds zero value in terms of functional rehabilitation.

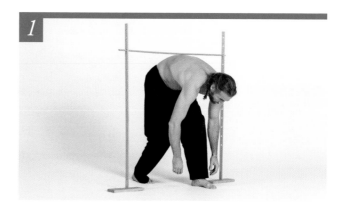

2   A more efficient approach is to first Hip Hinge, keeping your head up so you can look forward. Your spine is elongated behind your head and slightly beneath head level. Once your head has cleared the lower surface of the obstacle, you know that your spine will follow safely if you maintain that position far enough to clear the obstacle entirely as you regain a vertical stance. You also need to bend your legs and walk forward using cautious and relatively short steps, so it's relatively slow and energy-consuming.

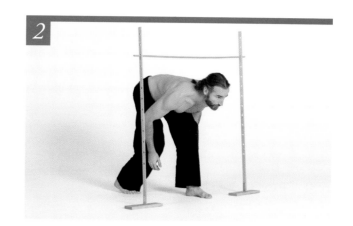

Sideways

If the space underneath the obstacle is wide enough—at least as wide as the length running from your sacrum to your forehead—and short enough, then stepping under with trunk rotation is the most efficient option. You can pass the obstacle in only two steps while keeping your back and spine safe, staying visually alert, and moving very swiftly.

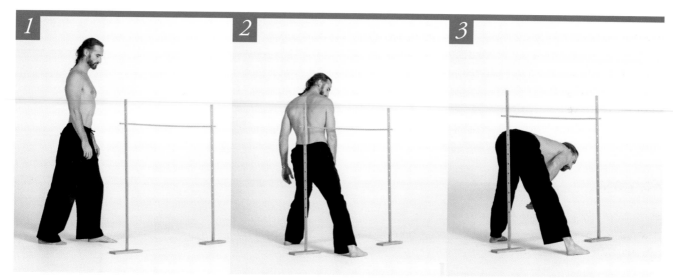

(continued on next page)

1   Approach the obstacle from the side.

2   Shift your weight onto your back foot and reach with your front leg to slide it underneath toward the far side of the obstacle, then place the foot of that leg on the ground. The ideal base of support is neither too narrow or too wide.

3   While maintaining a straight spine, bend your torso forward by folding at the hips and centering your weight over both feet, which brings your hips directly under the obstacle. As you're doing so, keep the back of your head slightly above your spine to make sure that it never comes in contact with the obstacle. Ideally your center of gravity, the obstacle, and the middle of your base of support are vertically aligned at this point.

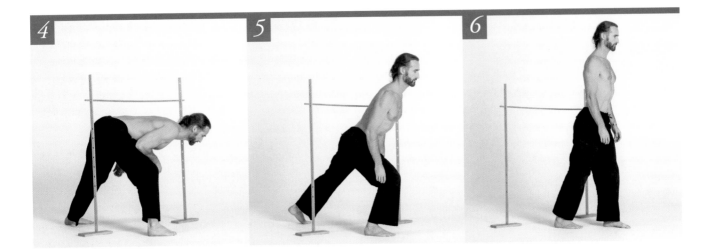

4   Swing your torso under the obstacle so that it clears the far side of the obstacle; begin to shift your weight onto the foot on the far side of the obstacle.

5   Once your torso is fully clear of the obstacle, stand erect and turn to face the direction you're traveling. Shift all your weight onto the forward foot, bringing your hips out from under the obstacle.

6   Pull your back leg completely out and transition to a regular standing walk.

TECHNIQUE TIP

If the obstacle is at an angle, place your head toward the higher end and your hips toward the lower one.

Stepping Through

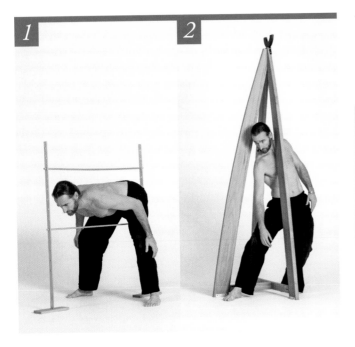

1   Stepping Through Horizontally (over-under): This variation requires enough space for your torso to pass and spatial awareness both above and below your trunk.

TECHNIQUE TIP

A technique I use for variation 1 when the space barely allows me to pass through is to entirely deflate my lungs, which flattens my rib cage and creates extra space.

2   Stepping Through Vertically: When practicing this variation, try to stay very relaxed but also move quickly while avoiding touching the obstacle. In most cases, lightly rubbing against the sides of the obstacle is not an issue, but rubbing or bumping them with force can be a problem.

Stepping Over and Out

You need to step out or over whenever an obstacle presents itself, and it's not possible or practical to go around it. Good examples include stepping across a stream, crossing a gap over a deep ravine, going over a fallen tree or a hole, or traversing a slippery, wet, or thorny area. Such obstacles are mostly passed either with a forward or sideways orientation; you use a backward orientation more rarely. The technique to step over and out has a lot to do with the following general principles, regardless of the kind of obstacle you're clearing:

- A sideways orientation of the body fits wider gaps or more elevated surfaces as it allows you to take wider steps than a forward orientation. Once the front foot is also on support and stable, a forward orientation can be regained by rotating your hips and pivoting on the balls of your feet.

- Start the movement with impeccable position and joint stability of your back foot and leg. Your balance during this temporary single-leg phase determines the accuracy of your foot placement as well as your stability during the phase where you're supported on both feet. Plus, if the step is wide or long, you might have to let gravity pull you off balance forward until the front foot lands, making your "off-balance balance" crucial.

- Once the front foot is grounded, as long as you aren't exceeding the range that makes stepping forward possible, you want to push off the back foot first to create forward momentum and to facilitate pushing off the front leg to finish clearing the obstacle.

- When you're stepping over an elevated surface without hand assistance, the height of the obstacle should ideally be a bit lower than the height of your groin area (otherwise you'll have to briefly assume a Straddle Sit position).

- When the distance you're stepping over is nearly the maximum distance you can cover, you need to predict that stepping will be within range. Keep your gaze focused on your lead foot until it's effectively grounded.

- If the surface where your lead foot steps is small or otherwise challenging, keep your gaze focused on where your lead foot is stepping until it's effectively grounded.

- Anticipate the stability and friction (or lack of it) of both the surface supporting your rear foot and the surface supporting your lead foot so you know how reliable they are. Surfaces may move, collapse beneath you, or be slippery, which can make you lose balance or land uncomfortably on your groin area.

- Your stepping should be accurate and enable you to land on the ball of your foot first—rather than on your heel—to establish a more stable foothold. Though it may seem more stable, stepping on your heel may make you slide forward and fall; by extending your ankle to point your foot forward, you can land farther if needed than if you try to land with your heel first.

- Keep your arms relaxed and resist the temptation to exaggeratedly use them for counterbalancing and as a compensatory strategy for lack of stability in the lower joints.

- Maintain ample and relaxed abdominal breathing.

- Never rush stepping out and over anything when there's potential danger, such as falling down a crevice, falling in water with strong current, and so on.

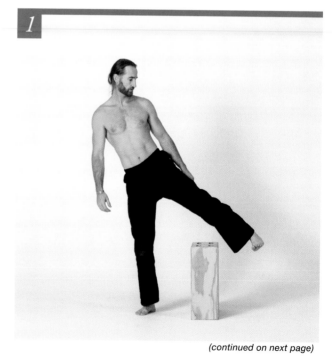

(continued on next page)

1 Stepping over forward sideways

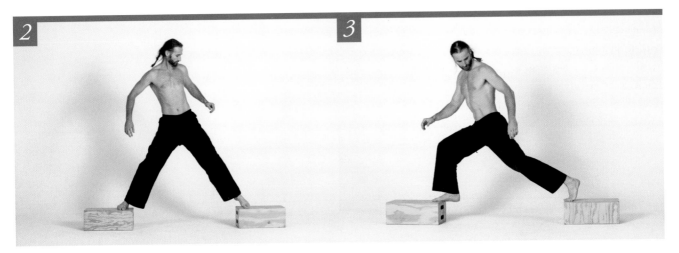

2   Stepping out/over sideways gap-crossing

3   Stepping out/over backward gap-crossing

Stepping Up

Stepping up implies that the lead foot is raised onto an elevated surface. This can be done progressively in a step-by-step motion when walking up an inclined terrain, but it also happens when you encounter a sudden and sharp change of elevation. You might be able to step up on such an obstacle with walking momentum, or you might have to come to a stop, ensure stable footing, and then step up from a static stand. It can be a single event as you step up onto a raised surface, or it can be a repetitive pattern when you climb a steep slope covered with big rocks (or you're simply walking up some stairs).

Obviously, stepping up cannot be reduced to a single context, such as walking up stairs, which involves a flat, linear, stable, even, highly predictable environment that uses relatively short steps, uninterrupted momentum, and perfect visibility, which means each step is replicated the same way. This is nowhere as challenging as having to step up from a static standing position with no momentum onto a significantly raised surface that is uneven, small, inclined, slippery, or unstable, especially if you need to temporarily balance on a single leg before you can figure out where to step next. There are many modifications you can make as you step up that depend on the surfaces where you step, the height and width of the area on which you're stepping, how much momentum you have prior to stepping up, how fast you're going, and the direction your next step has to be.

Stepping down is the same. There is a huge difference between swiftly stepping down a low, flat step to flat ground and stepping slowly down a height on a single leg, with the supporting foot resting on an uneven or challenging surface.

Although momentum and speed can make stepping up faster and easier, there are times when you might have to do it without momentum—slowly, carefully, and accurately in the most balanced and controlled manner. This is the most challenging and unforgiving form of stepping up, and if we can determine what makes it efficient, then less difficult, more dynamic forms of stepping up will be made extremely easy.

Your primary concern is naturally producing enough force to oppose the pull of gravity by accelerating your body. Your second concern is ensuring single-leg stability without counterbalancing with your arms, just like when you balance. Of course, you might be wondering why you can't simply use your arms to assist the movement. The practical reason is very simple: Your arms may be busy and unable to assist (imagine that you're carrying a young child). From a skill development and functional perspective, intentionally preventing your arms from assisting increases your level of single-leg joint stability, which has benefit to other single-leg movements, such as in walking, balancing, running, and single-leg jumps or landings.

I address stepping up before I talk about stepping down because most of what I tell you about stepping up also applies to stepping down. Imagine that you are stepping only once, from a standing position (so you don't have any walking momentum) onto an uneven surface that is also higher than what's shown in the photos. You need to stay stable and balanced on a single leg, even if you are stepping up slowly, before you can either stand on top or step somewhere else.

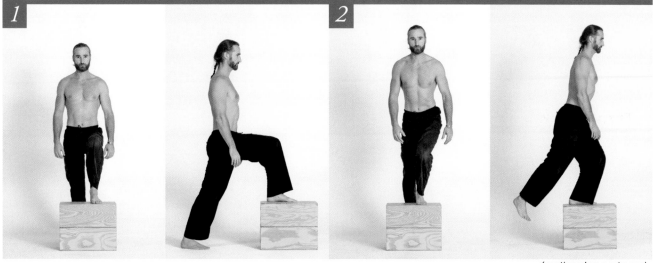

(continued on next page)

1 Face the elevated surface straight on with a forward orientation, then place your forward foot flat on top of the surface. You may stand about one step away, or you can bring your rear foot closer to the obstacle. Your knee is vertically aligned with your foot or slightly in front of it depending on the height of the obstacle, but your center of gravity is not (although it's not too far off). If your lead foot is higher than what's shown in the photo, it would become even more essential that you move your rear foot toward your lead foot to align your center of gravity as much as possible with your lead foot. The reason is simple: As you step up, you switch from a two-foot base of support to a one-foot base of support. If you start with no momentum, there's less possibility of pushing with the rear leg because it's already extended, you have greater knee flexion in the lead leg, and you have greater vertical distance your center of gravity has to travel before it reaches above your foot to balance your top position, so you'd better minimize the horizontal distance your center of gravity has to travel. Therefore, it's best to have your center of gravity fully aligned with the anticipated base of support (your lead foot).

2 Keeping your spine straight and your hips level, push off with your rear foot to shift your body weight onto the lead foot. Keep your knee vertically aligned with your foot (it might very slightly shift outward as a reflex to prevent it from caving inward, but it shouldn't shift significantly). Your knee does not align itself with the body's midline and center of gravity; your hip moves sideways toward the supporting knee and foot to align your midline and center of gravity with your one-foot base of support.

TECHNIQUE TIP

A sideways orientation is possible and useful when the surface is really elevated because you might be able to place the lead foot higher and flat onto the surface, whereas the forward orientation only allows you to place your heel on the surface. The choice of the sideways orientation may also have to do with what's best or doable in a given environment, including considering where you want to step next.

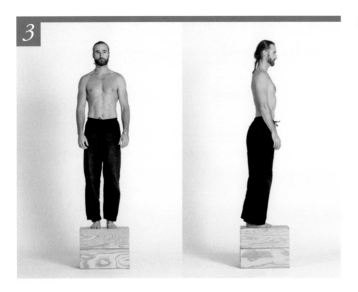

3 Fully extend the front leg as you bring your trailing leg up and onto the surface in a stand, with your center of gravity and midline vertically aligned with the center of your two-footed base of support. If your knee had moved vertically on the outside of your foot (inward or outward), it naturally moves back to a vertical alignment. However, you should have been able to maintain vertical alignment from start to finish. Although your hips might have had to move slightly sideways, your torso should not have needed to lean or twist sideways, which enables you to maintain a vertical torso without unnecessary movements.

Faults

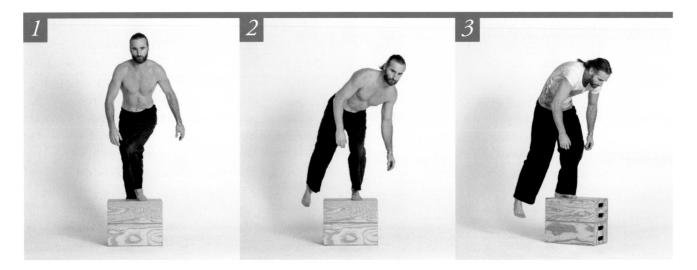

1 Allowing the knee to shift inward (or outward) outside of vertical alignment with the foot creates an unstable and weaker leg position.

2 Leaning your upper body in the direction of your stepping leg makes you unstable and can even throw you off balance.

3 Bending your back to hunch over and look down. This too can throw you off balance and/or prevent you from swiftly or accurately transitioning to your next move.

Other issues include trying to step up without a slight hip hinge, which keeps the torso too vertical and prevents your center of gravity from effectively moving forward toward your base of support; this results in either a slower movement or being forced to step back down.

The most challenging version of stepping up is when your lead foot is stepping onto the highest surface it can, your lead leg is in full flexion, and your rear leg (and maybe even your rear ankle) is fully extended with very little ability to push and create upward momentum, which makes the step-up a movement pattern that closely resembles the demands of the Single-Leg Squat Get-Up. What you learned by practicing the Single-Leg Squat Get-Up gives you great insight of how to create the strongest position to produce strength and maintain balance in a strictly vertical elevation of the body, regardless of speed of motion, and in the absence of prior momentum. In the bottom single-leg position, the foot, ankle, knee, and center of gravity must be vertically aligned. The same applies to stepping up (no momentum, full flexion or close to it) for the following reasons:

- You can step up without momentum and with little to no push from your rear foot. If your center of gravity is outside of vertical alignment, gravity keeps you stuck at the bottom.

- Producing force to elevate all your body weight vertically through single-leg extension starting in full flexion is more efficient, especially if you start without momentum.

- You can control the speed of the leg extension. If you're outside vertical alignment, gravity pulls you off balance and back down if you slow down or don't generate enough upward acceleration to shift your center of gravity to vertical alignment.

- You can switch from dynamic to static joint stability and stop at any point of the extension to hold a partial flexion. If you're outside vertical alignment, gravity pulls you off balance.

- Your knee remains vertically aligned with your foot from start to finish. If you start with it outside vertical alignment, your knee naturally comes back to vertical alignment as your leg finishes extending fully. This motion, in addition to being unnecessary and avoidable, might deviate your center of gravity from a vertical path and make you unstable. If you are stepping up continuously, as when you walk up stairs with an inward or outward knee position relative to your foot, your knee is basically wobbling with every single step you make, which is not an expression of joint stability.

The only way you can get away with having a starting position with your knee and center of gravity out of vertical alignment is when your lead foot is not too elevated so you have only partial knee flexion, and when you benefit from the push and body-weight shifting from your rear leg that gives you upward momentum. In that case, you don't need to push very hard on your lead leg, and you can vertically align your knee and center of gravity with your supporting foot as you move to the top position. The best situation is to start in a real power position and allow modification to these principles only when there is no other choice.

Following are the main reasons for allowing the knee to move outside of vertical alignment:

- **Direction of movement:** When you're in a forward orientation, your knee may slightly move forward beyond vertical alignment to slightly shift your center of gravity forward to help you avoid being pulled off balance backward (especially if you're carrying a loaded backpack). If you're concerned about stressing your knee, remember that in most cases you're not loaded (or not significantly loaded), that you don't start with your knee in full flexion, and that the push from your rear leg gives you upward momentum. If you're carrying a load to the front of your body, your center of gravity shifts forward more, which definitely helps you prevent the backward pull. When you're going upward but also sideways, your knee moves out of vertical alignment toward the movement direction after sufficient force and momentum have been produced rather than at the start of the movement, unless the direction of the movement goes sideways significantly.

- **Stepping friction:** When vertical alignment is not the position that ensures the most friction at your foot, a slight lateral position of your knee, usually outward, might help prevent foot slippage, such as when your foot and ankle are at an angle because of an inclined surface.

- **Obstacles:** An obstacle in the way of your knee prevents vertical alignment.

Fixing Single-Leg Instability

If you're having trouble with single-leg stability and balance when stepping up, here are several movement drills you can do to help. These drills benefit any single-leg movement, including stepping down or stepping over and out. Perform the following movements while maintaining vertical alignment of your knee and foot, a straight spine, controlled abdominal breathing, and relaxed arms. There are also many single-leg movement drills in Chapter 26, "Balancing Movement," that transfer to greater single-leg positions at ground level.

- **Partial knee flexion and extension:** From standing, lower your center of gravity as low as possible in a Single-Leg Half Squat, hold the position several seconds, stand up, and then do the same again. Switch legs.

- **Hip rotations:** From a single-leg stance with a partial knee flexion, rotate your hips in both directions by opening your free leg fully to the side and then bringing it back; then move it toward the front so that it crosses your body in front of your supporting leg. You may rotate your torso and neck as you rotate your hip, and you can add arm reaches and multidirectional positions of your head and line of vision.

- **Step-ups and step-downs:** Practice stepping up and stepping down very slowly with full positional control and without relying on momentum and speed to be effective and stable.

- **Balancing practice:** Numerous techniques and movement variations involve single-leg stances that improve single-leg stability.

- **Carrying:** Carrying while walking is a skill-mix that combines bipedal locomotion and the manipulation of an external load. This movement is obviously more challenging than regular walking, and it increases single-leg stability, especially when you do it on narrow or uneven surfaces.

Stepping Down

You can step down on a decline slope, on a staircase, or on a relatively small obstacle in a continuous walking fashion. This movement uses forward orientation most of the time, and there's little effort beyond extending one leg forward and down and shifting your center of gravity forward to use the pull of gravity. The amount of time spent in the rear, single-leg stance is very brief, and the amount of force to produce the movement—before your foot lands, that is to say—is close to none. All you need to do upon landing is to ensure the accuracy of your stepping if you're landing on uneven ground.

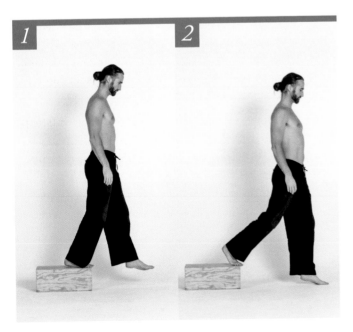

1 From standing at the top of the elevated surface, look down at the landing surface if you have a concern about stepping accurately on a specific area for safety, or gaze forward in the direction you're going. Push off your rear leg to shift your body weight forward as you extend your lead leg forward and down. Extend your ankle to present the ball of the foot toward the ground.

2 Contact the ground with the ball of your foot first to absorb the downward force smoothly. After decelerating through that single leg, pull and extend your trailing leg forward to continue walking, using the stored elastic energy to bounce off to the next step. Alternatively, you could bring the trailing foot down to the ground in a stand or jump off the landing leg.

Faults include stepping on your heel, on a flat foot, or with a stiff knee, which makes the landing heavy; letting your knee get out of vertical alignment; moving forward far beyond your foot (unless you are transitioning to a Half Kneel on the ground); stiffening all over; or losing positional control (with any other unwanted movement of the body occurring upon landing). The unwanted movement of your lead knee upon landing, either inward or outward, is the biggest issue because it can throw you off balance and hurt your knee. If you're changing direction upon landing—such as to move sideways—your knee should move out of vertical alignment after decelerating the body as it extends again; it shouldn't move during flexion where it needs a reliable position to ensure efficient deceleration.

Stepping Down Sideways

If you are stepping down from a high surface and need to land softly, accurately, silently, or simply in the most balanced manner possible, you must step down in a slow, controlled fashion with a sideways or backward (facing opposite to your movement direction) orientation, which allows your lead foot to reach much farther than a forward orientation does. Positional efficiency demands that your center of gravity, hip, knee, ankle, and foot remain vertically aligned at all times as when you step up in the absence of momentum or speed. It's the same movement pattern as Stepping Up but in reverse, with eccentric effort (generating deceleration) instead of concentric effort (generating acceleration). If your center of gravity shifts beyond vertical alignment with your supporting foot, you'll be pulled off balance, which could mean that you're not stepping down exactly where you need to, and you could fall.

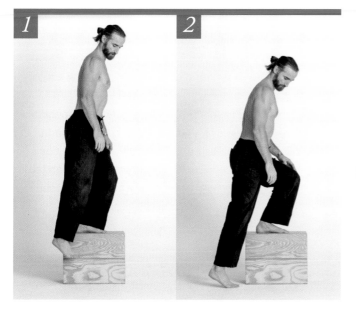

1   From standing on top of the surface, turn your head slightly to spot and maintain a gaze on your landing target. Shift your body weight onto your rear foot (the one that's furthest from the edge) with a slight knee flexion. Before you extend the other leg lower in the void, make sure that you are balanced with your center of gravity, knee, and foot aligned.

2   Maintain vertical alignment as you lower your lead leg, so you can control the speed at which you lower your body. This way you can always come to a stop or even step back up if needed. Keep looking at where you need to land your lead foot and extend the ankle to lower the ball of your foot to reach farther down or to step more accurately.

The Next Level: Stepping Accuracy

Walking is versatile. The ability to adaptively step forward, backward, sideways, or to step out, over, through, up, and down is an essential component of walking competency that enables you to pass obstacles in your way without discontinuity or with little waste of time.

If you're still not fully convinced that walking is a real skill that you can train, improve, and make more efficient and adaptable, just look at the walking speed and relaxation of an adept mover compared to an untrained person (including people who hike frequently but only on trails and who avoid obstacles as much as they can) on a complex environment such as the rocky bank of a stream. In addition to having great, fast positional control, joint mobility and stability (especially in the ankles and knees), and foot strength, the faster walker has great peripheral vision, spatial awareness, and rapid exteroception (the feedback from your feet every time you step, especially on uneven, unstable surfaces). This is especially impressive knowing that skillful movers can do so barefoot and yet be significantly more agile and faster than unskilled walkers who are shod. Trained "Natural Movers" are confident and accurate with their stepping, and they can recover quickly when they get unstable, without gazing directly at the difficulties of the terrain. As trained movers walk, they might not need to look down as they step because their vision and brains are already ahead of their feet to calculate the next move. Of course, with less difficult and more predictable terrains, looking straight forward is easy, but the challenging terrains and surfaces considerably slow down hikers who lack adaptability. The following drills basically teach you to watch your steps...without looking.

Stepping Accuracy Drills

- Start with a short distance and look where you intend to step from a distance. Start walking with an erect torso and head (without leaning forward and looking down); only let your eyes gaze down. Do your best to step as accurately as you can, then do it again increasingly faster.

- Repeat the exercise while keeping your line of vision at a 45-degree angle, and then do it again while looking straight ahead. The point is to develop greater peripheral vision and maintain stepping accuracy while not looking straight down at your feet and terrain.

- Once you have become comfortable doing this, you may walk on new terrains; as you do, look straight forward and only briefly glance down from time to time without tilting your head. By now you should have switched from looking down most of the time to looking straight ahead most of the time and using intermittent, quick looks down so you can foresee more challenging steps that could lead you to stumble.

- Another beneficial practice is to look at a particular obstacle or location several steps ahead of you, and to estimate how many steps you need to take before you step on that spot, even predicting which foot, left or right, will step on it.

Variations and Adaptability in Walking

Walking faster and/or for a greater distance is clearly an important part of Natural Movement practice, but intensity and volume alone aren't the only way to expand your walking practice and competency. There are other walking variations and transitions you can practice.

For instance, many balancing movements that you can do on narrow surfaces, such as the Cross Reverse and Pivot Reverse, also can be done when you're walking on the ground. In addition, you can include lower positions, such as the Deep Squat, and get-ups as part of your walking motions. Similarly, walking on unpredictable surfaces such as small unstable rocks where you need to "claw" your feet (flex your feet and toes) to increase friction and stability is a way to blend gait and balancing.

Skill-mixes such as walking and carrying something or throwing or catching while walking also should be part of your practice. Last, you want to practice walking in ways that adapt to increasingly more complex environmental demands, which can naturally be done in nature but also by using simple props that replicate some of the variables found in the real world. Wood sticks, PVC pipes, or thin ropes placed horizontally replicate branches and obstacles to be stepped over; simple lines drawn on the ground, pieces of tape stuck on the floor, or pieces of board on the ground replicate gaps you must clear by stepping out and so forth. With a little imagination, you can create many diverse ways to make walking and stepping engaging, challenging, beneficial, and fun. A hike in nature is naturally challenging and energizing to the body and mind.

Running

Run for your life! In most life-threatening situations, running is the most vital of all movement skills.

Many people believe that because running is something natural that everyone starts doing in childhood, the way you run must be a matter of personal style or preference. Yet running is just like any other Natural Movement ability: It can be efficient or inefficient, and it can be methodically improved using technique.

While slight individual stylistic variations in gait are always possible (because of the anatomy, age, health, or even emotional state of the person), it's essential to understand that the laws governing movement are the same for everyone, and there aren't individual ways to run efficiently.

Later in this section, I list inefficiencies, which you might previously have thought of as running "styles." You can run effectively for long distances with those inefficiencies, but this comes at a cost for your energy reserves, performance, comfort, and even body. (Conversely, you can run efficiently without having the stamina to run quickly or for long distances, so it's essential to separate those two aspects of running.)

Any of the inefficiencies could be necessary, momentary adjustments of your running form that you must make to remain effective and efficient. Running—just like any other natural movement—is a highly adaptable skill. The evolutionary ability we have for such diverse temporary variations of running gait stems out of a biological necessity to adapt to the context where the movement is taking place, which enables us to navigate through complex and changing environments. It's not about a concern for individual stylistic expression. Most of the time, in the absence of significant external variables, you should use a form that is neutral and consistent in pattern and levels of efficiency.

I prefer to talk about a "neutral" form rather than "perfect" or "pure" running form, which doesn't exist. The neutral form applies only to linear, flat surfaces that aren't subject to changing or unpredictable contextual demands. Trying to maintain the exact same running form regardless of environmental variables is absurd, and your "perfect" form will go down the drain the moment you hit the wild. However, overall principles do rule running efficiency, and you should learn and assimilate them to the point that they're so natural you revert to them whenever you can.

If your current form is different than what I describe, you need to be open to experimenting with a different approach. It's challenging to change patterns that are deeply ingrained. You might have been running with your current style for many years and miles, which means your technique is deeply ingrained in your brain and body. Modifying your pattern might at first feel unnatural, but with practice it will become more comfortable.

If you already have a certain amount of metabolic conditioning, with better technique you will improve distance, speed, and comfort. If you don't run at all because you've never enjoyed the ordeal (which is made worse by bad form), you'll discover that running can be made so much softer and physically enjoyable.

Repetitive Impact, Injury Risk, and Orthotics

Repetitive impact sounds like something that hurts. The truth is, repetitive impact can make you strong, or it can hurt you. Repetitive impact is determined by external and internal parameters, including the following:

- The type of ground (hard, soft, smooth, uneven, flat, or angled)
- Your footwear (if you're not barefoot)
- The position of your foot, ankle, knee, hip, and back at the moment of impact
- The speed at impact
- Volume (number of strides, duration of the run)
- Individual body weight
- Existing conditioning of your tissues to a given type of impact (including the listed parameters)
- Health levels and ability to physiologically recover

Our tissues are conditioned to certain intensity, volume, and frequency in relation to particular positional patterns in movement. There also is a certain "loading" pattern or physical and physiological impact on your tissues called *mechanome*, which affects the body in good or bad ways. A certain type of running that remains unchanged induces a specific "impact pattern," which is part of the overall individual mechanome. Changing several variables, or even changing a single variable, of this loading pattern can be tremendously beneficial in some cases; in others, it's detrimental.

Let's take a conventional heel-strike runner who can run a daily 5k comfortably at a slow speed on concrete wearing conventional running shoes (positive, thickly cushioned heel) and who does not sustain any running-related ailment or injury. What would happen if this person decided to take on a challenge to get stronger at running and changed a single parameter overnight, such as one of the following:

- Run barefoot (or with thin, minimal shoes) without modifying running form
- Run with the same footwear but with a forefoot-heel-forefoot landing
- Run on a rocky trail or on a sandy beach
- Run twice as fast
- Run loaded with a 20-pound backpack
- Run the same distance downhill
- Run at the same slow speed but go twice the distance (10k)

It is likely that instead of adapting without any noticeable consequence other than unusual soreness, the runner will experience discomfort or pain within days, if not the very next day. Eventually, if the runner were to persist with the change, they could sustain injury. The reason is not because repetitive impact has suddenly become "bad." It's because the runner didn't make the change progressively. The change was too significant and too rapid; it was simply too brutal on the body. The truth is that the runner could adapt to any new demand, and to greater levels of repetitive impact, but the change can't happen overnight.

So, you first need to make your running form biomechanically efficient. This will induce a change in the loading pattern of your body upon each stride, which can cause you discomfort, pain, and even injury if you're not very cautious and if you don't make a progressive transition. Efficient form can hurt you not because the new mechanics aren't right for you but because you are stressing your body through movement and loading patterns that are new to it, and you're not paying attention to progressions that let your body adapt healthily. For instance, changing your running gait from heel-forefoot landing to forefoot-heel-forefoot landing while maintaining all other running variables (intensity, duration, frequency, recovery time) could potentially fix any current running-induced injuries or issues, but the change might also bring other running-induced injuries. The more variables you change at once (technique, footwear, terrain, volume, speed, recovery time, and so on) without progression, the greater the chance that you'll have to deal with detrimental consequences. Patience and progressiveness are keys to being successful at making this change in running movement, technique, and training.

Adapting to minimal footwear and then switching to running barefoot is the next step. It's a good thing to practice your technique while wearing minimal footwear as soon as you can. You can keep the volume and intensity relatively low at first. You also can even run barefoot if you run on smooth and slightly soft surfaces (while still keeping the volume and intensity low in the beginning). Learning efficient running while unshod is a very effective method because the feedback from your feet is totally unaltered. Of course, practicing all Natural Movement while barefoot nicely conditions your feet and ankles to better sustain a change in running mechanics and footwear.

Five Easy Steps for Running Efficiently

Learning efficient running shouldn't be achieved through a complicated series of isolated drills. In fact, "overdrilling" might confuse you and make you mentally and physically tense.

Another problem with isolated drills is lack of transfer. For instance, doing "butt kicks" (kicking your heels toward your rear while standing in one spot) is not the same as pulling your heels higher and faster toward your rear when you run faster. In the context of running, elastic energy and hip extension contribute to the action of the lower leg winding up toward the rear beyond the contraction of the hamstrings.

Depending on your current running form, the approach to running I present here may represent a limited change, but for most people the change will be enormous. Therefore, instead of trying to change aspects of your running pattern by bits, I want you

to go through a series of short, simple drills as if you know nothing about running. These drills support a better perception of what running efficiency should feel like. From there, you should work on any aspect of your running form that you want to address or improve through actual running practice rather than in isolation.

NOTE

Before going through the following drills, go outside with a watch and, without changing anything about the way you normally run, count how many steps you make in one minute. Ideally, you would film yourself running, so you can later compare your "before and after" running forms.

Start with abdominal breathing and a neutral spine, your shoulders down, your chest open, and a forward line of vision. We now know that abdominal breathing supports spinal alignment, but it's also my assumption that the abdominal compression that stems from abdominal breathing helps limit the internal bouncing of organs and may prevent the occurrence of side stitch.

Feel that your spine is as long as possible in a "tall stance." Many natural movements you've done or are doing will help you tremendously with a perception of a neutral spine and make the position reflexive so that you start to transport your "tall posture" with every stride. In any case, you cannot run efficiently if you can't maintain spinal positional control; yet being able to maintain positional control while standing does not guarantee that you can maintain it while you're running. In any case, don't wait to run, or exclusively rely on running to build a strong core and spinal positional control.

Drill 1: Leg Pushing and Leg Pulling

Leg pushing: Start standing, push your body off one leg and land on the opposite leg, and then push off the landing leg immediately after landing. Keep doing this for a minute or so. Pay attention to the muscular effort in your legs: You must decelerate the body on a single leg upon landing, and then the same leg must push the body off the ground again before the opposite leg can take over.

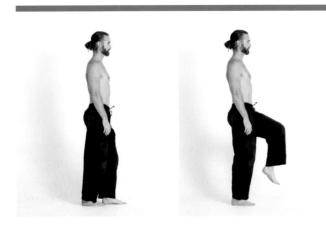

NOTE

This is pretty much how it feels when your idea of running is a succession of single-leg forward pushes or jumps. You try to push hard on your back leg and extend your front leg far; landing on it feels heavy, but you must push the same leg forward again. If it feels strenuous when you do it on the spot, think of how much energy you spend doing it as you move forward for miles?

Leg pulling: From the standing position, pull one knee up at about hip level or just below and then lower your foot to the ground; a brief moment before that foot contacts the ground and starts supporting your body weight, swiftly change support by having the opposite foot move up and off the ground (you're swiftly lifting the knee to hip level). You'll be briefly airborne after each step. Do this for about a minute. You should feel that the effort comes from your pelvic and abdominal area rather than your legs, especially if you do it fast. You need to quickly mobilize the muscles responsible for lifting your leg the moment you change support from one foot to the other. This pattern feels much more sustainable than the first one, doesn't it? Even though running involves some "push" upon landing to restore elastic energy, you want to replicate this sensation when you run and make the leg-pulling action dominant whenever possible.

If you were asked to choose between doing the leg-pushing drill and the leg-pulling drill for 20 minutes without interruption, which one would you choose and why?

Drill 2: Air Rope Skipping on the Spot

Pretend that you're rope skipping on the spot. Keep a straight back, and don't sway sideways. You may keep your forearms to the front of your body just above hip level instead of mimicking a circular motion on the sides of your body.

Would it make sense to land on your heels? Would that feel right? The answer is no because it would feel hard and painful. So, why would you want to run by landing on your heels?

If you've ever tiptoed without letting your heels contact the ground, you probably have realized that it's hard on your Achilles tendons and tends to make your feet stiffer. So, as you're rope skipping, make sure that every time you land on the ball of the feet with both feet, your heels come all the way to the ground and gently tap it before you return to the ball of your feet and become airborne again. It may take a few seconds or longer before you get this movement right, which is nothing but an upward jump to a low height.

After you feel comfortable air rope skipping with both feet, alternate your feet, landing on the ball of your foot, then your heel, and then the ball of your foot as you slightly pull your knees up in front of you. It should feel pretty much like you're gently running in place, with a leg-pulling sensation that's like the leg-pulling drill, rather than a leg-pushing feeling.

NOTE

By the way, have you noticed that I do not use the term *strike* when I talk about how the foot contacts the ground? That's because even though the landing of your foot should generate enough ground force reaction to load up your foot and leg and generate elastic energy, you should also land as lightly and smoothly as possible. You might call the way the foot lands foot *touchdown* rather than *strike*.

Drill 3: High Cadence

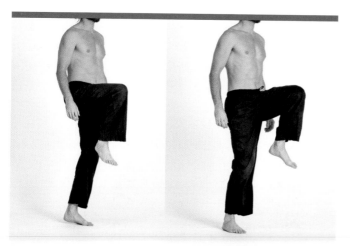

Keep skipping rope on the spot with alternating feet, just make sure that you are stepping about 180 times per minute. That's right—that many times. It means each foot will land on the ground 90 times within a minute. You can look at a watch and count your steps, use a metronome, or clap your hands three times per second. Jump for a full minute, rest another minute, and then do it again until you've memorized the tempo in your head and body.

Drill 4: Backward Jogging

This is as simple as it gets. Just make sure the space behind you is clear so you can keep gazing in front of you without having to twist your body to look where you go. Start slowly running backward. Notice that you might be intuitively doing the following:

- Slightly leaning backward with your whole body (without arching your lower back), which allows you to maintain a tall posture.
- Making small, quick steps without trying to push hard on your legs and make large steps.
- Contacting the ground on the ball of your feet first, bringing the heel flat to the ground, and then moving your heel off the ground as your foot returns to the ball before it takes off entirely.
- Letting your arms be relaxed enough so they swing naturally because of your running motion.

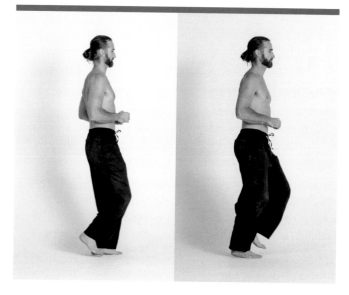

In a nutshell, this is exactly what you need to do in the reverse orientation when you run forward. What is especially noticeable is how soft each step feels. Landing on your heel first after a wide stride, even when wearing well-cushioned footwear, is one of the main reasons why your knees, lower back, and even neck feel stiff or painful after running (along with other possible issues).

Focusing on the feedback and memorizing the sensations from all four aspects I've listed can greatly help with establishing the same pattern and efficiency for running forward.

Drill 5: Air Rope Skipping with Whole-Body Lean

Now get back to skipping rope on the spot at a high cadence. What prevents you from moving forward isn't that you're not pushing hard enough on your legs. You may try to push on your legs, but you remain on the same spot as you did with the leg-pushing drill. Unless you lean forward, you're not going anywhere.

But how should you lean forward? If you bend at the hip, your trunk leans forward, but you're not necessarily shifting your center of gravity forward beyond a vertical line with your feet/base of support, in which case you keep skipping on the spot while being bent over. Think about what made you jog backward. Did you have to bend your back to the rear? No, you just needed your whole body to slightly lean backward. So, what about only flexing your ankles a tad so you can slightly lean forward? Eureka. It's all you have to do. By letting your ankles bend a little as you keep the rest of your body aligned, you are generating a gentle, almost unnoticeable forward whole-body lean that slightly shifts your center of gravity forward beyond your base of support. Gravity immediately takes over and slowly pulls you forward. (This is called gravitational torque.)

Simply lean your whole body forward as you maintain your rope-skipping motion, keep your spine straight, land softly on your feet, keep your body relaxed, and notice that you're inevitably stepping forward at a slow pace, effortlessly, or at least without any additional effort. You're basically jogging forward. That's it; that's running!

This is the neutral running form you're looking for. It looks and feels like slow backward jogging in reverse. Instead of pushing yourself forward through your legs and feet, you get a head start when gravity pulls you forward, and you can keep using the same forward momentum as long as you maintain the lean and replicate the exact same leg sequence in a cycle. Magic!

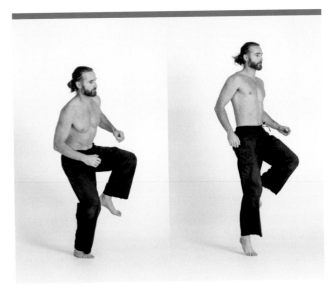

Because the lean is so slight and you're stepping at such a high cadence, you can easily maintain balance without any impression or fear that the pull will accelerate beyond control. It does not, and should not, feel like a "fall." While technically the shift of your center of gravity beyond vertical with your base of support is the very early stage of a fall, thinking of running as a "constant fall" can easily put you off and make you tense. Worse, it might make you automatically bend at the hip because that's what we unconsciously do to avoid or minimize a forward fall. Instead, think of the forward lean as a slight "whole-body lean."

You don't need to try to go fast at this point. Don't try to widen your stride or push hard on your legs. Your only task is to maintain this slight forward lean and keep pulling your feet as if you were rope skipping. Avoid any unnecessary positional modifications, such as trying to push off your legs to reach farther. Instead of pretending that your arms are swinging a rope with small circular movements, now let them gently swing forward.

Landing Foot Position

An additional, but important, technical detail of the foot touchdown is to first land on the lateral forefoot—in other words, closer to the outside edge or outer border of the forefoot rather than directly under the big toe—before the whole forefoot (followed by the heel) comes flat on the ground. This adds extra range of motion and dissipation of impact forces upon landing, but also keeps the ankle more stable. What we named "forefoot-heel" landing for the sake of simplicity is actually a "lateral forefoot-forefoot-heel" foot touchdown.

Staying Relaxed

The best form or pattern, from an external standpoint, is not the best if you are full of unnecessary internal tensions. The primary kind of relaxation you want to address is mental. There is no physical relaxation without mental relaxation. In the beginning of learning running efficiency, you might be tempted to overthink, which makes you mentally tense, which in turn leads to physical tension. You could also have a natural tendency to be tense. The mental checks you should regularly do relate to such or such aspect of your form, but they should always start with checking that you're mentally and physically relaxed. Resetting your breathing before you run, or whenever you notice a tendency to tense as you run, can help with both mental and physical relaxation. A few steps on the spot to keep your neck relaxed and your arms completely loose also can help because tensions in running are typically located in the neck, shoulders, and arms.

Recap

Now look at the three photos on the next page, which show the side view: three steps, two strides. The running is at a medium speed. Everything remains consistent, with only positional changes that are necessary to ensure the motion.

Notice the following things:

- One leg is bent and elevated.
- The other leg is supporting the whole body, with the knee bent—but not in an exaggerated way—and the ankle bent to ensure the whole-body lean.
- The head, neck, shoulders, back, hips, and supporting foot are aligned. This is a whole-body lean. The angle of the body's forward lean remains consistent. The head stays horizontally level or very close to it.
- The shoulders are relaxed. The elbows are bent at about 90 degrees. The arms are close to the ribcage and move slightly straight ahead and back at that speed.
- The rear foot is pulled up underneath the hip. Because the speed doesn't change in this sequence, the position of the legs stays the same regardless of which side is supporting the body. The center of gravity is horizontally ahead of the base of support: the back foot. As the center of gravity keeps shifting forward, there is a quick change of support with the front foot going down and the back leg being pulled up swiftly. Between the moment the front foot reaches the ground and the moment the back leg reaches the front, the body is airborne and traveling forward.
- Though you can't see it in the photos, the positional sequence of the foot upon landing is lateral forefoot-forefoot-heel, then forefoot again as the supporting foot is pulled up (otherwise called the *push-off*).
- While Natural Movement techniques rely on position/breathing, sequence/timing, and tension/relaxation, we could simplify the pillars of running as follows:
  - Position/breathing
  - Cadence
  - Relaxation

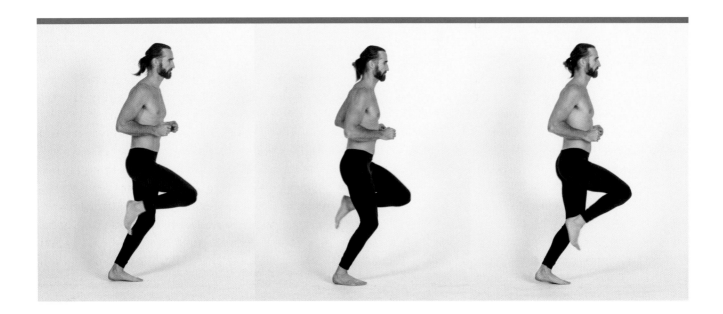

Practicing Inefficiencies

Practicing running inefficiencies is, in my experience, one of the most potent ways to fix ingrained habits and improve form and efficiency. Let me explain. While you are trying to run with efficient form, you're probably dealing with some ingrained inefficiencies that keep showing up as if they're on auto-pilot—because they are. You can easily find yourself over-drilling, overthinking, getting tense, becoming frustrated, and not getting where you want.

Addressing and tackling your inefficiencies one at a time is a great strategy because it allows you to first remove from your form what you shouldn't be doing. There are many more "don'ts" than "dos." When you can identify, as you run, what you tend to do constantly or intermittently that is counterproductive or superfluous, then you can start avoiding and removing those inefficiencies from your automatic running pattern. By tackling one inefficiency at a time, you're steadily "purifying" your form more effectively than if you try to achieve the "perfect" form at once.

Now, it can be quite tricky to perceive patterns that, despite being inefficient, have been ingrained in your movement memory for so long that they feel natural and go unnoticed. Reading about inefficiencies or having someone point them out will not fix the issue. You need to experience the problem and get sensory feedback that is strong and convincing enough for you to acknowledge it as an issue and be willing to address it.

Look at the diverse, common faults in the photos. You might go to a local park to observe casual runners, and you'll spot similar patterns. You'll even spot some runners who display several faults, such as running with long, jumping strides; landing on the heels; using exaggerated arm movements; and shifting their heads forward as if they want to look as athletic they can. Another runner could be running with short, slow strides; landing on the midfoot; bending at the hip with almost no flexion at the knees; rounding the back and hunching the shoulders; wobbling the head side to side; and using zero movement in their arms. Others pull their knees to the front and heels to the back or swing their arms as high as they can as if they're sprinting, even when they're just jogging. Others display a healthy forefoot-heel-forefoot landing pattern, but they run with their torsos leaning back. The possible combinations of inefficient running form are countless. If you didn't know, you could think that everyone's running form is fine and just a matter of personal style.

However, you want to do more than look at inefficiencies. You need to practice each of them to consciously experience how counterproductive and unnecessary each of these inefficiencies feel. By practicing the inefficiencies, you will experientially realize that they are indeed issues. Practicing inefficiencies is especially effective for helping you become aware of inefficiencies you didn't know you have.

I have ordered inefficiencies in the following list from the bottom of the body up—starting in the feet and legs, moving through the hips, and going all the way to the torso, arms, neck, and head. What happens in the feet, legs, and hips is the most important. You want to fix those issues before you address lower-priority issues. If your upper body is straight and relaxed but your hips, legs, and feet are doing a messy job, you're in more trouble than if the situation is the other way around.

Practice each of these inefficiencies, one at a time, for about 30 seconds, or until you really can't stand it anymore. Exaggerate them to the point that they look and feel either uncomfortable or plain absurd. If they feel that way when exaggerated, then even a "lighter," less pronounced or noticeable version of the issues can't really be a good thing, right?

Remember that any of the faults I've shown has the potential to be an actual, necessary adaptation to environmental or situational circumstances. The more complex the context becomes, the more likely that your "neutral" form will undergo a variety of positional modifications. Such changes are not only possible; they are mandatory to preserve efficiency. Heel striking becomes a good thing when going downhill, leaning backward becomes a good thing if you run beneath low tree branches, and so on. Clearly, this wouldn't be a fault; it's an adaptable motion. However, in the absence of necessity, any disturbance to a neutral form is an inefficiency. It's a good idea to film yourself running and play the footage in slow motion, so you can get visual feedback of your running form and be able to realize inefficiencies you normally can't see that you have.

TECHNIQUE TIP

Make sure to practice the neutral form in between experimenting with each inefficiency, so that you return to a form that feels good, relaxing, and efficient.

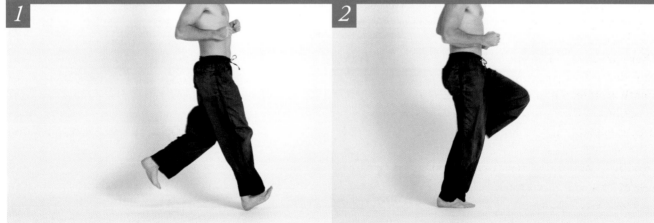

(continued on next page)

1 Heel striking: This makes landing hard on your whole body, and it slows you down.

2 Knees pulled way too high in relation to a slow pace: The same can be true of the heels being pulled up way too high toward the rear at a slow pace. Sometimes both your knees and heels are raised high, which looks like you're riding a bicycle. This unnecessary movement of the leg wastes energy.

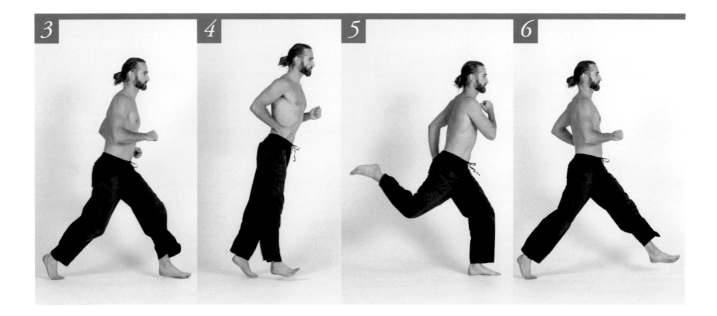

3 **A form of leg pushing run with no lean, midfoot landing, almost non-existent airborne moment:** While this style does minimize impact and makes running feel softer, this is closer to wide-step walking than running, and it fully relies on pushing off the quadriceps. Because you're keeping your feet low and close to the ground, you're not using your hamstrings to pull your heels up toward your rear, so the effort of bringing your leg forward is entirely left to your hip flexor muscles. This style is also slow, and you can't go fast with this technique if needed.

4 **Stiff legs, lack of flexion at the knees:** Knees are designed to bend upon landing to enable leg muscles to absorb impact and prevent a shock wave to stress your knees, hips, and back at every step. Preventing your knees from flexing forces your feet to work more than they should to absorb some of the impact if you land on the forefoot first and to keep pushing forward. Not bending your knees enough leaves all the effort to your feet, ankles, and calves, which stresses these areas more than necessary.

5 **Striding out:** Running with big, long strides forces you to push hard on your leg muscles to propel yourself far and to extend your lead leg far (making the back leg trail behind). This forces you to land on your heel, which increases the impact. The time it takes for your center of gravity to move forward so it's vertically aligned with your supporting foot is increased, which means the supporting foot must stay grounded longer. It absorbs the impact over a longer time, losing most of its ability to store and transfer elastic energy. It looks and feels as if you are "sitting" back on a single leg every time you land. The supporting leg has no other choice but to push forward with force again; rather than maintaining momentum, you basically re-create it with each step. This is not only extremely energy-consuming but it slows you down. Revert to much shorter and quicker steps any time you find yourself striding out.

6 **Striding out with extended leg and ankle:** This is another unconscious strategy aimed at avoiding a forward lean and maintaining a vertical, or even leaning-backward, torso as you attempt to step relatively softly. This style relies mostly on your hip flexor muscles to swing the leg forward without benefiting from the forward momentum from leg flexion. Also, extending the ankle early with the forefoot that is pointing forward all the way from the back to the front creates unnecessary tension at the ankle.

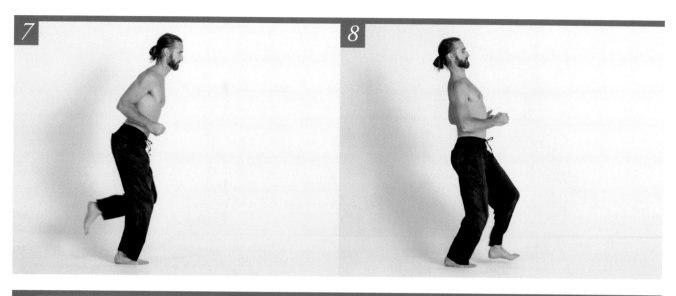

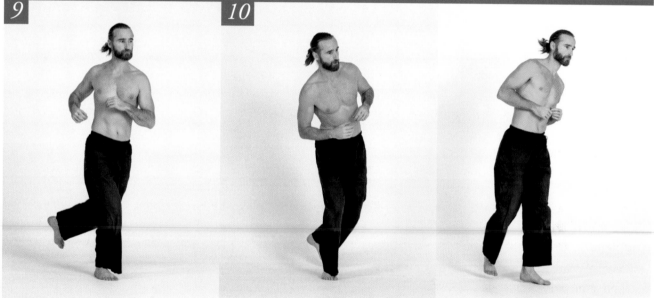

(continued on next page)

7 Bending at the hip, trunk leaning forward: You think that you are leaning forward and indeed you are, except that you are folding yourself in two or bending under a heavy load on your shoulders. This position in running stresses your lower back and lessens your ability to generate forward momentum because of gravity.

8 Trunk leaning backward: This style shifts your center of gravity behind your base of support. Although this backward lean would be great if you were running backward, in this case it prevents you from taking advantage of the forward pull of gravity, which increases your energy consumption, slows you down tremendously, and prevents you from going fast when needed.

9 Exaggerated hip and trunk rotation: This style makes your torso twist and your trailing leg rotate internally. The rotation can be mostly generated by your trunk or hips. Rotational motion of your hips is necessary in running, but it's limited and doesn't generate positional disturbance.

10 Trunk leaning/swaying from side to side: This upper-body motion wants to pull you sideways. On top of using energy necessary to stabilize your body, it diverts your kinetic motion from where it needs to be directed, which is forward.

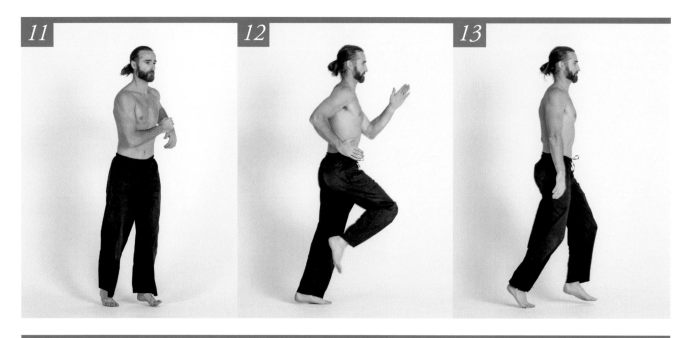

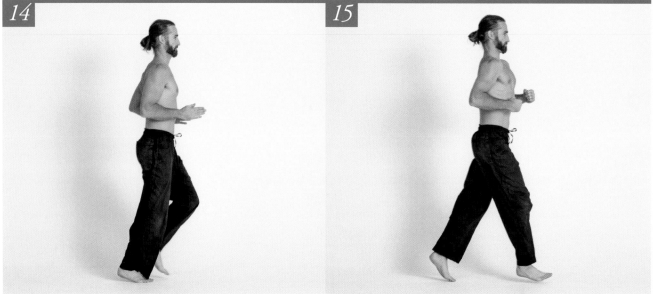

11 Arms are actively swung sideways across the body: Your arms should move forward and back similarly to your legs. When your lead leg moves forward, your opposing arm should move forward as well (to counterbalance the action of your leg). Your arms shouldn't move perpendicularly or at a pronounced angle.

12 Active arms: Arms are intentionally swung with great amplitude despite running slowly. How much your arms swing is balanced with your speed; it's not an independent motion. Ample arm swinging can be momentarily used to assist acceleration as you run uphill; otherwise it's a waste of energy.

13 Overly relaxed arms: Your arms are supposed to be sufficiently relaxed to enable a natural motion that counterbalances the movement of your legs, but your arms shouldn't be dead weight. In this photo, it's good that the shoulders are relaxed, but you need just enough tension in the biceps to keep your forearms up to the front just above hip level.

14 Tense arms and hands: The arms remain in a set position. This is unnecessary tension.

15 Tense, stiff upper body (neck, shoulders, arms, fists): This is unnecessary tension.

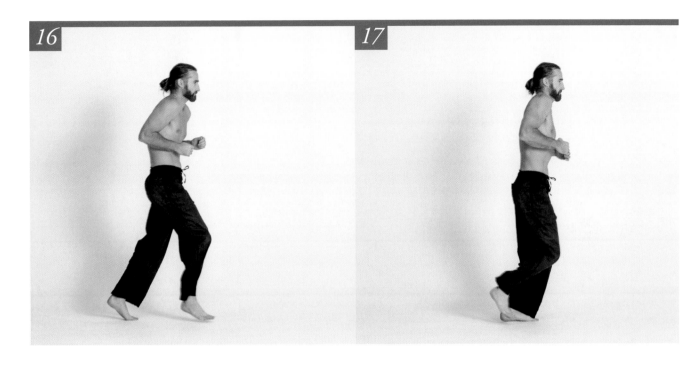

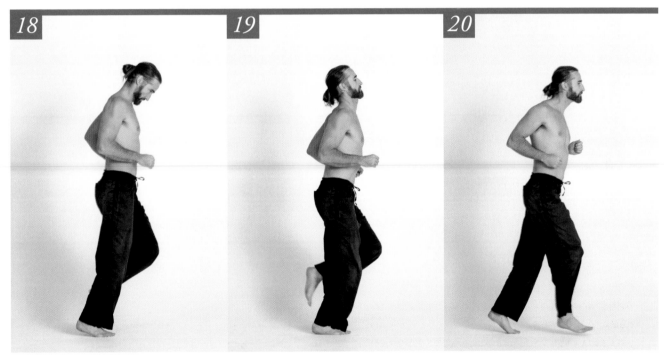

16 Hunched shoulders, flexed upper back: This is unnecessary tension.

17 Shrugged shoulders: This is unnecessary tension.

18 Head tilted down: When you have unnecessary tension in the neck, you end up with a rounded upper back, and your line of vision is restricted to the ground.

19 Head tilted back: This is unnecessary tension.

20 Head thrust forward ("head-chasing"): This is unnecessary tension.

The preceding list covers the most common ineffi-ciencies. The following are some other inefficiencies:

- Tiptoeing. If you don't let your heel gently tap the ground after you've landed on your forefoot, you're not using elastic energy because the range of motion in your ankles and the stretch in your calf muscles is limited, preventing your feet from "loading up" as they contact the ground. You are instead forcing your feet, Achilles tendons, and calves to maintain constant tension. You should tiptoe only when necessary. For instance, in certain contexts tiptoeing could help you im-prove frictional force and stability for a very short distance as you forcefully accelerate from a Foot-Hand Crawl to sprinting.
- Running with splayed feet.
- Wobbling your head.
- Swinging a single arm outwardly, leaning to a single side, or any imbalance and lack of symme-try (caused by habit or compensation for a recent or old injury).

Cadence Versus Speed

Are you running yet? Yes, you are! The five fundamen-tals of improving your efficiency were using a slight forward whole-body lean, emphasizing a pulling leg motion, landing on the ball of your feet first, keeping a rather short stride and a high cadence. If you're not at all a runner to begin with, and you normally don't enjoy running because it feels hard on your legs and body, you should feel liberated that this new running pattern feels so light and easy.

You might be tempted to quickly try to run faster, especially if you're are a runner already. The prob-lem is that greater speed might have you immediately revert to inefficient habits. So, we need to talk about running faster (but not sprinting) while maintaining the same form and pattern you've just established.

First, though, I want to explain high cadence and why it matters for running efficiency. In running, ca-dence (also called rhythm, tempo, or turnover) is the frequency at which you move your legs to stride and step, regardless of your running speed. Your running speed is the distance you cover relative to time, re-gardless of how many leg movements (strides or steps) you perform. So, cadence has to do with the number of times (the rate or frequency) at which your feet hit the ground within a set amount of time. Just like your pulse or heart rate is the number of times your heart beats per minute, cadence is evaluated as the num-ber of times per minute you step. Therefore, you can cover the same distance by running relatively slowly at a high cadence with short strides or running rela-tively quickly at a low cadence with long strides. You also can run quickly at a high cadence or run slowly at a slow cadence—and anything in between.

A high cadence doesn't necessarily imply that you're running fast if you keep your forward lean very slight and your strides short. Do you want proof? Think about the high cadence drill (drill 3, page 323). You were able to do very short, quick steps (180 per minute) while staying on the spot as long as you kept your center of gravity vertically aligned with your feet and avoided any forward whole-body lean. Clearly you can independently control your running cadence and your running speed.

Typically, an unskilled runner who's jogging dis-plays a low stride rate—or, if you prefer, a low ca-dence—of about 130 to 140 steps per minute without a significant increase of cadence when they run faster. Instead of mostly increasing cadence, unskilled run-ners accelerate by increasing stride length with wider steps, which makes it challenging to increase cadence. The problem is that running with large steps demands much more energy. With wider strides, you must first push hard off your leg to make the opposite foot land way ahead of your center of gravity. This usually re-sults in your body moving not just horizontally but also overly vertically in an up-and-down fashion that resembles the elliptical airborne trajectory that's typ-ical of jumping. I'm not saying that there's no vertical propulsion in running, but it should be limited. When you add significant vertical momentum to your move-ment, you add more airborne time, which is a reason why you paradoxically might go slower even when you're trying to go faster. Also, the front leg, which is landing from a greater elevation than necessary, must absorb the heavier impact, usually after the heel lands first with a hard landing. You must wait for the rest of your body and center of gravity to move forward be-fore you can push off your leg again. Meanwhile, your foot spends a significantly longer time on the ground supporting your body weight, and all muscle elasticity normally stored upon landing dissipates long before it can be transferred to the next step. The heel-first landing pattern, although it occasionally can be sustained depending on context, has a braking effect on your landing, with greater impact forces, increased ground time, and reduced elastic energy storage, which participates in slowing you down and tiring you early.

In a nutshell, you waste a lot of precious energy in the process. On top of consuming much more energy than needed, this pattern creates unnecessary levels of stress on your joints—your knees especially—and supports a much greater risk of pain during or after running sessions.

Conversely, short and rapid strides or high cadence keep you "elastic" at a much lower cost, with your feet landing right under your center of gravity and your supporting leg being able to immediately transfer a lot of stored elastic energy toward the next step. Both the time your body spends airborne and your feet spend grounded (which is as little as one-tenth of a second when you're running really fast) gets much shorter. It's much less tiring to cover a long distance with short, quick steps than to cover the same distance with long, slow steps. This difference in energy-consumption is something that you have already somewhat experienced with the leg-pushing and leg-pulling drills that you performed on the spot.

Is There a Magic Number?

So, what cadence is best, and for what speed? It's often said that the best running cadence is 180 steps per minute regardless of speed. That's about three steps per second, which might sound like a lot, but leg movement in running is faster than you think when you make sure to keep your stride short. At that cadence, you can fully, consistently benefit from both muscle-tendon elasticity in your feet and legs and ground reaction forces. Running with a low cadence of about 130 to 150 steps per minute is a sign of an unskilled runner who is striding out all the time.

Another advantage of short strides is that it's much easier to maintain a forefoot-heel-forefoot landing pattern and to land with your center of gravity right above your supporting foot, so you're ready to be immediately pulled forward by gravity.

The "best" cadence of 180 steps per minute is an average determined after evaluating elite marathoners who were running at a racing speed. Does that mean that cadence should become the norm—a one-size-fits-all cadence for all runners at any running speeds? Of course not. Cadence has to do with pace and variations in running speed. When jogging, especially for short distances, your cadence can be as low as 160 to 170 steps per minute. If you normally are a low-cadence runner who takes about 130 steps per minute, a cadence of 160 to 170 steps per minute represents a significant increase in stride rate of about 30 percent. As you accelerate to become a faster runner, your cadence should increase to around 180 steps per minute, so you sustain greater speed without widening your strides. Now, if your average cadence was 130 steps per minute and you increase your cadence to 180 to 190 steps per minute, you've increased your stride rate by about 50 percent. Clearly, the only way you can achieve a higher cadence is by making what might feel like fast "baby steps" if you are used to wide strides.

A sprinting cadence ranges from 220 to 240 steps per minute. That's about a 70 percent increase in stride rate compared to a low 130-steps-per-minute jogging cadence! Could you seriously almost double your stride rate while also significantly widening your stride?

Relative Speed Versus Absolute Speed

There are factors that can decrease or increase your velocity even if you're not deliberately modifying your speed. Have you ever run on a treadmill so that you're running on the spot despite running fast? Your relative speed may be high, but your absolute speed remains close to zero. You get the idea.

For example, a slight incline in terrain (uphill) can slow you down even when you aren't decelerating, and a slight decline in terrain (downhill) boosts your speed even if you don't accelerate. Low-friction surfaces or footwear or changes of direction also tend to reduce your velocity even when you maintain the same cadence and speed.

Going Faster

Now that you know that running with short and fast strides is good for efficiency, how do you run faster without having to revert to pushing hard on your legs in long, bouncy, jump-like, lower-cadence strides? It's relatively simple: increase your ankle flexion. Remember doing short and quick steps on the spot without leaning and doing short and quick steps with a very slight lean so that you were jogging? What happens if you increase the lean?

Increasing ankle flexion increases your whole body lean and accelerates your forward momentum. As a result, you need to pull your legs forward faster. To do so, you need to use your hamstrings more to lift your heels toward your rear faster, which pushes your knee forward and helps you pull it forward faster. What this means is that the range of motion of your legs increases in amplitude, so you can conserve your balance as you lean forward more and make your forward momentum accelerate more through it.

Another important aspect that makes you go faster is lengthening your stride, but doing so without widening your steps. Let me explain.

Striding out is making long strides by widening your leg movement with the front foot reaching far forward. The stride length I'm talking about is the horizontal distance that your body covers between each step, not how wide your legs and feet are apart whenever your feet hit the ground. As your body leans at a greater forward angle, gravity accelerates how fast you move forward, which, without changing your stride rate, increases stride length. You're running faster in part because your cadence increases, but also because a greater whole-body lean angle accelerates forward momentum and the distance covered in between steps, even without widening your leg movement.

Running Uphill and Downhill

Running uphill and/or downhill requires that you modify the neutral running technique and running effort, especially as the grade increases. Uphill and downhill running are normally imposed by topographical changes in the environment, but when available they also can be strategic options when you're using them as shortcuts. Even though they're more energy-consuming options or not as safe as running on flat terrain (the risk of injury is much higher when running down a steep grade and difficult terrain), an inclined route might represent a faster alternative and choosing to go up or down a hill might save overall time and energy compared to running on a flat but longer route.

NOTE

Contrary to appearances, and distances being equal, even running downhill is costlier in terms of energy consumption than running on flat terrain.

Uphill

Even though you'll do your best to maintain a pulling pattern, as the grade of the incline increases, it becomes evident that you do need to push harder on your legs.

To accommodate for the grade of the incline and place your lead foot higher on the ground, your knee must drive upward higher than on flat terrain at the same speed. Because the ball of the foot is higher than the heel, your heels may not even touch the ground any longer (unless you momentarily step on one spot where the surface is horizontal, such as rock, or unless you are running up a stairway), which demands more strength and stability from your foot and ankle. The muscular effort becomes mostly concentric, with much less benefit from stored elastic energy. You must actively swing your arms upward—but not backward—and with more amplitude to generate additional momentum that you can transfer to whole-body momentum. You swing your arms in a contralateral fashion with the supporting/grounded foot with impeccable timing.

Because of these changes in pattern, you must give more attention to the relationship of tension and relaxation. You want to maintain a stable lower back and tight core and avoid rounding your upper back, swaying side to side, and other similar positional disturbances unless they're necessary. As always, you should maintain impeccable abdominal breath control even when the effort is so intense that you also breathe through the chest as well.

Those are a lot of aspects to consider while being rapidly fatigued by the intensity of the effort running uphill represents.

The good side of running uphill, though, is that shock absorption is much less a factor, and the risk for injury is very low compared to running downhill.

Downhill

When you run downhill, gravity obviously is accelerating forward and down much faster, which you must deal with very carefully. While the assistance of gravity enables you to accelerate very quickly without effort, you can absolutely lose control of your speed, become unable to change direction, or find it difficult to slow down to avoid obstacles, which means you might crash.

Although you want to preserve a technique as close to the neutral form as you can, as the grade of the decline increases, the degree of forward lean decreases to prevent uncontrolled acceleration and speed, to the point of having to literally lean backward if the slope gets really steep. The degree of leg pull isn't as pronounced as in general running technique. Instead, the leg extends downward to a lower surface of support.

Because you're stepping down, you need to disperse greater impact forces upon landing, with your leg muscles working eccentrically and staying on support a little longer than on flat terrain to ensure deceleration. Even if you maintain short strides, the eccentric contractions required for downhill running might cause you soreness in the thighs the next day if you aren't accustomed to it.

With steeper inclines, you need to revert to landing first on your heels to better decelerate and also to ensure greater ankle stability upon landing, thus protecting yourself from a potential ankle twist or sprain.

Another reason you flex your ankles rather than extending them is because landing on the forefoot first when going downhill can easily make the foot slide forward and could even result in breaking toes when the foot slides and bumps onto a rock. The reality is that when you're running downhill on steep grades and difficult terrains, such as when it's rocky, your neutral form is completely disrupted because you have no choice but to continuously adjust position and cadence to the demands of the terrain to maintain balance and safety. Overall, the potential for a traumatic injury is real when running downhill.

However, if the ground is clear of obstacles and the grade of the decline isn't steep, you can introduce more forward lean so you can elongate each stride. You may occasionally allow yourself to take strides longer than on a horizontal terrain, with a lower cadence, making sure to stay relaxed as you maintain a tight core.

TECHNIQUE TIP

It's best to practice uphill and downhill running with lower grades first and with surfaces that are clear of obstacles. For a very fun yet very intense training, run downhill toward an uphill slope and use the momentum you gain to reach greater speed as you run uphill.

Deceleration *or* Stopping

It's a good thing to know how to quickly decelerate, which can be necessary to simply keep control of your balance or avoid running too fast when you see surfaces coming that can be risky for your feet and ankles. Sometimes you just need to stop immediately (for example, because of a change of situation, upcoming gap, or unexpected obstacle). The way people usually come to a stop resembles what is normally seen as running inefficiencies: striding out and landing on the heels. Those techniques are also inefficient when decelerating because they're hard on the body and don't stop you that quickly.

If you just want to reduce your speed, simply reduce your whole-body forward lean and transition from a very high cadence (well over 200 steps per minute) to a high cadence (around 180 steps per minute). It's that simple. If you do need to abruptly stop yourself (which takes place over several strides), you literally want to lean back as much as you can, which makes the balls of your feet (not your heels) act as brakes on the ground.

Running Variations, Adaptations, *and* Progressions

As I've pointed out, you should be able to adapt your running form in many ways to preserve effectiveness. While running variations are not as efficient as the neutral running form in terms of energy cost, they are the only way to maintain effective performance level in a given context. The idea of a one-size-fits-all running form, when exposed to the diverse demands of contextual complexity, rapidly becomes mere dogma. For instance, instead of being brief, the time you spend with your foot in contact with the ground can increase considerably proportionally to the gait cycle (such as when you're running uphill on steep terrain, when you're carrying a load, or when the ground is muddy and sandy). Airborne time can also increase when you're striding out to clear an obstacle. Those are just some examples.

In the absence of actual contextual demands, you have the possibility of imagining such demands to physically create the movement behaviors and efforts they generate. For instance, both Side Shuffle and Cross-Stepping enable you to run laterally in a direction while still being able to turn your head in directions that a forward orientation would not enable. Those patterns could be employed as well for the obvious reason of having to go through a narrow passage. It's a great approach to running competency to regularly practice these variations and make yourself comfortable with them.

See the following examples of running variations.

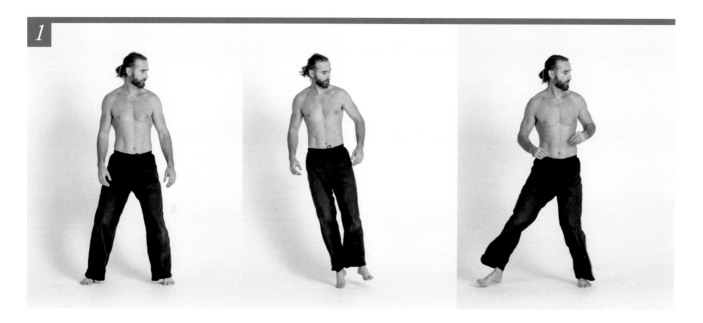

1   Side Shuffle

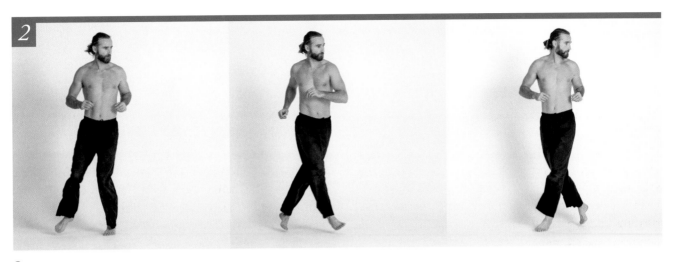

2 Cross-Stepping

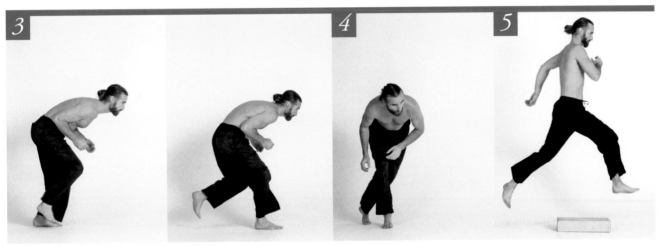

3 Crouched

4 Cross-Stepping Crouched

5 Striding out

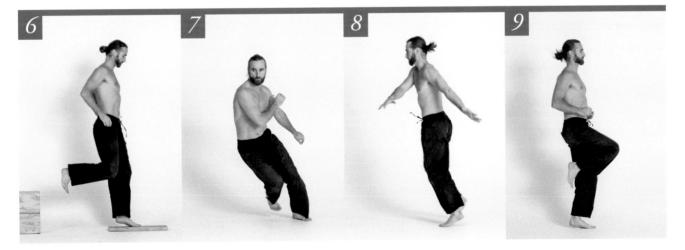

6 Stepping down

7 Directional change

8 Orientation change (to keep running in the same direction while facing the opposite one)

9 Leaning backward

Examples of additional variations include the following:

- Changing foot position and sequence upon landing: heels (hindfoot, rearfoot), ball of the foot (forefoot), internal or external side of the foot.
- Trunk leaning sideways.
- Having your feet land in line or wide apart.
- Stepping up, down, over, through.
- Half-turn/reverse.
- Full-turn/reverse.
- Accelerations and decelerations.
- Frequent changes of pace (which is known as *fartlek*).
- Running with a loaded backpack (If the load and/or running speed is significant, your weight upon landing increases significantly and will easily exceed your plyometric strength and endurance in your feet and calves, forcing you to land on the midfoot or even on the heel, which can be hard on your lower back.)
- Adjusting start positions (lying, kneeling, squatting, and so on).
- Stepping accuracy; learning to step precisely where you intend to (small rocks, stumps, ledge of sidewalk).
- Transitioning from skill to skill (crawling to running, jumping to running).
- Running on varied surfaces (flat, uneven, stable, unstable, soft, hard, smooth, rough, inclined, declined, hot, cold, frozen, dry, humid, wet, muddy, icy, snowy, rocky, sandy, gravel, vegetation, wood, concrete, metal, plastic/synthetic).
- Skill-mixing (running and throwing, running and catching, running and carrying, running and balancing, running and lifting).

Of course, there are endless adaptations, some of which I've previously described as inefficiencies, but they can be temporary, necessary adaptations in a specific context.

Most running variations are completely instinctive and don't necessitate technical instruction beyond the fundamental principles of breathing and staying as relaxed as possible. However, some simple tips can go a long way in immediately making some of these variations much more efficient. Here are some examples:

- Generally speaking, your arms play an active role in helping you maintain balance, change direction, or propel you over obstacles. Pump your arms (swing them actively) when you're running uphill on steep slopes or when you transition from a ground position to sprinting to make you accelerate and reach top speed faster.
- To decelerate faster when you're sprinting, stride out and lean backward (you may even heel strike). That's exactly what you don't want to do when you're running economically, but this is the way to efficiently stop yourself when you run fast.
- When you reverse your orientation (while you keep running in the same direction) swiftly turn your head before you rotate your hips.
- When changing direction a sharp 90 degrees to the side (for instance, after a tree or cutting a corner in a street), step with the front foot opposite the direction you're turning, then rotate your head and hips toward where you're turning to swiftly pivot on the ball of the foot. This is more efficient than making smaller steps.
- When you run through wooded, leafy areas with flexible branches, don't slow to pull and hold branches with your hands. Simply extend your arms forward, internally rotate your arms to point your palms out, and push the branches away from your face and torso.
- Never take any step for granted. Anticipate the type of surface (soft, hard, wet, dry, stable, unstable, slippery, or providing friction) and how it might alter your foot position, gait, balance, and speed. Use visual input and pay attention to anything noticeable that indicates there potentially will be an issue when you step. For instance, mud or stone can have a certain shine or darkness to it that indicates it will be slippery or soft.
- When you run on soft surfaces, attempting to conserve a neutral running gait can be inefficient and unsafe for the ankle. The ground reaction force is low, and landing on the ball of the foot generates a delayed input of when and how much to bend the leg and load the foot; once loaded, the foot might slide back. It puts a big stress on the Achilles tendons and feet as they struggle to stabilize on a ground that's unstable. In this case, landing on the heel or on the midfoot becomes more efficient. The heel starts compressing the

ground enough to provide more stability for the ankle and load the leg, then the ball of the foot comes down with a stabilized ankle and the forefoot can compress the ground to help stabilize on the surface before the push off, which reduces the tendency of the forefoot to slide back. Because the surface is soft, landing on the heel first is relatively comfortable. On the one hand, this technique is less energy-efficient because it requires that you bend the leg more to load it; that you do it more slowly, so you spend more time with your foot on the ground; and to push off the leg more. On the other hand, it's more energy-efficient overall because you avoid "backpaddling."

- When you're unsure of the stability or friction of a surface where you intend to step, don't fully commit all your body weight as you step on it. Don't load the landing foot and stay light to minimize the risk of slippage on the surface or of making it move under your foot.

- Pick up your toes (keep them flexed/raised) when you go downhill or on horizontal but slippery surfaces. If your foot slides forward into an obstacle, you will bump the ball of the foot beneath the toes instead of spraining or even breaking your toes or having to slow down or step to the side at the last second, which might put you on a surface that is worse.

- Picking up your toes also is helpful when you're running on terrains with tall vegetation or shallow water when you can't see where you step or when the terrain is rocky, but you can't spend your time always looking down. In this case you want to pick up your toes and swing the foot, lifting it a little higher than you normally would, and keeping it tucked/flexed until it extends forward and down. The worst-case scenario if you can't see the obstacle is that you bump underneath your toes and the ball of your foot, and you might stumble and fall but without hurting your foot. You can use this tip to prevent hurting your feet even when obstacles are visible but abundant, such as when running on rocky terrain.

Running variations are not just natural occurrences when you run in nature. They also should be part of your running practice—not something to avoid by choosing predictable, linear, smooth terrains and routes. You should include variables in your regular practice. The benefits to your overall running competency are obvious, but the fine-tuning of your motor skills and physiological adaptations that stem from their development transfers to overall movement competency, which makes your tendons stronger, your balance and agility better, your footing more reliable, your stamina and recovery time better, and so on. Those improvements are useful in many sports.

So, don't wait to find yourself in a natural context to start practicing running variations. You can reproduce some of the natural variables in urban environments by running around the block, along the edge of a sidewalk, striding to step on paint marks on the pavement, going up and down streets, accelerating and decelerating, changing direction abruptly, and so on. It's also a good idea to punctuate your run with intermittent short periods of other diverse other natural movements (crawling, balancing, jumping, and so on). This approach to running practice makes a difference in your overall physical preparedness, and it also makes your running practice more challenging while keeping it motivating and satisfying, compared to always running the same way on the same type of surface. This is true whether you're a Natural Mover, or you're primarily or exclusively a runner. Don't be a specialist within your own specialized practice. Just remember to be sensible about your practice because the more brutal the changes in movement patterns, footwear, intensity, duration, and distance, the more susceptible to injury you become.

Last, the acquisition of efficient technique cannot compensate for a lack of conditioning or a lack of progressiveness. Training progressions in running involve environmental complexity (including diverse weather conditions), intensity (fast variations in speed and direction), volume (distance and duration), and the ability to run barefoot (if you want to develop such ability).

28
Airborne Movement

"Jump, and you will find out how to unfold your wings as you fall."

—Ray Bradbury

Jumping is a very particular movement ability that enables us to propel ourselves into the air for a brief time. The human body doesn't go airborne exclusively when jumping. Airborne movement also occurs when you're running, and it may occasionally happen when you're crawling fast or climbing. However, the most significant airborne movement does take place when you're jumping.

Jumping can be viewed as a gait—just like running—in which the entire body is temporarily airborne, but there are several aspects that clearly distinguish jumping from running—for example, the momentary nature of jumping, the relatively long duration of the off-ground phase, the nonhorizontal angle of the launch, the parabolic trajectory before landing (in most cases), and the high diversity of possible jumping and landing patterns and surfaces. For all these reasons, I prefer to specifically categorize jumping as an airborne type of gait.

Humans jump for practical reasons to pass obstacles that are in their way—such as when there is no way around it, when finding an alternative path would take too long, or when clearing the obstacle using another movement would be more dangerous or slower. Jumping can be risky and energy-consuming, so for that reason it's used only momentarily as a way of locomotion. However, when jumping is the only effective movement option in a given environment or situation—or when it's the most efficient option—you need to be skillful at it. Jumping is occasionally used for combat, either as a defensive maneuver to avoid blows or as an offensive move that's often combined with kicking or punching. Jumping also can be used in the form of sprawling (ground movement) to avoid projectiles.

Young humans practice jumping instinctively through movement play because it's naturally exhilarating. Occasionally, children attempt jumps that are risky relative to their size to push their limits. This natural drive to jump has found many outlets for expression. Jumping was used extensively in many ancient activities, and it's still used extensively in modern physical activities and contests ranging from highly specialized jumping patterns in athletics (the high, long, or triple jump and hurdling) to many team sports, such as basketball and volleyball. Martial arts and movement disciplines (such as gymnastics, dance, capoeira or parkour, and fitness programs) incorporate jumping. Regardless of pattern, activity, or cultural context, there is no doubt that jumping is highly rewarding for the performer and an impressive and entertaining feat for the viewer.

As with other skill categories, Natural Movement rejects cultural or sports conventions, or even aesthetic considerations, primarily emphasizing the practicality of jumping and how it adapts to highly diverse environmental variables. Whatever the form or purpose behind the movement, jumping is phenomenal at giving us intense sensations, especially with the airborne, weightless, "gravity-free" moment it provides.

Icarus had a dream of flying in the air, which humans can achieve only with the assistance of non-biological technology external to the body. Jumping to propel oneself into the air and moving through space above ground, even for only a short distance and a brief duration, is the closest thing to flying humans can experience by natural means.

Even though we may use the term "flight" to name the phase where you're off ground, jumping and flying are not technically the same. To jump, you need a surface that is solid or firm enough to create a reactive force so that you can apply power or transfer momentum to propel yourself away from it into an airborne moment. This is how we turn ourselves into living "projectiles" that follow a flight path or trajectory through space as a function of time. As you're above ground, you're not subject to significant aerodynamic forces for very long before you land, and you can't change the direction, speed, distance, or duration of your trajectory; you can change only your body orientation.

The initial jump conditions fully dictate your trajectory, except when you can push off a surface while you're airborne, such as in vaulting. Even flying squirrels don't actually fly; they're only using evolutionary anatomical adaptations to glide, extend the range of the jump post-launch, and change direction.

Comparatively, birds may initiate flight with a jump so that they push off a substrate (ground, water), but after they're off ground, they're able to modify not only their body orientation but also their direction, speed, the distance they cover, and the time they're aloft. They even use aerodynamic forces to their advantage. Even the best human jumpers will never get close to what birds can do. Sorry, folks. Flying is a natural movement that belongs to other species—not humans. But jumping is an amazing Natural Movement skill, and you're going to learn a lot about it.

Jumping Sequence

Regardless of the technique used, jumping is a sequence that's always made of three components or phases that are closely related: the launching generates the airborne trajectory, which in turn ends up in a landing. Too often most of the attention goes to the airborne phase, and little or no attention is given to the landing. In Natural Movement, we are highly aware of how strongly these three phases influence each other.

The Launching

Except for the very particular case in which jumping is initiated by releasing one's grip when hanging, launching is the movement that either produces power, transfers momentum, or combines both actions to create a takeoff. You can jump either from a steady position like a stand, Deep Knee Bend, Squat, or even a balancing position, or you can jump after a movement, such as walking, running, crawling, balancing, and even hanging or jumping.

A jump launched from a static position is done in a single movement that relies on power, gravity, or a combination of both. For instance, jumping downward with little or no horizontal distance involved requires little power at the launching and relies on gravity for most of the distance to be traveled. Such downward trajectory makes the launching quite easy and energy-efficient (with the landing that follows being usually more difficult and energy-costly in comparison). Conversely, an upward jump requires significant power to oppose gravity with an energy-costly launch (with the landing that follows being usually light and energy-efficient in comparison). A jump launched from a static standing position on the edge of an elevated surface aimed at reaching the greatest distance possible relies on both power and gravity. Jumping from a stationary stance is not always a choice; you might have to do it because there is no space before the launching surface to create momentum, because the launching surface is too challenging or not reliable enough to be used with additional momentum (such as with an unstable ground or when you're balancing), or because the landing is technical and jumping from a static position helps you better control the landing.

Compared to a Power Jump launched from a static position, the amount of power necessary for a jump that follows forward momentum to cover an equal distance is not as great. This is because some of the velocity and kinetic energy produced before taking off, such as when you run fast, is transferred to the jumping action, which reduces the overall amount of muscular power required.

Velocity can be needed when you're in a hurry or you're being chased, if you don't have a reason to come to a stop before jumping, or simply if the distance you need to jump exceeds that which muscular power alone could produce. You may want to create as much velocity as you can to jump as fast and as far as you can. But the presence of great velocity, or even any momentum at all prior to jumping, is not always necessary or even an advantage, and the lack of it might not be an issue or a disadvantage. It depends on the context. For instance, you might want to significantly decelerate your run before jumping to ensure a soft and accurate landing. When you don't slow down, you sometimes land very heavily or even miss the surface where you should land, and there's a clear risk of injury.

How much power you need to generate from static positions, and how much momentum and power you need to use from moving, has everything to do with the distance you need to cover, the direction you're going, and how you will land. For instance, you need less power and/or momentum when you launch a jump from an elevated surface and land at a lower level than you do to cover the same distance with the launching and landing surfaces horizontally leveled.

Conversely, you need more power and/or momentum when you launch a jump from a lower level and are going to a more elevated surface. I talk about this more in the next section about trajectory.

NOTE

Velocity and power can be combined to produce more significant jumping speeds and distances than jumps that rely solely on power generated from static positions.

Even though ultimately the trajectory of a jump can go in any direction—forward, upward, downward, sideways, and even backward—a certain level of vertical velocity must exist to elevate the body's center of gravity upward and enable a takeoff. The combination of upward and forward velocity creates a launch angle. The launch angle of your jump also plays an important part in determining both your trajectory and how much power or momentum you need.

For instance, if you're standing still on both feet and want to use a Power Jump (commonly known as a broad jump) to travel the maximum horizontal distance you can, then a 45-degree forward angle is the best (see the nearby Note), along with the maximum power output your muscles can generate.

You can lean forward only so far at launching; beyond a certain lean angle, you're guaranteed to land in a Front Sprawl or Front Roll instead of landing on your feet. But if you want to use the exact same jumping technique and pattern vertically to reach as high as you can above where you stand, then you don't want to lean forward at all and your launch angle is zero-degree (but you still want maximum power output).

NOTE

For a similar amount of power generated, a launch angle between roughly 40 and 50 degrees results in about 90 percent of the maximum horizontal distance traveled, with a 45-degree angle resulting in maximal distance.

You can create vertical and horizontal velocity from a static position by muscular power alone, but if horizontal velocity precedes the jump, such as when you run before the launch, then part of the horizontal velocity must be turned into vertical velocity to reach a greater distance.

The angle at which you launch a jump and the power and velocity you use to take off determine the height and distance you cover during the trajectory. On the other hand, it's the trajectory necessary for the most efficient landing that dictates how much power you need to generate, how much velocity you want to transfer, and what angle you want to use. Last, but not least, the instability or slipperiness of the launching surface (or making a bad step when moving) can rob enormous power during the launch or make you lose balance, which renders the jump completely ineffective even in the presence of great velocity and power. At best it makes the jump much less efficient and challenges both the intended trajectory, the body position during the trajectory, and the landing.

The Trajectory

Once the launching is done, the takeoff occurs, which means you no longer have any points of support and initiate the airborne phase or "hang time." While airborne, all your attention should be focused on optimally preparing for the landing. How you jump determines your "flight path" or airborne trajectory.

As I previously mentioned, once you've launched the jump, there is nothing you can do to alter the speed, distance, and duration of your trajectory unless you can push off a solid surface before landing, as when you vault. During the airborne phase, you can modify only your position. This is tremendously important to understand: The launching is entirely responsible for the trajectory that your body will follow and your speed, which in turn determines where and when you land. However, how you position your body during the "flight" also plays a part in how you land based on the surface where you land and/or the movement you want to immediately transition to upon landing. For instance, in a Downward Jump, you may want to be upright before you land on your feet to a balanced stand, or you might want to lean forward while airborne to facilitate a smooth transition to a Front Roll when you land. You might position your feet in a square fashion for a Square Landing or in a

staggered manner for an "in-line" landing. You might fully extend your body upward to reach out with your arms and land in a hanging position. Depending on the context, you might have several options for how you land and consequently how you position your body while airborne, or you might have no options.

It's often said that a jumping trajectory follows a parabolic path, which is mostly true when the launching and landing surfaces are horizontally leveled. Otherwise, the trajectory of a jump is, in most cases, curved—remember that the body must be propelled both forward and upward to elevate the body's center of gravity and reach a greater distance—but not necessarily parabolic.

NOTE

A *parabola* is a mirror-symmetrical curve.

How deep and far or how high and far you need to reach while jumping creates a variety of ratios that change the shape of your flight path. If you're jumping down and away from where you're launching the jump, you have a depth-distance ratio; you're traveling down and forward. You may jump down a little depth and try to jump as far forward as you can, or conversely you may jump down a deep distance without trying to reach forward by much.

If you're jumping up and away from where you're launching the jump, you have a height-distance ratio; you're traveling upward and forward. You may have to jump nearly vertically to reach a high-elevated surface by launching the jump from close to the bottom of the obstacle, or you might bridge a broad gap while having to land just slightly higher than where you're launching the jump from.

Other possibilities involve a certain distance-height-distance ratio, which occurs when you're jumping over an elevated surface at a distance or want to touch something elevated with your hand(s) that is both above and away from you, before landing at a certain distance. In these cases, you create a certain elevation of your trajectory to reach high enough, and that's greater than if you only had a horizontal distance to cover. If the landing surface also was below the launching one you'd have a distance-height-depth-distance ratio.

Consequently, your airborne trajectory always presents a curve (except for a purely linear, vertical trajectory in the case of a downward jump launched from a motionless hang or a strictly vertical upward jump), but it won't necessarily be "mirror symmetrical." Even when you're taking off from an elevated surface to jump down or you're jumping up to an elevated surface, your trajectory won't be strictly linear, but it will be far from a symmetrical curve that resembles a parabola. This is another reason why you must absolutely consider these ratios of distance, height, and depth, as well as what the landing should be like, to give you a sense of what the shape of your airborne path should be even before takeoff.

To summarize, the following are true at equal launching power and velocity:

- When the takeoff and landing height are at the same horizontal level, the time between the takeoff and the *peak* of your trajectory (the highest vertical point it reaches) is identical to the time between the peak and the landing. The trajectory is parabolic.

- When the takeoff height is higher than the landing height, the overall airborne time and distance are greater (than when the takeoff and landing height are at the same horizontal level), with the time and distance between the peak and the landing greater than between the takeoff and peak. At equal power and/or velocity employed in a jump, a jump launched from an elevation and landing lower than the launching surface will travel a distance greater than when the takeoff and landing height are at the same horizontal level.

- When the takeoff height is lower than the landing height, the overall airborne time and distance are shorter (than when the takeoff and landing height are at the same horizontal level), with the time and distance between the takeoff and peak greater than between the peak and landing.

AIRBORNE MANEUVERS

Cats are famous for their ability to land on their feet even after falling upside down. This airborne balance reflex is known as *air-righting reaction*, and it can be trained for both intentional movements, such as jumps, and involuntary movements, such as falls. Although you cannot change the direction and speed of your trajectory, you can maneuver your body to modify its position and orientation while you're airborne by moving your arms, head, hips, or legs. A simple example is to horizontally spin in the air while maintaining a vertical position so that you land standing but oriented facing a direction different than when you jumped. Many other maneuvers are possible, ranging from simple and practical to complex and acrobatic.

The Landing

The landing happens when you reconnect with a surface of support. Although it's the last part of a jump, it's the most important. Anyone can launch a jump with power, but not everyone is competent in regaining balance safely upon landing. The launching and positional control during the airborne phase create the best conditions for avoiding collision and landing efficiency, but the landing still can be inefficient. Knowing that, in Natural Movement, very few jumps will conveniently land in a soft sandpit, the efficiency of your landing is paramount. It doesn't matter how powerful, technical, or stylish the launching was if it results in an unnecessarily hard landing or leads to a fall and injury. No jump is good if the landing is bad. It's ultimately the quality of the landing that separates the skilled jumper from the unskilled one. How confident you are in your landing is what makes the very brief, "weightless," airborne phase a moment of either pure bliss or pure fear.

> **NOTE**
>
> A collision is an uncontrolled landing with no positional control and very little or no dissipation of impact forces. Most of the time, a collision is damaging to the body.

While the launching precedes the landing, and in most cases plays a significant influence in the landing's efficiency, it's how you expect to land that has the most influence on how you launch the jump. In short, landing should not be dictated by how you launch the jump; how you launch the jump should be dictated by how you intend to land. Unless you're going to rebound into another jump upon landing, landings are always "skill-to-skill" transitions from jumping to another position or a movement. The moment you reconnect to a firm surface, you're exiting the airborne phase to be on a support again, which means you're both exiting jumping and entering another type of position or movement.

The type of landing you use has a lot to do with the surface where you land, your technical ability, the level of impact forces, and the kind of movement you have to transition to upon landing. As always, the context is a big factor in determining landing, and there's an enormous difference in the following situations:

- Landing in a stand on a stable, wide area when the launching and landing surfaces are horizontally level
- Landing in a Dive Roll after a jump involving depth-distance and preceded by a run
- Landing balanced on a narrow and unstable surface after a vertical jump
- Landing on your feet and hanging by your hands on a wall after a depth-distance trajectory
- Landing hanging from your hands after a distance-height trajectory

Another example is that although it's best to land on the foot opposite the one you used for launching or to land on two feet, you might have to hop and land on the same foot and leg you used for launching to make a particular landing effective or to ensure a transition to stepping in a particular direction.

How much impact forces have to be dissipated when you land is a factor of several variables, including the following:

- Your own body weight plus additional weight you're carrying with you.
- The trajectory's velocity.
- The trajectory's direction. The more upward you travel, the less the force of impact. Jumping from a greater height and going more downward increases the impact forces.
- The position or movement upon landing in relation to the landing surface.
- The firmness or softness of the landing surface as well as the type of footwear you're wearing (if you're not barefoot).
- The stability or instability of the landing surface.

How well you handle such impact forces has to do with all the listed variables as well as your technique, physical condition, specific training, and physical state when you land. The biological structures of your body—muscles and tendons and, to a lesser extent, ligaments, bones, and cartilage—possess properties for the storage and release of energy but also for its dissipation, which participate in absorbing impact forces upon landing. All other conditions being equal, how conditioned your tissues are to handle such levels of energy dissipation makes a very important difference in your ability to land efficiently.

Another element that plays a role in efficient landing is the "neurogenic effect," which is the brain's ability to anticipate the shock of impact and fire the muscles responsible for the dissipation of impact forces. Multiple variables play a role in assessing the impact, including the distance, depth, height, and speed of the airborne phase, the body position upon landing, the hardness of the landing surface or of your footwear, and the external weight you're carrying. In other words, with practice your reflexes upon landing are both faster and more accurate at responding to the impact and make your landings more efficient, smoother, and more graceful, which is ideally what all landings should have in common.

Landing should be as light and stable (and even as silent) as possible, and, of course, you want all landings to be safe. Depending on the context, even the most skilled and seasoned natural mover doesn't always land well. However, with consistent, technical, mindful practice that combines diverse ways of launching jumps, trajectories, and landing surfaces and strategies, anyone can vastly improve landing ability.

Putting *It* All Together

Regardless of how much power you possess, learning to use the right jumping technique at the right launch angle with the right amount of kinetic energy—whether from muscular power alone or a combination of power and velocity—in the appropriate way for the context (the type of launching surface, airborne trajectory, landing surface, and follow-up movement transition) is important to your jumping competency.

Your jumping ability can't be learned through mental analysis or mathematical calculations. It's developed by accumulating experience with a great variety of jumping patterns that launch from different surfaces, use different trajectories, and end with a landing on different surfaces. By practicing in many different situations, you'll develop a quick eye that enables you to assess the situation and jump and land in the most efficient way possible without actively thinking about it. (That said, it's a good idea to take your time before jumping whenever possible.)

So, if you ever thought that a single jumping pattern done on a single surface—such as jumping to and from a wooden box without much regard for technique—would prepare you for any of the limitless combination of variables, you're unfortunately quite mistaken. You're in no way prepared for any kind of launching and landing, and your sense of jumping competency is at best completely flawed. You have become adapted to doing many repetitions in a row of a specific, limited jumping and landing pattern, which isn't applicable to any form of real-life jumping and landing pattern. What will happen if you have to perform a single jump that's different from the way you've trained, especially if you know that you have only one shot at it? If you now understand this major difference in approach, I advise that you seriously reconsider the SAID principle (refer to principle 7, "Adaptable") and immediately prepare to expand your jumping competency, starting with landing skills.

Once you have established fundamental techniques, keep expanding your jumping adaptability by exploring many combinations of launching, trajectories, and landings. You can launch from sitting, hanging, crawling, balancing, or in any awkward fashion. You can create variation in trajectory direction and body orientation while airborne. You can alternate landing patterns and surfaces. In addition, you could practice skill-mixes, such as carrying something as you jump or throwing or catching something while you're airborne. A whole world of Natural Movement possibilities awaits!

Landing Techniques

It makes lots of sense to address essential landing patterns before shifting the focus to how to launch jumps. Too often in physical training the emphasis lies on the intensity of the jump, how far or high one can jump, and how to strengthen to develop more power to jump farther and higher, whereas landing is taken for granted and is usually done on a flat and stable surface without variability. Neglecting landing mechanics can create quite an issue because, if you can't do it soundly, chances are that you'll end up strained, in pain, or injured.

In this section, I cover several fundamental landing strategies: the Two-Step Square Landing, the Two-Step Split Landing, the Extended Two-Step Split

Landing, the Square Landing, and the Foot-to-Hand Landing. Previously I described another important landing strategy—the Dive Roll—in Chapter 24, "Ground Movement 1." The Back Roll also can be useful with downward trajectories when your body is oriented backward. I also address strategies to handle higher levels of impact forces, such as with downward trajectories (or Downward Jumps).

Greater environmental complexity, such as landing on uneven or smaller surfaces, as well as particular skill-to-skill transitions—such as jumping to balancing or jumping to climbing—create specific landing demands that are beyond the scope of this book (although I do address the landing from Power Jump to climb up position later in this section).

Landing progressions—in terms of intensity (distance, height, depth), environmental complexity (wide/narrow, stable/unstable, even/uneven, flat/angled, soft/firm), and movement complexity (simple or complex technique)—must be approached carefully, gradually, and as a safely as possible after you've acquired enough competence with fundamental launching and landing techniques. Once you've acquired such fundamental landing competency, you need to expand your landing ability and repertoire by practicing the following progressions:

- Increasing the intensity of the landing with greater impact forces by increasing the intensity of the jump launching (aiming at and reaching greater distance, height or depth, or a combination of those, by adding power and/or velocity).
- Increasing the technicality of the launching, which might challenge the trajectory and consequently the landing.
- Increasing the complexity of the landing surface(s), which demands impeccable launching to ensure impeccable positional control during the trajectory.
- Improving your ability to combine and switch between varied launchings, trajectories, and landings, at diverse levels of launching intensity and landing intensity and complexity.

Let me give you an example with some of the progressions listed above applied to the Split Jump technique:

- Distance Standing Split Jump: Increase intensity to reach greater distance.
- Distance Standing Split Jump to Balancing Landing on a 2x4 board: Increase complexity by making the landing surface more challenging.
- Distance Standing Split Jump to Balancing Landing on a narrow and rounded surface: Increase complexity by making the landing surface more challenging.
- Distance-Depth Standing Split Jump to Balancing Landing on a 2x4 board: Increase intensity by adding depth to distance and increasing complexity by making the landing surface more challenging.
- Three-Step Distance-Depth Split Jump to Balancing Landing on a 2x4 board: Increase the intensity of the preceding jump by adding velocity to the launching, which adds intensity to the launching and landing.
- Distance-Depth Running Split Jump to Dive Roll: Increase the intensity of the jump by adding significant velocity and intensity to the launching and significant intensity and movement complexity upon landing.

I could provide many other examples that combine all three phases of the jump at diverse levels of intensity and complexity. Where you choose to practice and how you choose to practice—in terms of the intensity, volume, complexity, and frequency—affects the specificity of programming progressions while managing safety. It boils down to individual objectives, personal ability, and response to training.

Leg Swing Jump to Two-Step Square Landing

With this combination, you're going to conveniently learn both a simple, low-intensity jumping technique and a landing technique that are a perfect match for each other (and they're a perfect point of entry to jumping and landing techniques for the beginner natural mover). Practicing the Tiptoeing and Single-Leg balancing movements will greatly help your stability when you're standing on a single foot and swinging your leg. That practice also will help your efficiency upon landing.

The Leg Swing Jump is a technique done from a standing position that relies equally on power from a single supporting leg and body-weight transfer generated from the swing action of the other leg. It's useful for short distances when you'd have to step out too far or it's too risky to step out; it helps you generate additional distance with the most accurate level of kinetic energy to ensure a smooth, light, and/or accurate landing. It's perfectly combined with the Two-Step Square Landing for maximum lightness and accuracy upon landing, especially on small, narrow, or unstable landing surfaces, which makes it a great option when you're landing in a balancing fashion. Of course, the Leg Swing Jump is not necessarily always followed by a Two-Step Square Landing, just as the Two-Step Square Landing can be preceded by any kind of jumping launch.

The Leg Swing Jump is a form of *leaping*, as you launch from one foot and land on the other foot, even though the trail foot immediately lands next to the front foot. Once you're reaching the maximum distance that can be produced with this technique, you'll find it very difficult to land in any other way than two-footed, which makes the jump an *assemble jump* (in which you launch from one foot and land on

two feet). So, this technique is similar to (but not exactly like) a Stride Jump in which the trail leg travels forward upon landing instead of landing next to the front foot.

The Leg Swing Jump uses the momentum created by the free leg swinging forward as much as the power of the supporting leg, which enables you to reach a greater distance—or to use less energy to reach an equal distance—than if you push off a single leg. The distance gained is not enormous (because power is always the primary generator of distance); however, you can gain a solid foot of extra distance if you do the technique with enough velocity and amplitude when swinging the free leg.

Another significant advantage of the Leg Swing Jump compared to pushing off a single leg from a standing position is that you don't need to lean forward as much to launch your jump and reach maximum distance, which allows you to decrease the launch lean and conserve a more erect position and better control of your landing. If you lean forward a lot to generate distance, you might end up landing on a single foot as in *striding*, and the landing of the trail foot is delayed, which makes the landing heavier and less balanced.

To start giving you a sense of relevance of using the Leg Swing Jump technique in relation to distance, you want to first draw a line on the ground or floor as a starting point.

While standing on a single-leg with the toes of your supporting foot placed just before that line, see how far you can step out in a controlled and safe manner (which means that you're able to push off the front foot to a standing position). Immediately beyond that distance starts your leg swing "zone."

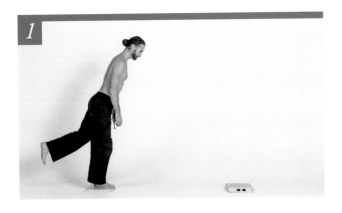

1   Stand straight or slightly lean forward, as your body reflects your intention to move forward and cross a gap. Get a mental sense of how much energy you need to generate to be able to reach the landing surface without pushing too hard or landing heavily. Shift your body weight to a single foot, bend your knee slightly, and pull the other leg behind your body as your upper body leans forward with a slight bend at the hip. Maintain a straight posture,

keep your arms relaxed, and look at your landing target. Your neck may very slightly extend forward for better visual input, but you should never stretch it forward in a "head-chasing" fashion.

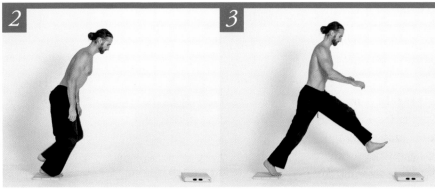

2   Load your supporting leg by bending more at the knee and swiftly start swinging your trail leg forward in the direction of your landing surface to generate and transfer momentum to your whole body.

3   As your trail leg passes to the front of your supporting leg and extends forward, strongly push off your supporting foot and leg. Look at where

your front foot is going to land. Your arms should stay to the front of your body; they might have a very gentle swing motion, but they shouldn't have highly active movement in any direction.

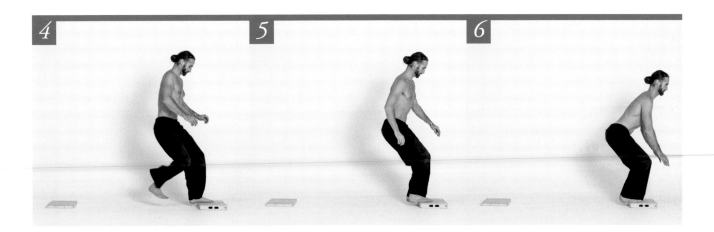

4   While you're airborne, rapidly pull your trail leg toward your front leg. Your front foot should land less than a second before your trail foot. You should feel a "tap-tap" vibration and rhythm in your feet as both feet land nearly simultaneously.

5   The landing of both feet takes place on the ball of your foot first, then your heels lower to a square, horizontal foot position if there is enough space for your heels to be supported by the landing surface. If the landing surface is big enough, always allow both feet to come flat after landing on the balls of your feet because it makes for a smoother landing and greater stability. As you land, bend your knees and hinge slightly at the hip to disperse impact forces, but make sure to keep a tall back.

6   If needed, you may ensure a stable landing by bending your legs a bit more to stabilize your body fully before you stand up. For the purpose of practice, don't immediately step off the landing surface. Instead, come back to a fully erect standing position for a few seconds. This way you can assess whether you really have the ability to regain perfect balance upon landing.

Regressions

If the knee of your supporting leg is unstable, and you lack overall stability when swinging the free leg, you may limit the movement to the single-leg stand and swinging the free leg back and forth. First use just a little speed and amplitude so you can ensure positional control. Increase the speed and the amplitude of the leg swing while maintaining positional control until you feel ready to jump and land.

Progressions

First develop sufficient control and efficiency by working at ground level and jumping short distances (shorter than three feet). From there, progressively increase the distance. When you've reached the maximum distance you can reach with this technique, you shouldn't try to modify your form and push to greater distances, as more powerful jumping techniques are available for greater distances. You can increase complexity by working with different elevations and narrower, uneven, or unstable surfaces. You also can land in an in-line fashion or practice the Leg Swing Jump sideways.

Square Landing

Because most jumps are launched and landed from a standing position, the Square Landing pattern is one of the most frequently used, and you should fully master it. It's a preferred landing pattern when you have to stabilize to a standing position—for instance, when you're landing on a relatively narrow surface and are at risk of falling off it, such as when you land on a rock surrounded by water, the ledge of a wall, or a fallen tree trunk. Choosing this option means that another landing option is not available, a fast transition to another movement or position is not necessary, or a transition is too risky to be done without establishing standing balance first.

The pattern of the Square Landing blends impeccable sequence and timing with great positional control and eccentric contraction power. Indeed, you will land standing on both feet simultaneously and bend your legs in a squatting fashion, which stretches your leg muscles and disperses impact forces through only your own power. Depending on the intensity of the jump—say you launched a Power Jump with maximum power output or used a fast run-up in the case of a Split Jump—the distance and speed of the trajectory might demand great eccentric power to be landed in this fashion. If depth is added to distance and speed,

the eccentric power required to land might reach a level where you might have to choose landing alternatives—such as the Dive Roll—that help disperse greater impact forces. However, when you jump upward to land on surfaces more elevated than the launching surface, the amount of impact force to be dispersed is less, which makes the landing less energy-costly and lighter.

Doing the Square Landing efficiently is more demanding than it looks, and it requires great motor control. Although eccentric strength is required from your legs and lower body, the landing doesn't rely only on leg flexion; it also requires hip hinging to deflect impact force.

I find it convenient to break the landing down into separate drills to ensure the progressive and effective acquisition of the right positional control, sequence, and timing. Don't underestimate the value of these progressions. If you can't perform such simple movement drills efficiently at low intensity, what do you think will happen when you attempt more difficult jumps? Your landing will likely look and feel horrible. Trust the process of progressive skill acquisition, and don't skip elementary steps because you're overconfident.

TECHNIQUE TIP

Find a piece of board that is thin and flat, about 2x1 feet. You can also tape a box on the floor, draw one in the dirt, or even make a simple straight line with a piece of tape. You can practice without this confined surface, but using a restricted area for launching and landing helps you assess your balance and accuracy.

You simply can't learn to land well if you can't Hip Hinge and Squat well.

Square Landing Drill 1

This first drill doesn't involve an actual landing because your body is always grounded. However, its value relies on the swift elevation and lowering of your heels and the swift squatting-down motion, which have the potential to throw your balance off at first. This drill helps you start to get a feel of the deceleration and eccentric tension required in your lower body, starting in the feet, to prevent your rear from reaching your calves before your knees must absorb the impact, and it helps you have positional control despite the dynamic movement. You may practice this drill slowly first; then do it as dynamically as you can.

NOTE

Though it makes landing harder and stiffer, landing with flat feet isn't going to make you fail your landing because 2 to 3 inches of ankle flexion alone aren't responsible for the bulk of the deceleration necessary for an effective Square Landing.

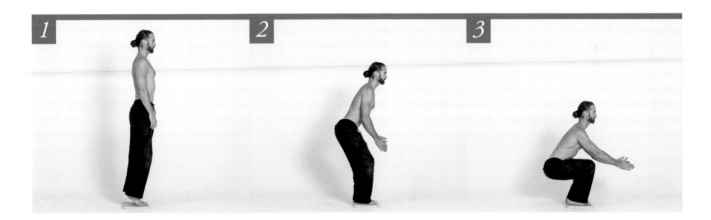

1   Assume a tall, relaxed, focused standing position, and then swiftly elevate your heels while maintaining your tall posture and balance. Keep your arms relaxed on each side of your body.

2   Swiftly bring your heels down as you move your arms forward, hinge at hip level, and start flexing your legs. Enter a squatting movement the moment you feel that your heels are on the ground.

3   Keep moving your arms forward as you lower your center of gravity to a Half-Squat position with your legs bent at a 90-degree angle and your rear horizontally aligned with your knees, or slightly below. The moment your arms stop moving coincides with the moment you've reached your deepest position. A slight extension of your neck is not an issue at all; it's better than looking down or letting your head slightly lean down, which holds the potential to make you go off balance forward. Mark a one- or two-second pause before you stand up and repeat the sequence.

Square Landing Drill 2

In this drill, you add a short vertical jump, but you're keeping it low impact and focused on efficiency. The point here is twofold:

- The launching must be controlled so the landing is accurate and stable. If you're off balance in any direction upon landing, it's very likely that your launching is the culprit;
- You're now dealing with an actual landing and need to disperse greater impact forces while you maintain positional control and balance.

TECHNIQUE TIP

The reason for swinging your arms forward might not be apparent to you at this low-intensity stage, but it helps both with dispersing impact forces and stabilizing your body. If you try to do the same drill while keeping your arms in a set position from launching to landing, you should feel a difference. Rest assured that once you are jumping far forward and dealing with greater impact forces, you'll want to use your arms to facilitate a smoother landing rather than keeping them in a set position.

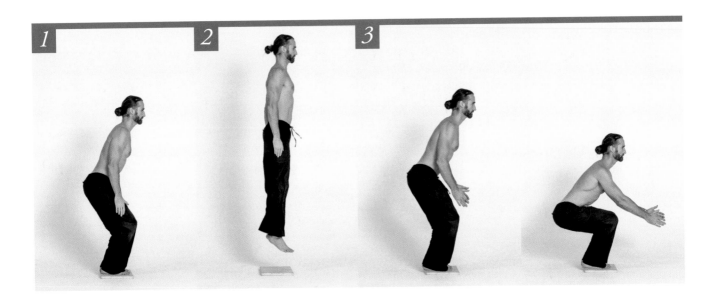

1   Assume a tall, relaxed, focused standing position. Bend your knees, slightly Hip Hinge, and load your legs so you're ready to jump up. Keep your arms down and relaxed.

2   Jump 1 to 2 inches high at first; don't go higher than that. While launching and while airborne, keep your whole body vertically aligned and your arms relaxed. Any angle during the launch causes you to land in the same direction of the angle. Look straight ahead and refrain from looking down. Extend your ankles to present the balls of your feet toward the landing surface.

3   Your extended ankles enable you to land on the balls of your feet first and give you full range of motion at the ankles to start decelerating the body. This part is like the previous drill except that you're connecting to the ground from an airborne position. Paying attention to the moment the balls of your feet connect with the ground is essential to have the best timing with this sequence. For practice purposes, don't immediately step off the landing surface, but come back to a fully erect standing position for a moment. This way you can assess whether you regained perfect balance. Imagine that

you're landing within an environment that would not allow you to hold on to anything to secure your position and where stepping off the landing surface would mean falling from a great height.

Faults

Look at the photos below. You may identify some of your own issues. If you're not sure, maybe you could film yourself to get a visual evidence of your current form. You might discover elements of inefficiency you did not even suspect you're doing. Again, remember that unless inefficiencies are addressed at this stage, increased intensity or complexity will only magnify the issues rather than fixing them.

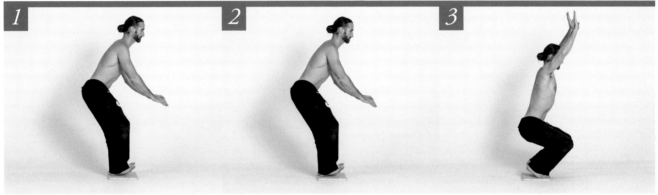

(continued on next page)

1   Landing on your heels first, which makes landing heavy and hard. Don't bypass the balls of your feet if you want a soft landing. Landing with your feet flat is better but still not as good as landing on the balls of your feet.

2   Landing on the balls of your feet without allowing your heels to come down. This makes for a potentially harder and less stable landing for two reasons: letting your heels come down to the ground contributes to deceleration, and you're more stable with your feet flat on the surface (when the landing surface is big enough, of course) than when you tiptoe.

3   Like photo 2, only you try to counterbalance with your arms. Instead, let your heels reach the ground and relax your arms.

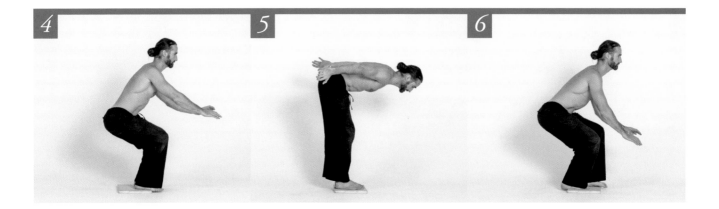

4   Off target. Check out the perfect verticality of the launching and body position during the airborne phase.

5   Leaning forward during launching or while airborne—perhaps because you tried to look down before landing—and attempting to correct it upon landing, which isn't possible. Your feet might land on target, but you're pushed forward and must step out and forward.

6   Landing with staggered feet, either because you didn't keep your feet assembled or you let your body rotate while airborne. Keep your legs assembled and your body's orientation forward while airborne, and keep your feet square upon landing.

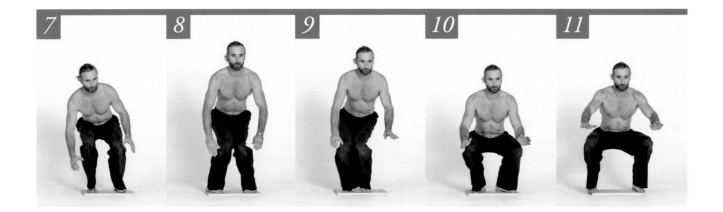

7   Off balance sideways. You leaned sideways during launching, while airborne, or upon landing (or all of that).

8   Knees cave in (knock-knees) upon landing, which generates a very weak position that might hurt your knees.

9   Like the preceding issue in terms of being a positional control issue except both knees move in the same direction.

10 Externally rotating your flexed legs to try to prevent your knees from caving in, which is not a strong landing position.

11 Using a too-wide stand. A wider stance makes you feel more stable, but it also reduces your range of motion and the depth of your squat, so when intensity goes up you feel very stiff when landing as more deceleration and dispersion of impact forces have to be achieved with less range of motion.

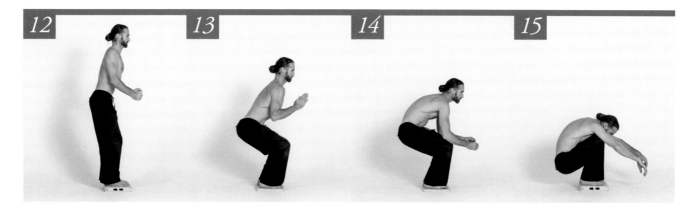

12 Lack of flexion at knee level, which makes the landing hard, heavy, and likely to be unstable.

13 Overall stiffness upon landing that's visible in the tension in the arms. Perhaps your arms were already in the front of your body before the landing, and maybe you were holding your breath as well.

14 Not lowering your center of gravity enough and rounding your back.

15 Lack of tension or delayed reaction upon landing, which leads to a "collapsed" position upon landing with the potential of hurting your knees.

If you encounter any of these issues (or more), reset your movement and position pattern by reverting to lower intensity. Make sure that you're barely taking off the ground at first and add height to your jump only if all aspects of efficiency are present at low intensity.

If all is going well (sequence, timing, balance, positional control, relaxation), then start adding more power to your jump. The higher you reach, the more time you spend airborne and the more challenging it gets to maintain balance while airborne. Also, it becomes more challenging to land in a balanced manner while conserving positional control. Always aim at the height that you can handle upon landing rather than going for the maximum height that you can jump.

Progressions

Progressions for becoming better at the Square Landing involve intensity with greater distance, which can be created with jumping techniques that can create broad distances, such as the Power Jump or the Stepping Split Jump. You can increase intensity when using the Square Landing after a downward trajectory, as you will see later when I discuss the Downward Jump. The same effect can be reproduced to some extent by jumping as high as possible on the spot. You can combine distance and depth to make it as challenging as possible. Last, you can add complexity with uneven, unstable, or smaller landing surfaces. Conversely, the Square Landing is made easier when reaching an elevated surface is the goal; significantly lower impact forces are involved in landing to an elevated surface when launching takes place below the landing surface, and you may land with your arms already to the front of your body.

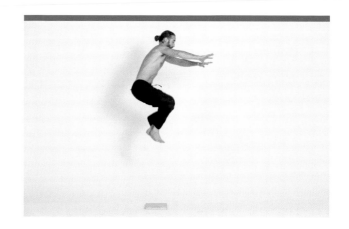

NOTE

An increase in hardness of the landing surface is most noticeable after a Downward Jump. Also, a reduction in friction levels of the landing surface affects forward jumps the most.

Precision Square Landing

One of the major variations and progressions that you need to learn and practice is the Precision Square Landing, which is when you land standing on both feet on a surface that's too small for the entire surface of your feet to come flat, such as on the edge of a rock, wall, or tree branch. There is a small yet essential technical detail here that makes landing on the edge safer. Because you land on a small surface with not even half of the surface of your foot, you're dealing with two main risks. First, if you come a bit short and land on your toes, you won't have the support you need to land, and your feet will slide down, which causes you to fall forward. Second, if you land a little too far back (on your midfoot or heel), and the surface is short (such as the edge of a wall), there might be too little friction to decelerate your feet, which causes your feet to slide forward and your body to fall backward. Even if you land with your feet right where they need to be but on a low-friction landing surface or with a low-friction footwear, the risk of forward slippage of your feet followed by a fall is high.

Immediately after your forefoot lands on the edge, you need to use ankle flexion the same way you do when you land on a bigger surface. The difference is that on the smaller surface you let your ankles flex so your heels go below the level of the surface of support, which enables your midfoot to act as a brake to the forward momentum and prevents slippage.

You also want to consider the two following risks:

- When the distance before landing is far and the trajectory goes downward, the risk of ankle hyperflexion is real. It causes pain in the front part of the ankle (the ankle crease with the upper foot). You want to strengthen your feet and ankles for this kind of landing by progressively increasing the intensity. Ankle hyperflexion can even make you bounce off and miss the landing so you fall.
- The risk of ankle sprain is much higher if you land on the edge of a surface that is unstable and can flip under your feet.

Downward Jumps

Downward Jumps are often referred to as Depth Jumps or Drop Jumps. Those terms are fine, too, but they indicate only that a jump follows a downward trajectory and no more. Indeed, you can enter a "Depth Jump" or jump downward in different ways, such as by stepping out, running, performing a Power Jump, pushing off your hands from a sit, sliding down a slope, sliding off a cliff that ends in the void, or releasing your grip from a Dead Hang or hanging swing. A downward trajectory can be intentional but totally reckless, or it can be an actual fall that leads to lethal consequences from which no landing technique or training could save you.

You can use several landing strategies, such as Square Landing, Split Landing, Foot-to-Hand Landing, and Dive Roll. You could go into water either feet or head first. You also could land in a Double-Hand Hang or a Foot-Hand Hang position; these types of landings normally follow a Downward Jump that's launched from a position opposite to the direction where you're jumping. With all the possible ways a downward trajectory can start and end, there are a lot of possible combinations. Which one is *the* Depth Jump? Clearly there is not a single Depth Jump—just many variations of it. "Depth Jump" doesn't describe a technique; it describes a downward trajectory that can use diverse launching and landing strategies.

In the absence of the necessity to cover horizontal distance, downward trajectories require close to no strength to launch. A simple step forward, and you're airborne and descending. Once you're airborne, if the vertical distance before landing is sufficient, your speed continues accelerating until it reaches "terminal velocity," which is the highest speed attainable by an object falling through air: about 122 miles per hour or 54 meters per second. Such speed is attained in

15 seconds, and I hope you never reach it unless you are equipped with a parachute and have enough time and height to open it to decelerate fully before contacting the earth again. You reach *half* that speed after only 3 seconds in the air. The airborne duration of a jump from a height of 2 meters is only 0.6 second, and only 0.9 second from 4 meters because velocity increases exponentially with height, which explains why a fall from 100 meters of elevation lasts only 4.5 seconds before you land.

The speed of your body falling and the acceleration rate are not affected by your mass (body weight), so a heavy person doesn't fall more rapidly than a lighter one. However, the greater the height from which you jump and the heavier you are, the higher the energy at impact (or the greater the impact forces upon landing). For example, jumping from a height of 2 meters generates twice the impact forces of jumping from 1 meter, and a person who weighs 200 pounds will have to handle twice the impact forces compared to a person who weighs 100 pounds. Although it might take little effort to initiate a big drop, the forces necessary to dissipate impact forces can become rapidly enormous. Obviously, jumping from heights must be taken very seriously.

When you jump from this height...	Your speed at impact is...
5 feet	12 miles per hour
10 feet	17 miles per hour
15 feet	21 miles per hour
20 feet	24 miles per hour
25 feet	27 miles per hour
30 feet	30 miles per hour

As long as you jump from a sustainable height (that is, one that won't kill you) and you are sufficiently healthy and functional, how well you handle the dispersion of impact forces when landing vertically on your feet in a Square Landing relates mostly to your strength with eccentric contractions and your body mass index. Being overweight clearly doesn't help, but even someone who's not overweight will suffer

if untrained to this specific kind of physical demand and response compared to someone who might be a little overweight but who is specifically trained for such landings. The only variables that might decrease impact forces are the softness of the landing surface and of your footwear (if you wear any). In any case, it's just best to learn to handle impact forces through technique and physical conditioning rather than moonboots and crash pads

If you don't land correctly, even diving in water will feel like you're diving into concrete. With practice, it becomes easier to anticipate how much impact forces you will have to handle for a given height, even though it's always a better mindset to anticipate greater impact forces upon landing than to underestimate them.

Downward Jump to Square Landing

A Downward Jump that lands in a Square Landing is what is commonly considered *the* Depth Jump. The most typical way is to launch forward, but you also can launch sideways and even backward before the path turns downward. It's a convenient strategy when the height from which it's launched isn't high, and it becomes a costly but fast strategy when climbing down a relatively high surface or finding an alternative route would take too long; sometimes it's just faster and simpler to use gravity to travel downward fast.

Unless you must go fast or must clear horizontal distance in addition to going down, you normally want to reduce your speed as much as possible before you jump down to reduce forward momentum and impact forces upon landing. If you're standing still, you use just enough kinetic energy to step in the void, so there's no need to swing your arms forward. If you need or want to reduce impact forces a little more, you may even do a Deep Knee Bend first so that your center of gravity is closer to the ground compared to a standing launch. While in a Deep Knee Bend, you could even drive your hips forward to bring your knees forward and downward before you launch the jump, which makes the landing a little bit softer. However, with greater heights, these minor strategies become less relevant.

The vertical downward trajectory combined with a Square Landing is a phenomenal way to develop eccentric power in your legs and lower body. (Also, developing greater lower-body strength, such as through heavy loaded squats, supports a better ability to dissipate impact forces.) Part of the benefit to strength is because such practice shocks and excites muscles, which makes eccentric contraction (and even plyometric contractions, if you bounce off after absorbing the impact) much faster and more reflexive.

However, the Square Landing after a downward trajectory involves significant eccentric-contraction effort, which stresses your muscles and joints. It's not recommended that you train downward jumps too frequently, unless you employ techniques such as the Dive Roll. I also don't recommend high volumes (more than ten to twenty repetitions), but how sustainable a given volume is depends on many variables beyond height. Trained natural movers can handle many repetitions if they train for this specific type of endurance.

Knowing what depth a beginner can handle requires safe trial and error "from the bottom up." The best progression is to step on top of a surface that's 1 foot high, jump, land, and assess form and sensations before you carefully and progressively increase the height (and consequently the depth of your jump). If you don't want to measure the height you jump from, you can start with a height as tall as your knees, move to hip height, and then increase to chest height. The ability to land an efficient downward jump from a height that's equivalent to your shoulders or the top of your head is a good goal, though the depth you should be ultimately able to handle is a very individual consideration. Although you can train to land a Depth Jump from higher than your shoulder height, as height increases it becomes less and less sustainable to use the Square Landing, and you'll have to start using other landing strategies.

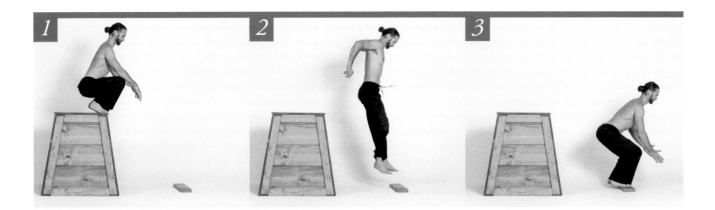

1   Start in a Deep Knee Bend on top of an object. Stand as close to the edge as possible. Fix your gaze on your landing target (if there is one).

2   Shift your weight forward and gently push off with your feet to create sufficient clearance without generating too much forward momentum. Immediately extend your legs with your feet pointing downward as you reach with your forefeet. In the photo, you'll notice my feet are horizontally slightly in front of my hips, and thus in front of my center of gravity; that's because a little forward distance is involved. Otherwise I would keep my feet straight under my center of gravity. Compared to a forward Square Landing, the downward

Square Landing requires an extremely fast muscular response, so while I'm airborne I'm highly focused on the "trigger signal," which is feeling my feet contact the ground. You may also keep looking down with your head up or slightly tilted forward, your chin in, and your eyes looking down.

3   The landing is like the Square Landing except that the levels and rate of force development of eccentric strength are much higher. If you're landing on a narrow surface where your heels cannot come flat to the ground, then the levels of foot strength and ankle stability required are also much higher.

Progressions

Beginners should start without a target and use low heights. However, once efficient technique has been established, using a target for landing precision provides an additional challenge and benefit for a similar amount of training time and energy. An interesting progression is to immediately bounce upward upon landing, which helps you develop great plyometric strength and is quite useful when you need to immediately bounce to a standing movement transition after landing rather than sticking in a balanced position.

Faults

Even from low heights, beginners tend to lack consistent positional control during the downward trajectory, which throws your balance off while you are airborne and results in faulty landing.

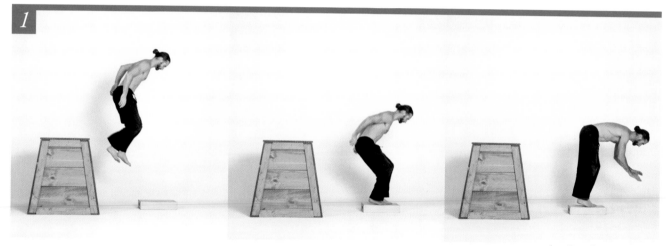

(continued on next page)

1   Leaning forward with your center of gravity forward of your feet. Beginners frequently do this when they lean forward with their heads down because they're trying too hard to look where they'll be landing, or they unnecessarily put too much forward power in the launch. You may save the landing with a Foot-to-Hand Landing if there's enough surface in front of you; otherwise, you fall off. Keep your center of gravity above your feet, or slightly to the back if there's a little forward distance. Spot your landing before launching; do not lean forward to look at your feet.

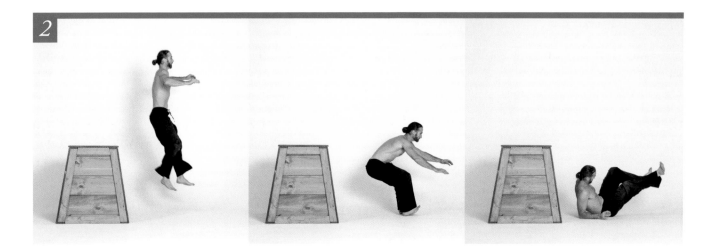

2 Leaning backward with your center of gravity behind your feet. In the absence of forward distance, leaning backward even slightly upon launching might result in landing off balance backward, potentially landing hard on your heels, your rear, your back, and sometimes your head. It also can make your rear travel all the way down, causing a full and hard knee flexion that is harmful to your knee joints. Keep your feet directly under your center of gravity from beginning to end. In the presence of forward distance along with the downward path, your feet should more or less extend to the front of the center of gravity, but not overly so.

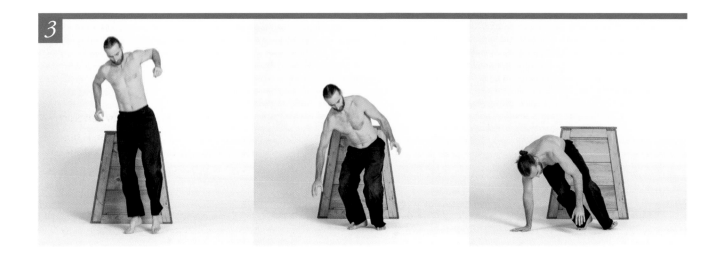

3 Leaning sideways with the center of gravity to the side of your feet. You will land harder on one foot and fall toward that side. Again, keep your feet directly under your center of gravity.

4 Keeping the knees in a slight flexion while airborne reduces the range of motion needed for optimal deceleration upon landing (not shown). You should keep your legs fully extended.

Foot-to-Hand Landing

The Foot-to-Hand Landing is a form of two-step landing in a quadrupedal fashion, even though you might be on all fours very briefly. This landing converts some of the downward momentum into forward momentum by enabling your feet and legs to absorb only part of the impact forces; you lean forward so that some of it can be distributed toward your arms and upper body.

The landing surface must be big enough to allow space for your hands to land to the front of your feet, of course. You use the Foot-to-Hand Landing when the Square Landing is not sustainable or is too energy-costly, if there's additional forward momentum upon launching, or if the intended transition upon landing is sprinting or crawling and the body position should be leaning forward to facilitate a quick transition.

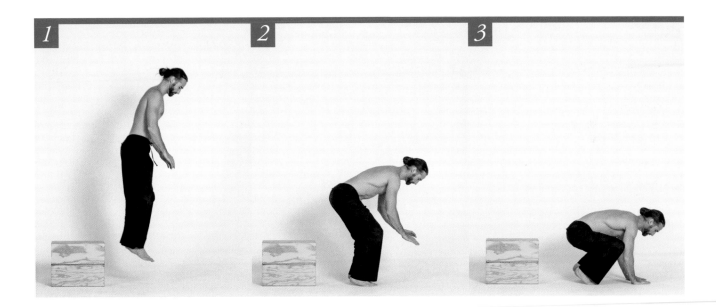

1 Begin in a relaxed stance on top of an object. Fix your gaze on your landing target. Step off the object with your torso leaning forward slightly. Keep your legs extended below your hips, and reach with the balls of your feet.

2 As your feet contact the ground, shift your center of gravity beyond your base of support to the front and start dispersing the impact by entering a Deep Knee Bend, bending at the hips with your torso leaning forward and your heels off the ground. Keep your hands to the front and look down at where your hands are going to land.

3 As your hands contact the ground, they should be vertically aligned with your shoulders. Keep your elbows inside your legs between your knees as you absorb the impact through your arms and upper body. Bending your arms may push your elbows out to help keep your knees out rather than going straight down. Your back is naturally slightly rounded. Depending on the transition, either stay low in a crawling position or immediately push off the ground with your hands to come back to a standing position or movement, using the elastic energy stored in your legs and arms upon landing.

Downward-Forward Trajectory

Sometimes with a downward trajectory, you might also want to travel forward a certain distance. You may use power, forward momentum, or a combination of both to achieve the additional distance. It's important to remember that the laws of physics enable the jumper to reach a greater forward distance when landing at a level below the height at which launching is done compared to a jump done with the same kinetic energy and the launching and landing occurring at the same horizontal level. Knowing this is important because the depth-distance ratio of your jump determines how you need to launch it, how much velocity you need, and at what angle you should take off.

For instance, if your maximum distance in a Forward Power Jump is 8 feet at ground level using maximum power, you know that if you jump from some elevation with an equal amount of power, you'll reach a greater distance, which implies that if you want to reach a distance of 8 feet from the same elevation, you need to use less than maximum power.

LANDING QUICK SUMMARY

Use the Square Landing as long as it is sustainable for you (you have the ability to handle impact forces in that manner) or if there is no ground in front of you to use for a Foot-to-Hand Landing or a Dive Roll.

Use the Two-Step Square Landing or Split Landing if the landing surface is narrow, small, or unstable or if you're not confident in a Square Landing.

Use the Foot-to-Hand Landing if the Square Landing is not sustainable for you or is too energy-costly. You also can use it if you have additional forward momentum upon launching or your transition move is sprinting or crawling. Of course, always make sure there's enough surface to the front to accommodate this type of landing.

Use the Dive Roll if you are launching the jump from a significant height or if there's a lot of forward velocity added to a downward trajectory. This is another landing that requires adequate ground distance in front of you.

Launching Techniques

This section covers the diverse techniques employed to travel greater airborne distances. First you learn how to generate power from standing positions. Second, you learn to convert forward momentum and combine it with power to create even greater levels of velocity.

Power Jump

For the Power Jump technique, you first must Hip Hinge and then powerfully "triple extend," which means you extend your hip, knees, and ankles. The triple-extension is a fundamental, powerful pattern employed in lifting techniques as well. Acquiring this pattern through power jumping supports learning the lifting techniques that use the same pattern, and the power gained through training this pattern in heavy lifting supports greater force production in jumping. It's a win-win combination. When you use the triple extension for jumping, all body segments that are not grounded are accelerated upward to generate velocity and takeoff.

Arm Swing

Additional, segmental momentum (or body-weight transfer) from the arms contributes to whole-body momentum and increased ground reaction force, and overall acceleration and velocity contributes significantly to the total force produced at takeoff, which increases the maximum distance that can be jumped. The arm swing is a fundamental part of the Power Jump technique.

Like other forms of body-weight transfer, the arm swing occurs briefly before the primary movers (the main muscles producing force) extend. If the goal is to reach the greatest distance, the greatest momentum is generated with maximum amplitude (range of motion at the shoulders) and velocity in the arms. It's also important to fully extend your arms and keep them straight instead of keeping them bent (which is a common mistake in athletic people) because straight arms generate more segmental momentum. The more you flex at the elbows and the closer your arms are to the body's center of mass, the less acceleration and momentum you produce.

Zero Arm Motion Drill

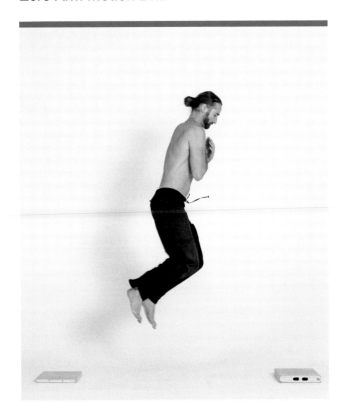

To get a sense of the importance of the arm swing upon launching, it's a good idea to experiment with power jumping without using your arms so you can feel how awkward it is. Choose a medium distance that you feel you can comfortably jump and land, wrap your arms across your chest or clasp your hands behind your lower back, and then jump. Jumping with zero arm motion should naturally feel very counterintuitive; you instinctively want to use your arms. (If you did the drills for the Square Landing, you probably already experienced the awkwardness of landing without arm motion.)

NOTE

A very effective way to experience the importance of the arm motion in jumping is to try the Downward-Upward Rebound Jump.

Back-Front-Back-Front Arm Swing Sequence Drill

I've discussed that you want to swing your arms forward upon launching as well as upon landing if you're using a Square Landing, which is often the case after a Power Jump. But what happens between swinging your arms forward for the launching and bringing them forward again for the landing? Clearly, a piece is missing.

You need to pull your arms back down and to the back while airborne to make it possible to swing your arms forward a second time for the landing. You are reloading your arms for a second forward swing. If your arms stay stuck to the front, then they can't participate in efficient Square Landing. The complete arm sequence, especially doing it with perfect timing, can be really confusing at first, especially if you're entirely absorbed in generating the most powerful takeoff without thinking too much of the landing and what your arms must do while airborne.

The pattern of this drill is a "mini" Power Jump that replicates the entire Power Jump–to–Square Landing sequence on the spot, which teaches you perfect arm sequence and timing without the intensity normally attached to the Power Jump. It's a great entry drill for learning the actual Power Jump because all you must do is increase flexion, acceleration, and forward lean to Power Jump.

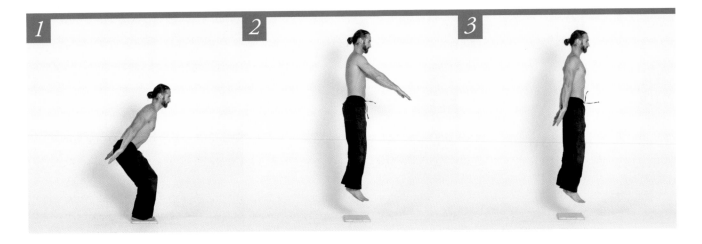

1   Assume a tall, relaxed, and focused standing position. Bend your knees and slightly Hip Hinge, loading your legs as if you're ready to jump upward. Pull your arms behind you, hands level with your rear or a bit higher.

2   Start swinging your arms forward, aiming for a 45-degree angle, and immediately push off your legs. The arm motion slightly precedes the action of your legs and hips even though the time difference is barely perceptible at first. Jump about 2 to 4 inches high at first. Your arms should reach a 45-degree angle at the same time your feet reach their maximum elevation.

3   While you're still airborne and your body is descending with gravity, quickly pull your arms back just behind your rear and have them ready to move forward upon landing, as you have done in earlier drills. Keep your whole body vertically aligned. From there, you're ready for a Square Landing, with your arms starting to swing forward again the moment the balls of your feet connect with the ground.

The lower you jump, the less high you need to swing your arms, which means that they travel less distance, but you also have less time to pull them back. The higher you jump, the farther your arms travel, and the more time you have to pull them back. This is a sequence that demands perfect timing. Issues that usually occur are that you don't pull your arms back fast enough while you're airborne (or don't pull them back at all), so upon landing you either swing them forward partially or can't swing them forward at all. You also might be so focused on pulling your arms back while you're airborne that you start swinging them forward only after you have reached the Squat position, which is too late.

Forward Power Jump

The first progression to the Forward Power Jump is done at ground level. You do it at low intensity like you just did the Back-Front-Back-Front Arm Swing Sequence Drill.

All you need to create forward distance is a bit of lean (launching angle). Resist the natural temptation to attempt to jump far right away. Instead, make sure that the power and distance that you produce matches your ability to land efficiently.

Start with a very slight angle at launching and jump at most one or two feet forward; assess your technique, positional control, and landing efficiency.

If you encounter any issue, you haven't earned greater intensity, even if you have the physical potential for it. Aim at three successful, efficient repetitions in a row before you increase intensity and distance by a half-foot or so. When your progressions are going well, you may use large pieces of board, tape rectangles on the floor, or draw a target in the dirt to create a more realistic sense of context with visible distance and landing accuracy. Keep increasing the distance progressively, making sure to always stay within the limit of efficiency based on how your body responds and feels with the increased intensity and volume.

TECHNIQUE TIP

There are several technical aspects you want to pay attention to if you want to increase intensity and distance:

- Generate the maximum power output you can, including from your feet. You generate a significant amount of power by the forward hip drive.
- The farther the distance, the greater the launching angle. A 45-degree angle generates the greatest distance. A 35- or 55-degree angle, however, allows you to reach 90 percent of your maximum distance for the same power output. Beyond 55 degrees, it becomes more and more challenging to be able to land on your feet, and you will start sprawling.
- Swing your arms forward more vigorously to add to whole-body momentum.
- Pull your heels toward your rear and drive your knees forward explosively immediately after taking off.

A nontechnical way to increase power and distance (regardless of the direction of your Power Jump) involves resistance training, which is done with specific manipulative movements such as explosive lifts.

TECHNIQUE TIP

After a Forward Power Jump in which you land on a surface with low friction and there's a risk that you'll slide forward, you may make your trajectory reach a little more upward than you otherwise would need to as long as the distance you need to jump across is shorter than the maximum distance you can jump. Increasing the upward trajectory helps you land from a more vertical point, which reduces your forward momentum and the risk of slipping.

The following photos show the positional sequence of a Forward Power Jump from launching to airborne trajectory to Square Landing.

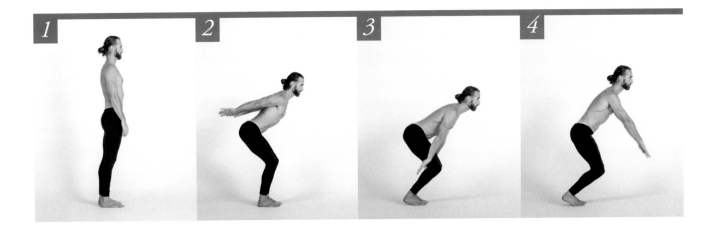

1   Stand tall and relaxed. (Experimenting with diverse launching positions has shown me that the distance that can be covered with a Power Jump is relatively the same regardless of the positional set employed.)

2   Hip Hinge with bent legs and pull your arms behind your back with full extension and internal rotation, so your palms are facing up. If you aim at reaching maximum distance, you may increase the stretch reflex by swiftly swinging your arms backward, which helps make the forward arm swing swifter and adds a little velocity to your jump.

3   Start swinging your arms forward as you bend your legs more to load your legs and feet. Lean forward at a 45-degree angle. Your heels start to slightly elevate off the ground.

4   Your arms have swung to the front of the body and are pointing down at about a 45-degree angle while your legs and hips start to forcefully extend to generate power. Your feet and calves must participate through a solid, powerful ankle extension.

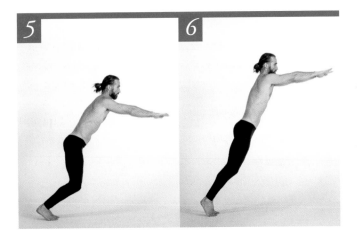

5   Your arms continue to swing forward and are now close to parallel to the ground. Your legs and hips are now about halfway to full extension.

6   Your arms have reached maximum amplitude, so they're pointing slightly above horizontal. Your legs, hips, and feet are fully extended. The launching part of the sequence is over as your whole body is about to become airborne.

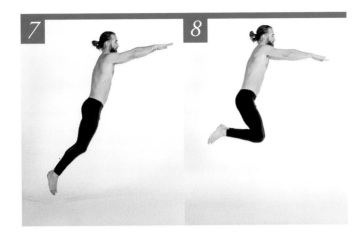

7 At the moment of takeoff, your feet are leaving the ground and beginning the "flight" phase or parabolic trajectory. Your hamstrings fire to swiftly pull to kick your heels toward your rear, which supports the hip motion and abdominal effort that drives your knees forward and up. Sometimes one leg kicks a little before the other, which often has to do with the level of friction or foot position at launching. Symmetry is best.

8 About midway through the trajectory, your body has reached its maximum elevation and maintains impeccable positional control and balance while airborne. Your heels have kicked up enough to bring your knees slightly to the front of your body with both legs bent and perfectly assembled. Your feet and knees are close to level.

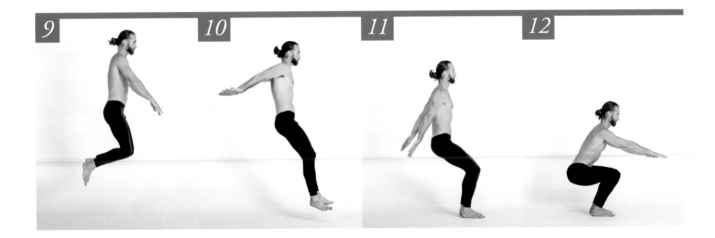

9 As your body starts descending during the second half of the parabolic path, your hips have moved forward, which allows the body to position itself more upright. Your head, torso, hips, and knees are nearly in vertical alignment. Your feet and arms start moving down.

10 Your hips have continued moving forward slightly to the front of your body with a slight backward lean. Your arms are fully pulled back, and your legs are extending to bring your feet forward and downward. Your feet are pointing down ahead of the rest of your body, preparing the balls of your feet to contact the ground.

11 The balls of your feet have landed. Your heels immediately land next, and your legs are bending. Your arms are swiftly starting to swing forward the moment you feel the balls of your feet connect to the ground. Your upper body has regained a vertical position as it keeps moving forward toward the base of support.

12 Your body finishes landing and disperses impact forces by decelerating through a squatting movement. Your arms fully swing to the front of your body, and your center of gravity moves forward until it's vertically aligned with the base of support.

Alternatively, you can use diverse bipedal positions to launch the Power Jump, such as the Deep Squat or the Deep Knee Bend, as well as modified standing stances. Through experimentation, I've observed that using varied modifications of the standing stance (examples are given in the following list) with maximum power output doesn't reduce the maximum distance reached.

- "Sumo" stance with feet a bit broader than shoulder width
- Narrow base (feet/ankles touching)
- Narrow base with feet pointing out at 45 degrees; heels touching each other
- Narrow base with feet pointing out at 45 degrees; heels touching each other and knees outside vertical line with the feet
- Having a rounded back
- Using too much or not enough power output in relation to the trajectory intended.

Faults

Inefficiencies can occur during a Power Jump at any of the three stages of the jump. I previously described some landing issues; other issues relate to launching and positional control during the trajectory.

Common launching issues include the following:
- Starting in the Hip Hinge position rather than standing reduces power output because the stretch reflex in the lower body can't be generated in a swift transition from standing to the Hip Hinge position, which enables the lower-body musculature to recruit more total muscle fibers during the eccentric loading phase, and that leads to more power output. This phase could also produce extra stored elastic energy thanks to ground force reaction because of the downward force in the feet when you Hip Hinge.
- Lack of Hip Hinge amplitude or velocity reduces power output.
- Lack of leg flexion reduces power output
- Keeping your feet flat until take off and not loading the feet reduces the power output. The only exception is if the support surface is unreliable and keeping your flat feet ensures stability and power output.
- Loose, repeated back-and-forth arm swing before takeoff, which usually disturbs your upper-body position.
- Using too much or not enough speed or amplitude in your arm swing in relation to the power generated or to the trajectory intended. Tense arms may prevent your arm swing from being swift enough or ample enough.

Common trajectory issues include the following:
- Leaning sideways, even slightly, makes you land off balance sideways.
- Swinging arms all the way upward. For a Forward Power Jump, your arms don't need to be elevated much beyond horizontal. Swinging your arms too much also makes it difficult to pull your arms all the way down and back before you land.
- Flailing your arms around, usually to the outside and in backward circles. This issue often has to do with either attempting to keep your body balanced while airborne or exerting too much power at launching, so you vainly try to decelerate using your arms to avoid landing beyond a targeted landing surface. Moving your arms changes your trajectory, but it prevents you from pulling your arms back before you land.
- Keeping your arms completely to the front during the whole airborne phase or pulling them back too slowly and partially before landing.

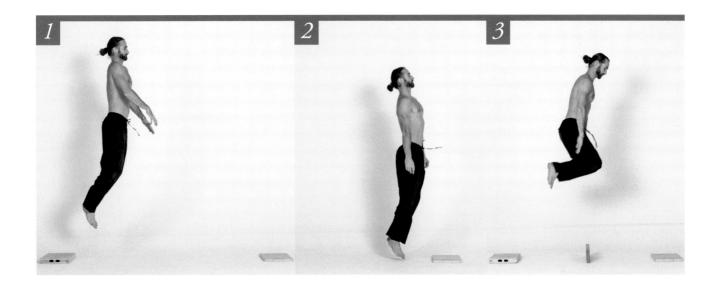

1-2 **"Freezing" fault:** This issue occurs when the whole body is kept fully extended and in an almost completely vertical position with your legs hanging and your feet staying low. Your arms aren't following the swing sequence. It's as if your body freezes after takeoff. This pattern can appear independently of the arm sequence being done correctly, but often there's also a lack of amplitude in the arms and rigidity in the whole body. This issue can happen even when the launching position, sequence, timing, and angle are on point. This issue might have to do with the jumper's nervousness, an inability to mentally follow through with the parts of the sequence following the launching, or an inability to fire the hamstrings and abs to lift the feet and tuck the knees forward. There are two negative consequences to this issue. First, the body doesn't reach a slight backward lean during the second half of the airborne phase, which means the feet are straight below the body until landing instead of moving forward past the body and to the front, which makes the feet land not as far as they should. Second, the center of gravity is already vertically above the base of support the moment the feet reach the ground while there is still some forward momentum going on, and the legs are already extended. This usually makes for a shorter, stiffer, and less stable landing. Pulling your feet higher gives you more time and latitude to place your feet accurately upon landing.

If the Power Jump is new to you and you're doing several of them for maximum distance, keeping your hips and abs working properly and explosively to tuck your knees "blasts" your abdominal muscles, and they should be on fire the next day!

3 **Self-correcting fix:** Place a slightly elevated obstacle midway through the intended trajectory. It shouldn't be high enough for your feet to hit it, but unconsciously you will make sure to pick up your feet to avoid it. To make your feet go over the obstacle, you pull your heels toward your rear and bend your knees, which also brings your knees to the front of the body and helps drive your hips forward enough to create a slight backward lean starting after the midpoint of the trajectory. This gives you the most efficient position for a smooth landing. Another alternative is to practice a few upward Power Jumps to an elevated landing at a medium height, which inherently forces you to tuck your knees forward and up and to lift your feet high.

Power Jump Variations and Progressions

Aside from adding intensity to your Power Jumps (making them more explosive, travel farther, and go higher), some progressions to the Power Jump include both movement and environmental complexity. Practicing such variations as part of practicing progressions challenges and stimulates motor control and helps to expand your jumping repertoire and competency. You will learn all the minor positional adjustments required to be effective and efficient and develop the "eye" necessary for your brain to determine the adequate and optimum movement for a given set of environmental variables.

Launching Variations

- Start from a Deep Squat or Deep Knee Bend position
- Start from a standing balancing position or Deep Knee Bend
- Start from diverse surfaces (uneven, angled, or slightly unstable)
- Move from stepping to Power Jump

Trajectory Variations

- Vary distances and angles.
- Add slight height or depth to have forward-downward and forward-upward trajectories. These variations help you realize that for the same power output you travel more or less distance depending on whether the greater elevation is at launching or landing.
- Put an elevated obstacle in the middle of your flight at varying distances from the launching or landing spots, so you must jump not only far, but a bit higher than you would normally need (photo 1).
- Change position while you're airborne.

Landing Variations

- Precision Square Landing (small surfaces, edge of the support surface).
- Landing on diverse surfaces (uneven, angled, or slightly unstable), which makes landing riskier so you must approach it mindfully, wisely, and progressively. Make sure that the landing surfaces won't slide forward or flip under your feet as you land (unstable rocks, rotten bark, spinning surfaces, and so on). To avoid making your ankle unstable and suffering an ankle sprain, it's sometimes safer to use a heel-first landing on slippery surfaces (or land on your midfoot) rather than landing on the forefoot first.
- Land in a Deep Knee Bend, Deep Squat, Foot-Hand Crawl position, and so on.
- Perform skill-to-skill transitions from the Power Jump to balancing, climbing, and so on.

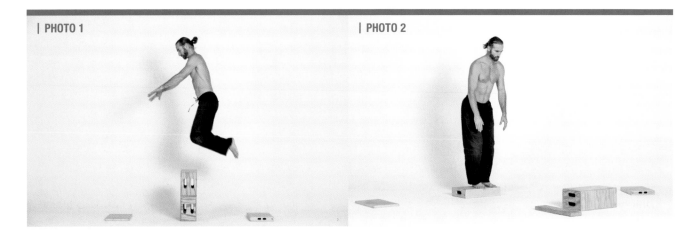

| PHOTO 1 | PHOTO 2

A fantastic training strategy is to vary launching position, surfaces, distances, angles, and trajectories as well as landing positions and surfaces with each jump (see photo 2 on age 370). These variations develop your ability to spontaneously adjust your movement in terms of launching, trajectory, and angle. It helps you develop a faster ability to adapt to changing environmental variables.

You'll certainly be able to figure out more variations than I can possibly list. If you feel like challenging yourself at an even higher level, don't control your practice environment and get outside to confront yourself with real obstacles that may involve greater elevations and danger, slippery surfaces, lack of light, wind, and harsh weather conditions. You can even do it barefoot. But make sure you have established competency and efficiency at lower levels of intensity and complexity. (This is a MovNat/Natural Movement golden rule; it should be your golden rule as well.)

Split Jump

The Split Jump is a single-footed jumping technique that uses power, body-weight shifting, body-weight transfer, and, in most cases, velocity. It usually ends in a Square Landing. The interest of this technique lies in achieving greater forward or upward distances by adding forward velocity to the launching with either wide and swift walking steps or fast running strides. Another advantage of this technique is that you don't have to come to a stop before the takeoff, which saves energy and time.

Because this jump launches on a single leg—with a hinge at the hips unless the forward velocity is high—with the free leg swiftly swinging forward, balance and coordination can be easily challenged and greatly reduce the efficiency of the pattern. This is why it's best to begin practicing at ground level from a stationary Split Standing position, as shown in the photos.

If you launch from a stationary Split Standing stance with good technique, you generate as much forward distance as the Forward Power Jump. Achieving equal distance with the Forward Power Jump is an effective way to assess the efficiency of your Split Jump technique before you add stepping or running.

Although you may begin practicing without a launching and landing surface, it's a good idea to use them as long as they present very little elevation (no higher than an inch).

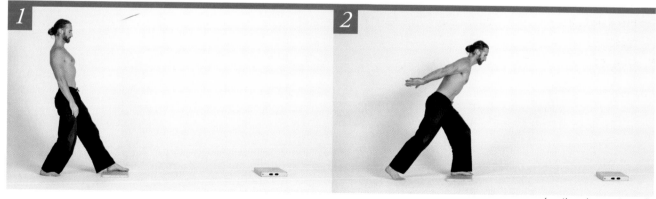

(continued on next page)

1 Begin in a Split Stand with your forward foot accurately positioned on the surface you're launching from. Shift your body weight backward onto your rear foot with a slight backward lean of your torso.

2 Quickly shift your body weight forward onto your front foot to initiate body-weight shifting momentum and greater ground force reaction while you swing your arms backward. Also hinge at the hip.

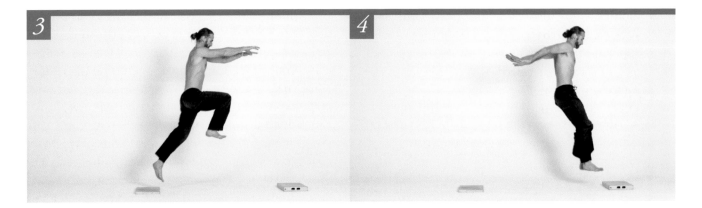

3   Immediately swing your arms and free leg forward to generate body-weight transfer momentum, and then immediately drive your hip forward and push off with your supporting leg to generate power. Your free leg is flexed with your knee tucked forward, and your torso regains a close-to-upright position.

4   Bring your trail leg forward toward your front leg to assemble them, and extend both legs toward the front so that both your feet are side by side as you approach the landing surface. Depending on the length and duration of the trajectory, assembling legs and feet fully may take place after mid-distance—and even just before landing. Also, pull your arms back to prepare for a Square Landing.

Faults

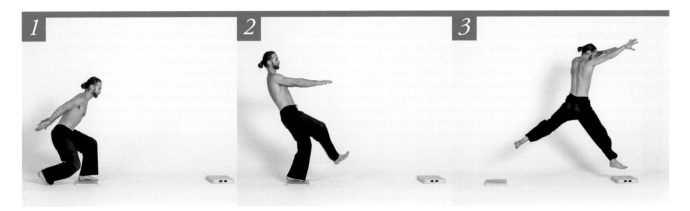

1   Distributing your body weight evenly between both feet in a Split Squat and bending your knees excessively to push off both legs simultaneously.

2   Swinging your free leg while leaning backward. You're fighting your own momentum, which will make the jump short with the possibility of losing balance backward.

3   Not assembling your legs while airborne and leaving the rear leg trailing. If you let your rear leg trail, you leave the absorption of impact forces entirely to the front leg, which makes landing heavy and difficult. There's also a risk that you might initiate a rotation of your body while airborne toward the inside of your front leg, which makes the landing very unstable and potentially unsafe.

Other faults include the following:

- Keeping your torso strictly vertical in the absence of significant forward velocity. The Hip Hinge allows your hips to powerfully drive forward at launching, which adds to momentum.
- Stepping with the front foot aligned with the back foot, which is unstable and might make the launching directionally veer off toward the inside of the front leg.
- Overstepping the launching surface, which causes you to topple forward and fall.
- Swinging your arms too early or too late, rendering the motion useless.
- Leaning sideways upon launching or while airborne, which creates an imbalance upon landing.

After you've mastered the Split Jump from a stationary Split Standing position, you can add one step at a time. Learning to use spatial awareness and peripheral vision to step faster and with more accuracy has been addressed in Chapter 27, "Gait Movement." The principle here is similar, but its importance is even greater because overstepping means you immediately fall forward and down. Because of the inherent risk and danger, it's best to train stepping accuracy at ground level; take a single step at first, use a small launching surface, go at a slow pace, and watch the placement of your foot as you step.

If you must perform this jump in real conditions, it's best to stay on the safe side and make sure to not step on your midfoot or with your toes reaching beyond the edge of the launching surface. If you do

that, the result is that as you intend to shift body weight to your forefoot (the ball of your foot), it will find no support, and you'll topple and fall forward because you're unable to transfer momentum, produce force, and conserve balance.

Make sure to alternate your front foot with each repetition to develop equal skill on both sides. Depending on efficiency, you may add one, two, three, or more steps. The more steps you add, the wider and faster the steps need to be. Learn to keep your steps equal in distance and pace, and to predict what leg will become the supporting one and which one will be the swinging one at launching. You may ultimately run toward the jump at greater speeds, with the challenge of turning horizontal momentum into vertical momentum to reach greater distance (hence this jump usually being called the "long jump"). In the real world, a fast run-up doesn't necessarily imply that you'll launch with full power for maximum distance. For instance, if the distance of the particular gap you must clear is shorter than the maximum distance you could jump over, you won't decelerate during the run-up because you're in a hurry, but you will decrease the velocity you transfer to the jump at launching to reduce the distance you reach. With running and the velocity produced, arm-swinging and Hip Hinging become less relevant because the distance traveled will be mainly generated by the velocity you're able to generate with the run-up. You may conserve a more erect position and keep both arms to the front upon launching.

Vaulting

Vaulting is a way to jump when you use one or more points of support on a firm surface during the trajectory to modify its direction, orientation, distance, duration, or speed. In most cases it happens while your feet, legs, and whole body (except your hands) are airborne. The support (on one or both hands, plus sometimes one or two feet) may be so light and brief that it looks like your body is bouncing like a ball off

the support; alternatively, the support from the surface can be more pronounced and the time spent on support a bit longer, with the body briefly balanced above the surface. The mid-trajectory support, even when it's short and light, could be seen as a form of rebound that uses the existing momentum to launch another jump.

There are multiple ways to vault; the method you choose depends on the context, the way a jump is launched before the trajectory, whether there is an airborne phase before the vault itself, the surface used for support, the position used during support, and the direction and body orientation intended for landing. The fastest vaults that have a long airborne phase before you contact the support are the most challenging, impressive, and intimidating.

Vaults are highly practical (and there are more types than I can cover in this book), but it's important to know when and how to employ them. For instance, the Front Vault is a vaulting technique where the body is facing the obstacle straightforward; the arms land apart on the support while feet and legs pass through the arms over the obstacle to land on the other side. This technique is effective and definitely worth learning, but it's also technical and risky to beginners because you can clip your toes on the surface and fall forward over the obstacle head first. Unless the space to vault through is very narrow, you can achieve the same effective result with other vaulting strategies than the Front Vault, without the risks.

NOTE

When you practice, you can involve the type of blind vault I just described because you'll know what's on the other side of the obstacle, but in real-world situations you can't be sure what's on the other side.

Once you have committed to a vault, you can't change your trajectory at all. Therefore, when the height of an obstacle is too low to actually justify vaulting over it, simply stepping up onto the same surface and continuing to run would be as fast, safer, and much more energy-efficient, and you'd still be able to change speed or direction at any time while on the obstacle.

Let's focus on the most practical ways to vault, starting with a relatively easy technique called the Tripod Vault, which is the best vault technique for those unfamiliar with vaults because it uses the support of a leg, can be done very slowly, and is easy to break down.

Tripod Vault

The pattern of the Tripod Vault is like the Tripod Get-Up I cover in Chapter 25, "Ground Movement 2," except you apply it dynamically to an elevated surface. This vault is mostly used to pass over a low to moderately tall obstacle that is either horizontal or at an angle. The Tripod Vault is particularly safe because you can perform it at a slow, controlled speed, and you can remain stable, even when the obstacle is not.

The Tripod Vault is the vault of choice if stepping on the top surface of the obstacle or down on the other side of it is potentially unsafe. You also might use it when you're carrying a relatively heavy load behind you or if one arm is busy holding an object.

The real convenience of this technique is how you can control speed (except in the presence of great velocity before launching) and how you can pause by balancing on top of the surface to check out the landing area before you jump off. What differentiates the Tripod Vault from the Tripod Get-Up is that in the vault there is a moment after launching where the whole body is airborne before the foot and hand land on the obstacle, or at least both feet are off the ground with one hand on support on the obstacle. Without that airborne moment, you just have a Tripod Get-Up applied with a vertical and horizontal distance over an obstacle.

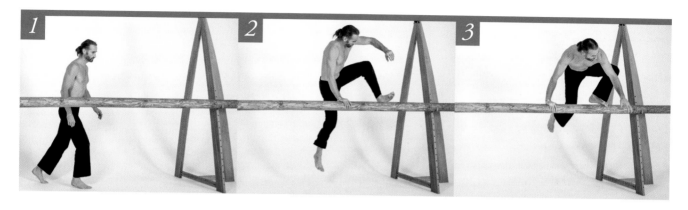

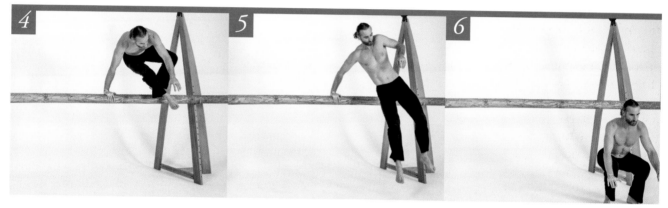

1 Approach the obstacle at an angle (or straight on) by stepping toward it with your front leg closest to the obstacle. Your front hand and trail foot become your points of support for the vault. If the edge of the obstacle is inclined, your supporting hand should be higher than your supporting foot.

2 A safe but slow option is to first place the hand that's on the same side as your lead leg on the surface; then push off with your lead leg to pull your trail leg forward and up so you can place your trail foot on top of the obstacle. A more dynamic option is to transfer the stepping momentum to a jump with an airborne phase before your lead hand and trail foot land on top of the surface. With the more dynamic option, your hand lands just a little before your foot does. With either option, your upper body leans sideways toward the lead hand. If the obstacle isn't too high, your supporting arm is already in the locked-out position; otherwise, enough elevation must be attained through momentum to allow your supporting arm to lock out.

3 Place the ball of your foot on the surface for better positional control and safety, and lock out your arm (if it isn't already locked out) to establish a stable base of support between the hand and foot.

4 With all your body weight on your supporting hand and foot, begin pushing off your supporting leg to elevate your hips and center of gravity, creating clearance so that you can bend and pull your trail leg up and through the space between your points of support. Use your other arm for balance if necessary; otherwise, keep it relaxed.

5 Push off the supporting leg to release the support foot and propel your body forward and down while you extend your free leg in the direction where you want to land. Your supporting arm keeps pushing and guiding your body while ensuring clearance with the obstacle, which is now behind your body. Your hand may stay in the same position from beginning to end, or it might slightly pivot before your body moves to the other side of the obstacle.

6 Bring both legs together and transition into a Square Landing. (Other types of landings and transitions are possible, of course.)

TECHNIQUE TIP

When the obstacle is high, you need to generate upward momentum, with both hands extending toward the upper surface of the obstacle to start pressing up as soon as they reach it, which assists with the elevation of your center of gravity until the knee of one leg can tuck up and your foot can reach the top. When your foot is established on the surface, you can release your inner hand in a position similar to the Tripod Get-Up.

Faults

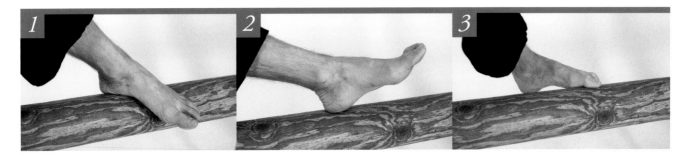

1   Incorrect foot position. Placing your foot flat gives little range of motion to change the position of your foot as needed for balance or direction. Your foot also might slide sideways and lower your base of support.

2   Incorrect foot position. By placing your heel on the surface, it's very likely it will slide forward and place you in an uncomfortable or unsafe position.

3   Incorrect foot position. If your foot is too short with only the toes on support, it might slide back with the same result.

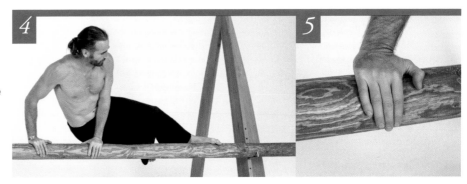

4   You place your foot, or let it slide, too far from your hand with a very wide and low base of support. This position makes it impossible to elevate your hips sufficiently to bring your trailing leg through. Conversely, you could place your foot too close to your hand, making the position compact, narrow, and less stable. Another issue arises when your supporting arm is not in the lockout position, which lowers the base of support and makes it unstable as well.

5   Improper position of your hand. Your fingers, instead of your palm, are on top of the surface, and your wrist isn't aligned with your palm, which compromises the position of your wrist and turns your hand into a weak point of support.

NOTE

The photos show the faults being performed with two hands on the support, but the faults are the same with a single arm.

Tripod Vault Beginner Drills

Warm up with the Tripod Get-Up on the floor to start getting a good feel for base and points of support, joint alignment, and shoulder stability. If the vault is new to you and intimidating, choose a practice surface that's relatively low and has a flat top, such as a wood box. First perform a regular Tripod Get-Up from standing, slowly stepping down on the other side, which you may do with two arms instead of one.

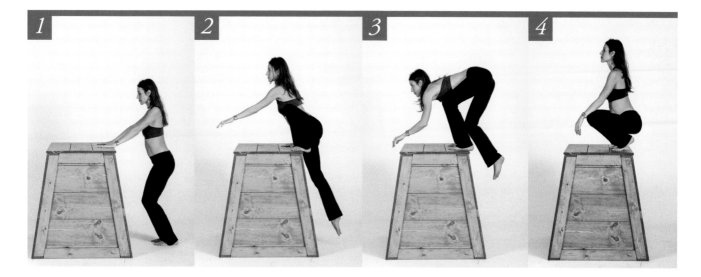

1   Begin standing facing the box; your feet should be together. Place both hands on top of the box and decide which foot will move up as you shift your body weight to the opposite hand.

2   Using assistance from your hands, jump up and replace one supporting hand with the foot on the same side. This places you in a Single-Leg Deep Knee Bend assisted with the opposite arm in the lockout; your trail leg is extended down.

3   Push off the supporting foot on top of the box to elevate your hips enough to bring your trailing leg up and place it on the box, between your supporting foot and hand.

4   Release your supporting hand and transition into a Deep Knee Bend. From here, you may get back down in a Tripod Get-Up fashion or jump down either on the side where you started or on the other side of the box.

TECHNIQUE TIP

Practice the complete movement as described, but do it more dynamically. Then practice the movement on slightly higher and more narrow surfaces. Eventually approach the obstacle at increasingly greater speed.

Double-Handed Side Vault

The Double-Handed Side Vault doesn't use any support from your foot, and it enables you to clear similar obstacles as the Tripod Vault but with more speed. The Single-Handed Side Vault enables you to be even faster still.

As with the Tripod Vault, you can do this vault slowly from a stationary standing position, but you must have sufficient momentum to do it, and you can't stabilize and pause above the obstacle. You can do this vault during a run so that you clear the obstacle and resume running upon landing.

Using both arms provides a strong base of support, and it maximizes the use of upper-body strength to support the elevation of your center of gravity and the effective passing of the obstacle, which is especially useful if the obstacle is much above your center of gravity and there is little to no momentum at launching. If the obstacle is about level with your center of gravity, you can use greater speed during the run-up, and your body will clear the obstacle with brief and light support from a single hand.

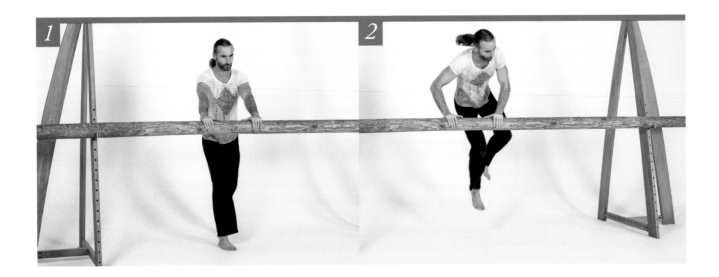

1   Face the obstacle straight on with your hands shoulder width apart on the top surface. In the photo, the obstacle stands well above my center of gravity; in that case, you must elevate your center of gravity high enough to generate enough power with your legs to launch an upward jump before transferring your body weight to your hands.

2   Push off with your lead foot and swing your trailing leg up and to the side to generate additional momentum. Optionally, you can start with your feet squared to the obstacle, in which case you push off both legs simultaneously. Your feet are airborne, your center of gravity is above the top of the surface, and you're shifting body weight to your arms.

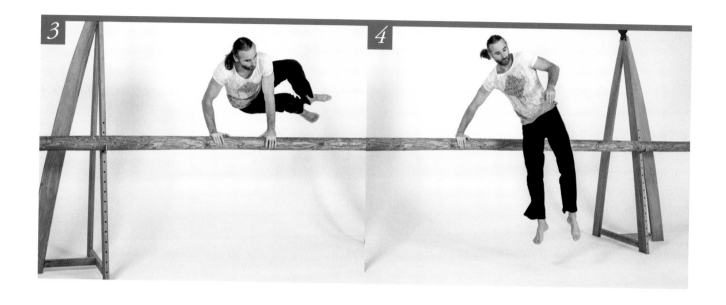

3   Extend both arms by pushing down on the supporting surface to keep transferring and generating more upward momentum. You're elevating your center of gravity to create clearance for your legs. Bring both legs out to the side with your knees bent.

4   Release your inside hand (the one that's on the same side as the legs) to allow your legs to pass over the obstacle; push off the surface with your other hand to push your body away from the obstacle and guide it in the direction where you want to land. As your legs pass over the obstacle, extend them to the ground.

TECHNIQUE TIP

As you increase the speed of the vault, you may generate a take-off and airborne phase with both feet and hands off the ground while your body and arms are extending toward the surface of support. You may also modify your support to the Single-Handed Side Vault. The technique is the same as the Double-Handed Side Vault, but you do it with only the arm that's opposite to where your legs are going. Use this variation when power and momentum are greater, which reduces the need for strong support with both arms.

29
Climbing Movement

"Identifying and overcoming natural fear is one of the pleasing struggles intrinsic to climbing."

—*Alex Lowe*

We climb to reach higher grounds or surfaces or lower ones. Humans naturally climb for a variety of reasons, such as to look for food, seek shelter, get to a safe place to rest, scout surroundings from an elevated point, take a shortcut, or reach areas that are only accessible through climbing. I like to say that climbing is (most of the time) a form of vertical crawling.

Young children often start climbing by crawling up stairways. From a Natural Movement perspective, climbing movements involve ascending, descending, or traversing any kind of steep and elevated natural or man-made surfaces such as cliffs, boulders, walls, trees, ropes, bars, poles, platforms, ladders, bridges, and so on. In most cases, Natural Movement climbing practice is done without any specific gear, although you can do it with safety equipment, such as crash pads or harnesses and ropes, when the elevation and danger involved merits it.

Apart from rescue climbing, modern forms of climbing are done mostly for recreational purposes. These climbing types have become specialized activities named after the type of surface or environment where they're performed, such as bouldering, rock climbing, mountaineering, ice climbing, canyoneering, pole and rope climbing, and buildering (climbing on the outsides of buildings). In most cases, these types of climbing use gear that's specific to the surface and activity. Such gear makes climbing much safer.

However, even in the presence of equipment, climbing mostly relies on Natural Movement patterns that were developed through evolution and arboreal locomotion. Indeed, science suggests our ancestors at some point of our evolution mostly lived in trees, which means they extensively moved in trees before they became primarily bipedal—including needing to brachiate as is suggested by our relatively elongated upper limbs, flexible shoulder joints, and fingers and hands that are well-suited for grasping. These physical characteristics probably allowed our ancestors to test the reliability of supporting surfaces ahead; to cross gaps; to reach resources such as fruits, nuts, or eggs; to brachiate; and to do pretty much anything in a tree related to survival, such as finding shelter, resting, hiding, or scouting the environment around and below. Arboreal locomotion is still practiced by many hunter-gatherers, and brachiating is a Natural Movement activity that healthy children cannot resist doing whenever "monkey bars" or low-hanging branches are available.

NOTE

Brachiating is a form of climbing locomotion in which one hangs, swings, or leaps by hanging with both arms or each arm alternately. The word comes from Latin brachium, which means "arm." Maybe this explains why many people are "dendrophiles," which are people who love trees and forests.

Climbing doesn't necessarily start from the ground. You can climb down from elevated ground to reach a lower surface, make a jump landing in a climb position, switch from balancing on a narrow horizontal surface to hanging from it, or start and end in a fully horizontal traversing movement. You can exit a climb in diverse ways; jumping, balancing, or crawling are possible transitions. Climbing can be a short transition between jumping and running or balancing, or you can transition from jump to jump. Climbing can last a long time when you're ascending high and challenging surfaces. It can be as easy as climbing up a ladder, as scary as climbing up a cliff, as unpredictable as climbing mud walls, or nearly impossible when you attempt to climb surfaces completely covered in thick ice.

While on a climbing route you may be briefly balancing, jumping, or even vaulting, such as when you're moving through large trees or from tree to tree. Even when you're climbing surfaces such as boulders and walls, jumping can be briefly part of a climbing action when you generate power to move upward or sideways with the body partly airborne. You also might climb down in a jump-style way, relying on gravity as your feet leave the support to become briefly airborne as you use your hands to keep hanging onto the surface of support. Because of such great diversity in practical goals, surfaces, and routes, many body parts

can be involved beyond feet and hands; you might be able to hold positions or generate movement with your forearms, elbow and knee creases, heels, shoulders, armpits, groin, seat, back, and belly.

With the presence of verticality, elevation, steepness, narrowness, or instability of the supporting surface, losing your base of support completely while climbing results in an immediate fall like you might experience with balancing. However, the difference is that, in balancing, all points of support are below your center of gravity, and your body weight rests on or is pushed from the supporting surface, whereas in climbing the points of support are either split between being below the center of gravity (resting on the supporting surface) and being above the center of gravity (hanging and pulling from the supporting surface) or all the points of support are above the center of gravity as you hang from the surface of support. The latter option negates any risk of toppling, which means that, in some cases, hanging is a more effective and safer option than balancing for traversing a surface. When you completely lose balance from a balancing position, a fall is guaranteed, whereas losing balance in a hanging position just makes you swing as long as you can maintain your grip; gravity will naturally restore your balance. In any case, climbing absolutely demands a great sense of balance, and losing balance may precipitate a disastrous fall.

Hanging

Most of us immediately think of hanging as having the whole body suspended in the air as we hang by the hands with straight arms. Even mainstream fitness—in which hanging is rarely involved—shrinks its scope to that exclusive position of hanging with straight arms by the hands only, with the unique purpose of developing core and upper-body strength. You're about to discover how extremely oversimplified this image of hanging is and how Natural Movement and a knowledge of real-life contextual demands vastly expands the range of hanging positions and movements.

A realistic and accurate definition of hanging is that the body is fully or partly suspended, which means that some or all of the points of support we

hold a position from are located above both the center of gravity and body weight. Such suspension can be done in a variety of ways, and you can hang by your hands as well as by your elbows, forearms, upper thighs, back of the knees, and feet.

You can have one, two, three, four, or even up to six points of support in a contralateral or ipsilateral fashion, and your body can be in a (potentially inverted) vertical or horizontal position. Even when your body weight is mostly supported by your feet and your center of gravity is above the lower points of supports, such as when you're climbing up a tree or boulder, hanging is involved usually with the hands preventing the body from falling backward, which implies a certain degree of suspension. On some surfaces and routes, climbing can be achieved in a purely hanging fashion without using any points of support below your center of gravity.

The supporting surface can be thin, thick, vertical, angled, horizontal, even or uneven, smooth or rugged, stable or unstable. Clearly, that many variables create an impressively versatile repertoire of dozens of hanging positions that is incredibly more diverse than hanging only with straight arms. This repertoire also constitutes the necessary lead-up for a vast number of complex climbing movements on diverse surfaces and going in various directions, which takes your climbing scope and competency way beyond linear upward movements such as pull-ups.

Gripping Friction, Real-Life Environments, and Practical Movement Reality

You might suppose that hanging is a relatively relaxed and easy activity, but this is far from the truth. Hanging is work, and there's no such thing as a "passive hang." Any amount of muscular tension makes a position "active," and even the most relaxed hangs involve a certain level of muscular tension.

We wouldn't call a stationary standing position with both legs fully extended a "passive stand," and the same standing stance with both knees mildly flexed would be called an "active stand," right? Of course not. The same way a total absence of tension when standing would make you collapse to the ground, a total absence of tension when hanging signifies losing all frictional force, which precipitates a fall. The only way that a hang can be "passive" is if you're tied up with a piece of rope by your wrists, ankles, or neck!

However, whenever possible, hanging should certainly be done in the most relaxed manner possible and with the least amount of work. In other words, once the minimal level of "activation" or tension required to generate the level of frictional force necessary to sustain the position has been reached, all body parts or muscles that are not involved in holding the position can be as relaxed as possible.

Depending on the context, the same position may be held with minimal tension, or held with additional tension, with both positions being "active" anyway. For instance, with a "double-hand" hang (commonly known as Dead Hang) you can securely hang from a thin, non-slippery round surface with a Hook Grip with tension in only your forearms while the rest of your body is mostly relaxed. However, to ensure that you can sustain the same hang position from on a thick, round, and somewhat slippery surface, you must use an Open-Hand Grip and have additional tension in the lats, scapular area, and abdominal muscles. This simple change of surface increases environmental complexity, which necessitates adjustments to positional control through additional tension to modify the pull angle and increase frictional force in your hands. Making and keeping the hang effective is the primary reason for additional tension. With a thinner surface, your hang position is a little bit lower, more vertical, and relaxed; with a thicker surface, your hang position is slightly higher, at an angle, and not as relaxed. Both are active positions.

Additional tension may be used as a strategy for protecting your joints—usually the shoulders—when they're not healthy by reducing the amount of stress that's placed in these joints. Regardless of the situation, unless you have a practical reason that demands additional tension, you should conserve optimum relaxation. Remember, though, that optimum relaxation does not mean complete relaxation.

Selective tension is an issue with beginners who tend to create too much tension in the muscles that handle the production of frictional force, and superfluous tension in those muscles that don't even participate in such force, which generates early fatigue and shorter hanging time. Beginners may include individuals who are otherwise seen as fit, including people who can perform several Pull-Ups in a row; if they're not familiar with positional diversity and demands or don't have the particular strength required to hold various hangs on varied surfaces, they're beginners when it comes to climbing.

I've witnessed fit individuals who can perform many Pull-Ups in a gym setting but find themselves barely able to hang from a thick, rounded, slippery surface, for the simple reason that their hanging practice—and therefore their ability to hang—is exclusively restricted to regular pull-up bars.

Grip strength is commonly seen as being exclusively related to the hands, but it actually extends to grasping and hanging actions with any body part. For instance, hanging from your forearms demands grip strength as well, except that it isn't located in the hands. Grip strength has to do with the ability to generate the friction necessary to hold the hanging positions regardless of what the position is. The stronger the gripping, the more friction, and the more reliable the hang positions, which makes them fully reliable for movement involving power and momentum. Indeed, the strength grip required for strong hangs isn't limited to holding stationary hangs.

While hanging, you can produce dynamic motion, such as pulling upward with power or generating swinging momentum. If holding a stationary hanging position is already challenging to you, then controlled ascents, descents, or traverse movements that involve hanging will be an even greater challenge. For this reason, a beginner approach to climbing should involve a lot of hanging that develops the grip strength and positional control required to hold positions steadily on both vertical and horizontal surfaces.

Hand Grip

Recent studies suggest that millennials have significantly weaker hand grips than young people from three decades ago. The explanation has a lot to do with movement behavior because younger generations have spent much more time indoors—sitting and playing with electronics—than being physically active outdoors, which usually involves a wide range of movements, including climbing and object manipulation or manual work that all contribute to hand grip strength.

The first problem is that weakness in your hands is a symptom that reveals deficiency in overall physical strength and function. Grip strength is literally linked to life expectancy and is a more reliable predictor than blood pressure. Studies have shown that levels of grip strength in elderly populations are predictors of admission rates in hospitals and that elderly patients with greater grip strength generally are released from the hospital significantly faster than people with lower grip strength. This implies that your level of grip strength might indicate more than your levels of strength and function; it might be an indicator of the overall status of your health, vitality, and mortality.

The second problem is that you can't expect to just practice isolated hand grip drills to remedy the overall issue. Fortunately, Natural Movement skills such as climbing and manipulation efforts (lifting, carrying, throwing, or catching) contribute to strengthening

your hands and your whole body because in those movements your hands and the rest of your body are tightly connected as you perform the movement.

In short, in such movements the stress and effort in your hands can't be disconnected from the stress and efforts in your body or the other way around. Similarly, you can't expect to develop full hand grip strength by practicing a single position or movement—for example, hanging from the hands or deadlifting. With about thirty muscles in the hands and forearms, hand grip strength is supposed to adapt to many kinds of positions and efforts. The grip strength necessary for hanging from open hands or from a finger hold isn't the same, and the hand grip necessary to massage someone or use a screwdriver must adapt to a particular forearm, wrist, and finger movement (position, amplitude, intensity, duration, and volume).

NOTE

You can find more information about the studies of grip strength at the following web pages:

- **Hand grip among millennials:** www.ncbi.nlm.nih.gov/pubmed/26869476
- **Grip strength and life expectancy:** https://fhs.mcmaster.ca/main/news/news_2015/handgrip_study.html
- **Grip strength and hospital admission rates:** https://academic.oup.com/ageing/article/44/6/954/81109
- **Grip strength and length of hospital stay:** www.ncbi.nlm.nih.gov/pmc/articles/PMC3723742/

Efficient hand grip is not only about strength. There's no need to routinely "crush" whatever surface you're holding when you climb or manipulate an object; you need to do that when you feel that it's the only way to ensure your grip. You can easily fatigue your hands and forearms if you systematically employ as much tension as you can in those areas, and when you get fatigued you must rapidly abandon the position or the task. Whereas you may always let go in training, releasing your grip isn't always possible in real-life situations. In climbing, how much grip strength you need isn't just a factor of your body weight in relation to the surface you're climbing on; it also has to do with your overall position. A slight adjustment in body position angle can cause you to fatigue your forearms and hands more quickly.

Your hands are highly sensitive body parts that have the ability to automatically increase tension when they sense that your hold becomes unreliable with less tension. Such *reactive grip response* also works when you manipulate handheld objects. Usually, it's a good idea to start hanging with a little more tension than you need for safety until you sense that you can lower tension while keeping your hold sustainable. Aspects of hand grip specific to manipulation are covered in Chapter 30, "Manipulation Movement 1."

Regardless of finger position, there are three main hand orientations in hanging:

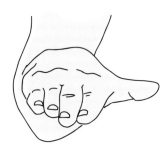

PRONE, IN WHICH THE HAND IS IN FRONT OF THE SURFACE OF SUPPORT, PALM POSITIONED ON TOP OF THE SURFACE OF SUPPORT AND FACING DOWN

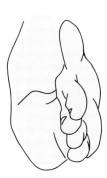

SIDEWAYS, IN WHICH THE PALM FACES TO THE SIDE, EITHER INTERNALLY OR EXTERNALLY

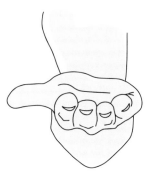

SUPINE, IN WHICH THE HAND IS BEHIND THE SURFACE OF SUPPORT, PALM POSITIONED ON TOP OF THE SURFACE OF SUPPORT AND FACING DOWN

NOTE

The prone grip is often called "overhand," whereas the supine grip is often called "underhand," which is a misnomer. The reality is that, to provide hang support, both grips must be prone or "overhand" with the palm placed on top of the surface of support and not under it, regardless of whether you place your hand or hands in front of or behind the supporting surface. However, it's convenient to use the terms "prone" and "supine" to mean the palm facing out and facing toward you, respectively.

By default, arm hangs done from horizontal surfaces (such as a horizontal tree branch) use a prone grip. A supine hand position is rarely used for two main reasons:

- A supine grip provides less gripping friction on thick surfaces because it's difficult to get your palms far enough onto the surface.
- When you pull upward, you're forced to travel your hand beneath the supporting surface from behind to in front of and over it, which is very inefficient.

It's good to know that a supine grip is possible, but for practical purposes, it's inconvenient or plain inefficient when used on horizontal surfaces. On the other hand, the prone grip allows you, if necessary, to "hook" your hand higher and more forward over the supporting surface so your palm can be pressing down, with your wrist bent at an angle (up to 45 degrees, with your hand aligned perpendicularly with your forearm).

Another aspect of the hand grip relates to the position of the fingers on the hand, especially the position of the thumb in relation to the hand and other fingers. The Hook Grip, which is also known as the Power Grip, implies that the fingers (as well as the palm, when the surface is thick) clamp down on the surface with the thumb creating counter pressure. It's a very strong grip with many purposes: hanging in arm or arm-leg hangs, climbing, or manipulating objects. But in hanging or manipulation, the Hook Grip is only possible when the surface held is thin enough. Beyond a certain thickness, it's best to hook the thumb together with the other fingers over the surface instead of under it. Such an Open-Hand Grip (known as "False Grip," although there is nothing "false" about it) is basically the only option you have when the surface you're holding is thick, which in the real world is most often the case.

NOTE

Although with the Open-Hand Grip the thumb can't exert counterpressure opposite to the other fingers and palm, it still can exert pressure down on the surface and against the index finger, which keeps the grip quite effective. The position of the hand and fingers in the Open-Hand Grip is either at an angle, curled, or rounded.

Aside from lianas (woody climbing plants), ropes, cables, and pull-up bars in a gym, you will be hard-pressed to find surfaces that are narrow enough yet strong enough to enable you to use a Hook Grip, especially in arm hangs where all your weight depends on such a surface of support. Most real-life surfaces are too thick for a Hook Grip. Your training mindset and practice should take this limitation into account and progressively accustom you to thicker surfaces, so you can strengthen your prone Open-Hand Grip significantly and feel secure even when swinging momentum is involved.

When the palm and fingers are aligned horizontally, I use the term Flat Grip. This grip is the position your hand is in when you're hanging from flat surfaces, such as from a board or the edge of a platform.

Last, a hand grip sometimes relies on finger grip or fingerholds only. In these cases, the points of support are limited to one finger or more, and the surface generating friction is even restricted to the tips of the fingers.

Finally, hand grip strength is an issue when your palms are sweaty because of exertion, weather, or fear (and chalk is not always handy). A simple trick (aside from wiping your hands on your clothes) is to grab a handful of sand or dirt and rub it on your hands. Last, the natural thickening of the skin (known as *keratoderma*) that occurs when you practice a lot of hanging not only protects the skin of your hands (especially when climbing on natural surfaces), it also increases gripping friction.

Benefits of Hanging

I show you many hanging techniques in this chapter, and all hold practical movement value. If you try to bypass any, you'll miss out on some great assets to your movement competency and preparedness.

I've already mentioned some benefits of practicing a wide range of hanging positions, but here's a brief summary:

- From a practical movement perspective, hanging is a prerequisite foundation to the ability to perform diverse climbing movements and transitions from and to such positions, on diverse surfaces and in varied directions.

- Hanging practice develops gripping strength and endurance not limited to hands and forearms and involving many muscles and body parts.

- Hanging improves joint function and health. Depending on position, the benefits aren't limited to the wrist, elbow, and shoulder joints; the thoracic spine and hip can benefit, too. Like ground positions where gravity and body weight push joints into optimal range of motion, gravity and body weight pull joints into optimal range of motion when you're hanging. It's especially the case when hangs rely on only hands and the rest of the body dangles below in a fully relaxed fashion.

SAFETY NOTE

Hanging also places a higher demand or stress on joints, and some individuals with unhealthy joints might not be able to practice hangs, especially if they're not strong enough to create additional tension to protect them while holding the positions. Hangs involving the legs shift part of the body weight toward the leg and away from your wrists, elbows, and shoulders, making hang positions more sustainable.

Hang Practice

Unlike the earlier movement skills, I'm not introducing all hanging positions before I describe all climbing movements. You may locate all stationary climbing positions and practice each of them to develop stability before you attempt any climbing movement, or you may start with particular positions relating to particular climbing patterns on particular types of climbing surfaces.

With the Push-Pull Hang, your practice can begin in the easiest way without involving any elevation; simply hang with one or two hands gripping a wall, a fence, or a small tree with your feet resting on the ground.

Pull Hangs involving the hands or arms and the legs hooked over the surface of support are another good starting point, before you transition to more challenging hangs that involve the upper body with no assistance from the lower body.

Progressions

Hanging positions that don't have any support below the center of gravity are more challenging than those that have support from both above and below the center of gravity. In addition, hanging positions with fewer or more challenging points of support are more difficult to hold than those that involve more points of support and more reliable ones. For instance, hanging from the hands is easier if your feet can rest perpendicularly against a vertical surface than if your feet are strictly in the void, and hooking a leg over the supporting surface when hanging by the hands is easier than a Double-Hand Hang.

I have structured the hangs in this chapter in a way that follows this progression in level of difficulty. However, you don't necessarily need to postpone practicing Hand Hangs (hanging only by the hands).

Beyond the progression in gripping strength level or difficulty of holding the position due to the position itself, progressions may involve the following:

- Longer holds. You may start holding a position a few seconds and aim at holding it a whole minute or longer.
- Raised hangs (often known as "active hangs"), which involves pulling from your shoulder/scapula area, arms, or legs to elevate your center of gravity and position (without changing your base of support).
- More challenging surfaces, such those that are thicker or smoother.
- Additional external weight (such as a weighed vest).
- Some body-weight shifting or swinging momentum while holding the position.

TECHNIQUE TIP

Apart from the progression involving longer holds, which requires more gripping endurance, all other options demand higher levels of frictional force, which means they require more muscular tension and greater gripping strength, so it's likely you'll want to reduce the duration of your holds at first. The good thing is that an increase in gripping strength increases your gripping endurance.

SAFETY NOTE

Be particularly cautious when practicing on natural surfaces that might not be reliable. When you're climbing trees and stepping on and pulling from branches, it is important to get a feel for the strength and reliability of the surfaces. (Honestly, this is true for any surface.) Generally speaking, larger branches are stronger than thinner ones and live limbs are stronger than dead and dry ones. Other considerations, such as the type of tree, the presence of moss, humidity, or even rotten bark, will change friction and make a difference in strength and reliability. As a rule of thumb, place your feet and hands as close as possible to the trunk instead of away from it, try to distribute your body weight on more points of support, place less body weight on areas you believe aren't reliable, and always be prepared for a sudden breakage.

Push-Pull Hangs

The Push-Pull Hangs are the most common in climbing. They partly rely on points of support above the center of gravity—usually the hands—that handle some of the body weight by pulling from the supporting surface, and partly rely on points of support below the center of gravity—usually the feet—that handle some of the body weight by pushing on it. Whenever possible, most of the body weight should rest on your feet, and climbing upward should rely on a pushing effort from your legs, while you minimize tension and effort from your arms and upper body as much as possible. The loss of all points of support from below your center of gravity might not entail a fall as you can turn the position into an Arm Hang. However, if all points of support above your center of gravity were lost, there's a greater chance that your center of gravity would be pulled back out of alignment with the base of support to precipitate a fall, unless you're able to lean the upper body forward enough to avoid it.

Therefore, when you're climbing in Push-Pull Hang positions, the priority focus is always twofold: shifting as much body weight to your feet and as much of the effort to your legs while ensuring reliable gripping from the points of support above your center of gravity in case your feet slip. You can use these positions on a boulder, a cliff, a tree, or an urban wall to rest, collect yourself, and transition to the next move.

You can easily and safely start practicing Push-Pull Hang positions with most of your body weight shifted on your feet resting on the ground. To increase the challenge, you may modify your position to progressively increase the hanging effort from your upper body, such as moving your center of gravity away from the surface of support and pulling up with your arms or hanging with a single arm; finally step up with your feet resting on the vertical surface rather than flat on the ground. You may also modify the positions of your shoulders, hips, spine, legs, and feet while holding the hang to create different loads on as many joints as you can.

Depending on the type of surface, the direction of movement can be upward, downward, or sideways in a traversing fashion, generally with an alternation of three and four points of support—all fours, two feet and one hand, one foot and two hands—because holding a position with only two points of support can easily destabilize you and create a risk. The position can be compact, vertically extended, or horizontally wide, with the body close to or farther from the supporting surface, and your center of gravity vertically centered, either lower and closer to the feet or higher and closer to the hands or arms.

You can elevate your body either by pushing off your feet or pulling from your hands or arms. If the surface is wide, such as a rocky surface or wall, you can move in a traversing fashion sideways or at an angle. In the presence of a surface that's flat and wide enough, you might be able to place your forearms on the surface for support, such as when you reach the top edge of a wall. There is too much position and movement specificity to list all options, so I'll start with the main positions.

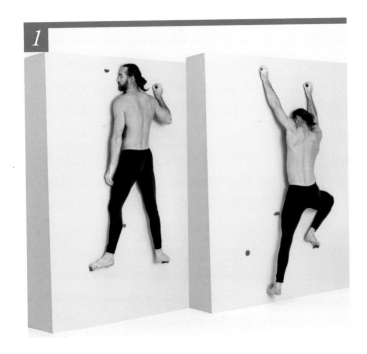

1   Push-Pull, Single-Hand Foot-Hand Hang: Most of your body weight is supported by your feet. If you lose your footing, you have a chance to maintain a Single-Hand Pull Hang and hopefully a Two-Handed Pull Hang. However, if you release your single handhold, you fall back and down.

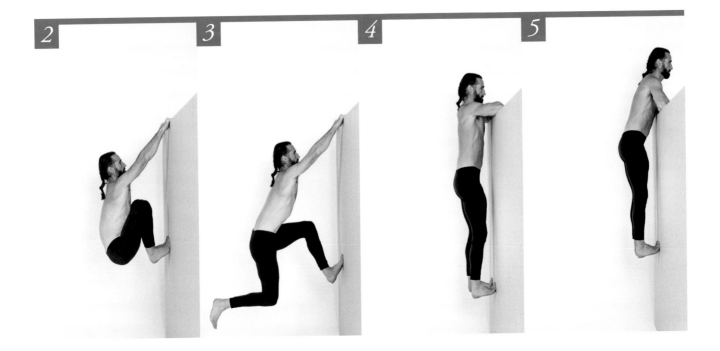

2   Square Bent Extended Arms Foot-Hand Hang

3   Single-Foot Extended Arms Foot-Hand Hang: A similar position can be held with a single hand in a contralateral fashion (using the foot and hand on opposite sides of the body) because a same-side foot and hand is very unstable.

4   Extended Legs Neutral Foot-Forearm Hang

5   Extended Legs High Foot-Forearm Hang

There are more variations of similar positions (especially hand positions) than I have room to show you in this book. For instance, fingerholds can be in a C-shape curly position, in an L-shape straight-angle position, or in a curled and spread out position. Handholds can be made of a flat hand, round hand, or fist stuck in a crack of a rock. The position of the hand can be overhand (pressing down), underhand (pressing up), or sideways (pressing to the side). As long as pulling from the upper points of support is required to handle some body weight, maintain position, and prevent gravity from pulling your body down to the back is required, you're in a hanging position.

SAFETY NOTE

When the surface is narrow, smooth, or round, such as a pole or tree trunk, only upward or downward movement is possible, although you still can change your body orientation by moving around the surface of support. A surface without handholds or footholds—which is especially challenging when the surface is smooth and slippery—gives frictional force, which is generated by positional control, something that's enormously important. Climbing in that situation also demands more balance because the base of support is very narrow; in certain positions, your body might be pulled off balance into a sideways swing. Controlling the descent is also more challenging when there's greater likelihood that you'll lose balance or slide down uncontrollably.

Some of the positions shown in the next set of photos are quite like the same positions on a wide vertical surface, but I've adapted them to the specificity of the supporting surface. You should step up from the ground and practice holds close to ground level before you attempt to reach a height. Upward motion is nearly impossible if you struggle with simply holding the positions. Managing gripping friction and positional control efficiently is the name of the game.

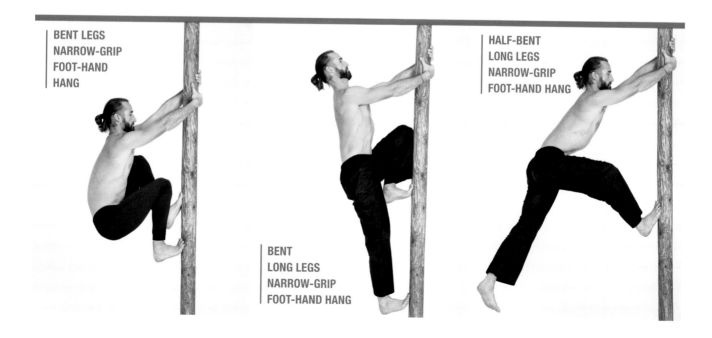

BENT LEGS
NARROW-GRIP
FOOT-HAND
HANG

BENT
LONG LEGS
NARROW-GRIP
FOOT-HAND HANG

HALF-BENT
LONG LEGS
NARROW-GRIP
FOOT-HAND HANG

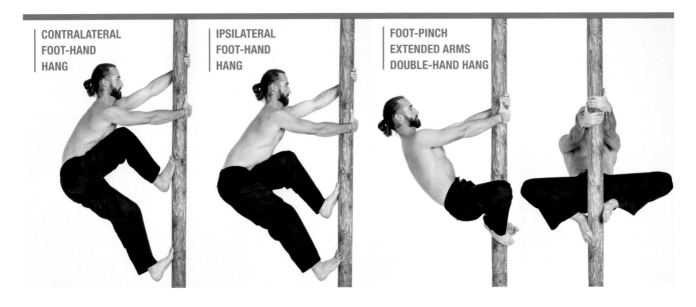

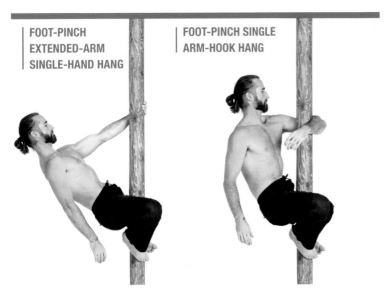

Push-Pull Movements

Foot-hand and foot-forearm hangs can be positions you use to move sideways, up-ward, or downward; you both push off the feet and pull from the hands or forearms. The simplest and easiest form of push-pull climbing patterns is used to scale a ladder or climb a tree that has "perfect" branches that provide easy and reliable horizontal sup-port for the feet and hands. Another relatively easy form of a push-pull climb is scram-bling up or down a not-too-steep slope. However, using this type of climb on a slope often implies a slippery surface such as grass, moss, gravel, sand, or unstable stones. As a surface gets more vertical, the surfaces for you to push or pull from get smaller and more slippery, which means the climbing gets more difficult. Of course, the farther apart vertically the handholds and footholds are, the more difficult it is to ascend. (In most cases, descending is more difficult, too.)

On Wide Vertical Surfaces

You can traverse a surface, such as a wall, rather than going upward or downward, by hanging from its top edge, pushing off your feet to step sideways, and pulling from your hands to move them in the same direction, alternately. You can do this with your arms fully extended or with them bent. You mostly bend your arms to increase frictional force and gripping strength when necessary.

The Push Power-Up technique is usually a final climbing action to exit climbing and enter another movement as you reach the top edge of the climbing surface, but that technique also can allow you to elevate your body enough to grasp higher handholds.

When you do the Push Power-Up explosively, you can do an upward jump with a high arm reach.

You can do the Push Power-Up on either natural or urban walls. Climbing over a tall wall often seems like a daunting, impossible mission for beginners. First you need to reach the top edge and grasp it with your hands; you can do that by either climbing or jumping.

Push Power-Up

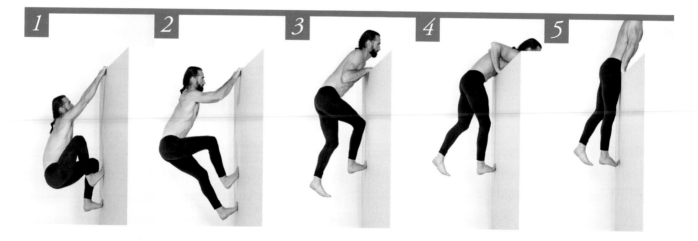

1   Start in a Split Bent-Legs Foot-Hand position.

2   Strongly push off your legs and, when you reach close to full extension, strongly flex your arms to pull from them to generate enough upward momentum to elevate your center of gravity quickly.

3   As you pull strongly with both arms in full flexion to reach close to maximum pulling elevation, swiftly slide your hands forward to a flat grip as you press down on the top supporting surface. As your body elevates, your lower foot naturally is released from providing support.

4   Without losing momentum, keep pulling up and forward with your modified hang grip until your elbows have raised above your hands, so you're transitioning from a pulling motion to a pushing motion. Keep pressing away from the vertical edge by pushing off the ball of your foot, which helps your balance.

5   Press up to a Vertical Hand Press position.

On Narrow Vertical Surfaces

The other push-pull climbing movements I want to explain are specifically for narrow vertical surfaces. Such surfaces can be either natural or man-made; they can be angled or completely vertical, thick or narrow, flat or rounded, even or uneven, stable or unstable.

Natural surfaces are thicker at the bottom and become thinner as they get higher, and they're not attached to anything at the top. As a result, your body weight may make some of these surfaces sway more and more as you climb higher, to the point they can bend under your weight. Man-made surfaces are often more stable because they're made of materials that don't bend and are sometimes attached to something at the top.

If the surface is at a slight angle, there's a greater risk that your feet will slip or you'll lose balance and go into a spinning swing, similarly to what would happen if you're moving in a balancing Foot-Hand Crawl on a narrow inclined surface. However, if your position does get inverted, you might be able to transition to an Arm-Leg Hang by curling your feet around the surface to create gripping friction similar to the position of your hands and turning muscular effort in your feet and legs to a pulling motion rather than a pushing one as you keep climbing. (As a matter of fact,

when approaching a narrow vertical surface that isn't at an angle, you have the option to climb from below in an Arm-Leg Hang fashion from the start, as I describe later in this chapter).

Of course, there's a limit to how thick the surface can be. Greater thicknesses reduce the space between the points of support and the front of your body, which reduces the range of motion of your limbs and demands much greater hand-grip strength for positions to be held. Thin and soft surfaces, such as ropes, must be approached with specific leg and foot positions that allow frictional force to be applied in the feet. Otherwise, climbing would be entirely left to upper-body power. Space in this book doesn't allow me to cover all techniques, so I'm focusing on the Foot-Hand Climb and the Foot-Pinch Climb. The Foot-Hand Climb is a "child" of the Foot-Hand Crawl pattern I discussed earlier in the book. As with the crawling version, you can do the Foot-Hand Climb in a four-three point of support pattern that alternates ipsilateral and contralateral positions, or in a four-two point of support pattern in either the ipsilateral or contralateral positions. With the Foot-Pinch techniques, your feet are level with each other, and you simultaneously move both legs.

4-3 Foot-Hand Climb

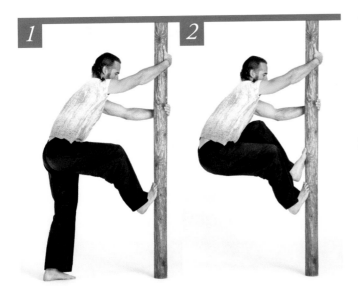

1   Stand in front of the vertical surface, reach out to it with both arms extended and vertically split with about one foot between them, and curl both hands around the surface. Center the ball of one foot on the surface where it's about level with the knee of the supporting leg. Keep the lead leg half flexed.

2   Shift your body weight onto the foot that's on the surface and push and control your balance as you release your trail foot. Place it just above the foot that's already on the surface in a contralateral Foot-Hand Hang. Find a position where you feel your body weight is nearly equally distributed among all four points of support.

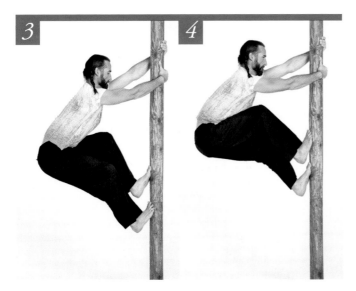

3 Release the lower hand (trail hand or inside hand) and reach up to regrip the surface. You'll briefly hang with three points of support as you do this. What was the lower hand is now the upper hand, and your position is now ipsilateral. If you instead were to move the trail foot upward first, you would end up in an uncomfortable, overly compact position.

4 Release and move the trail foot opposite to the hand you just moved and place it just above the upper foot. You'll briefly hang with three points of support as you do this. Your position has returned to a contralateral position on the side opposite from where you started.

TECHNIQUE TIP

If you place the lead foot higher when you step into hanging, the trail foot would have been positioned below it in an ipsilateral position. Because this is a 4-3 pattern, it doesn't really matter which of the two positions you start in. What matters the most is how balanced your position is at all times, and you should avoid positions that are too compact or too stretched. A rounded lower back is normal, but a rounded upper back usually indicates a position that's too compact or that there's a lack of tension in the scapula and shoulder girdle, which affects friction at the hands. The space between your feet should be nearly the same as the space between your hands and should be consistent as you climb; the space between your feet and hands will slightly narrow and widen as you move your feet and hands alternately, but the range should remain as consistent as possible.

The flexion in both legs should also remain consistent except for momentary modifications to ensure friction and balance. Your supporting arms should remain as extended as possible in a hanging fashion, to let your legs handle most of the upward motion as they extend. Bending your arms in a pulling action mostly creates early fatigue of the upper body. It could force the legs to extend, shifting your center of gravity forward and upward. This applies downward force and reduces friction in your feet, which increases the risk of foot slippage as well as the fatigue in the hands and arms. Unless the surface of support is such that you have to continuously rely on arm pulling and strength, you flex your arms only occasionally to reposition and ensure friction; when you do, make sure to maintain force in your feet perpendicular to the supporting surface.

An alternative foot position is the open foot, where the midfoot is on support at an angle with the surface of support. Depending on the surface, this position might allow greater friction and reduce the risk of foot slipping.

Open Foot-Hand Climb

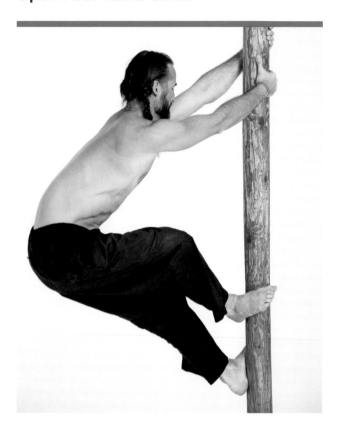

The Open-Foot-Hand Climb is a variation of the Foot-Hand Climb. The difference is that the feet are externally rotated on the surface of support. The advantage of this alternative foot positioning is to improve friction at the feet when a forward positioning isn't as reliable and could cause the feet to slide to the side and off support. The disadvantage of such positioning is that range of motion at the feet and ankle is reduced, which reduces the extension of the legs and forces smaller steps. It's useful whenever you want to pause and rest in the Foot-Hand Climb or to transition to the Foot-Pinch Climb (or from the Foot-Pinch Climb back to the Foot-Hand Climb). To transition from the Foot-Hand Climb to the Foot-Pinch position, you first transition to the Open-Foot-Hand Climb stance, level your feet, and then bend your legs or lower your knees to the Foot-Pinch Climb position.

Faults

The next two photos show the main inefficiencies with the Foot-Pinch Hang. Neither of these positions is sustainable.

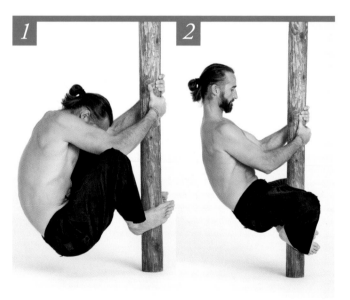

1   Your back is compact and rounded, and your arms are bent. The knees are high with only a narrow space between them. If you extend your arms, your hand grip becomes really difficult to maintain, and you might lose your grip. If you bring your hands higher or your feet lower, downward force is applied on your feet without an opposite force; your feet will slide down, and your body will follow and fully extend downward.

2   Opposite force is applied through your feet against the surface, which is an improvement on the first position, but your arms remain flexed unnecessarily, which wastes precious strength.

Foot-Pinch Climb

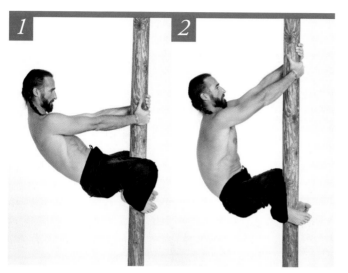

1 Establish the Foot-Pinch Hang on the surface.

TECHNIQUE TIP

You can enter the Foot-Pinch Hang by grasping the surface with your hands and then stepping or jumping into position. Advanced entries include climbing into position from another elevated surface (tree to tree, for instance) or landing in position after a jump from a distance.

2 Move your hands higher while keeping them extended, which causes your torso to be more vertical.

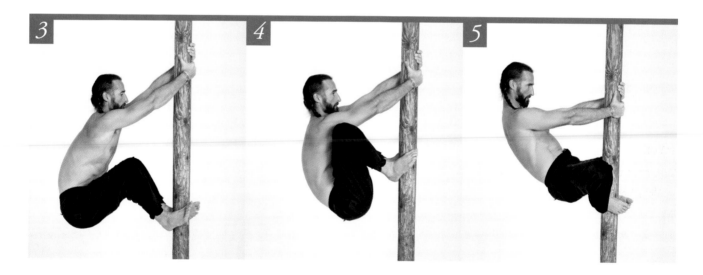

3 Push through your legs, driving your hips away from the surface to create space for your leg to move up.

4 In a swift motion, tuck your knees all the way up to bring your feet from below rear level to about sternum level. Make sure that you keep your feet pointing out enough (with your heels close together) to ensure stability and prevent slipping. Your body should be in a compact position, with your knees at shoulder level and your legs close to your body with little space in between your legs and body.

5 Pull from the scapula/shoulder girdle while keeping your arms lengthened to drive your hips up and forward while opening your legs and lowering your knees on each side to create optimum frictional force in a more stable and efficient Foot-Pinch Hang. From here, repeat the same sequence to keep moving up the surface.

NOTE

Sometimes while in the Foot-Pinch climb you may find yourself off-balance and pulled to a sideways spin. This type of motion is dictated by the environment, and it naturally brings you back in a balanced position, just with a little different orientation. Once such motion is triggered, it's nearly impossible to stop and takes an enormous amount of strength if you try to. It is best to go with the flow and not resist it.

Climbing Down

Climbing down can be tricky because it's easy to not pay attention and be pulled into full-body extension so that you slide down with little control. You're safe from a fall if you can maintain a hang as you're sliding—for instance, by wrapping both arms and legs around the surface—but this can easily cause you to be badly scratched or burned because of kinetic friction. Following are the key points for a controlled descent:

- Don't attempt to move down too fast.
- Foot-hand "strides" should not be significantly longer than when you move up. From a stable Foot-Pinch Hang, don't let your feet move down too far, or you'll extend your legs and body too much and too vertically, which increases vertical force onto your feet and makes them slide down to a point where gripping friction is lost; then you lose gripping friction force in your hands.
- Move your hands down very rapidly after you move your feet, so you can quickly replicate the Foot-Pinch Hang a little farther down.

NOTE

Some people living in exotic areas have maintained tremendous ability to quickly scale coconut trees using mostly the Open-Foot Foot-Hand Climb with their bare hands and feet, which demands great skill, strength, and mental fortitude. They also traditionally use some kind of strap or rope tied around their feet in a loop, which prevents their feet from slipping out of support and facilitates friction at the feet, enabling the climber to move faster with a more extended body and longer strides.

Pull Hangs

Now it's time for me to address hanging positions and movements entirely based on points of support located above your center of gravity, regardless of the body parts used for support: hands, feet, or something else. There's no pushing from points of support located beneath the center of gravity; these positions and movements are strict hangs or "pull hangs." This is normally the case when the supporting surface is horizontal or at a slight angle, and it's narrow, such as a tree limb, a rope, a cable, or the edge of a platform with a void beneath it.

Pull hangs can have two different body orientations:

- The side hang in which all points of support are hanging from the same side of the supporting surface
- The front hang in which points of support are hanging from both sides of it

For practice purposes, to enter pull hang positions (either arm hangs or arm-leg hangs), you need to practice on a surface that's elevated enough for you to hang from your hands without your feet touching the ground, but it shouldn't be too high for you to reach it relatively easily. The height should be safe and not intimidating. You might have to jump up a bit or step up onto something for your hands to reach the surface. The latter option is the easier and safer one for beginners.

However, in the real world, you might have to start in a Double-Hand Hang without the option of stepping up on a raised surface, maybe after jumping upward to a High Hand Reach to grasp the supporting surface—such as a high-hanging branch—then to be able to hold this position with 100 percent of your body weight hanging only from your hands (and sometimes only one hand before you can place the second hand) before you can elevate your legs to establish a three- or four-limbed hang. Beyond the benefits of developing upper-body joint strength and mobility, the ability to hold strong arm-hangs is extremely important for a practical reason because, in most cases, it's a necessary transition to establishing arm-leg hangs.

This is the progression I'm taking you through:

- Arm hangs and sideways arm-hang movements.
- Strategies to transition from arm hangs to arm-leg hangs.
- Arm-leg hangs and sideways arm and leg movements
- Upward arm-leg hang movements

I finish this chapter with the most power-demanding upward arm-hang movements.

Arm Hangs

Some climbing positions are "side" hangs, which means the orientation of your body is parallel to the surface; other hangs are "front," which is when your orientation is perpendicular to the surface.

By default, arm hangs are "low" in the sense that you are using only the minimal level of tension required to maintain the hang and avoid falling off the support surface, letting gravity pull your center of gravity farther down and away below your base of support. However, additional tension may be necessary to elevate your position, which raises your center of gravity closer to the base of support. For this reason I occasionally specify the height of the elevation of a given hang position as low, mid, or high.

The base of support of an arm hang can be narrow, neutral, or wide depending on the space between the points of support.

Here are some practical examples of the pros and cons of particular positions, which show that choice of position is contextual and depends on the physical action you intend to perform and/or on the surface where it is done :

- A wide grip in a side Double-Hand Hang is not efficient for upward movement, but it's efficient for ample and fast side-swing traversing if gripping friction is reliable.
- Scapular activation isn't necessary in an arm hang unless it helps with gripping friction, if it's part of transition to another movement, or if you need to protect your shoulder joints.
- You can't Side Swing efficiently in a Forearm Hang, but you can move upward (pop up).
- You can't Front Swing Traverse efficiently in a Double-Arm-Hook Front Hang, but you can Front Swing to establish a Double-Arm-Hook Foot-Pinch Hang.
- A Double-Armpit Hang is great for resting, but it doesn't enable you to pull upward.

You should develop an understanding of the specific role of each arm-hang position and practice holding them all with sufficient strength and control.

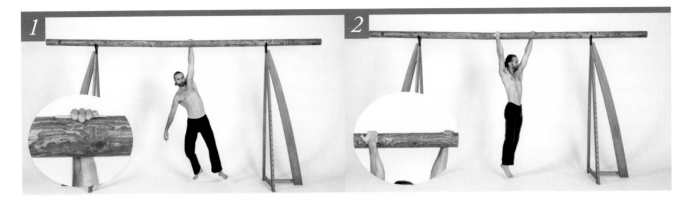

1 Single-Hand Hang: The body tends to rotate until it stabilizes itself in a side position. Hanging with one arm usually happens statically after a High Hand-Reach Jump or dynamically with a swing to reach up or out with the other hand.

2 Neutral-Base, Double-Hand Front Hang: Your hands are about shoulder width apart. This hang is mostly used for Front Swing Traversing.

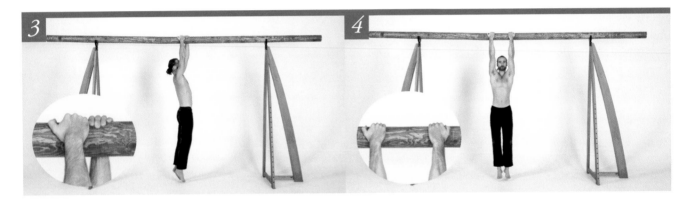

3 Narrow-Base, Double-Hand Front Hang: This hang is normally used to secure a strong grip before you elevate the legs to an arm-leg hang. You can interlace your fingers to add friction to the grip.

4 Supine-Grip, Neutral-Base, Double-Hand Side Hang: The base width is typical, but the hang grip is unusual because usually a prone grip is used.

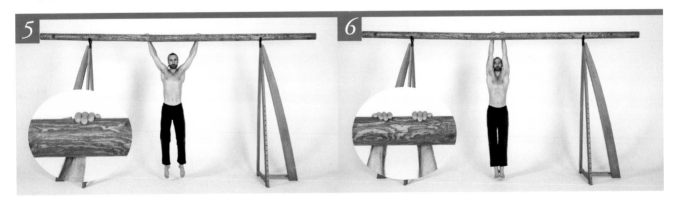

5 Wide-Base, Double-Hand Side Hang (Dead Hang): This is inefficient for upward movements, but it's efficient for Side Swing Traversing.

6 Narrow-Base, Double-Hand Side Hang: You use this hang when it helps secure frictional grip or as a transition in arm-hang traversing.

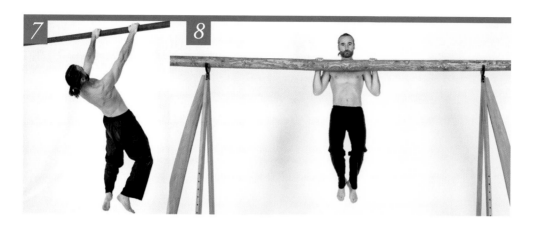

7   **Scapular Pull Double-Hand Hang:** Use this hang with tension or back lean to strengthen gripping, protect shoulder joints, change your line of vision, or prepare for an upward motion.

8   **High Double-Hand Side Hang** (called Mid Side Arm Hang when there's half flexion): You can use this Raised Hang when you must perform a transition from a low Double-Hand Side Hang to a Double-Forearm Hang (or the other way around) slowly or with caution.

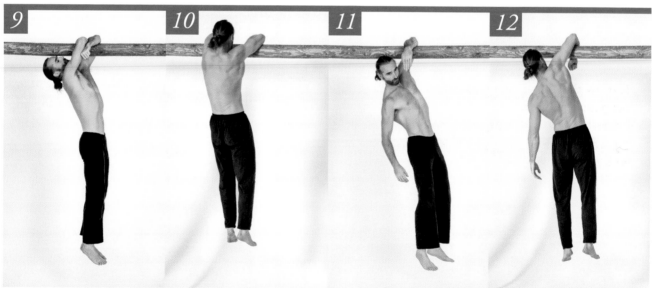

(continued on next page)

9   **Double-Arm-Hook Front Hang:** You can use this hang to transition to an arm-leg hang or to secure an arm hang when hanging from the hands isn't possible. You also can use it as a rest or recovery hang.

10 **Double-Arm-Hook Side Hang:** Same as above.

11 **Single-Arm-Hook Front Hang:** In this hang, your head is on the opposite side of your supporting arm.

12 **Single-Arm-Hook Side Hang:** In this hang, your head is on the same side as your supporting arm.

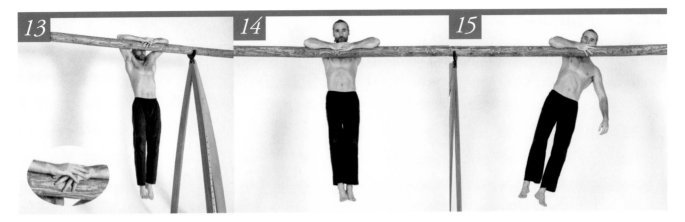

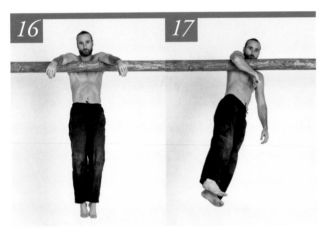

13 Low Double-Forearm Side Hang: This position precedes the Pop-Up (upward) or after you lower the body from a High Double-Forearm Hang. You also can use it as a transition to or from an arm-leg hang.

14 High Double-Forearm Side Hang: You can use this hang to elevate your hips to facilitate hooking a leg in an arm-leg hang.

15 High Single-Forearm Side Hang: You usually use this hang to securely transition from the Double-Hand Hang to the Double-Forearm Hang or the other way around.

16 Double-Armpit Hang: This is a rest or recovery hang.

17 Single-Armpit Hang: Same as above.

SAFETY NOTE

Safety in arm hangs is enhanced mostly by an increase in muscular strength—mostly in grip strength and shoulder girdle strength—which naturally develops as you hang more frequently for longer periods of time on thicker support surfaces or as you move more dynamically while hanging.

Sideways Arm-Hang Movements

You can use double-hand hangs to move sideways using either power or gravity and momentum. Because they rely only on the hands, the hangs become more challenging as more momentum is used, the surface of the support becomes thicker, or the surface becomes more slippery.

Slide Side Traverse

The Slide Side Traverse is an entry arm-hang traverse that's straightforward and requires no technique and little strength because it's done with minimal body swing and no arm flexion. Therefore, it's conveniently used by people who don't have enough strength to perform other arm-hang traverse techniques yet. You may also alternate the Side Swing Traverse with a Slide Swing Traverse as long as you intentionally keep increasing the otherwise slight side swing the Slide Swing Traverse naturally generates.

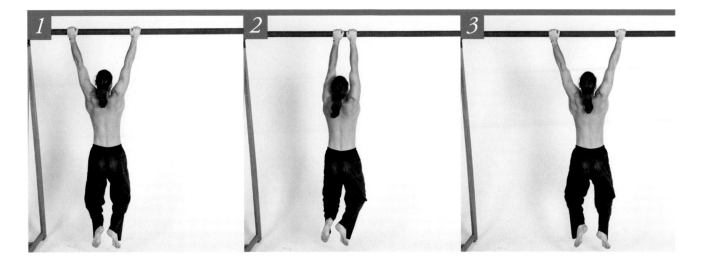

1 Begin in a Wide-Base Double-Hand Hang.

2 Release your rear hand to slide it forward and place it next to your other hand, which puts you in a narrow-base hang. As you move your rear hand, your front hand becomes the main point of support for your body weight, which helps your center of gravity shift in the direction you're heading. Keep your shoulder blades retracted, which is easy because the supporting surface is used as a guide for the hand, arm, and shoulder position.

3 Release your forward hand and slide it forward to reach it as far forward as possible if you have great frictional grip; otherwise, shorter distances are safer.

Side Swing and Side Swing Traverse

The Side Swing is a dynamic, pendulum-like approach to traversing that's energy-efficient and requires no power. However, it does demand great grip strength—especially if the support surface is thick—because a swing momentum is involved with full body weight briefly supported by a single hand as the other hand slides over the supporting surface to move forward. You also must have the ability to keep your upper body and lower body tightly connected through your core to maintain positional control and balance.

You will maintain the same body orientation parallel to the surface of support at all times. You can reduce or increase both the amplitude of the swing and the width of the base of support, which makes the level of difficulty of the movement easily manageable. When the surface is rounded, the movement becomes ineffective past a certain thickness. When that happens, or if the surface is slippery, it's best to opt for a Power Side Traverse or even an Arm-Leg Hang Traverse.

The Double-Hand Hang Side Swing is involved in this technique, which means you should first learn it as a separate, stationary drill (see the next section) so you can create more swing momentum and amplitude through the combination of muscular action and the pull of gravity while still maintaining positional control. The Side Swing also is useful to efficiently transition to arm-leg hang positions from the Double-Hand Side Hang.

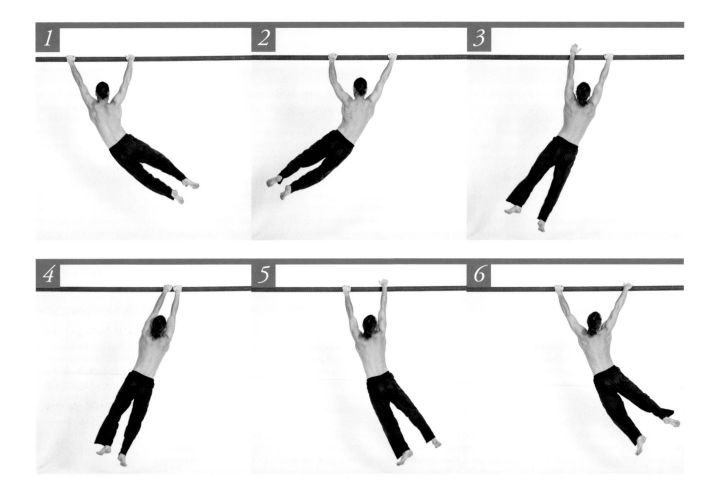

1   Begin in a Neutral-Base Double-Hand Hang. You can make the base a little wider, depending on your grip strength and how ample you want your movement to be. Keep your shoulder blades retracted and your arms extended and raise your hips and legs to one side, contracting your obliques to initiate the movement. You don't need to force your legs to elevate too high; you can progressively gain greater elevation through several Side Swing motions. You should entirely generate the swing momentum through the lower body without active assistance from your arms.

2   Allow gravity to pull you back down and swing you up on the other side. As your legs start to elevate on the other side, you may assist the momentum by contracting your obliques to keep elevating your hips and legs a little higher. You don't need to pull on your arms to generate momentum. Your rear arm may passively bend slightly because of the elevation of your center of gravity; otherwise,

both arms remain in the lockout position. You may swing forward and backward one more time if you feel that you need more momentum, or you can do it as a practice drill.

3   As your legs reach the top of the back swing and as the momentum makes your rear hand feel light, release your rear hand. The forward swing immediately accelerates as your base of support suddenly shifts forward while your center of gravity is high at the back, so your center of gravity is pulled down and forward very swiftly.

4   Before your legs return to center, put your free hand back on the supporting surface as close as possible to your fixed hand in a narrow-base hang.

5   As you enter the front half of the swing, release the front hand and extend your front arm forward.

6   Place your front hand farther on the supporting surface as you reach the top of the swing. From here, let your body swing back and resume the motion from step 4.

TECHNIQUE TIP

You may use upper-body strength and pull with the arms at any point during the Side Swing Traverse to tighten your grip if you feel that it's unsure. Losing your grip means immediately falling. Otherwise, keep your arms relaxed whenever possible.

You may also intentionally drive the Side Swing motion entirely through the arms with two benefits: teaching you the difference between driving the Side Swing motion from the lower body and driving it from the upper body and building upper-body pulling strength.

Stationary Double-Hand Hang Side Swing Drill

Combine steps 1 and 2 from the Side Swing Traverse in a repetitive sequence. You can use this drill to learn to control a stable and efficient hanging Side Swing position and motion (see the faults later in this section) or to warm up for the Side Swing Traverse.

(An alternative drill involves generating the Side Swing motion by flexing your arms to build upper-body strength that is useful in the Power Side Traverse).

Faults

- Generating the swing by pulling down the arms.
- Leading the sequence through your arms instead of allowing the Side Swing to determine the timing of your arm sequence, which disrupts the rhythm of the technique.
- Generating too much or not enough swing amplitude in relation to the width or the base of support. The amplitude of the Side Swing should match the width of the base of support. Use less amplitude with a narrower base, and more amplitude with a wider base.
- Lack of positional control with hip rotation that results in altering the direction of the swing and your balance.

Arm Hang to Arm-Leg Hang Transitions

To transition from arm hangs to arm-leg hangs, you must be able to elevate your legs all the way to the surface of support. The types of hangs you use depend first on how reliable a given arm-hang position is on a given surface and your level of strength at a given moment. Other factors include your body orientation in relation to the supporting surface (which relates to the movement you want to do after the transition), your level of strength, and how fast you want to do the transition. Contrary to common belief, relatively little upper-body strength is required for these transitions, but a certain level of abdominal strength is essential. In the absence of the minimum level of strength required, even the easiest methods are out of reach.

The most efficient way to do the transition starts in a Narrow-Base, Double-Hand Front Hang. You use body-weight transfer through a Front Swing to reach a Double-Hand Foot-Pinch Hang. From there, you can establish a more elevated arm-leg hang. The next strategy is to start in a Double-Hand Side Hang and use a Side Swing to reach a Double-Hand Single-Leg-Hook Hang. Both strategies are the prerequisite to being able to do a Swing Up.

Beyond those two methods that use momentum, you can make similar transitions by relying only on strength to elevate the legs toward the surface of support, which is faster but more energy costly. It's also a good idea to avoid the swing momentum if gripping friction in an arm hang is challenging—for instance, if the surface of support tends to be slippery. However, you should develop the ability to perform these transitions either way with the same level of ease, and training both is mutually beneficial: The swing momentum–assisted approach helps develop greater abdominal strength, and the strength-based, no-momentum approach develops greater abdominal and core strength, which makes the swing-momentum method even easier and more effective. In fact, the abdominal strength gained through those drills is also essential for upward climbing movements from a Double-Hand Side Hang, such as the Pop-Up, Power-Up, or Roll-Up.

Drills

When the supporting surface is horizontal, your feet or legs must move 45 degrees from an arm-hang vertical position to become points of support in an arm-leg hang horizontal body position. The higher you elevate your hips and legs, the more horizontal your body position becomes.

If the supporting surface is at an angle, your hands or arms should be higher than your legs; otherwise, an inverted position becomes less and less sustainable as the angle increase and the legs are at a higher level than the hands or arms. This holds true for techniques such as the Swing-Up and for the traversing arm-leg hang techniques. The greater the angle (closer to a vertical surface), the shorter and easier the transition in terms of abdominal strength (although the greater the demand on hand grip strength), which can be a better approach for beginners who lack the abdominal strength needed for a horizontal surface.

Drills should be done with swing momentum first; then you progress to doing them without momentum as you build strength. The most difficult progressions don't use momentum and are as explosive as possible to build power.

Following is a list of drills that are components of transitions, in which you elevate your legs progressively higher.

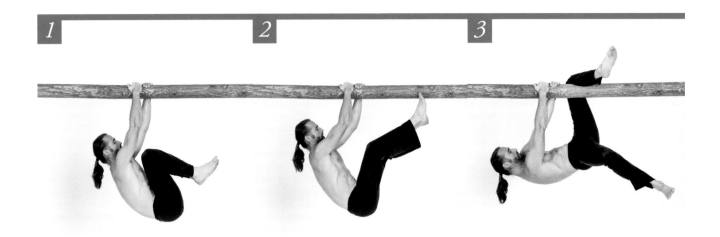

1   Knee tucks as high as you can

2   Feet to hand level (touch the surface of support)

3   Single-leg hook from a side arm-hang

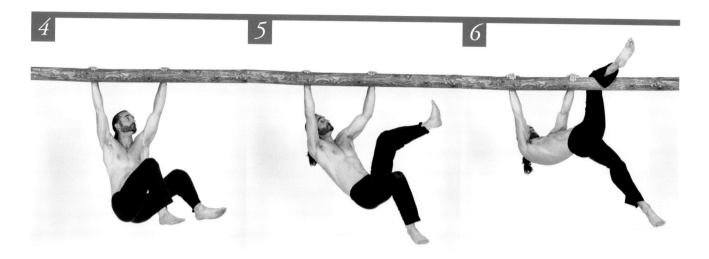

4 Side knee tucks

5 Single-side foot to hand level (touch the surface of support)

6 Single-leg hook

Arm-Leg Hangs

Arm-leg hangs are stronger, more secure, and more reliable than arm hangs, which is especially import-ant if you're dealing with an added load (for example, light equipment, clothing, or heavy footwear) or if you're already fatigued. You can hold an arm-leg hang for a relatively brief time to rest before returning to an arm hang or as a transitional position to achieve more elevated positions above the supporting sur-face. Most arm-leg hangs are front hangs because they use points of support on each side of the supporting surface, which means you can use only traversing movements. Side hangs, in which all points of sup-port are on one side of the supporting surface, enable upward climbing movements, such as the Swing-Up.

The positions in the next set of photos display pro-gressively more elevated points of support, which is not related to the level of difficulty or importance of such-or-such hang. Only through practice can you discover what positions are more difficult for you and what practical value is attached to each position.

TECHNIQUE TIP

Approach arm-leg hangs with the same attention to variety I've mentioned before. Switching from position to position can easily make for a grueling "workout."

SAFETY NOTE

Holding a horizontal hang with your back facing down is not as safe as hanging by your hands with your feet close to the ground. Safe practice means starting with low heights and thin surfaces; you need to be ready to let go of your feet or legs before letting go of your arms so that you regain a vertical position prior to releasing the hang entirely. A crash pad or person to spot you is very handy.

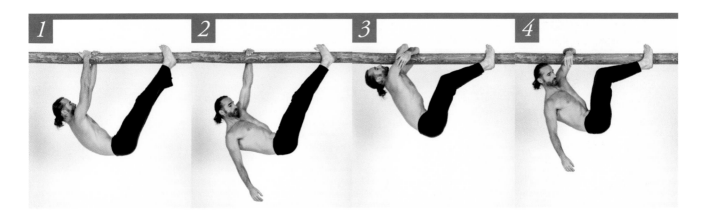

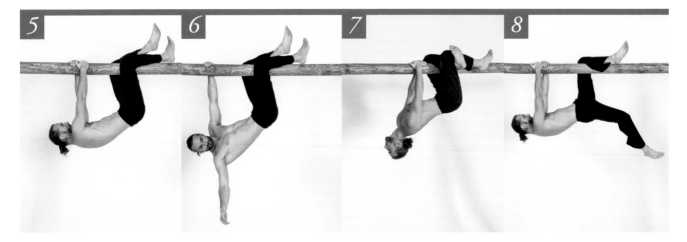

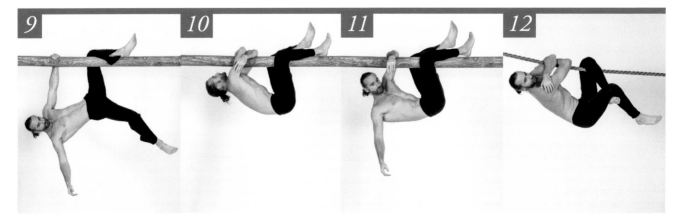

1   Double-Hand Foot-Pinch Hang

2   Single-Hand Foot-Pinch Hang

3   Double-Arm-Hook Foot-Pinch Hang

4   Single-Arm-Hook Foot-Pinch Hang

5   Double-Hand, Double-Leg-Hook Hang

6   Single-Hand, Double-Leg-Hook Hang

7   Double-Hand, Triangle-Leg -Hook Hang

8   Double-Hand, Single-Leg-Hook Hang

9   Ipsilateral Single-Hand, Single-Leg-Hook Hang
    (also possible in a contralateral position)

10 Double-Arm-Hook, Double-Leg-Hook Hang

11 Single-Arm-Hook, Double-Leg-Hook Hang

12 Double-Arm-Hook, Triangle-Leg Hook Hang

13 Contralateral Single-Arm-Hook, Single-Leg-Hook Hang

14 Contralateral Single-Forearm, Single-Leg-Hook Hang

15 Ipsilateral Single-Forearm, Single-Leg-Hook Hang

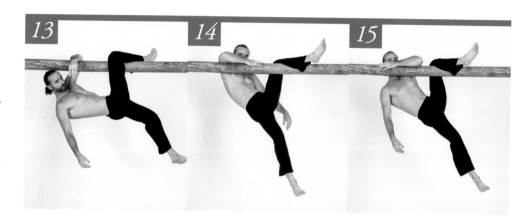

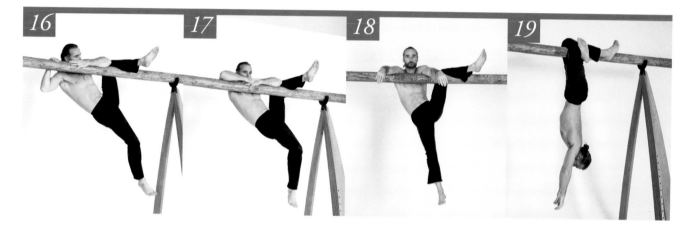

16 Single-Hand, Single-Forearm, Single-Leg-Hook Hang

17 Double-Forearm, Single-Leg-Hook Hang

18 Double-Armpit Single-Leg-Hook Hang

19 Triangle-Leg-Hook Hang (inverted vertical position)

Arm-Leg Hang Traverse Movements

Traversing a horizontal surface (a long tree limb, a metal pole, or a rope) by balancing on top of it may-be impossible, very unsafe, or just too slow, especially when the surface is narrow, rounded, slippery, or unstable. Those problematic factors can be made even worse if strong winds are blowing, if it's raining and dark, if you're fatigued and lack mental sharpness, or if you're carrying a load. The Leg-Hook Traverse can be a more effective and safer way to deal with such environmental variables.

The Leg-Hook Traverse is an effective alternative to all the problems with balancing. If you unintentionally go into an arm-leg hang after losing balance, you may resume movement in a hang instead of going through the effort of re-establishing a top balancing position. The Swing Leg-Hook Traverse is another arm-leg hang technique that's faster than the Leg-Hook Traverse, but it works only with great gripping friction, such as when you're hanging from a rope.

The direction of the movement in such inverted hang positions can seem counterintuitive, as going forward means that you're going in the direction of your head and going backward means you're moving in the direction of your feet. Going forward in the direction of your head is more intuitive and easier and always preferred to moving backward in the direction of your feet, unless you're climbing down a declined surface of support. Indeed, when the surface of support is at an angle, the more efficient positioning is with the hands holding on the higher side of the surface with your legs on the lower side, regardless of whether you're going upward or downward.

Leg-Hook Traverse

With both arm and leg points of support on both sides, the Leg-Hook Traverse enables you to traverse the supporting surface with a pattern like the Foot-Hand Crawl. The Leg-Hook Traverse is a 4-3 points of support sequence, but it's in an inverted, hanging position. It's slower than its swinging counterpart, but it's stronger, safer, and more economical.

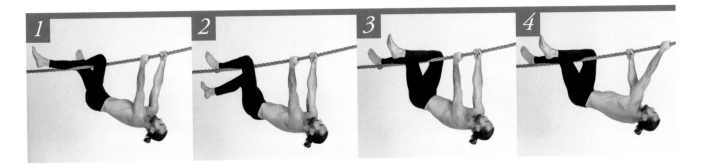

1   Assume a contralateral Double-Hand, Double-Leg-Hook Hang. On one side of your body, your leg and hand are relatively close to each other, whereas they're more distant from each other on the other side. Your front leg is more securely hooked at a close angle (it's more perpendicularly angled with the surface, and your foot is slightly below the knee of the same leg) than the rear one; the front leg is the point of support while you release the rear leg as you move. There must be sufficient space between the front leg and rear hand so that the rear leg can be positioned between the two without creating a stiff, compact position. Keep your arms straight whenever possible.

2   Shift your body weight more to the front leg so you can release the rear leg and slide the rear leg off the rope. A quick release of the leg or an unstable surface might cause your center of gravity to shift and make you slightly swing. In this case, you may use the momentum created to move the free leg forward slightly toward your hands.

3   Hook the moving leg over the supporting surface in front of the supporting leg and behind the rear hand, securing the point of support in your kneepit (the back of the knee). At this point you're in a hanging ipsilateral position, but you're also more secure with four points of support.

4   Release the rear hand and reach it forward overhead to return to the starting contralateral position but on the opposite side. From there, repeat the sequence on the other side to continue traversing forward.

TECHNIQUE TIP

Start practicing on a horizontal surface that provides a strong grip for your hands but is gentle on your kneepits (such as a metal bar that's two or three inches in diameter) and isn't too high so you can easily get into position and step down. Progressions include surfaces that are thicker, unstable, and more slippery.

Optionally, you can hook your arms around the surface. You can use the arm-hook option when the surface becomes less secure or as a position for a temporary recovery. This option is slower because it shortens your arm reach (how far you can extend your arms to create a further point of support), but it's easier to prevent the hooked arm from sliding off the surface than it is to prevent your hand from losing its grip.

Another option is the Heel-Hook Traverse, but that movement works only with boots that accentuate the back of the heel and allow enough friction for it to become a point of support.

Swing Leg-Hook Traverse

This technique provides a very fast method of traversing a rope, but it requires great frictional grip in the hands, great abdominal strength, and impeccable positional control and coordination to replicate the sequence with flawless timing. In short, even if you possess the strength required for the movement, you can become confused easily if your technique isn't sharp. Once you've mastered it, you might feel like a pirate on his way to board another ship.

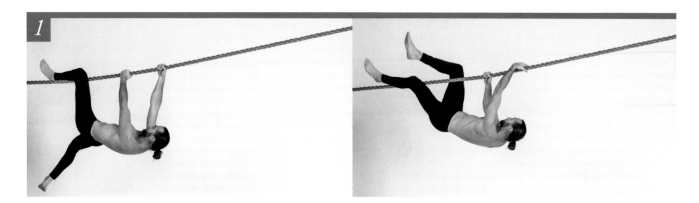

1   Begin in a Double-Hand, Single-Leg-Hook Hang with your free leg fully relaxed and extended beneath you. Swing your free leg up toward the rope. At the top of the swing, the momentum of the swinging leg causes your weight to

lift off the supporting leg, which enables you to simultaneously release that leg. Using a contralateral pattern, bring the hand opposite the swinging leg forward, and grip the rope as far forward as possible.

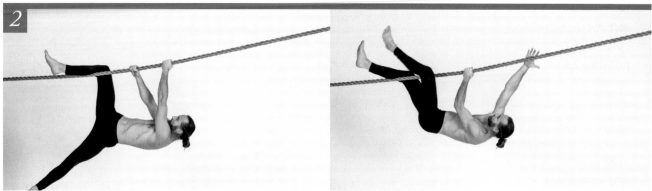

(continued on next page)

2   As you hook the swinging leg around the rope, pull yourself forward by bringing your arms toward your hips so that your shoulders are directly under your hands. Allow your free leg to hang beneath you in full extension. Repeat the pattern on the other side by swinging your free leg up toward

the rope. Again, as your weight shifts off the supporting leg, release it and simultaneously reach the hand on the opposite side as the swinging leg as far forward as possible, pulling yourself forward along the rope with the other arm.

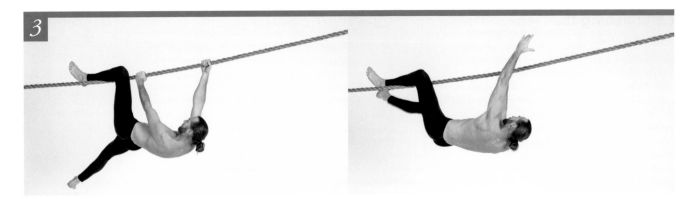

3 Hook your swinging leg over the rope and finish in a Double-Hand, Single-Leg Hook Hang. Continue along the rope by repeating steps 1 and 2.

Faults

Faults in the Swing Leg-Hook Traverse are usually like the faults for the Leg-Hook Traverse except that they tend to be magnified by the swinging momentum of the movement. Re-establishing a reliable leg position is the most important part of efficiency in this technique. What also often happens is that when you reposition the leg, it's easy to pull it too high and shrink your position or to not move the trail hand as you reposition the hooked leg, which ends in entangled legs and hands.

Arm-Leg Hang Upward Movements

Establishing a balanced position on top of a horizontal surface of support starting from a Double-Hand Hang, without jumping momentum or pushing off anything with your feet, is not only a practical skill; it's an incredibly rewarding—even exhilarating—experience the first time you achieve it. This can be done with no less than six techniques, three of which are arm-leg hang movements. The three others are arm-hang movements.

The arm-leg hang upward movement techniques are called *swing-ups*. Interestingly, the upward movements from arm-leg hangs are skill-to-skill transitions to balancing in the sense that the top position is basically a balancing position.

I start with the most approachable movement that employs the easiest strategy, which is the Sliding Swing-Up. (Keep in mind that *easiest* does not mean *easy* in any way.) Although the method relies a lot on technique, it also relies on a fundamental level of strength that no amount of technique can replace. One of the big challenges that beginners face is being able to establish the arm-leg hang from the Double-Hand Hang without assistance—no jumping into position or pushing with the feet on a vertical surface. Therefore, all the necessary stages and transitions involved can be broken down into simpler, specific drills to help you build the strength, stability, and confidence you need to perform the entire sequence effectively.

The fastest way to transition from the Double-Hand Hang to an arm-leg hang is to simply pull yourself directly into it.

However, such a transition requires strength that you might not have developed yet. So, before I describe the Sliding Swing-Up per se, I show you the transition from a Double-Hand Hang to an arm-leg hang called the Double-Forearm, Single-Leg-Hook Hang that's more accessible to those who lack strength. This transition combined with the Sliding Swing-Up represents the easiest method to mount to the top of a horizontal support surface from a Double-Hand Hang without assistance.

Establishing the Double-Forearm, Single-Leg-Hook Hang

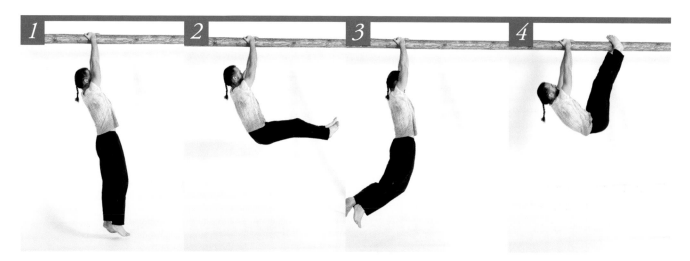

1   Assume a stationary Narrow-Base, Double-Hand Front Hang. You may interlace your fingers for better hand grip.

2   Initiate a Front Swing. Optionally, if you lack abdominal strength but possess some upper-body strength, during the Front Swing you could flex your arms to help your feet elevate.

3   Allow your legs to swing behind you.

4   Use the momentum of your legs as they swing forward again to lift your feet all the way to the surface, so you can grip it with your arches to establish a Double-Hand Foot-Pinch Hang.

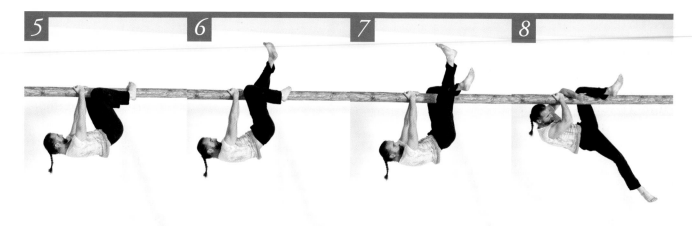

(continued on next page)

5   Keep your arms extended, and pull from your feet to elevate your knees to the surface and grip it in a knee pinch.

6   Slide one leg up and over the top of the surface, and bend your knee to form a leg-hook. From here you may pull up with your arms to arm-hook the arm that's on the same side as the leg-hook. Otherwise, use a swing momentum from your leg to help transition to the arm-hook.

7   Extend your other leg straight up.

8   Swing your extended leg down to generate momentum and immediately pull up with your arms.

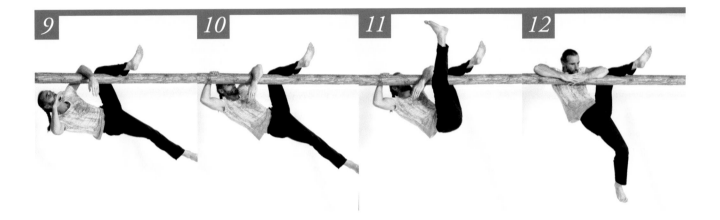

9 Keep your free leg and hip relaxed. Release the hand of your free arm, which puts you in an ipsilateral Single-Arm-Hook, Single-Leg-Hook Hang.

10 Place your free hand on the support on the same side as your hooking arm and leg using a prone grip.

11 Lift your free leg straight up in front of you on the side opposite your hooked leg.

12 Swing the free leg down swiftly to generate momentum and enable your lower arm to come on top of the surface at the top of your pull. Establish a Double-Forearm, Single-Leg-Hook Hang.

TECHNIQUE TIP

After you've worked through the steps to establish an arm-leg hang, you're in a position that enables you to mount to the top. Regardless of the variation of the swing-up you're using, remember that because you're hooking only one leg to the side, all variations are unilateral movements. Therefore, you must practice on both sides (alternating the leg you hook) to develop equal ability on both sides.

If the support surface is inclined at an angle, the hooked leg must be on the side lower than your arms and upper body.

SAFETY NOTE

Unstable horizontal surfaces can easily throw off your balance the moment you swing your leg to create momentum, so they're the most challenging surfaces on which to practice swing-ups.

Sliding Swing-Up

You start the Sliding Swing-Up by hanging with both armpits and a single leg hooked on the side. You do the movement mostly with body-weight transfer that you generate with the legs, and you do almost no pulling from the upper body. The Sliding Swing-Up is a great entry to the swing-up variations; because you can't pull from the upper body at all, this movement teaches you to use your legs and to maximize body-weight transfer efficiency through the leg swing, which is important with every other variation of the swing-up.

TECHNIQUE TIP

Because your chest remains in close contact with (even rubbing against) the supporting surface, the Sliding Swing-Up can be an uncomfortable movement. For that reason, women could opt for a hybrid version that mixes the Sliding Swing-Up pattern with the Forearm Swing-Up pattern that's shown next.

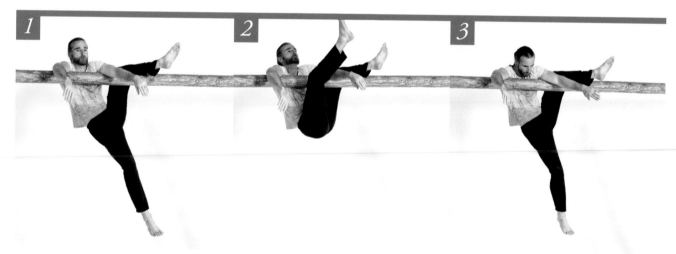

(continued on next page)

1 If the supporting surface is not already positioned under your armpits, push down on the supporting surface with your forearms to elevate your chest just enough to slide your position onto your armpits. Both arms should be extended in front of you and relaxed. This is the base position for the Sliding Swing-Up.

2 Bring your free leg up in front of you in preparation for another swift leg-and-hip swing.

3 Swing your free leg down swiftly and with amplitude.

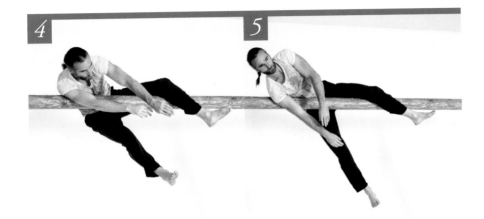

4   As your hips rise in the back, pull down on the supporting surface using your hooked leg, and lean toward the side of your swinging leg to get your armpit on the side of the hooked leg clear of the supporting surface and above it. Maintain downward pressure through the supporting arm to keep elevating your center of gravity.

5   As your hips and center of gravity have raised to their highest point, you're exiting a hanging position to enter a balancing position. The pull motion of your hooked leg turns into a push motion, which pushes your torso to extend to the side along the supporting surface until you reach full extension. Maintain balance over the supporting surface. Elevate your hips and upper body a little more until you've shifted your center of gravity vertically above your base of support.

TECHNIQUE TIP

Beginners tend to try to secure their position with their hands and arms by grasping the top of the support surface. This is an inefficient reflex because your balance on top does not rely on tension in your arms; it relies on your center of gravity being well balanced above your base of support. If you feel that gravity keeps pulling you backward, you should pull through your hooked leg and press down with the inside of your upper arms.

When you're in a balancing position on top of the surface, you may place your palms down on the surface to extend your arms and torso to a Tripod Get-Up or slide your supporting arm out to the other side to a Prone Lying or Straddle Sit balancing position. The first time you get to the top without assistance, you will probably feel ecstatic!

TECHNIQUE TIP

The leg swing is critical to generating the momentum required to elevate your center of gravity high enough before you pull from the arms. If the leg swing lacks speed or amplitude, momentum is not produced at a sufficient level to do this. Your leg doesn't necessarily have to be fully extended before or during the swing. What matters most is that the motion at the hip is strong; however, the extension of the leg supports a swifter hip motion and greater levels of segmental momentum through your leg and hip.

Faults

Once the base position has been established, the following faults occur frequently:

- The supporting leg isn't hooked correctly; the leg is supported on the calf rather than behind the knee. Sometimes, there's too little tension in the hamstring for the position to be secure. When the leg isn't hooked correctly, the position is too weak to handle and transfer the momentum of the leg swing, and an effort to recover a stable position becomes more important than the elevation of the position.

- The leg swing lacks velocity, amplitude, or both. The body swings back but not high (or not high enough).

- Bringing the swinging leg back to the front will shift the center of gravity forward and down.

- Not pulling from the hooked leg after the leg swing.

- After the leg swing, the body goes upward first, then upward and sideways, and finally sideways. Trying to elevate the body upwardly only instead of sideways ends up with gravity pulling the body back down.

- Not pushing off the hooked leg prevents you from pushing the body sideways to finish elevating the center of gravity to a balancing position above the surface of support.

Forearm Swing-Up

This variation of the swing-up enables a faster upward transition that elevates the body to a higher balancing position. It requires more upper-body strength to pull from the forearms, which can be specifically developed thanks to arm-hang movements such as the Forearm Pull-Up and the Pop-Up and will greatly facilitate the Forearm Swing-Up. (You can find these movements later in this chapter in the section about arm-hang upward movements).

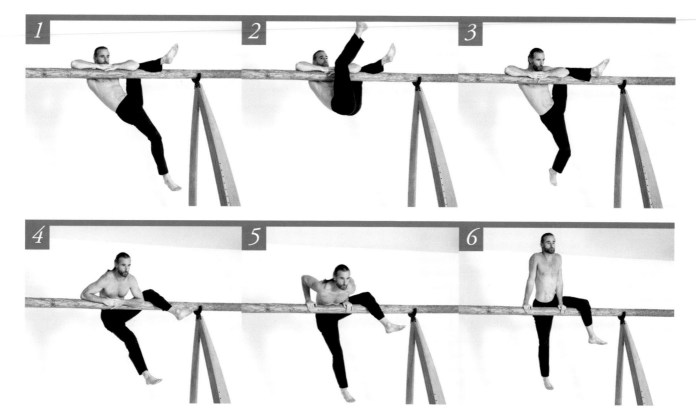

Faults

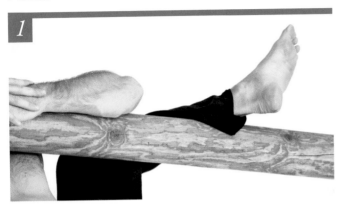

1 Improper leg hook

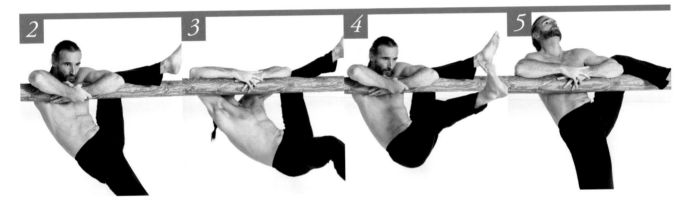

2 Low Double-Forearm Hang where your shoulders are below forearm level and you have a rotated hip position. The low hang makes it more difficult to achieve the top position because you start pulling from a lower position and must generate more power and cover more distance. The outward position of the hooked leg and hip deviates the swinging leg and momentum from a front axis that's more efficiently transferred to upward direction.

3 Improper arm position with the inside of your upper arms on support. This creates several issues: It reduces the range of motion from your arms and reduces the height that can be reached by your body as well as the power that you can generate when pulling. It also brings your chest closer to the supporting surface, which makes your chest bang on the surface and pushes your torso back instead of up. Finally, it creates unstable support that tends to slide forward upon momentum, which worsens the problem.

4 Bringing your swinging leg back to the front shifts your center of gravity forward and the position down.

5 Directing the momentum and pull only upward instead of forward. Your upper body is rapidly pulled to a back lean and back down away from the surface.

Other faults not shown in the photos include the following:

- Raising the Double-Forearm hang too high, which reduces the range of motion and power of the pull.
- A leg swing that lacks velocity, amplitude, or both. Your body swings back, but it doesn't swing high (or not high enough).

Arm-Hang Upward Movements

You mostly use side arm-hang upward movements to achieve a skill-to-skill transition to balancing on top of the supporting surface (such as establishing a Vertical Hand Press position) or to reach and grasp a higher handhold.

Although a certain level of technique is required for these movements, this kind of physical performance demands significant levels of upper-body power. You must realize that such power is developed only through dedicated, systematic training. If you were able to achieve a successful upward movement from an arm-leg hang—such as a swing-up—you'll get even greater exhilaration the first time you're able to achieve a Pop-Up or even a Power-Up by pulling exclusively through your arms. In most cases, there are more economical alternatives available to achieve the same result of establishing a top position on the surface of support, but they're not as fast, and, in some circumstances, speed is vital. Therefore, the acquisition of these techniques and the development of power is essential for having a broader real-world physical preparedness.

Pull-Up/Pop-Up/Power-Up/Roll-Up

The way you develop the fundamental levels of grip strength, arm strength, and core strength is to start with diverse forms of arm and arm-leg hang positions, transitions, and movements. By doing this, you improve your ability to link your whole body together and prepares your joints and tissues, which is required to develop the ability to perform Pull-Ups. Otherwise, attempting a Pull-Up for the first time without preparation and progression is not only daunting, it's also healthy. Reverting to hanging position and movements practice is not a "regression"; it's just common sense and a natural progression that children follow naturally; adults may use the same progression as effectively.

Scapular Pull-Up

Scapular Pull-Ups are about achieving a slightly raised Double-Hand Hang. They're good for people who have trouble activating their shoulder girdle and lats (which should be the first motion of an efficient Pull-Up). The ability to hang with straight arms and then pull your shoulder blades down your back is an excellent way to learn how to initiate a Pull-Up with your lats and make your back stronger for pulling. Flexing your biceps is the next phase to performing a Pull-Up. You also can use the Scapular Pull-Up to help generate forward momentum from hanging because the movement causes your center of gravity to move forward. When you properly time the movement and add forward motion of your legs as needed, it's an effective way to drive forward swinging. This movement also helps you learn how to initiate the pull for the Double-Hand Foot Pinch or the Double-Hand Single-Leg Hook hangs.

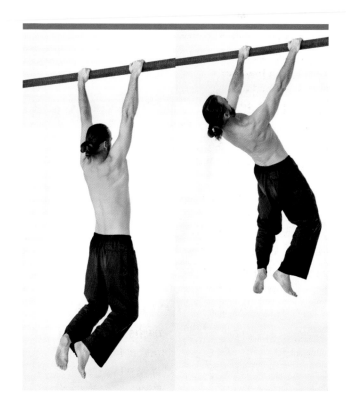

Double-Hand Side Hang Pull-Up

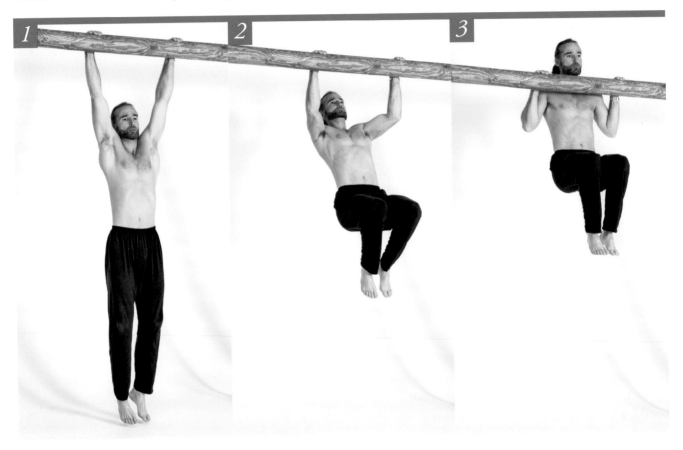

1   From the Double-Hand Side Hang, start generating tension in the lats, torso, and shoulder girdle through scapular pulling.

2   After starting to raise your hang from the scapula, immediately start flexing your arms, keeping a straight spine to present your chest toward the bar while keeping a vertical position.

3   Maintain tight tension to preserve a stable spine, shoulder, chest and arm position and movement all the way to the top. Keep flexing your arms and elevating your position as high as you can. Keep pulling your elbows all the way backward, which results in your shoulder blades being brought closer to each other as your chest goes forward; it also supports the linear alignment of your spine (refer to the reverse-view photos).

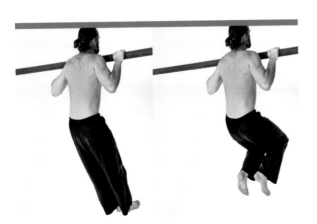

Faults

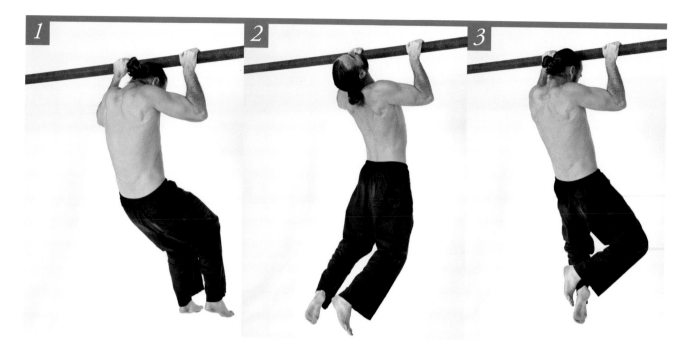

1   Your head is tucked in, with the top of it reaching the support surface. Your upper back rounds, which collapses your chest, shifts your elbows toward the front, and keeps your body away from the bar. Even if you were to keep your head up, the inefficiency of the position, compact upper body, and distance from the support surface make you lose velocity and prevent you from finishing the movement with your chin reaching bar level or higher. On top of preventing you from reaching a higher elevation, you can't see where to reach with your hands next and could even bang your head. Don't turn this natural movement into a mindless strength drill; keep a realistic mindset as if you were actually intending to climb.

2   The backward head position is a fault unless it's an adjustment necessary if the surface above you extends backward or if you want to reach with your hand both above you and toward the back.

3   Pulling up with crossed legs is a very bad habit. You never want to keep your legs in a set position. You can expect to have to extend one foot (or both feet) to be a point of support, or you might have to suddenly land on both feet. You must keep your legs free and ready to adapt to whatever happens.

TECHNIQUE TIP

Keep a realistic mindset as if you are in a climbing situation rather than turning the Pull-Up into a mindless strength drill.

Progressions

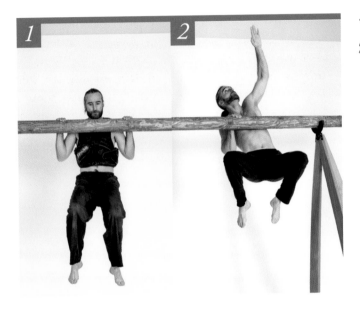

Following are some other progressions:

- Diverse grips (finger holds, rope, and so on), including thicker surfaces that challenge grip strength more
- Unstable surfaces
- Raising your position and holding static holds
- Slow negatives (moving from the high position to slowly come down to the Dead Hang)

1 Weighted Hand Pull-Up

2 High Hand-Reach Pull-Up: This pull-up helps you develop the explosiveness and stability necessary to reach a higher handhold (as well as performing Power-Ups). You can do it by extending a single arm or both arms (in which case it creates a brief upward airborne phase). When you're reaching with a single arm, your position becomes a unilateral static hold, which means that your base of support is reduced to a single point of support, and your center of gravity must shift toward vertical alignment so you don't go off balance. Keep the upper body tight/compact with your elbows in as you pull; the reason is not only to keep a position that generates more power but to anticipate the release of a point of support (the reaching hand) and the change of base of support that induces a shift of center of gravity. By keeping your elbows in, you can maintain balance until you grasp the target or your hand returns to its previous hold level because you're keeping your center of gravity in closer vertical alignment with the single point of support.

Side Hand Pull-Up to Mid-Raised Double-Forearm Hang
(Or the Slower Active Single Forearm Hang to Active Double Forearm Hang)

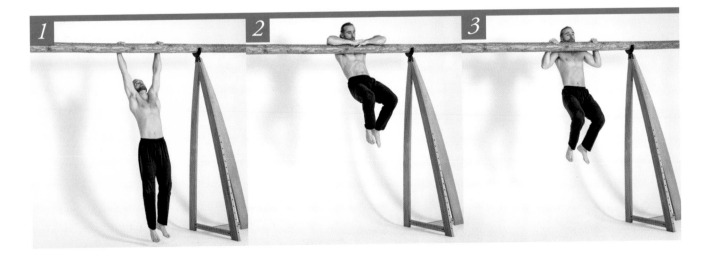

Double-Forearm Hang Position—Close-Up View

Performing a Pop-Up is more than just a matter of muscle power; it's also requires good technique for specific positional control in a Double-Forearm Hang. The position of your arms on the supporting surface is essential to your stability, balance, and range of motion when applying force. Without it, you won't be able to develop as much power as you possess.

The details of this specific positional control apply to the Forearm Swing-Up as well. Training the Forearm Swing-Up helps you with the specific positioning of the Double-Forearm Hang Pull-Up and the Pop-Up, and training those movements in turn makes your Forearm Swing-Up base position and pull much stronger and more efficient.

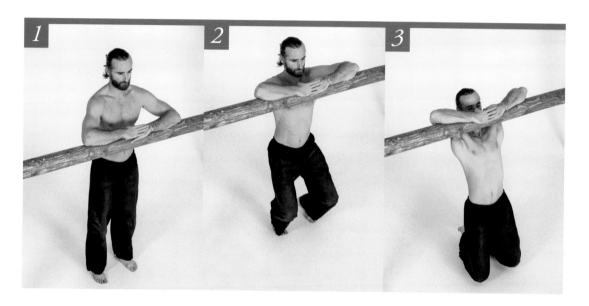

1 Stand facing the supporting surface, and place both elbows on the supporting surface at a width a little greater than shoulder width. Lower your forearms onto the surface of support. Your hands should be stacked with your fingertips pointing toward the opposite elbow and aligned at the wrist of the opposite arm. Your thumbs or knuckles are aligned with your midline.

2 Lower your center of gravity in a half flexion of your legs while pressing down on your forearms. You should feel your body weight shifting onto your forearms, and your elbow joint moving off the surface of support to be slightly above it. Start to activate your lats (back muscles) and scapula.

3 Shift all your body weight onto your forearms, releasing your feet and applying much greater tension in your back so you're in a low Double-Forearm Hang. Your elbows move out and back in a slight external rotation.

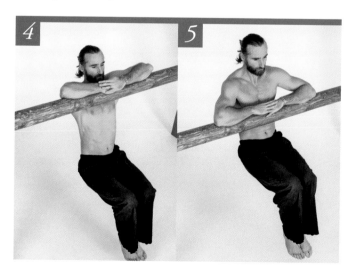

4 Test the reliability of your base of support as well as your levels of strength by raising your position so your shoulders are aligned with your forearms or the surface of support (or a little below). Your knees are tucked to the front. Maintain abdominal breath control.

5 If you can, elevate your position by raising your shoulders above the surface of support and hold the high hang for a few seconds.

TECHNIQUE TIP

You can make holding this position at all three levels a stationary, isometric drill that develops the specific strength needed. You also can do slow, short-range-of-motion but stable Pull-Ups or slow negative Pull-Ups (a controlled descent from the high position), until you can do several full Forearm Pull-Ups from the low position to where your shoulder and hand are level.

Faults

You might hold the following hang positions briefly in a climbing situation, but they become faults when you apply them to a Pop-Up.

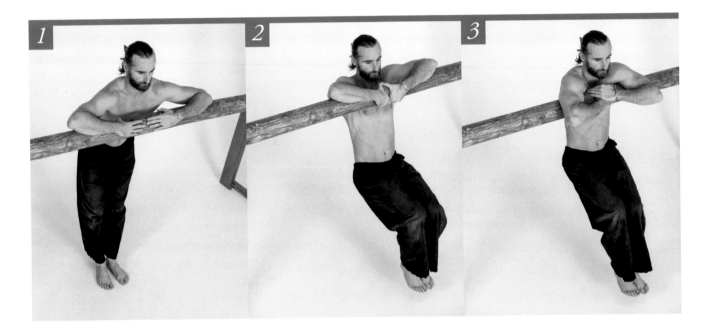

1   Base of support is too wide. It reduces your range of motion, how much power you can generate, and your balance at the end of the movement.

2   Grasping the supporting surface tightly with your hands. Unless the supporting surface is slippery, this is superfluous tension that tends to distract you from the task of power generation.

3   Using your armpit or upper inside arm for support. This position means there's no distance from the supporting surface for your chest to clear it. Also, you don't have any range of motion and can't generate power. This is a frequent fault in beginners who don't possess the strength to hold an actual Double-Forearm Hang. You can hang and rest in this position, but you can't move unless you either slide your forearms backward onto the support surface or hook one leg to the side.

Pull-Up to Double-Forearm Hang Transition Drill

Once you know how to correctly position your forearms on the surface of support, can hold the position, and even can perform a few forearm Pull-Ups, you must train your ability to transition from the side Double-Hand Hang to the Double-Forearm Hang through a Pull-Up.

There are two variations for this transition. The first, easier variation is to pull up and place one forearm on the support and then place the other arm on the support. The second variation necessitates a Pull-Up that's explosive enough to place both forearms on the support simultaneously.

Whichever variation you're able to use, this is a necessary transition you must be able to perform to position yourself for the Pop-Up. Note that training the variation with simultaneous positioning of the forearms helps develop the same pull-up power needed to perform the Power-Up.

High Forearm Pull-Up

Once you have developed enough strength to do a handful of Forearm Pull-Ups in a row, you're ready to work on developing actual power. Performing explosive Forearm Pull-Ups is the prerequisite to the Pop-Up. Aim at one to three repetitions in a row maximum, and accelerate as fast as possible upward each time with the intention to both go as fast as possible and reach as high as possible. A knee tuck motion assists the generation of power through body-weight transfer. The photos show the highest elevation you can reach before the Forearm Pull-Up turns into an actual Pop-Up.

Pop-Up

The Pop-Up is a Power-Up that starts in a Double-Forearm Hang. When you do a Pop-Up explosively, it can transition directly to the Vertical Hand Press similarly to the Power-Up that's done starting from a Double-Hand Side Hang. You can do a Pop-Up with a tuck or a swing.

Tuck Pop-Up

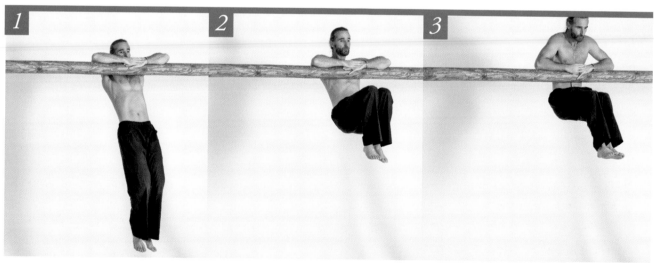

(continued on next page)

1 Start in a Double-Forearm Hang with your shoulders at forearm level (although you could start in a lower hang). Your hang must be solid all the way through as when you're doing Double-Forearm Pull-Ups.

2 Initiate a "tuck" that generates body-weight transfer from the lower body toward the upper body. You do the tuck by kicking your heels toward your rear, which swiftly elevates your knees and legs, which are followed by the hips and the rest of the body.

3 Immediately start pulling from your arms while maintaining a vertical position.

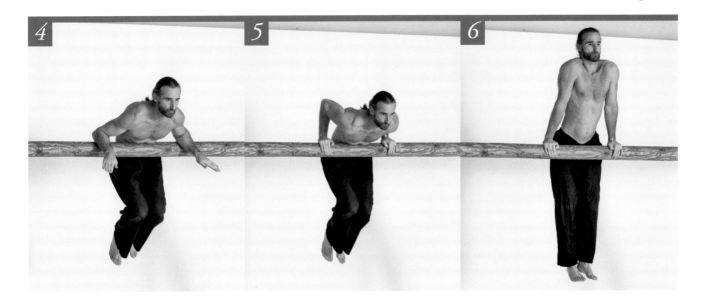

4   As you're finishing the pulling motion, lean your head, shoulders, and chest forward to shift your center of gravity above your base of support. Maintain balance, and externally rotate your arms as you anticipate placing your hands on the support. At this stage of the movement, you're in a balancing position more than a climbing position. Optionally, you could leave your forearms in the initial position if you want to balance and rest on them rather than extending your arms and elevating your position higher.

5   While briefly resting your abdomen on the support surface in a balanced position, place your hands on the support close to your rib cage.

6   Shift your body weight onto your hands and press up to reach the top position of the Vertical Press-Up.

Faults

If you possess enough upper-body power to achieve the Pop-Up without achieving it yet, the following are the most common issues:

- Starting the pull from a raised forearm hang, which reduces the range of motion you need to optimally accelerate upward
- Pulling too early—before or at the same time of the tuck
- Kicking the knees up and to the front as you tuck, which shifts the center of gravity forward and makes you lean backward, which throws off your balance
- Pulling forward too early before you've reached high enough, which means you bang your chest on the bar
- Not leaning forward immediately after your chest has passed bar level

30
Manipulation Movement 1

Object manipulation is generally defined as the skillful throwing and/or catching of a great variety of light objects (balls, clubs, hoops, poi, knives, nunchaku, or any ordinary object that is relatively light) primarily through the motion of the arms and hands, although any part of the body can be used. The most frequent purpose of this type of object manipulation is recreation and entertainment; it demands high levels of dexterity but a relatively low level of strength.

Many specialized sports are based on other forms of object manipulation. An Olympic lifter uses a single type of apparatus, using two techniques to lift the object from the ground to overhead, which requires enormous amounts of skill and power. A powerlifter focuses on three heavy lifts of somewhat limited range of motion, which demand enormous amounts of strength but little power (strength + speed). A bodybuilder manipulates barbells for the sake of gaining muscle mass, which requires strength but no significant movement skill. A javelin specialist might not be efficient at pitching a baseball, and a baseball player might not be good at throwing a javelin. An expert juggler might not be able to squat with a load equal to his own body weight, and a powerlifter might be unskilled at throwing or catching anything with accuracy. We can learn useful techniques and training methods that have been developed for each of these modalities, but except for "strongman" training that provides the most diverse and realistic display of manipulative skills and challenges, most manipulation activities are very standardized and limited in scope.

A Natural Movement perspective of the concept of object manipulation is broader and more practical, without concern for sport-specific rules. Natural Movement manipulation aims at moving any kind of object in any useful way necessary, from contact to release. A natural spectrum of manipulation will include a great variety of techniques and movement patterns with objects of varied shape, material, texture, and weight and displaced on diverse types of terrains. This inclusive approach to manipulation implies throwing and catching objects that aren't necessarily light, as well as lifting potentially heavy loads or voluminous objects off the ground, carrying them over a long distance or quickly over a short distance, and sometimes carrying an item in partnership.

The objects you manipulate are irrelevant: It is why and how you manipulate them that matters. The goal is not to develop elite levels of proficiency in a given, standardized manipulative discipline but to acquire the basic skills, strength, and work capacity required for real-life competency. Therefore, you should learn a large number of lifting, carrying, throwing, or catching techniques, which will help you develop greater levels of strength, power, and endurance of "work capacity under load."

Technique aside, strength, power, and endurance are highly desirable and necessary physical qualities one must increase and that are an integral part of MovNat training. However, developing such physiological adaptations requires specific training and programming that goes beyond the scope of this book but which follows some of the principles of progression delineated in Part 3, "Practice Efficiency."

I'm addressing Manipulation movement in two chapters. The first focuses on lifting and carrying; the second focuses on throwing and catching. The general concepts covered in this introduction apply to the skills of throwing and catching as well as lifting and carrying. With the comprehensive information I've provided, you will learn everything you need to know for efficient and safe real-world object manipulation.

The Basics *of* Manipulation Movement

The efficient manipulation of objects demands great positional control. Therefore, all the motor-control, physical, and physiological benefits you should have already gained through the practice of natural loco-motive skills, such as greater mobility, stability, balance, coordination, or strength, will prove to be a precious help to your progress in diverse manipulation techniques. The same way a lot of people who are movement-proficient would gain from developing greater levels of strength, a lot of people with great strength would benefit from moving better first.

Focusing first on efficient form at low intensity rather than insisting on how heavy you can lift, carry, throw, or catch might expose issues that prevent you from reaching the greatest levels of performance you could attain, which gives you a chance to resolve them. For instance, ankle, hip, thoracic spine, and shoulder mobility are fundamental to being efficient at lifting heavy loads. Can you assume a comfortable Deep Squat or perform an efficient Hip Hinge with optimal spinal position? If not, what do you think will happen as you load those movement patterns with heavy weights? It's important that you not immediately focus your Natural Movement practice on manipulation skills, and you especially shouldn't practice them at high levels of intensity.

Manipulation movements such as in lifting and carrying are not entirely new movement patterns;

they're movements you're familiar with for the most part, but you modify how you execute them so that you can sustain external loads. The Deadlift relies mostly on hip hinging, which is a pattern employed in the Power Jump and the Square Landing. Carrying implies locomotion with patterns such as get-ups, walking, running, occasionally crawling, balancing, jumping, climbing, and even swimming. You just learn to do it as efficiently as possible with a load. Learning to skillfully move your body around before you learn to skillfully move stuff around—not the other way around—is a wise approach.

Great technique does not "give" you strength that you don't have; it enables you to maximize the use of the strength you do have. So, after you've acquired efficient form in manipulative techniques, it's time to work on greater levels of strength and power as you simultaneously keep refining your skills continuously. You see, in an authentic quest for general and rather equalized movement competency, strength folks should consider their deficiencies in diverse areas of movement function and skill, whereas the proponents of "mindful movement" should consider their inability to handle heavy loads and intensity. After all, courage is about putting your weaknesses on the line, whatever those weaknesses might be.

Contact Event and Grip

Manipulative movement sequences are called *contact events* in which you first grasp, hold, or displace the object, and then you release it. *Grasping* happens when you first make contact with the object using your hands or another body part. You can grasp an object while it's still or when you catch a moving object.

After you've grasped the object, you can hold it or displace it to a new location. Last, the object is released by being set down, dropped, or thrown. Like climbing, grasping objects has a lot to do with gripping or the mechanical interface between your body and the load or object. Without an effective grip, all manipulation becomes ineffective.

The application of a gentle yet skillful grip is necessary when you're throwing light objects, whereas a very strong grip is required to lift a heavy load off the ground or to strike powerfully with a heavy handheld tool. You might use intermediate levels of tension in your hands and forearms as the load and movement require. Hand position varies depending on the shape or weight of the object or the technique used for manipulation. Sometimes *grip* means balancing the object on some part of your body—flat open hand, head, or shoulder—rather than grasping it with your hands. The good thing in manipulation is that losing your grip doesn't necessarily mean losing your balance or falling. Only the object or load should fall if you have released your grip before it compromises your position.

Combined Center of Mass

It's easy to hold a book at arm's length to put it on a shelf without realizing that your center of gravity has slightly shifted. However, you might notice a shift in your center of gravity if you carry a heavy bag of groceries with one hand as you walk to your car. Do you feel that you're pulling to the side with every step you make and that you have unusual instability in the way you step? You feel this way because the external load pulls your center of gravity in a given direction. Efficiently managing the combined center of gravity is an integral part of positional control that relates not only to the position of your body but also to the position of the object in relation to your body.

Regardless of the specific manipulative skill or technique, whenever you're handling an external load, its center of mass will alter the position of your center of gravity, resulting in a *combined center of gravity*. This is especially true as you hold the object farther away from your center of gravity and as the load gets heavier. The heavier the object gets, the more technically important it becomes to vertically align the center of mass of the load with your center of gravity and with your base of support to make the combined center of gravity more manageable. Even a slightly misaligned combined center of gravity affects your balance, movement, and work, causing unnecessary resistance and muscular tension. If the shift of the combined center of gravity farther beyond your line of gravity continues, you'll be forced to drop the object and maybe lose your balance as well. On top of losing your balance, you may also compromise your spine with a greater risk of injury. Efficiently managing the combined center of gravity, especially in the manipulation of significantly heavy objects with uneven weight distribution and on uneven terrain, reduces the necessary muscle force and compression on joints, and it keeps your body safer. In short, an efficient combined center of gravity ensures economy and safety in carrying.

The necessary management of the combined center of gravity, including the path it follows in a lift before being stabilized as a carry, also forces you to trigger faster compensatory responses in positional control, which is based on a higher sense of alertness. Because balance under load is more demanding than balancing without a load, a positive side effect of learning to manage the combined center of gravity is that it may aid in developing the righting reflex and greater balance when moving without a load.

Bone Density, Back Health, and Injury Prevention

Lifting and carrying heavy loads improves mineral density in your bones, regardless of age, which is essential to robust health. It makes sense that resisting the downward pull of gravity on the loads you manipulate requires bones to be strong enough to handle the stress of greater levels of muscular tension. Doing lifting movements correctly also makes your back strong, but doing them incorrectly can be a source of everything from a mild strain in the back muscles to a disabling back injury. Intervertebral disks (the fibrous rings that act as cushions between vertebrae) can bulge and even rupture because of the compressive forces of handling heavy loads, especially when you lift while your spine is in a compromised position. Since the central nervous system is made up of the spinal cord and brain, back issues may cause discomfort, acute pain, or even motor-control issues. If you get injured lifting, there isn't much movement you can do afterward, so ensuring safety in lifting is paramount.

To prevent injury, take the following considerations very seriously.

Neutral Lower Back

The better your technique, the less chance that you'll be injured. The single most important aspect of all manipulative techniques is to keep your lower back neutral, which you can learn before you begin lifting by doing other natural movements. Once you've acquired the neutral lower back reflex, adding a load both reinforces this reflex and strengthens the "natural belt" (the muscles that stabilize your spine) that protects it even more.

Although rounding, arching, and rotating your lower back are natural motions of your spine, excessively rounding, arching, or rotating—hyperflexion (including laterally), hyperextension, and hyper-rotation, respectively—your lower back as the intervertebral discs are compressed under load can squeeze the discs from the front, back, or side, which puts the spine at a serious risk of injury, such as a herniated disk. The middle and upper spine statistically suffer less injury incidence, but you should still keep them neutral to avoid any risk. Also, a neutral middle and upper spine support a neutral lower back. Maintaining a neutral spine from sacrum to neck is not only the most significant key to reducing the risk of back injury, but it leads to greater manipulative performance.

Symmetry

Symmetry has to do with distributing the load equally on both sides of your body as much as possible. Loading a single side of the body, such as in a Single-Hand Carry or Shoulder Carry, forces the back to lean sideways with the muscles on the loaded side shortened and muscles on the opposite side lengthened. If you don't do this with control, the result might be a lateral wedging of the disk (lateral hyperflexion), which places it at risk of injury. I'm not saying that you must avoid unilateral manipulative movements, only that you must approach them even more carefully than those with an even distribution of the load on the body. Also, it's essential that you train any single-side manipulative movement on both sides equally.

The weight distribution of the load is also important, as an object with a center of mass that moves tends to create more instability and asymmetry.

Mindfulness

Mindfulness always is key to ensuring good form. A single short moment of inattention may place your spine in a dangerous position, such as hyperextension, hyperflexion, lateral hyperflexion, or axial hyper-rotation. A moment of imbalance, foot slippage on challenging terrain, a lack of grip, or hand slippage can easily distract you.

The integrity of your back position should be your highest focus point from the moment you grasp the object to the moment you release it. You should approach every lift as if the weight you're going to lift is heavier than what it is so you reflexively assume a strong position. During the contact event, if you ever feel that your back position is compromised or is about to be compromised with little chance of recovery, you should be ready to drop the load. It's much wiser to pick up a load from the ground again than to risk a severe injury, isn't it? Even after you've dropped a heavy object, be mindful of getting your feet out of the way. Sometimes loads bounce back or roll off, hurting your toes, feet, or ankles.

Volume and Intensity

Even the best technique and being mindful won't protect your spine if the intensity, volume, or both are too high for your strength. Nurses who must lift heavy patients multiple times a day are taught to use efficient and safe body mechanics simply: "Keep your back straight; bend at the hips and knees."

However, even the best body mechanics in the world won't protect your back if the overall forces and stress placed upon your spine are too large and too repetitive, which will end up disrupting your form and placing your spine at great risk. Therefore, it's essential that, aside from having efficient form, you commit to respect sustainable intensity, volume, and individual progressions.

Progressive Complexity

Beginners should start not only with light loads but also with more controlled environments, including the type of load. You need to use objects with a secure grip and an even distribution of weight, and you should stand on an even, flat, non-slippery surface. Read more about this later in this chapter in the "Choice of Equipment."

LIFTING AND CARRYING

Lifting and carrying in MovNat are tightly related because the main practical purpose for lifting a load is obviously to carry it (sometimes throw it), not to drop it on the spot immediately after lifting it.

I show how lifting and carrying work together depending on the object you lift and how you intend to carry it. For instance, it makes sense to learn the various carry strategies that are already available immediately after the basic lifting methods—Deadlift or Lapping—rather than learning the significantly more complex Clean-and-Jerk technique first.

What you learn in this chapter also makes you better able you to throw objects that are relatively heavy and to better handle them after you catch them.

Lifting

When you lift, your aim is to cancel the inertia of an object to raise it vertically, which most of the time is necessary before the object can be carried, thrown, or lowered back to the ground. Lowering an object can be important for protecting the load, the surface below it, or the operator. Though we can't say that lifting and lowering are the same, they're related parts of the same practical goal: moving objects from one vertical position to another—either upward or downward. Indeed, you lift a heavy box full of glassware off the ground to hip level and then slowly and carefully lower it to the ground a few steps away with the same muscles and movement pattern; only the type of muscle contraction differs.

Raising a heavy piece of furniture off the floor and picking up a pair of socks from the floor are both lifting. While the latter is accessible to anyone with fundamental movement ability because of the lightness of the object, in the absence of technique and strength, the former becomes inaccessible.

The type of lift depends on many variables, such as the shape, texture, volume, and weight distribution of the object; its position relative to your body when you grasp it; the surface where you stand; and what you intend to do with the object after you lift it. Short-range lifting movements, such as the Deadlift, require strength, whereas lifting a load with the Clean-and-Jerk movement demands power and greater levels of technique. The higher you move the load vertically, the greater the chance you'll lose balance and the more important it becomes that you maintain a balanced combined center of gravity.

Setting

Setting is the part of positional control that happens before the lift to ensure effective and efficient lifting. It involves several aspects that are pretty much constant regardless of the lifting technique you're using. Setting becomes more important as the loads you're lifting become heavier.

Grasping and Body Position

Placing your hands on the object to grip it securely (*grasping*) is the first phase of the contact event in lifting, and it's a crucial one that you shouldn't rush. A strong grip matters mostly at the beginning of the lift when you're overcoming inertia and as you slowly raise the load. In more explosive lifts such as a Clean, the load becomes significantly accelerated upward after it leaves the ground, and with such momentum, the level of grip strength required rapidly decreases.

The weight of the object, the position of your hands or arms, and the level of surface friction where your hands grasp the object determine the level of gripping friction you need. For instance, you can lift heavier with a Hook Grip than with an Open-Hand Grip, but lifting something of equal weight with a Hook Grip when the surface you're grasping is slippery necessitates a much higher level of grip strength.

In the weight-lifting world, you will often hear that you must "squeeze" the handle you grasp as hard as you can before you attempt to lift a load, which makes a lot of sense if you are dealing with a load that's very heavy relative to your strength. It signals the muscles in the posterior chain that are involved in the lift to activate strongly as an intense effort is coming up; it also makes sure that the level of friction in your grip matches or even slightly exceeds what lifting the load demands. Indeed, if your grip is weak, you won't be able to lift the load even if the rest of your body is strong enough, and your hands will give in. Another advantage is that tightly grasping prevents latency in the gripping reflex at the very beginning of the lift. Your hands are ready even before the rest of your body is.

However, efficient gripping is not always as simple as "squeezing as hard as you can." There's no need to squeeze as hard as you can unless you're trying to lift an object that weighs nearly the maximum weight you can lift. Regardless of the weight of the load and grip position, the friction in your hands should match the gripping strength required to lift the load. Think of it this way: There's no need to squeeze a pet as hard as you can to pick her up, correct? You need to make sure, by feel, that the level of friction you create in the interface with the load (fingers, hands, wrists, and forearms) is enough to secure it while executing the lift. To be on the safe side, you might use slightly more friction than what is needed but no more than that.

Another important consideration is that grip strength doesn't always come only from your fingers; you might need to try a variety of handholds, some of them involving inward pressure from your arms, to assist hand gripping. Ensuring a secure grip and adequate levels of friction in the real world might require more than a strong Hook Grip because you usually don't get a handle narrow enough to wrap your fingers all the way around it. For instance, when lifting a log that's thick and rounded, you use an Open-Hand Grip, and although you'll apply some force from your fingers with no thumb opposition, you mostly apply force through the wrists, forearms, and the pectorals with your arms pushing inwardly to help squeeze the extremity of the log between your forearms.

Last, when dealing with unfamiliar and oddly shaped objects, and when you do not have an accurate sense of their weight, it's tricky to determine the levels of grip strength required for the lift. The strategy for producing the right levels of friction before lifting is to assume the bottom deadlift position and grasp the object. As you activate and tense your muscles by simulating an imminent lifting effort, feedback travels between the muscles in the posterior chain and those muscles at the front of the body that are handling the gripping. It feels a little as if you're pushing slightly backward on your feet and preventing yourself from falling backward by holding on with your hands. Such "feel" is a mutually regulating phase that tells both sets of muscles how much tension is required, which prevents latency in muscular contraction responsible both for the lift and the grip. Although such feedback might trigger positional modifications and muscular activation adjustments in the front of the body to secure the grip, it might also do the same at the back of the body to secure friction in the footing to "ground" the body. The process also ensures you have the best positional set to get a better sense of the combined center of gravity and facilitate efficient muscular synergy from start to end, which helps you avoid having your balance be disturbed. So, the level of grip strength you can apply also depends on your general body position. Finding optimal positioning of the hands relative to the body, and the other way around, might take several seconds. What matters the most is that you're in a strong position before lifting.

Upper Back and Shoulder Position

We know how important keeping a neutral lower back is, but establishing and maintaining a neutral upper spine is another critical aspect of efficiency in lifting and carrying as well. You want to keep a "big chest," which you do by extending your upper spine to push your chest forward and pull your shoulder blades backward to keep your shoulders neutral. The shoulder girdle and upper spine are strongly associated, and, in most cases, protracted (slouching) shoulders indicate a flexed upper spine, which under load is a very weak position.

Neck and Eye Position

As I explain in Part 2, "Movement Efficiency Principles," eye position can be beneficial or detrimental depending on the movement. During lifting or lowering, maintaining a forward or upward line of vision facilitates back extension and supports maintaining a neutral spine, and it keeps the position of the neck either neutral or slightly extended.

Preloading and Bracing

The last part of setting up for your lift involves creating tension and bracing. You want to start creating some level of tension in the muscles responsible for producing force and stabilizing your position just *before* you lift, not *as* you lift; indeed, being overly relaxed as you begin lifting can easily compromise not only your position—starting with spinal alignment—but also the whole lifting attempt.

"Preloading" necessitates that you develop a familiar sensation of contracting (or "loading") the specific muscles responsible for generating the force you want rather than generating unnecessary tension all over, especially in antagonistic muscles, because, as I've said before, selective tension with proper timing is a must for efficiency. Of course, preloading isn't exclusive to manipulative movement, but it is crucial in lifting heavy loads. Bracing hard is a fundamental part of creating tension before you lift heavy loads. The control of spinal alignment and stability is especially important when you're manipulating heavy loads as in lifting and carrying.

Bracing involves abdominal tension and a temporary abdominal breath-hold to increase intra-abdominal-pressure. The pressure inside the abdominal cavity acts on both the diaphragm and the vertebral column and supports positional control and stability of the pelvic-spinal-thoracic complex under load. It also helps you keep your trunk extended to a neutral alignment. Before you begin to lift, you need to inhale through the abdomen while keeping your abdominal muscles tight. You hold your breath in the first seconds of the lift until you've raised the load past your knees; then you slowly exhale. The goal is to keep the spine as stable as possible when it needs stability the most, which is when a large force must overcome the inertia of the load to create vertical acceleration. Often, you should hear yourself taking a strong breath before you lift.

Bracing is a reflex you must develop and activate before attempting any lift, even when the load is not your maximum. Bracing is also used when you carry heavy loads for postural control and also to regulate a high-intensity effort under load. When you brace while carrying, you don't hold your breath, but you maintain strong abdominal tension while also limiting the amplitude of your abdominal breathing.

Mindset

Last, approaching any heavy lift requires a confident, determined—even aggressive—mindset. Don't wait to start lifting before you realize that you need more willpower to achieve the lift. Be mentally strong before you lift so that you can create and maintain optimum muscular tension throughout the lift.

Center of Pressure

Something that is common to all lifts is the necessity to stay balanced over your base of support as you move the object upward. The best way to achieve such balance is to maintain an efficient combined center of gravity throughout the movement and have the load follow a vertical path as linearly as possible, minimizing any forward, backward, or side movement. Such motions of your combined center of gravity away from vertical alignment with your base of support would disturb your balance, potentially compromise your position, and decrease overall efficiency. Although such disturbances may not always be visually perceptible, you feel them in your feet right as you start lifting the load because it influences overall weight distribution, which combines your body weight and the weight of the object you're lifting, which you experience as pressure in your feet. Your goal is to establish an even distribution of the weight through your feet and maintain it throughout the lift; the center of pressure should be in the middle of your feet whenever possible, even though uneven surfaces might be more challenging in this regard.

It's often said that you should shift your body weight to your heels when you lift, but I don't necessarily agree with this. The goal is to be stable to lift in the most vertical way possible and to avoid having the center of pressure shift around through the feet, which you can do by controlling the upward, vertical path of the combined center of gravity. The result is that your feet are stable and connected evenly to the ground. Experiencing shifts such as feeling that the balls of your feet, your heels, or the side of your feet want to take off from the ground (or actually do) shows that you're unable to make the combined center of gravity follow the line of gravity from bottom to top. In a nutshell, it's not the stability of your feet that determines the stability of your body and the load while lifting but the other way around. Bottom line: ensure the vertically linear motion of the combined center of gravity.

Standing Position

The "top" position that's you achieve through the lift and must establish at the end of it is also something people often neglect. Strong lifts demand a powerful, constant contraction of the glutes, and it's essential to keep the glutes and the abdominals contracted while holding a load at the end of the lift to stabilize your lower back and keep it safe. Finishing lifts with the lower spine extended rather than keeping it neutral with a stronger glute contraction stresses the lumbar area unnecessarily. Last, strong positional control with neutral spine must be maintained as long as you're holding the load; only when you release the grip can you relax.

Lowering and Dropping

From a practical, real-world perspective, it's assumed that the object you lift should be immediately positioned onto the body to be held and carried.

In training, the object can often be immediately dropped after a lift. In fact, although learning to lower a load safely—for both the performer and the object—is necessary because in real life you might need to gently lower an object or person to the ground, it is recommended that you carefully drop the load when weight and intensity reach a high level because slowly lowering a heavy load is a liability to your spine.

When you lift something heavy, your sense of strength is boosted by the upward acceleration imparted to the load, but as you lower the same weight slowly, the absence of upward acceleration makes it feel heavier. It's more difficult to decelerate the load and the significant downward force gravity imparts to the heavy load.

Choice of Equipment

In Natural Movement practice, you may or may not use the typical equipment available for specialized manipulative discipline. There's nothing wrong with that equipment, just as there's nothing wrong with practicing with logs, stones, beer kegs, or any odd heavy object. The different types of objects that you lift and carry serve different purposes, and because they have both advantages and downsides, they all have their place in your practice.

The way you want to look at equipment depends on the following considerations:

- The technique you're training, and how much scalability you need to ensure methodical progressions. Sports equipment is highly scalable by design; odd objects are much less scalable.
- How realistic you want the practice to be. At equal weight, deadlifting a bulky round shape stone resting on the ground is much harder than deadlifting an Olympic bar.
- How much comfort or safety you need. A medicine ball keeps your palms smooth and your toes intact; rough stones might not.
- How much money you want to spend if you want to own your props.

My recommendation is that you start with controlled environments. Equipment that provides a secure, replicable grip, an evenly distributed weight that can be scaled down and up, and a flat, high-friction surface is best because it enables you to focus on efficient technique. The manipulation of an oddly shaped, less-predictable object on a complex, uneven, low-friction surface demands greater levels of adaptability, which might distract you from the more priority aspects of technique, and it can slow down skill acquisition.

You should do lifts on a flat, high-friction surface. A relatively light kettlebell is perfect because you can securely grasp the elevated handle. Another advantage is that it's a compact object, and its whole volume and weight fit between your feet. You can extend both arms between your knees, which is a convenient positional set.

Olympic bars—although their design is quite unrealistic from a real-world perspective—make it possible to place the load on the sides of the bar, which enables you to optimally manage the combined center of gravity without the volume or shape of the load impairing movement. Olympic bars also provide a very strong and secure handhold, and you easily can scale the weight. These characteristics mean Olympic bars are a phenomenal training tool for increasing strength and power.

I'm not suggesting that you must invest in pricey sports equipment; I'm only mentioning how convenient such tools are. If you don't own or plan on owning any particular equipment, you can practice with a variety of objects such as stones of different sizes, weights, and shapes and which you can get for free.

Lifting Techniques

The Deadlift and Lapping are the two most fundamental lifting techniques. The Deadlift is a core component of the more complex and dynamic Clean lifting technique, and Lapping enables a great number of carrying holds.

Deadlift

When you pick up a young child who's sitting on the floor or pick up a box full of books, chances are you executed a Deadlift. *Dead* in the name relates to the fact that whatever you lift has zero momentum; you need to overcome its inertia to raise it vertically.

The Deadlift is the most fundamental lifting technique; you lift an object from the ground to hold it at waist level or just below in a standing position, primarily through a Hip Hinge motion. From a practical standpoint, the Deadlift is used to free something stuck (that it is the object itself or something underneath it), check out what is underneath an object, toss an object to the side, or initiate a Waist Carry. It's also a big part of the movement pattern used for Lapping, and it's the first phase of the Clean, which is a more explosive and complex lifting sequence, so acquiring the technical skills of performing a Deadlift is a prerequisite to learning an efficient Clean technique.

You probably have heard people say, "Lift with your legs, not your back." Well, in *my* opinion, a better way to put it is, "Lift with your *hips* and legs, not just with your back." Although you engage the muscles of your back and legs in a Deadlift, the leverage you gain from a strong Hip Hinge motion is the most fundamental component to performing an efficient Deadlift while keeping your spine neutral and safe.

Deadlifting tremendously strengthens your back, improves your posture, and helps prevent back pain. As you deadlift increasingly heavier loads and lift more explosively, the strength and power you gain transfer directly to doing heavier Cleans, sprinting faster, performing greater Power Jumps, and gaining similar benefits to other locomotion skills.

SAFETY NOTE

In the examples, I do the Deadlift with a natural stone. If you're new to this technique or can't Deep Squat with ease (which makes it difficult to grasp with your hands at a level close to the ground), I recommend a light kettlebell or anything that enables you to secure a grip without necessarily reaching a Deep Squat position.

1

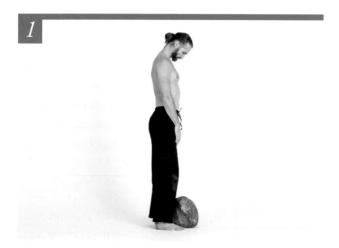

TECHNIQUE TIP

If you're using a kettlebell, skip step 2 unless you intend to lift the kettlebell without using the handle.

2

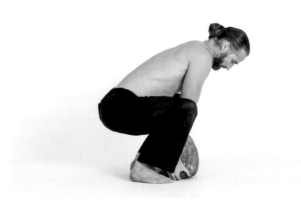

1 Stand with your feet close to the object on each side of it. Your feet should be about shoulder width, and your arms are relaxed. Look down and envision standing in the same spot as you hold the object at waist level or just below, with your arms extended, after you've elevated the object along a vertical path as much as possible. You should see your waist and hands vertically aligned with the center of mass of the object (or close to it). Since the object should end up in front of your body resting against your waist, and since the object's path should be as vertically linear as possible, a simple way to determine how close to the object your feet should be is to vertically align your waist with the close edge of the object or slightly beyond. Otherwise, if your feet aren't close enough to the object, the combined center of gravity is not optimal, your balance is challenged, and unnecessary stress is applied to your spine at the beginning of the lift until the load is high enough to be pulled back toward the center of gravity.

2 Squat down to grasp the sides of the object; get your fingers as far as possible under the object as they can go. At this point, you're getting a sense of grip on an odd object. You may slightly push it side to side with two advantages: You might be able to reach a little farther underneath the object for a stronger grip (make sure not to roll it on your fingertips and pinch them), and you can get an idea of its weight. The optimal grip isn't restricted to finger and hand position; it also involves arm position, and you exert inward pressure onto the object through your arms. Externally rotate both arms in the lockout position as much as possible.

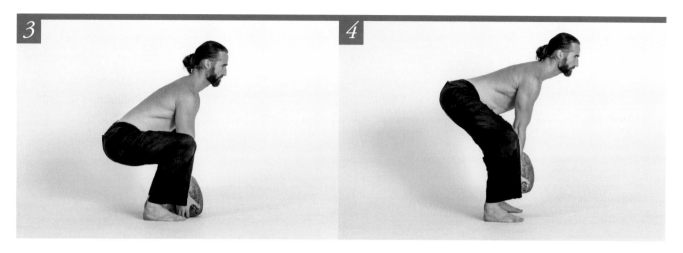

3 Now that you have a sense of grip, start assuming the positional set for the Deadlift. Load your legs and drive your rear backward in a Half Squat with your torso at about a 45-degree angle. At this point, your knees and hips may be level or your hips may be slightly above knee level, depending on the height of the grip or your physical makeup. Ultimately, as you start deadlifting, your hips will have to be higher than knee level. Both arms are fully extended. Your spine is in a mostly neutral line from lower back to neck or head; it's not rounded. A slight arch in your lower back is natural and may be maintained to help prevent flexion (rounding your spine), which is good as long as it doesn't turn into hyperextension. Your shoulders are straight and centered as well as vertically aligned with your knees, arms, and hands. You may very slightly tilt your head back to maintain a forward or slightly upward line of vision. In this positional set, the combined center of gravity is optimally aligned with the line of gravity and base of support.

4 Breathe in through your abdomen and brace (hold your breath) to increase intra-abdominal pressure to help stabilize your torso. Tightly contract your lats, lower back, abdominals, hamstrings, and glutes to prevent losing position and balance upon beginning the lift and throughout the pull. Slightly extend on your legs to elevate your hips a little above knee level. As you do so, your lower back extends in a slight, natural arch, and you should apply more strength through your hands to ensure grip friction. At this point, you have fully assumed the positional set for the Deadlift. Slowly but strongly start exerting force through your legs and rear, which overcomes inertia and starts elevating the object off the ground. It should feel through your feet as if you're pushing the ground away from you as much as it feels that you are elevating the load. As you keep your spine, shoulders, and arms straight, slowly exhale shortly after the load takes off. If you're concerned with grip friction, generate more pressure on the object by pressing it inwardly between your hands and arms to tighten your grip.

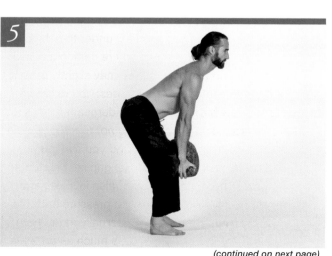

(continued on next page)

5 Keep extending your legs and, as your grip level reaches past knee level, start powerfully driving your hips forward while maintaining a neutral spine and a balanced position without being pulled forward or pushed back.

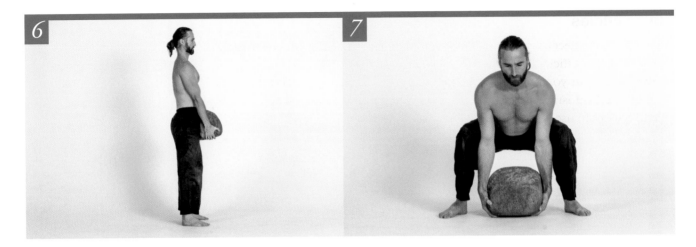

6 Finish extending both your legs and hips at the same time to end standing straight with your arms fully lengthened, shoulders down and neutral, and chest out. Contracting your glutes and abdominals helps you maintain a strong standing position, especially as the load becomes heavy. Your hips are in the lockout position, but since the mass of the object wants to pull you forward, adjust the combined center of gravity by driving your hips forward and extending your lower back very slightly (it's barely noticeable by the naked eye) while maintaining a neutral lower back. From here you want to either Waist Carry the object, Power Clean, lower the load, or drop it.

7 This view provides a insight about the width of your base of support when grasping, so your arms can extend fully and follow a path between your legs and knees. Your arms and hands are positioned to support optimum friction. Notice the lockout arm position and the possibility of a wider base of support.

TECHNIQUE TIP

When you're lowering yourself from standing to grasp a kettlebell, bend at the hips and knees in a Hip Hinge. Because the handle extends above the kettlebell, your hips will be slightly higher than the knee.

Lowering

How you bring an object down to the ground is a product of both practicality and effectiveness. You could have to drop a load. You also could quickly or slowly lower it with varying degrees of accuracy depending on whether the object or the surface where you're relocating it are fragile, whether you need to position the object a certain way, and whether you need to lower the object to a raised surface or all the way to the ground. Obviously, lowering the object should follow the same positional sequence as lifting, but it happens in reverse, with a hip flexion instead of a hip extension.

Whereas lifting a heavy weight demands that your muscles shorten to create an upward acceleration, lowering it means that the same muscles lengthen to resist a downward acceleration through eccentric contraction. This movement is significantly more stressful on your back, especially as your trunk approaches being parallel with the ground. The heavier the load gets, the faster you should lower it. As mentioned previously, when you practice with heavy loads, it's safer to carefully drop the object. Resisting the downward pull is mechanically easier close to the top position than the bottom position, which means that lowering a heavy load should be slow at the top and accelerated toward the bottom.

Inefficiencies

The Deadlift is a deceptively simple movement, and many inefficiencies may occur. Although not all inefficiencies may prevent you from effectively deadlifting the load, they do effectively put your lower spine at risk. You might manage a Deadlift inefficiently when the load isn't too high, but any inefficiency greatly compromises how much strength you can use.

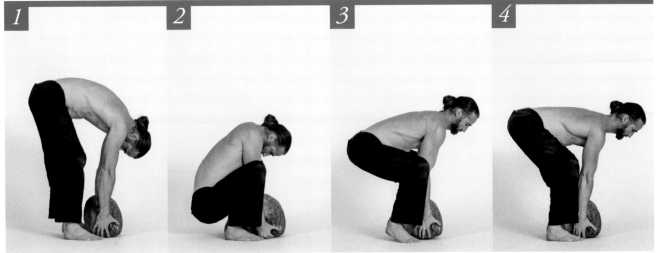

(continued on next page)

1   Your knees aren't bent; your torso and head are leaning down, and your back is entirely rounded. The intention is to pull the object using only your arms, which is a tendency that's typical of people who have no sense of lifting mechanics whatsoever.

2   The intention is to lift the object through your legs and arms only from a bottom squat position, without using hip motion. Notice the lowered head and shrugged shoulders. This position sets the combined center of gravity forward beyond the line of gravity, which keeps your lower back rounded throughout the lift and puts it in a very stressful and dangerous position. Deadlifting with low hips and an upright torso in a squat pattern with no hip drive may work with loads that aren't too challenging, but it doesn't work as the load becomes significantly heavy.

3   Raising the heels shifts your combined center of gravity forward and throws you off balance as you start to lift.

4   Your legs are too extended, which raises your hips too high and makes your torso parallel to the ground. Because your legs are almost fully extended, they won't assist much, which leaves all the effort to your lower back and puts great stress on it as the load starts to leave the ground. This position also increases the risk that you'll be pulled off balance forward. Your neck is overly extended to help maintain balance.

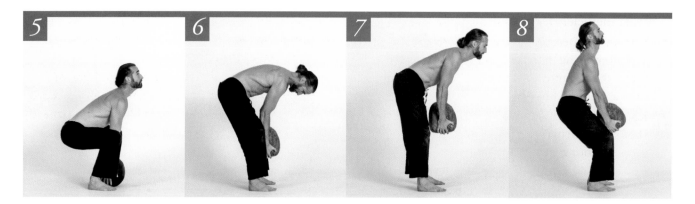

5 The positional set is good except for the hyperextension of the neck, which compresses the nerves in the area and potentially decreases overall levels of strength.

6 As you try to pull through your arms and extend your legs before driving your hips forward, you focus on the effort of your arms and get distracted from the position of your back, which becomes completely compromised. Your back rounds after the object leaves the ground. Unless the load is light, your arms aren't strong enough to raise it, and you may also hurt them.

7 Your legs are in the lockout position before your hips are finished extending, shifting your combined center of gravity forward and forcing great levels of unnecessary tension in the posterior chain and in your arms to maintain balance. This leaves your back responsible for finishing the pull in a stressful and dangerous position.

8 Your torso is too erect for this level of knee flexion with your hips trying to lock out before your legs. Your legs are not extended enough to allow your hips to move forward smoothly.

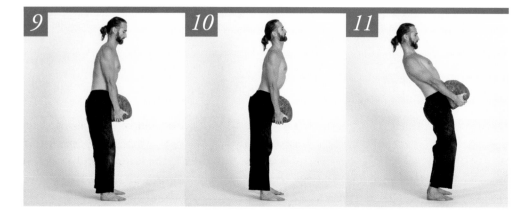

9 Your hips and legs have not reached the lockout position. Incomplete extension of your leg and hip causes stressful tension in your upper back and shoulders with your combined center of gravity not aligned with your base of support.

10 Your legs are in the lockout position, but your hips aren't, which results in hyperextension of your lower back and neck to compensate for the forward pull of the combined center of gravity that's not aligned with your base of support. You might have a false sense of positional control that is not at all efficient.

11 You have an exaggerated backward lean with a hyperextended lower back at the top of the lift. This issue often happens when you don't activate your glutes, but it also occurs when you have an exaggerated contraction and a false sense of strong top position.

Other inefficiencies include the following:

- Starting the Deadlift with a rounded low back and attempting to make it neutral after the object leaves the ground. Start neutral and stay that way throughout the lift.
- Keeping your arms straight but shrugging your shoulders. Shrugging your shoulders does not increase your grip.

- Breathing through the chest, exhaling just before or at the start of the lift, or holding your breath all the way to standing.
- Having a downward eye position and line of vision may facilitate a flexion reflex and compromise your spinal position. Look straight forward or slightly upward the moment you initiate the Deadlift.

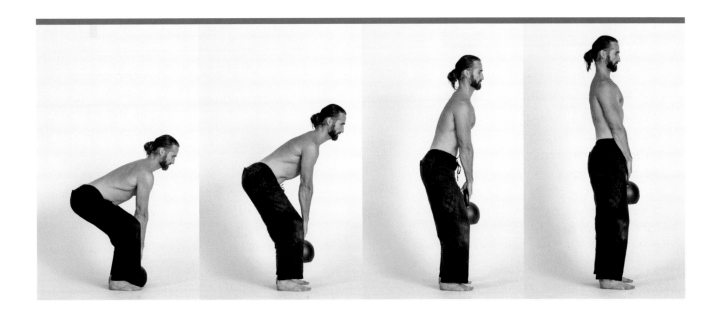

Progressions

Regardless of grip or stance variation, the two big takeaways regarding Deadlifts should be maintaining a neutral spine at all times and lifting through the hips. Practice this pattern whenever you pick up something, even when the object is light, so it becomes a second-nature reflex. Once your hip hinge pattern is efficient with a load, you may practice it on a single leg, which has a possible practical application while also helping to improve gait and standing balancing.

Lifting heavy, bulky objects that cannot be lifted by a single person is also a great way to work cooperatively.

Progressions naturally involve increasing intensity with greater weights to build higher levels of strength. As your strength grows, handling variables such as odd objects and uneven terrains becomes easier, but don't wait until you've reached power-lifting levels to explore complexity. The Single-Hand Deadlift is also a good practice; it strengthens your shoulder and grip. Make sure to alternate sides when you do it.

If you practice several repetitions of Deadlifts in a row for strength training, make sure you systematically lower the load all the way to the ground for the safety of your back to prevent unnecessary stress on your lower back. Lowering the load also gives you an opportunity to reset your position each time. If you're training with objects and surfaces that allow you to make the load bounce as it hits the ground, do not use the bounce to lift more and faster because using artificial momentum may prevent you from maintaining a safe back position.

Lapping

Lapping objects is an alternative to deadlifting when the object is too difficult to grasp with the hands and raise from the ground to hip level in a single motion—for example, when the object doesn't provide any form of handhold, has a low friction surface, is bulky, or all of the above. Compared to the Deadlift, the Lapping option shortens the vertical distance you need to raise the load. After you've brought the object as high as your knees, you can rest the object on your lap, and the effort is handled by your legs more than your back. The second great advantage of Lapping is that once the object is in your lap, you can adjust gripping or positioning of the object on the body before you carry it. This slow, step-by-step elevation of the load is especially useful when you can't lift it explosively. Alternatively, it might happen that you deadlift the load and reach a standing position but decide to lower yourself into a Lapping position.

Elite lifters, such as those who compete in strongman competitions, manage to lap very heavy and bulky loads such as Atlas stones with a rounded back from start to end. The main reason for a rounded back is that the volume of the object forces the arms to reach forward and down almost to the front of the object to enable grasping and gripping strength, which makes back flexion unavoidable. I don't recommend this technique for the casual lifter. If the shape, volume, or weight of the object is too much for your ability to maintain a neutral spine, it becomes quite too dangerous to your back health, and you should renounce attempting to lift the object. What you have learned from practicing Deadlifts will be very useful, as the positional set and start of the sequence are the same.

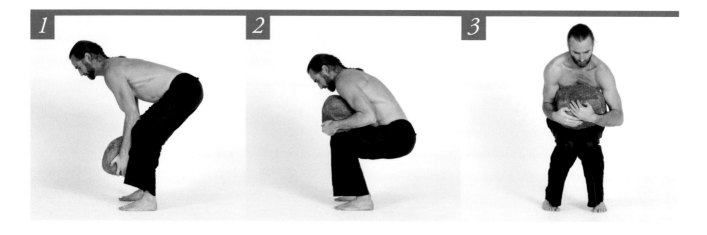

1   Grasp the object and start deadlifting it with a neutral spine. A bulkier object would require that you modify your position with a wider stance, with knees and feet pointing out to let your legs work. Your arms would reach more to the front and grasp the object not only with your hands but also by "wrapping" it with the inside of your forearms. As the load raises closer to knee level, initiate a slight pull with your arms.

2-3   Once the load passes knee level, and as you pull the object strongly toward your body, rotate both legs inwardly to have your knees contact and remove the space between them, providing a secure area for the load to rest. Because your combined center of gravity has shifted backward, let your torso lean forward so you avoid being pulled backward. Though this will make you round your back, it's not an issue because the load is resting on your legs. This is also where the movement starts if you grasp the object from a position raised above the ground at above knee or hip level.

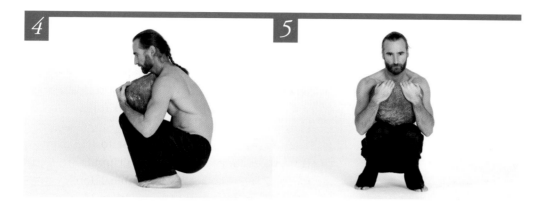

4-5 Depending on your strength, stability, or comfort, you may maintain a relatively high position, which demands great static strength in the legs, or you may transition to a Deep Squat to rest or recover your balance. From this position, you can manage your grip to transition to a Waist, Chest, or Shoulder Carry. To transition to the Waist Carry from the bottom squat, you have to push off your legs to elevate your position and rearrange your grip before your position gets too vertical to rest the load on your thighs. To transition to a Chest Carry, you need to make sure your arms wrap to the front of the object, so you can press it toward your chest as you stand up with it. You also can use the upward momentum to shift the object to your shoulder on your way up or wait until you're standing in a stable Chest Carry before shouldering it.

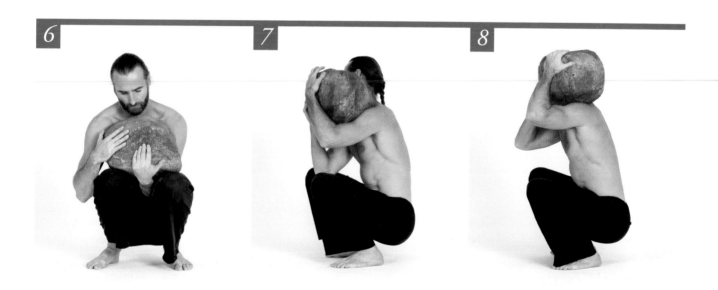

6-7-8 Alternatively, you can shoulder the load in the bottom position by sneaking one arm between your legs and underneath the object. You use that arm as well as your back to raise the object to your shoulder while maintaining balance before you stand up to a Shoulder Carry.

Carrying

The Deadlift and Lapping enable you to assume a large number of carrying holds, which I want to address before covering other lifting techniques. After all, in the real world, lifting is often immediately followed by carrying, and the goal is to initiate some form of gait to horizontally displace the load over some distance to relocate it.

Carrying can be done in many ways, both in terms of how you hold the load—various parts of the body can provide support for the load—and in terms of the locomotive pattern you use to carry it. Although carrying is most often done while you're walking, you can run, crawl, balance, climb, and swim with a load, as long as you can effectively maintain the load on your body.

As in every other manipulative skill, the gross mechanics of carrying are simple: manage the combined center of gravity as efficiently as possible over the distance you have to cover. It's always preferable to lower the load and lift it again to reposition the object efficiently on the body rather than continuing with a bad position. You don't want to waste energy with each step you make as you walk by holding the load in a miserable manner, do you? Keep in mind that this concern has to do not only with energy cost and economy but with the potential risk of injuring yourself if an inefficient way of carrying makes you stumble. Simply put, inefficient manipulation with the way you carry a load ensues inefficient locomotion. Once a grip or holding position has become inefficient, it's *already* unsustainable. If you can't fix your position without lowering the object first, then you must accept that lowering and lifting the load again might the best thing to do.

Grips and Holds

Deadlifting and Lapping enable you to assume a number of grip positions and holds without necessarily having to lift the object explosively or higher than hip level. The grip is restricted to hand positioning on the object, whereas the hold entails your grip as well as the position of your arms and the part of your body where the load rests. With certain holds, the hands grasp each other but not the surface of the load itself, whereas other holds might not involve any gripping or only minimal gripping if the way the load is positioned on the body and the way you wrap your arms around it minimize the need for gripping strength.

Choosing a grip and hold position is a factor of how sustainable it is in relation to the shape and weight of the object, the distance that you need to travel with it, and how fast you need to move. For instance, with the Waist Carry, you avoid having to lift the load higher than hip level while conveniently positioning the center of gravity of the load close to your center of gravity, which is stable and economical. In addition, you can help your walk with a slight forward hip drive when you step forward, which also helps support the load and gripping strength. But with loads involving objects that extend below the waist, the Waist Carry often prevents you from moving quickly on your feet if needed.

Comparatively and at equal weight, with a Chest Carry the combined center of gravity is more elevated and isn't as easy to manage, but you can accelerate rapidly on your feet in a second. Managing the combined center of gravity in the Side Shoulder Carry is highly efficient for long objects such as logs, but it's much more challenging with compact objects because they can easily roll off the shoulder.

The goal is always to manage an efficient combined center of gravity and find a hold that helps you avoid unnecessary tension in your arms while still being reliable.

You want to use a carry that enables the most efficient movement on your feet for the distance and speed you need to travel. For instance, in a Waist Carry, managing gripping that allows you to keep your arms extended is better than having to bend at the elbows. However, this is not always possible, and to ensure gripping, additional levels of tension in the arms, shoulders, and upper back are sometimes necessary.

Attention to grip and great grip response (the ability to automatically increase tension when you sense that your hold becomes unreliable) are very important. Letting a handheld object slip or changing position might mean you need to drop the object or compromise your position as you attempt to save your hold. In either case, it's a waste of your energy and time.

When you're in a standing position, an efficient combined center of gravity systematically requires some degree of positional adjustments and that you pay more attention to your midline/core stabilization:

- Your torso slightly leans to the side opposite of the load and your hip shifts slightly toward the load in the Single-Hand, Hip, and Shoulder Carries.

- Your torso slightly leans backward with your hip shifting slightly forward (without hyperextending the lower back) in the Waist and Chest Carries.

- Your torso slightly leans forward, and your hips shift backward in the Lumbar and Forehead Carries.

Following are most options available for holding a load. Other variations exist; the specific carry you use depends on the shape and volume of the object. For instance, with the Deep-Wrap, Wrist-Grip, Palm-Grip, Cross-Fingers, and S-Grip Chest Carries, the load can be supported from the bottom of the object, so object rests on the forearms and chest rather than being held with the arms wrapped to the middle and front and pressed in toward the torso. It's also obviously possible to hold more than one object at a time.

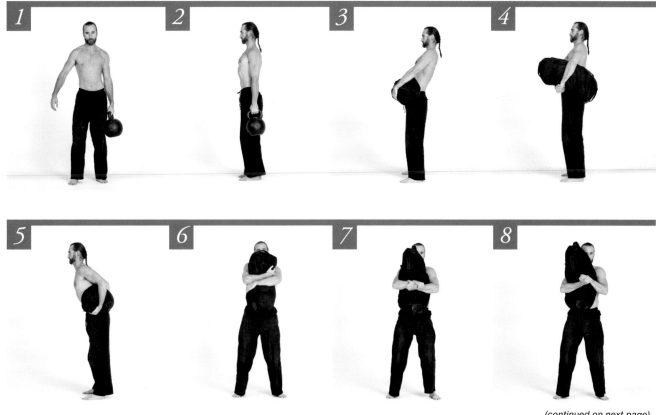

(continued on next page)

1 Single Hand Hold		**5** Lumbar Hold	
2 Hand Hold		**6** Deep Wrap Chest Hold	
3 Waist Hold		**7** Wrist Grip Chest Hold	
4 Hip Hold		**8** Palm/Gable Grip Chest Hold	

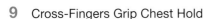

9   Cross-Fingers Grip Chest Hold

10 S-Grip Chest Hold.

11 Side-Squeeze Chest Hold.

12 Over-Wrap Chest Hold.

13 Under-Wrap Chest Hold (optionally, you can cross your forearms and position the load lower or higher).

14 Rack Chest Hold.

15 Shoulder Hold; you can stabilize the load with one or both arms, or you can carry the load without using your arms.

16 Forehead Hold; optionally, both arms can be relaxed.

17 Head Hold; you can stabilize the load with one or both arms, or you can carry the load without using your arms.

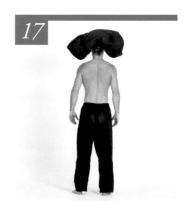

Carrying children can be done in diverse manners. The main point is to make sure that the hold is very secure and comfortable for the child first and for the adult second. Carrying a child can be challenging because young children tend to move in any direction without warning, which suddenly disrupts the combined center of gravity. Despite being a casual activity to any parent, lifting, holding, carrying, and lowering children multiple times in a day should not make us forget efficient mechanics, even though it will often place us in quite awkward positions and a suboptimal combined center of gravity, such as when having to place very young children in their car seats.

NOTE

Professional porters in the Himalayas and some African women have learned the Forehead Carry since a very young age and have developed highly efficient positional control specific to these kinds of carries. The load is not actually resting on the forehead but rather on the front top of the skull close to the forehead. Even though handling the load relies in part on resting on your back with your torso leaning forward, it nonetheless produces compression on top of your head with a strong protective contraction of the neck flexors, which increases compressive force on the cervical area. It's essential to prevent the hyperextension of your neck when compressed under load because hyperextension makes the central nervous system trigger a reflex to shut down muscular activity; you may fall because you're pulled backward by your load, a vital reflex designed to prevent damage to the nerves and disks in the neck.

Fortunately, your hands can assist and help prevent issues by pulling forward on the strap to keep your neck stable. However, if lots of force is required from your arms to ensure neck stability, this means that your neck is already at risk of injury. The Forehead and Head carries must be approached very cautiously, with very light loads in the beginning. Sound progressions will help build a healthy and strong neck.

Both carry methods are proven to be highly energy-efficient for traveling long distance. Another advantage is that you may free one or both hands to momentarily hold something and assist your balance or even to carry something else with your arms.

Regardless of the carry hold and grip you choose, once you've established an efficient combined center of gravity, it's time to move to relocate the object. To be an efficient motion, only your legs and (to some extent) your hips should move, and any positional disturbance should be avoided as much as possible otherwise. Your highest priority is maintaining a neutral spine or a very slight arch or side lean of the lower back, depending on the hold you've opted for. (Impeccable abdominal breath control tremendously helps with midline/core stabilization as well as economy of movement.) The initial positional set from lower back to head must remain as still as possible as you move. Depending on the weight of the load, it can be preferable to stop to a stand to rearrange either your grip or to switch your hold—to distribute the effort over diverse muscles—rather than attempting to do so while in motion, which can throw your balance off and compromise neutral lower back.

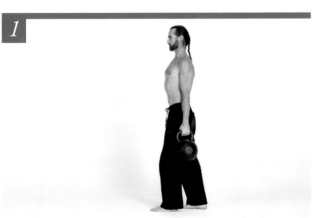

1

1 Hand Carry (also known as "farmer walk"): With an ideal distribution of weight, the combined center of gravity is perfectly aligned with the line of gravity and enables body joints from head to feet to remain vertically aligned.

(continued on next page)

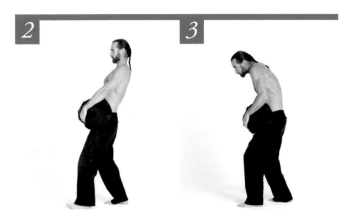

2   Waist Carry: In the swing phase (Single-Leg Standing with the opposing leg moving forward) your hips may optionally shift forward slightly more to push the load forward and rest the load a little more on the waist. Notice that the backward lean of the torso does not imply hyperextension of the lower back.

3   Inefficient Waist Carry

Clean (Squat Clean)

Cleaning in manipulation means lifting an object from the ground to shoulder level in a single, explosive, and rather complex movement, which requires great technique.

> **NOTE**
>
> The term *clean* comes from early times of Olympic weight lifting when touching the bar with any body part other than the hands before it reached shoulder position was forbidden.

Although the Deadlift and Lapping are done relatively slowly as weight increases, cleaning heavy objects is an explosive physical feat that relies on power to achieve the greatest vertical acceleration and momentum possible.

Great upward acceleration and velocity enables you to elevate the object to the maximal pulling height possible in the fastest way possible, so that your body can swiftly position itself underneath the object in a Deep Squat position and establish a hold at shoulder level to the front of the body, which is called the *Rack*. This movement is known as the Squat Clean because of the specific ending position. In short, it's a powerful move in which the object first rests on the ground with its center of mass below your center of gravity, and you pull it high enough to end up supporting it at shoulder level above ground, with the object's center of gravity above your own.

As with most objects, the greater the grip friction and the more even and stable the weight distribution, the more efficiently power can be used. That means

that cleaning becomes nearly impossible when the level of power required to produce vertical force exceeds the ability to generate sufficient levels of gripping friction. Although you might be able to raise a heavy, bulky object with no handles just high enough to lap it, there is no way you could clean the same object successfully because you can't pull it high enough and quickly enough. In a nutshell, although you might eventually end up achieving the same practical task, it's often the object itself that dictates the best, if not the only, movement strategy available.

In Olympic weightlifting, the Jerk follows the Clean, which means you raise the object overhead and then balance it for a moment with both arms fully extended. However, in Natural Movement, the practical reasons for the Clean are more diverse, including lifting overhead to stack the load on or toss it over a raised surface, keeping it at chest or shoulder level for a Chest or Shoulder Carry, or throwing it using a Push-Press Throw.

The Rack

The Rack is an essential part of positional control in cleaning, and without a strong Rack position at the end of the Clean, you might have to drop the load, which is a waste of a tremendous amount of energy and time. Before attempting to clean a log or any object, you must understand the mechanics that make the Rack position strong and reliable.

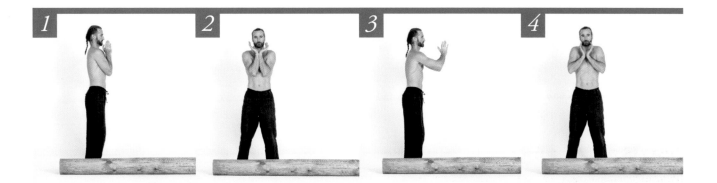

Photos 1 and 2 show optimal Rack position:

1 The elbows and triceps are resting and pressing against the chest. The combined center of gravity is close to the line of gravity, which provides strong support from the upper body for the arms and prevents the arms from lowering forward.

2 Elbows are in with the inside of the forearms and wrists facing and pressing against each other, which prevents the arms from lowering downward.

Photos 3 and 4 show inefficient Rack position:

3 Elbows are away from the chest. The arms have no support from the chest, which puts lots of tension in the shoulders and neck and pushes the combined center of gravity away from the body and makes it impossible to resist the pull of gravity. (This is the most problematic inefficiency.)

4 Elbows are out with the forearms separated, which makes it impossible to ensure enough tension to maintain the hold high. The hold might lower until it's entirely lost.

Experiment with the Rack hold and managing your combined center of gravity with diverse objects that require full support (as opposed to the log, which has one end resting on the ground) as you get up and down in a Squat or Split Squat fashion and as you hold the bottom Squat positions. Practicing helps you assess your stability, which is a key component of an efficient Clean. The type of object you lift is relevant to positional adjustments to the Rack position.

Logs won't move forward (unless they slide), so if your arm/Rack position is good and you engage close enough to it, a log won't pull you off balance forward or send you off balance backward (which might happen with objects and loads that you fully support—a sandbag, for instance).

Odd objects that are compact with a certain volume are more difficult to deal with. You must do what

you can to pull your head back or shift the object a little sideways with your head leaning in the opposite direction, so you can pull the Rack in toward you without getting the object in your face; pulling the combined center of gravity toward you the best you can is quite challenging. Olympic bars are designed to optimally align the Rack and weight the closest to your line of gravity, which makes managing the combined center of gravity and keeping a vertical body position easier.

The Clean starts the same way a Deadlift starts; therefore, I'm not describing that part of the movement pattern. As a matter of fact, if you've already deadlifted the object but marked a pause in the top position, you have the option to Clean from that position with a limited Hip Hinge (a movement called the Hang Clean). The particularity of the Deadlift when it's part of the Clean is that it has to generate upward acceleration greater than in a regular Dead-lift. Although you might not feel the acceleration at the beginning of the lift when you've just overcome inertia, you should start to feel it starting before your grip reaches knee level, and even more so as it passes knee level and your hips powerfully drive forward. However, it's important that you not try to generate speed right from the start of the lift-off. When a load is moving at a fast rate too early, it eventually decreases your ability to increase its upward velocity as you keep elevating the load. We could say that the goal is to "accelerate the acceleration" by starting to lift relatively slowly so you can accelerate the load more efficiently later in the movement.

As both your legs and hips approach full extension, the difference between the Clean and the Deadlift is that you also extend your ankles (raise your heels) to push off the balls of your feet and add vertical force. This movement is called *triple extension*. However, if maintaining friction at the feet (surface friction) and stability at the ankles (on uneven, unstable ground) is challenging, skip or minimize ankle extension for the sake of conserving maximum frictional force at the feet and ensuring a strong, balanced base of support.

As your body position becomes completely vertical, most of the upward force has been produced already, and it feels as if you're trying to Power Jump upward even though your feet shouldn't get off the ground. However, you still can amplify the upward momentum beyond that point to keep elevating the object (or where you grip it) to the endpoint of the pull. Now I can resume the description of the Clean technique.

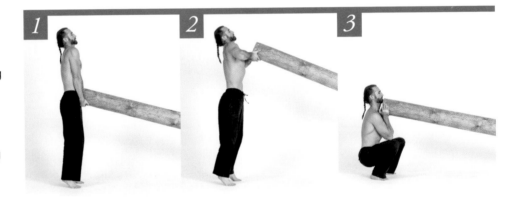

1 Upon full extension of your legs, hips, and ankles, shrug your shoulders to add pulling force to the upward momentum.

2 The velocity you've created keeps elevating the object and making it feel "light," which enables you to flex your arms to keep guiding the upward path of the load. Without forceful muscular action, pull your elbows sideways and as high as you can while maintaining your grip; you want to reach the maximum pulling height possible before upward acceleration drops to zero. Ideally, you want your elbows to be higher than your grip, but to maintain such a grip on a log you might have to keep your elbows and hands relatively level. The maximum pulling height depends on your power compared to the weight of the load, and you might not be able to elevate your grip higher than your navel. At this point, there is ideally zero or minimal force in your feet.

3 The moment the object reaches the vertical endpoint and for a brief moment it feels as if the object is suspended or even "floating," you must quickly change direction from upward to

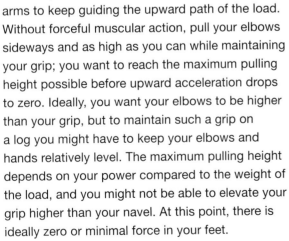

downward by dropping your center of gravity as low and as fast as you can to pull your body under the object to receive it in a squatting position. As you're moving downward, bring your elbows down and slide your hands down in the Rack hold position to receive the load smoothly and securely. Optionally, if the load is not too heavy and you generated sufficient vertical velocity, you could catch the load in the Rack in a position taller than the Deep Squat (such as a Half Squat), which is called a Power Clean. The Power Clean is convenient for people who lack the mobility to assume a strong, stable Deep Squat. However, the risk of catching the Rack too high is a compromise to your back position. However, it's good practice to train yourself to pull under the load as low and as fast as possible.

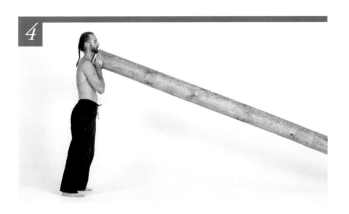

4 Get up to recover a standing position.

TECHNIQUE TIP

Because the Clean is a complex sequence that demands impeccable timing and positional control, it's great practice to break down the whole sequence into discrete drills to acquire proper timing, as I explain in Part 3, "Practice Efficiency." I describe the drills later in this chapter in the "Drills and Progressions" section.

NOTE

The gross mechanics of cleaning a log, a stone, or an Olympic bar are the same, with relatively minor positional modifications in the Grip, Rack position, and trajectory of the object.

Inefficiencies

Aside from the Deadlift faults that I previously covered, the following are inefficiencies for the Clean:

- Ankles, knees, and hips don't reach full extension simultaneously.
- No ankle extension (unless required).
- Early pull from your arms (bending at the elbows) with or without shoulder shrug before triple extension.
- Bending at your elbows (after triple extension) before shoulder shrug.
- No shoulder shrug.
- Not pulling your arms/elbows as high as possible.
- Kicking your feet toward the rear upon reaching the endpoint of the pull.
- Catching/receiving the object into the Rack position while standing or in a Half Squat, which is known as the "Power Clean." This might work with loads that are not excessive and save time when you're in a time-sensitive situation, but it won't work with heavy loads. This inefficiency could be the result of latency, letting your feet take off too high, kicking them backward, fear of receiving the load in the bottom Rack position, or

all of the above. It might result in your combined center of gravity being too much forward and dropping the object.

- The object shifts and pulls forward upon receiving the object in the bottom Rack position because the load moved away from your body (usually at the endpoint of the pull), the feet move backward which moves the base of support away from the load, or both.
- Upward acceleration is too slow. Most of the vertical force must be produced from lift-off to triple extension (ankle-knee-hip). Beginners tend to go to slow, thinking that they only need to lift the object high enough that they can pull it from hip to shoulder using only (or mostly) their arms. Another cause could be a lack of grip friction.
- Upward acceleration isn't steady. Upward momentum temporarily loses speed, usually upon the hip extension. Even though the object maintains upward momentum, the slower acceleration prevents you from reaching maximum pulling height, making it very difficult for the body to pull under.

Jerk

The Jerk normally starts after a Clean; however, you do it regardless of how you brought the object to shoulder level in the Rack position. The aim of jerking is holding and balancing the load overhead.

Holding an object overhead can be useful if you're stacking it or tossing over a height, passing it to someone who will pull it from a more elevated position, or holding it high to cross a deep stream while preventing the object from getting wet. The Jerk is the only way to efficiently shoulder a heavy log that has been resting on the ground. Even with enough arm and shoulder strength to push the load upward (Press) or with a push from the legs before pressing on the arms (Push-Press), with heavy weight you can't generate enough vertical force to achieve full arm extension. Instead, the strategy is to generate most of the vertical force from the lower body and to lower the center of gravity fast enough to be able to fully extend the arms from underneath the object as it still has upward momentum. Finally, you stand back up with the load balanced overhead.

The Jerk is a highly dynamic movement that demands equal amounts of power and technique. I first describe the Press and Push-Press techniques to help you better understand how they differ from the Jerk. All three movements start from the Rack, and, to the uninitiated, they may seem relatively similar.

- **Press technique:** From the Rack position in a stand, brace then push the load upward using only your arms and shoulders until you have full extension overhead. This movement relies entirely on upper-body strength. The center of gravity remains constant at standing level.

- **Push-Press technique:** From the Rack position in a stand, brace, slightly bend at the knees (also called the "dip"), and strongly push through your legs to immediately extend your arms until you have full extension overhead. This movement mostly relies on lower-body strength and on some upper-body strength. The center of gravity lowers and then elevates back to standing level.

- **Jerk:** This movement starts like a Push-Press, but you lower your body under the load until you fully extend your arms, and then you go back to standing. Instead of extending the load upward through your arms, you extend your arms away from the load as you lower your body below it. The center of gravity lowers and then elevates to generate upward momentum, lowers again to reach the Rack, and finally elevates back to standing level.

Push-pressing and pressing are useful both from a practical standpoint and from a strength training one. For instance, pressing enables a greater control of speed and elevation of an object, such as for stacking something or manipulating it above your head in a controlled fashion. It also develops valuable upper-body strength. The Push-Press pattern is also used to throw an object upward and at an angle; you simply release the grip at the end of the triple extension. However, although the Press and Push-Press work with weights that are not too heavy, it becomes impossible to achieve the same overhead result with heavy loads.

Jerking a log looks like this.

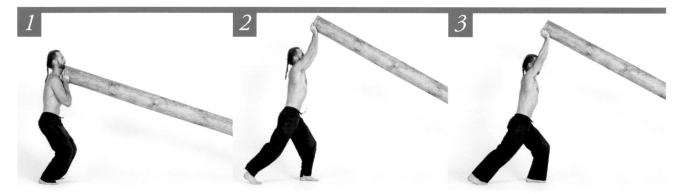

Unlike other objects that aren't supported on the ground at one of their extremities, the grip necessarily moves away from the body as the log elevates to a greater height, and while you raise it overhead, you do it at an angle instead of in a purely vertical manner. If the lifter fully supports the object without any portion resting on the ground or another surface, even a slight forward lean would force the load to fall forward.

In the next set of photos, I'm using a light load (a medicine ball) to show a Power Jerk (which means that I pull my body under the load just enough to catch the object with my arms fully extended).

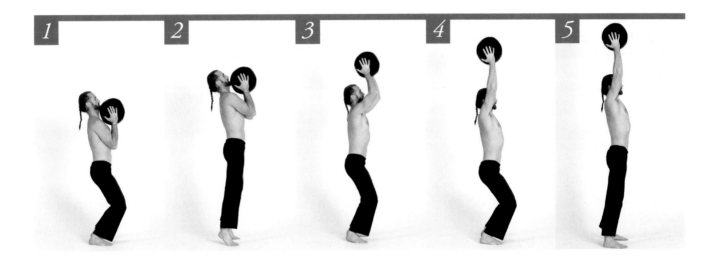

1   From a stand with your knees already very slightly bent (or unlocked) and holding the object in the Rack, lower your center of gravity and load your legs in a dip while maintaining a perfectly vertical stance. To help manage the combined center of gravity more efficiently and prevent any forward lean, keep your head back so you can drive your Rack in so it's more toward your shoulders and line of gravity.

2   Elevate your center of gravity a little higher than standing level by strongly extending your ankles and legs; immediately shrug your shoulders to generate as much vertical momentum as you can.

3   As the object accelerates upward, with zero force and no friction in your feet, swiftly dip again by bending your legs to lower your center of gravity. The reversal from an upward motion to a downward motion must be as brief and fast as possible.

4   Keep lowering your center of gravity until your arms fully extend. Despite what it looks like in the photo, you're not pressing on your arms to push the object up. Instead, you're extending your arms by lowering your body farther below the object until full extension before the object completely loses upward momentum.

5   After you've secured a balanced overhead hold, elevate your center of gravity back to standing level.

Once you've generated upward momentum of the load, how far you need to lower your body to reach the overhead position depends on how much vertical momentum you can generate in the load and how quickly you're able to lower your center of gravity. It's good practice to systematically train yourself to move under the load as quickly and as low as you can. In reality, you may "catch" (reach the overhead position with arms fully extended) it in a taller position (which is known as a Power Jerk) when the load isn't too heavy and you want to save energy and time. However, with heavier loads, lowering yourself all the way with the knee of the back leg almost touching the ground in a Deep Split Squat position will be the only way you can catch the load. Otherwise, you might not reach full arm extension and become forced to either drop the load or lower it to the Side Rack.

Repositioning the feet to a Split Squat means that you swiftly move one leg to the front and the other to the back at equal distance. The Split Squat position gives you two important advantages compared to a square position:

- It enables you to reach a lower position, which means more space and time for your arms to extend fully.
- The Overhead Hold with a grip as narrow as the Rack specific to the log is much stronger and more sustainable than a Deep Overhead Squat with such a narrow grip, especially with people who lack mobility in the thoracic spine and shoulder. My personal preference is a flexed-foot (back foot) position that helps me better control and stabilize my hip position.

Log Shouldering

No matter how you get the log overhead (Press, Push-Press, Jerk), the main purpose of the overhead position is to shoulder the log before you carry it. The distance you need to reach with the log must justify the effort of shouldering it. Otherwise, you may roll or pivot it on its base unless there isn't enough horizontal clearance (terrain, obstacles), in which case you might have to either raise it and topple it in the direction you want or drag it. (Those options are also available if you're unable to shoulder the log to carry it.) Side shouldering is a unilateral hold, with a single shoulder supporting the log's weight so you can balance it between the front and back of the body. This orientation is clearly more convenient than supporting it across the shoulders and upper back, which makes holding it harder on muscles and joints and also makes locomotion impossible if there's a lack of clearance on the sides, as in when you walk through a wooded area.

Side shouldering is an asymmetrical carry, both regarding position and force production on opposite sides of the spine. A slight side lean toward the side opposite the supporting shoulder ensures a balanced combined center of gravity. The core, back muscles, and lateral flexors on the supporting shoulder side (log side) lengthen, whereas they shorten on the opposing side. The lateral wedging of lumbar disks combined with compressive forces presents a risk of injury similar to the front wedging when flexing or back wedging when hyperextending the lumbar area under load. You can't maintain a completely neutral spine as you can with a symmetrical carry, and a slight lateral wedging is unavoidable. This doesn't mean that the side shoulder carry will hurt you. It just means that the risk of injury tends to be greater, which is especially the case if the load is heavy, you have issue managing the combined center of gravity, you can't strongly stabilize your core/midline, or you carry this way for a sustained period or over a long distance. In the latter case, a simple strategy to minimize the risk is to switch shoulders regularly.

Before you can attempt to shoulder the log, you need to position yourself by progressively elevating the log so you can move your body closer to the log's center of mass, as I describe in the following steps:

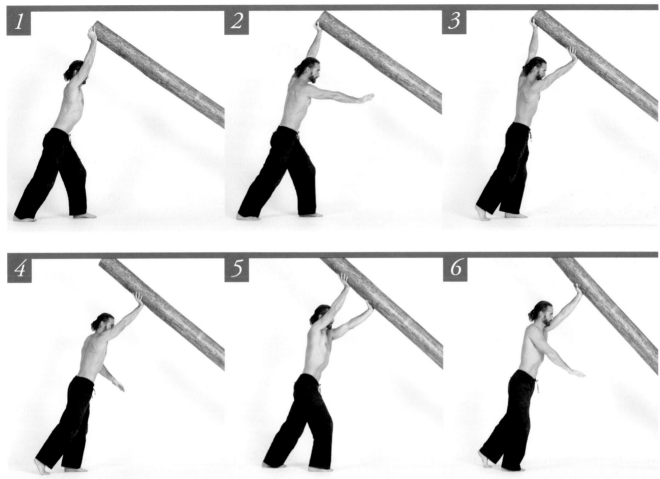

(continued on next page)

1 Start in a Split Stance in a strong, stable Overhead Hold position with your hands at the extremity of the log. Both arms are in the lockout position. Ensuring a neutral spine and midline stabilization by maintaining bracing at all times is very important. That doesn't mean you hold your breath throughout the whole sequence; just exhale partially to maintain strong, steady intra-abdominal pressure at all time. As you elevate the log, you have the options of supporting the log with both arms in a still stand so you can secure its balance or rest, lowering the log to a Side Shoulder Rack (which means that you'll have to jerk it back to overhead) or dropping it entirely to the side if your position becomes compromised. The objective is not to elevate the log as high as possible; you just want to raise it enough to move your hands down the log as it goes up to get your shoulder close to the center of gravity of the log.

2 Release the hand of the arm opposing the front leg and move it down and forward. Be very focused on stabilizing your position from palm to shoulder (in the lockout arm) to feet.

3 Push off your feet and have your back foot step forward just behind the front foot so your front hand can contact the log and create a point of support.

4 After establishing a strong and stable Single-Arm Overhead Hold with your front hand, release your back hand and start traveling it down and forward as you push off your feet again to step forward.

5 Step forward while reaching with your free arm toward the log to establish a strong Overhead Hold with both arms.

6 Push off your feet to let your back foot step forward behind your front foot as you push through the front arm and release the back arm to travel it down and forward toward the log.

7 Step forward again and establish a strong Split Stance and Overhead Hold with both arms.

8 With one more forward step and a switch of the arms, you're reaching the point where you might be able to shoulder the log. This is a crucial stage of the movement. Look up and down the log to verify that your hands are just a few inches below the center of gravity of the log. You may elevate or lower the log a little until you've ideally placed your hands. Assessing the log's center of gravity before shouldering it is rarely perfectly accurate. If you attempt to lift the log with the center of gravity too much to the front of your shoulder and body, the log will feel excessively heavy, and you'll need to press up the front part hard with your arms to manage to elevate the front part of the log off the ground. Even if you do manage to shoulder it that way, you might lose balance forward as you're pulled by the weight of the log, compromise your back position, waste great amounts of energy, and risk injury before you can adjust the combined center of gravity (if

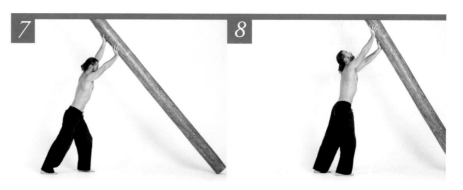

you can). Conversely, if you attempt to lift the log with its center of gravity too much to the back of your shoulder behind your body, it will feel very light and easy to lift the front part because gravity is pulling the back part down using your body as a fulcrum. Next, you either try to resist the pull of the back part of the log with your arms, or it just is too strong for you, and it pulls you off balance backward, with the possibility that you'll fall on your rear or back with the log on top of you, which is the worst scenario. When in doubt, it's always best to keep the center of gravity of the log in front of you. If you attempt to lift the log and it's too much to the front, you can use a partial Jerk to bump the log so you can slide your shoulder down a bit and get your shoulder closer to the center of gravity of the log.

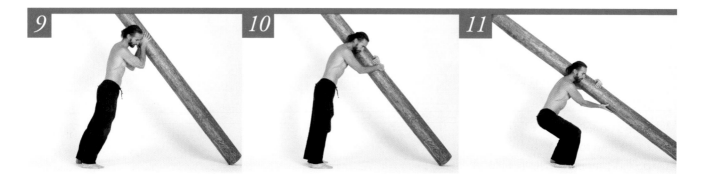

9 Once you have assessed where you want to place your shoulder on the log and what side of your body you want to shoulder it on, bring both hands to the same level. Lean forward to bring your shoulder in contact with the center of gravity of the log as you lower it as smoothly as possible toward your shoulder.

10 Establish contact with your shoulder, with the side of your neck and face pressing against the surface of the log. The arm on the same side as the weight-bearing shoulder wraps over the log.

11 Extend the arm opposite to the weight-bearing shoulder a little forward and bring your hand beneath the log to support it and push it upward. Then lower your position by bending at the knees.

12 As you lower yourself into a Half Squat, pull the log back with your top arm and push up with the bottom arm to assist the elevation of the front part of the log. As the front part of the log elevates, the back part lowers, which naturally facilitates reaching the combined center of gravity faster. If there's too much weight to the front and if the ground is slippery, the front extremity of the log might slide forward. In this case, you don't need to resist this motion; simply extend back up on your legs and step forward to maintain your hold on the log. As the log becomes more vertical again and its weight is pressing on its front extremity, it will stop sliding. This is often an indication that you need to move your shoulder farther down the log and closer to its center of gravity.

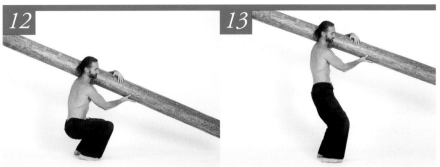

13 Get back up and keep paying attention to the motion of the log and its speed. The pendulum motion of the log should ideally bring it level. However, depending on how you have your shoulder positioned relative to the center of gravity of the log, you might have to push upward with your free arm if the front part of the log elevates too slowly. Alternatively, you might have to press down with the arm that's over the top of the log if the log elevates too rapidly. Both arms should be in a position to ensure either a pressing up or pressing down action onto the front part of the log.

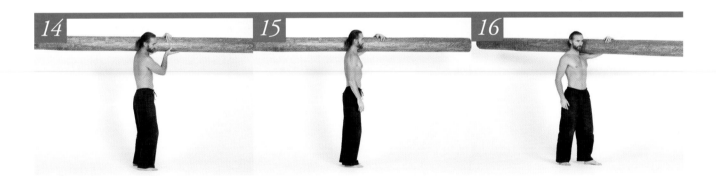

14 Stand up fully with the log horizontally level. A slight lean to the side opposite to the weight-bearing shoulder helps manage the combined center of gravity and prevents the log from exerting much tension against your top arm. Your body and shoulder are acting as a fulcrum onto which the log can pivot. If the front part tends to tilt down, you need to slide the log a bit backward; if it tends to tilt up, you need to slide it a bit forward. You can easily readjust the combined center of gravity by bumping the log in a Jerk and repositioning the log with your arms. You may move the center of gravity of the log very slightly to the back of your shoulder, which tends to elevate the front part of it, but which is counterbalanced by the weight of your arm over the log at the front.

15-16 When you have found a point of balance, you can release the arm opposite to the weight-bearing shoulder.

Loaded Squat Get-Up—Heavy Squat

While holding or carrying a load, you may have to partially or fully perform a Squat Get-Up, be it in the Clean, as you lift a body before using a Cross-Shoulder Carry, or to bring a load down. Technically speaking, a loaded squatting pattern, or heavy squat, is no different from the unloaded one except for the slight positional modifications necessary to hold the load and manage efficient combined center of gravity. The loaded Squat Get-Up may be performed in a square or Split Stance, and with a base of support that is relatively narrow or wide.

Several holds are possible: on a single shoulder, upper back, front shoulder Rack, and Chest Hold, for example. In the real world, it's unusual to have to repetitively squat down and stand up with a load on the spot, but it might happen after you've passed underneath low obstacles or if you have to lift and unload several objects over a short distance and in a short amount of time. However from a strength training standpoint, squatting several times in a row with a heavy load is a phenomenal way to develop high levels of strength and power in the legs and lower-body muscles (quads, hamstrings, glutes, back, and abdominals). That strength transfers not only to the ability to lift and carry heavier loads but also to greater power output in other natural movements, such as sprinting and jumping.

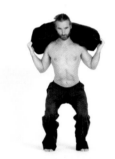 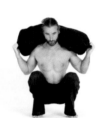 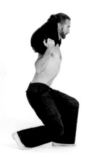 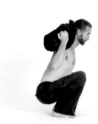

TECHNIQUE TIP

Following are some efficiency tips when squatting heavy loads:

- Focus on efficient positional control rather than load. If you don't have the mobility necessary to perform unloaded Squat Get-Ups, doing loaded Squat Get-Ups only magnifies your mobility issue. If you're new to strength training, don't overlook body-weight Squat Get-Ups; performing high volumes of them (up to 100 times a day) at high intensity (rapidly) increases strength endurance and vertical jump, and it's great for metabolic conditioning.
- Managing an efficient combined center of gravity when holding the load to the front of the body is challenging when the object is bulky, which is often the case with real-life objects and load. This tends to shift the combined center of gravity significantly to the front of the body and results in decreased force output compared to squatting holding an equal weight at the back. For this reason, the front rack is a great way to develop strength in the thoracic-spine muscles responsible for extending and stabilizing the back.

- Managing an efficient combined center of gravity is easier with the load on your upper back, but it tends to increase compressive forces on your spine.
- Manage an efficient combined center of gravity especially to prevent your torso from leaning forward (more than it needs) to use the back muscles to lift the load. Keep your upper body as vertical as the load allows, drive your torso up as much as possible, and use power from the hips when getting up.
- Using a base of support at least as wide as shoulder width or slightly wider, especially if you have mobility deficiencies, helps you maintain efficient bottom position and better recruit groin muscles for more force production.
- Keep a steady neck and eye position from start to end.
- Control the descent, which means resisting the load and preventing it from making you "collapse" under it, so you have better positional control and balance throughout the downward motion all the way to the Deep Squat. You can gently rebound on your knees at the bottom of your squat if your knees are healthy; otherwise, you might stop flexing your legs just before full flexion.
- "Spreading the ground" as if you want to make your base of support wider by pretending to slide your feet apart can be a useful cue when getting up from the Deep Squat under load. It helps engage the posterior chain, keeps the hips externally rotated, and keeps the knees over your feet.
- If you want to develop more power, you must explode up as swiftly as you can the moment you reach the bottom position and keep accelerating all the way to the top, as if you want to Power Jump with the load on your back. Speed, as well as acceleration or deceleration rates going downward and upward, can be varied to train adaptability of muscle contractions.
- Train the "pause," which is holding the Deep Squat for a few seconds while maintaining impeccable positional control.

Lumbar Carry

The Lumbar Carry, though it isn't only for carrying people, is mostly used when someone can't walk, when it's too hard for the carrier to elevate the person onto the shoulders, if the environment makes it difficult to stand tall while carrying a person, or as an active way to rest. In the Lumbar Carry, you place the carried person across the lower back and secure the person's position through your body position and arms. Because the weight of the body you're carrying is closer to your center of gravity, it allows you to carry a heavy person more easily and to ensure more stable movement on uneven grounds. The trade-off is that it might be relatively more challenging to secure a firm and reliable grip on the person's body, which tends to prevent running while carrying. Because of the transversal, "cross"-like position of the person's body relative to yours, this technique isn't suited for wooded or narrow areas; however, it works fine on open grounds.

Standing next to the person with one foot in front of him, use the hand that's away from the person to hold the wrist, lift it, and wrap the arm around your neck. Your other arm slides across the person's back so your hand can grab the back muscle (the lat) just below the armpit. You can optionally use this simple stance to help the person walk, which is known as the Support Carry.

> ⚠️
> **SAFETY NOTE**
>
> If one arm of the person is hurt, wrap the uninjured arm around your neck.

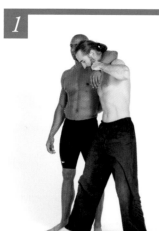

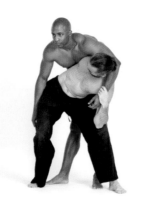

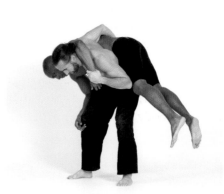

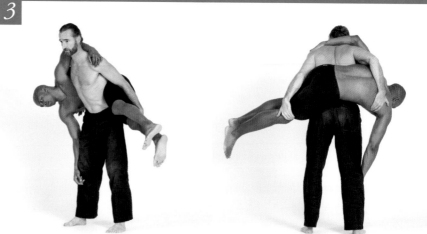

1   Step far forward in front of the person to establish a base of support wider than the person's base of support; drive and engage your hips far sideways while pushing the surface of your lower back against the person's abdomen area. Maintain a firm grip on their wrist, arm, and opposing armpit.

2   Bend your knees and lean forward in a Hip Hinge while pulling the person's body forward to load the person on your lumbar area. It's essential that you maintain a very firm grip with your arm gripping the person's back, so you can release the arm that grips the wrist and wrap it over both legs to reach and grip the back of the knee. The person's arm stays wrapped around your neck. Because you can't see the body, you must feel the position to balance the person's body weight on yours with an optimum combined center of gravity before you start walking. You can revert back to this position anytime as you walk and adjust the combined center of gravity by briefly bending and pushing off your legs to "bump" up the person; this leg action makes it easier to either reposition your waist, pull the person with your arms, or do both simultaneously.

3   While maintaining a neutral spine, drive your hips forward to regain a more erect position, but don't reach complete hip extension so you can maintain support for the person's body on your lower back.

Cross-Shoulder Carry

The Cross-Shoulder Carry (or the Fireman Carry) is the most emblematic of all body carries; it's a staple for first responders who regularly use it to carry victims or casualties to safety. This technique is a very efficient way to carry somebody because it keeps the body ideally balanced and stable on the upper back of the carrier, allowing them to jog if necessary or to cover a significant distance. You can secure the body with a single arm, so you can use your opposite arm to facilitate your balance or motion or to hold an object (gear, weapon, and so on). In most cases, the carry can't be done without first lifting the body with a Squat or Split Squat Get-Up.

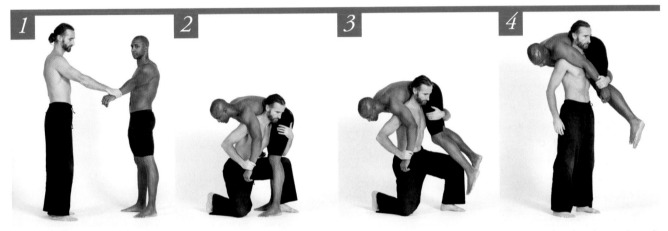

(continued on next page)

SAFETY NOTE

If one of the person's arms is hurt, grab the uninjured one.

1 Facing the person, grasp their wrist and lift their arm out.

2 Step forward in a Split Squat (a Tall Half-Kneeling, Deep Squat, or Half Squat are possible options) with your leg and arm opposite to the hand gripping the person's wrist between their legs. Pull their arm down to guide the torso onto your upper back as you slightly lean forward with your torso. While maintaining a strong neutral spine, press your shoulder and neck tightly against their belly while your inside arm wraps tightly around their leg, preparing for the lift.

3 Lean back (bring your posture up to an erect torso) to lift the person's body entirely off the ground. You may assist the motion of your back by pressing up onto the back of the person's thigh with your hand.

4 Stand up in a Split Squat Get-Up manner and establish a Square Stance. Bring the person's arm toward the arm you have wrapped around their leg to grasp their wrist with that hand, which enables you to free your opposing arm and tighten your hold.

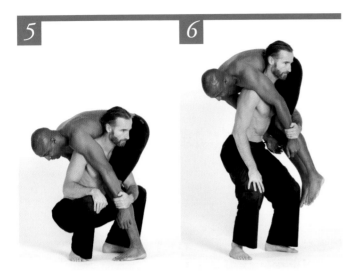

5-6 Alternatively, you could start in a Deep Squat with your arm wrapping between the person's legs and already gripping the wrist. With this technique, you're holding the person's body tightly before you lift, and you can even use your free arm to push off your leg to assist with getting up.

SAFETY NOTE ⚠

The lifting pattern for the Cross-Shoulder Carry can be used for defense—to swiftly lift and throw an opponent off balance.

Skill-Mixes

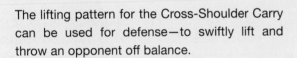

As mentioned at the beginning of this chapter, carrying is not solely done by walking and can be done using any locomotive movement, such as getups to begin with. With the real-world mindset of practical and adaptable physical performance, you'll open the doors to many ways to apply and practice the techniques you've learned with a diversity of contextual variables.

31
Manipulation Movement 2

Bipedalism has enabled humans to free their hands to develop both throwing and catching abilities to a level that's unique to humankind. Scientific evidence shows that early humans started throwing objects two million years ago. This enabled us to transition from being scavengers who threw rocks to defend ourselves from predators to being highly skilled throwers of handheld weapons, which turned us into successful predators in our own right. In fact, the transition from tree-dwellers to effective hunters on land and on foot has caused the anatomical structure of our shoulders to evolve to become more adept at throwing than at hanging from trees.

Although other primates also possess basic grasping and throwing abilities—as well as proportionally much greater physical strength compared to humans—their skill in those areas is nowhere near the level of expertise and performance humans can achieve in throwing and catching, especially when we have specific training. For instance, some athletes achieve a throwing speed of up to 90 miles per hour.

However, throwing is not only about power or the speed and distance that you can generate; it's also often about the accuracy and timing of the trajectory before it reaches the intended target. Such expertise exists in no other animal but humans, who can strike a moving target at a distance.

Today numerous recreational activities—ball games and competitive sports—are based on the skills of throwing and catching. Though such activities are far different from the original practical purpose of stopping targets at a distance or making them fall so that we can move close enough to grasp them, it's not surprising that modern humans have maintained an innate drive to practice throwing and catching skills in a different form.

Whereas some sports involve only the throwing aspect and only with the aim of throwing at a maximum distance—the javelin, discus, or shot put throw, to name a few—most sports involve both throwing and catching, with speed and accuracy playing a much greater role than power alone. For instance, in sports such as volleyball, you use hands and arms to catch and throw the ball simultaneously; in tennis, ping-pong, or squash, you use a racket for the same purpose. The object must be "caught" not to end its trajectory but to redirect it, which is a creative and highly entertaining way to bridge the gap between the actions of catching and throwing.

The Natural Movement approach focuses on the practical applications and outcomes of catching and throwing, even though those movements also benefit many of the structured games we play for recreation. The ability to throw and catch accurately—such as when exchanging a rope or a piece of equipment—is an aspect of physical competency that firefighters and rescue teams are well aware of. The benefits extend to brain function and emotional balance for several reasons, first because throwing and catching practice demands alertness and responsiveness and engages cognitive skills, and second because it's fun and often done cooperatively. Throwing hard may help release negative emotions, whereas striking, such as in chopping wood, is proven to dramatically increase testosterone levels, which is essential to functions in males.

While throwing accelerates an object to initiate an airborne trajectory, catching intercepts the object to decelerate and terminate its trajectory, and sometimes to deviate and redirect it. Both skills are obviously physically active; however, throwing is more active in the sense that we determine the trajectory of the object we throw, which in turn determines what our movement is going to be to ensure that trajectory, and usually we stay attentive to the trajectory of the object after we release it. Catching is more passive in the sense that we must be attentive to the predetermined trajectory of the object the moment we identify it, which determines our movement so that we can grasp it.

Throwing and catching are not necessarily associated in the real world or in practice. For instance, a catch doesn't necessarily follow a throw, and a throw doesn't necessarily precede a catch. However, throwing and catching have something in common in that both actions require an ability to anticipate trajectories and coordinate eyes and hands with accuracy and impeccable timing, sometimes with similar movement patterns done in a reversed sequence. Both skills require fine motor control and great levels of focus, alertness, reactivity, and accuracy to be performed efficiently. For this reason, they're often done in partnership. Practicing with a partner also develops a greater sense of cooperativeness and attention to others.

You can throw with one or two arms, and you can hold the object with a variety of grips. Most people tend to have and use a dominant hand, which is fine, even though ambidexterity is always highly desirable, and we train both sides in MovNat training. The most common approach to throwing and catching is to be in a standing stance, either in one spot or while moving, although you can throw and catch from other positions. The more body segments and muscles that participate in accelerating or decelerating the object and the greater range of motion we practice, the more effective and efficient we are at throwing and catching. This explains why these two skills are an effective means to learn to use the legs, hips, and midsection appropriately for producing powerful motion or safe deceleration of external forces; these movements improve health and mobility of the back, hips, and shoulders.

Throwing

Technically speaking, throwing is the action of launching an object into the air. You train throwing patterns to use them for a variety of practical reasons:

- To aim at hitting a target to damage, injure, or kill it (in which case the object becomes a "projectile") or make it fall
- To intimidate as a means of self-defense
- To pass an obstacle (such as throwing a bag across a stream)
- To enable someone else to catch something valuable or useful (such as food or a piece of equipment)

In Natural Movement, you grasp the object by hand and throw it without the help of any tool. You also can occasionally throw objects with your foot, but this strategy is inefficient compared to using your hand.

The Natural Movement throwing patterns are not limited to propelling objects to make them airborne; other throwing patterns include striking with the hands or fists in combative situations or striking with an object or weapon also for combat applications or with tools for work. The motion patterns that generate power are similar, except that in some cases the object remains handheld instead of being released into the air. Both throwing a punch and chopping wood with an ax are throwing patterns. By extension, explosive pushing or lifting movements aimed at fighting an opponent are throwing techniques and actions, yet we learn them in wrestling and grappling.

Although you should start learning all throwing techniques from stationary standing positions, you can add extra momentum by stepping or moving in the direction of the intended trajectory and target before the throw or by throwing your whole body off balance in the direction of the intended trajectory and target.

Because velocity is generated sequentially through diverse body segments, the continuity of the throwing motion is highly important with all throws of a certain intensity (either in terms of weight of the object, the distance of the trajectory intended, or both). You shouldn't pause after you've started the motion, just as you shouldn't pause after starting a lift or jump. Instead, focus on constant acceleration of the body. However, the goal is not always maximum distance or impact, for instance when you're trying to prevent damage to the object when it lands or to improve the chance that the catcher will receive the object successfully.

Following through is the last part of every throw. When you throw something, in most cases your goal is not just to get rid of the object you're holding; you expect a particular outcome, such as hitting a target. Maintaining focus on proper follow-through upon releasing the object eliminates the tendency to decelerate or to disturb your position in a way that would affect the precision of the intended trajectory or the amount of power you wanted to generate before releasing the object.

Catching

The practical reasons for catching are generally more protective than the reasons for throwing, such as grasping an object, decelerating it, and holding it firmly and securely to prevent it from getting damaged, lost, or even caught by someone else. Another possibility is to catch an object to pass it on to someone else by handing it off or throwing it to them, usually immediately after the catch is secured. By extension, the action of hitting an airborne object to deviate it from its original trajectory is a form of catching, but it doesn't include the grasping action. (Imagine an object is coming at you fast and unexpectedly with the potential to harm you, but you raise your hand or arm to deflect it.) Another technique is to catch an object with the arms as well as the whole body in a jumping action with the purpose of pressing down the object between the body and the ground.

Both throwing and catching rely on efficient gripping and the efficient management of combined center of gravity for heavier objects. However, the grip is especially important in catching because the interception of the moving, airborne object demands an extremely fast and accurate reactive grip response. You also need an extremely fast and accurate perception of the inertial force of the object—the force it exerts due to its motion—upon grasping it, so you can effectively decelerate it and end its velocity. A key aspect of efficient catching is to reduce impact to avoid injuring the body (especially the hands and back) upon contact.

Optimum positional control is key, including moving the body through space to catch from the best spot possible, but also in the most effective position. The heavier the object or the greater its velocity, the more it can produce a hard impact on the hands and body. To ensure a smooth deceleration of the moving object and make catching as efficient as possible, you must lengthen the displacement of the object upon contact, which means you rotate your body or take additional steps to increase the range of motion and your amplitude of movement as you grasp the object.

Catching has significant benefits to eye-hand coordination, which is the process by which vision guides the timing and movement of the body to enable the hands to grasp an object. Eye-hand coordination requires great mental alertness before the object is thrown, and great mental and physical responsiveness the moment the object starts its trajectory. Therefore, eye-hand coordination, positional control, and spatial awareness relative to the trajectory of the object are not the only aspects that matter in successful catching. You also want a minimum reaction time between the stimulus and your physical response, which is especially essential when the object is moving rapidly over short distances. The mental alertness and responsiveness you developed in catching practice are important benefits to brain function that carry over to many situations of life.

Equipment *and* Practice

The choice of equipment for training in throwing can be practically any object, depending on the application or outcome you're seeking. Objects used for catching are more of an issue; you should avoid using sharp objects for obvious reasons. Beginners should practice with relatively light objects that have an even weight distribution and that the thrower can grasp relatively easily. Medicine balls are perfect for both throwing and catching, and they're sufficiently cushioned to prevent injury in case uncontrolled contact with the body happens in catching practice. Strict beginners who lack technique, alertness, and responsiveness should avoid hard and heavy materials, such as metal or rock, because they can easily hurt their hands or crush their feet. Overall, it's best to start with objects that are easy to grasp, that are relatively soft with a smooth surface, and that are not too heavy. Advanced practitioners may train with heavy, rough rocks or any odd object that challenges grasping.

Note that you don't necessarily need a partner to train for throwing, but you always need a partner to train for catching! The beauty of this cooperative practice is that you train not just your technique but also your ability to stay focused, alert, and responsive.

If you're on your own, just use the throwing techniques. You can choose the distance, the weight and shape of the object, the level of accuracy, and the number of times you throw. However, when you practice with another person, you and your partner need to agree on these variables to make the practice is sustainable and enjoyable for both partners. The thrower becomes the catcher and vice versa every time the object flies in the air. The partners must be equally attentive to how they throw to each other, being mindful of being a good partner and helping the other practice in the best manner possible in a safe way. When practicing with a partner, throwing and catching techniques can be mixed—for instance, a thrower might do a Chest Throw, whereas the catcher might use a Rotational Catch.

Getting Started with Throwing and Catching

A simple way to start throwing and catching is to use small, light objects such as balls or dowels/sticks. This form of practice doesn't rely on physical strength or endurance, and it challenges the mind more than the body. The key points are to stay focused, breathe in a relaxed and ample way, and eliminate all unnecessary tensions while maintaining alertness, responsiveness, eye-hand coordination, timing, and accuracy. Although this practice is quite playful, it's also more than a game, as the ability to throw light objects with precision or to secure a quick and effective catch can be essential to certain situations, such as when you need to catch the end of a rope, a pair of keys, or a light piece of equipment.

Solo Practice

If you don't have a partner, begin with basic one-handed throw-and-catch practice. The goal is not to turn yourself into a master at juggling several objects at a time; you're just trying to get a sense of trajectory, timing, and accuracy in throwing and catching with both hands. Following are some of the variations you can use:

- Short distance, fast throw and catch between both hands, with an extremely brief contact event (the time spent grasping the object).
- Overhand (hand in supine position) and underhand (hand in the prone position) throw or catch.
- Swinging motions of the arm when throwing and catching.
- Spinning the object in the air.

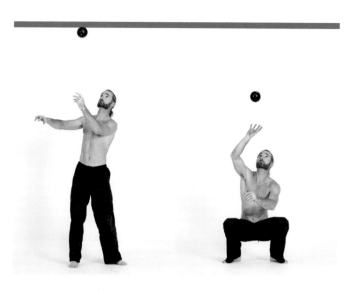

- Throwing and catching from diverse positions or change position (squat, kneel, lie down) each time you release the object and before you grasp it.
- Long vertical trajectories, catching with the same hand that threw the object or the opposite hand. While the object is airborne, add movements on the spot before you make the catch, such as spinning 360 degrees, doing side steps, going into a Front Sprawl and getting up.
- Throwing at a distance (forward, backward, sideways), running, and catching.
- Throwing a ball against a wall and catching it after it rebounds.

Partner Practice

Practicing in partnership is more realistic and cooperative than practicing alone. In the first few basic drills, the primary goal is to ensure a stable, predictable path of the dowel and a continuous, fluid, relaxed back-and-forth motion between partners.

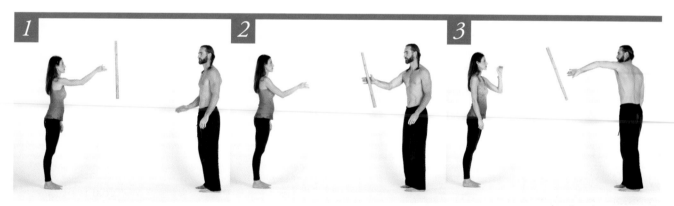

(continued on next page)

1. Stand a few feet from your partner. Your partner throws the stick with their right arm toward your right arm, which is called a Cross Throw. (Your partner could also straight throw from their right arm to your left arm.) Your partner uses a relaxed, ample single-arm motion, maintains good posture, and doesn't have unnecessary motion from the rest of the body. Their opposing arm stays down and relaxed. The goal is for your partner to help you catch the object by generating an elliptical (rounded) path that's aimed at your hand, with the dowel staying vertical. (It shouldn't tilt significantly.) As you see the stick going airborne, start raising your hand to catch with a relaxed arm.

2. Straight Catch the stick by grabbing it in the middle. (Optionally, you could Cross Catch it by grasping it with your left hand even though it's moving toward your right hand.) The softer and more accurately you catch, the better and quicker you're able to throw back the same way to facilitate an effective catch for your partner.

3. Optionally, you can internally rotate your catching arm.

4   In this photo, the dowel was thrown horizontally instead of vertically, with the same concern about ensuring a stable and predictable path.

5   When you're efficient at the basic drill, start looking progressively more sideways (downward or upward), relying on peripheral vision to both throw and catch accurately.

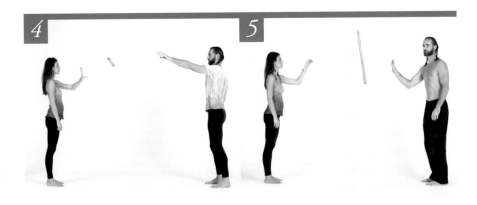

SAFETY NOTE

Make sure to start with a slight change of your line of vision; otherwise, you might catch the dowel with your face rather than your hand.

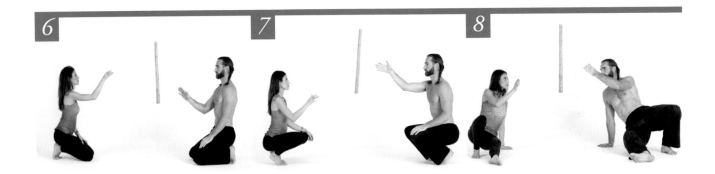

6-7-8 Throw and catch from diverse positions. Next, change positions without pausing and while maintaining a continuous, smooth back-and-forth throw and catch.

Progressions

Following are some suggestions for enhancing your partner practice for throwing and catching skills:

- Throw in unpredictable ways by varying timing (the catcher doesn't know when you will throw); trajectory (path of the object goes upward, downward, sideways, forward, or elliptical); and position (the object tilts or spins while airborne.

SAFETY NOTE

Never make the object tilt and spin forward, as it could hurt your partner's eyes or face!

- Spin around 360 degrees on the spot immediately after throwing and before you catch again. You also can Front Sprawl and get back up.
- Throw to the side to force the catcher to step sideways.
- Engage in a conversation, or ask your partner to perform basic mental math while both partners ensure smooth and continuous back-and-forth throw and catch, which stimulates very different parts of the brain simultaneously.

- Close the distance a little and throw back and forth quickly in a straight path for increased responsiveness.
- Widen the distance between you and your partner. Catching is easier at a greater distance, but efficient throwing is more challenging than when the partners are closer together.
- Run while throwing and catching.

Open-Arm Rotational Throw

Commonly known as an overhand throw, the Open-Arm Rotational Throw is the technique that enables the greatest acceleration of light objects, and you use it to throw for distance, precision, or both. (You also can use it for impact upon landing.) You use this throw when an object is too heavy to throw with an extension of the arm on the side, or it's too light to be thrown efficiently with two arms. The shape and weight of the object are essential for this particular throwing technique; the object should be compact and light enough for you to hold in a single hand. You also can use this technique with longer objects that can remain stable while airborne, such as spears. You can spin objects through a movement of the wrist to enhance their airborne stability. (This works best with nonspherical objects.) Practical applications of this technique include having to throw an object over an obstacle to prevent someone from grasping it, to toss an object to someone else, or to damage something by causing a heavy impact on it.

You can perform this throw from a standing position or while walking, running, or jumping. You can use other positions, such as while balancing or even swimming, but the efficiency might be compromised based on how much rotational hip power you're able to produce.

It's important to train this movement as a single, natural, fluid motion rather than trying to break it down. Before we consider the motion of the whole body in this throw, let's look at the two main upper-body and arm motions that should take place as you throw:

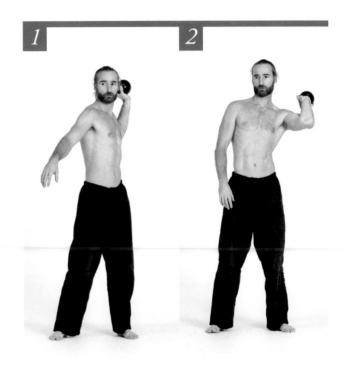

1 External rotation of the torso on the same side as the throwing arm

2 External rotation of the shoulder of the throwing arm

Start in a wide side stance facing perpendicularly to the direction of your throw; align your shoulders to the target or direction of your throw. Slide your front foot a few inches backward—enough to enable complete backward and forward rotation at the hip to ensure maximum hip power output; it also ensures your balance at the end of the throw in a shoulder-width Split Standing position. You also may lift the heel of the front foot to remove some friction and prevent any resistance to the hip rotation. Extend your back arm as you extend your front arm, making sure that your arms align in the direction of your throw. Your front foot is opposite to the throwing arm. The torso and shoulder should open in external rotation on the throwing side. Even though the arm action is not the primary reason for accelerating the load, with a longer arm action you can produce more acceleration. For the maximum distance or impact, pull the arm back as far and as dynamically as you can (to increase the stretch reflex) because the farther back you can retract the shoulder and the more you can rotate the arm externally, the more velocity you can generate.

Optionally, you may start with your shoulder in internal rotation with the arm bent, your hand and shoulder aligned, and your elbow at the back, which is known as the thumb-down position; then extend your arm fully before externally rotating your shoulder in a front-back-front swinging motion. It can be very useful if you swiftly rotate your hip, torso, shoulder, and arm toward the back before the forward throw because this movement supports the production of the greatest velocity possible by enabling the upper body's tendons and ligaments with a tremendous amount of stored elastic energy through the stretch reflex. If you're throwing on the spot without stepping momentum before you throw, you might want to use a back-to-front body-weight shifting motion to add power to your throw. If you're aiming at a target, keep a line of vision in this direction.

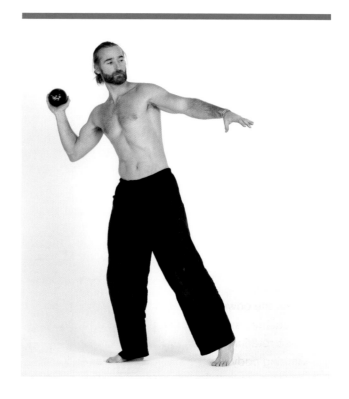

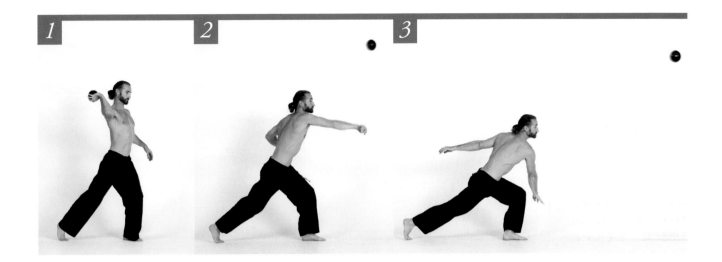

1   Once the power from the hip rotation has been unleashed, swiftly rotating the arm, shoulder, and torso rotation finishes producing peak velocity. Shifting body weight from the back leg to the front leg (as in the photo) also contributes to the velocity. As you produce rotational power in your torso as you swing your arm, you unleash all power in a whipping motion of your arm. Your elbow moves in toward the direction of the throw ahead of your forearm and gripping hand to generate a greater forward whipping motion as your throwing arm fully extends.

2   Finish fully rotating your torso while fully extending the arm in the direction of the throw. Release the object at a point and angle that ensures the trajectory you intend. If your aim is maximum distance, release your grip as your arm reaches a 45-degree angle. Don't forcefully swing your opposite arm to add power; not only does doing this not add power but it can easily throw your movement and balance off.

3   Follow through by watching the trajectory of the projectile and where it lands. If you have thrown with maximum power, your body keeps moving diagonally even after you've released your grip. You naturally lean forward at the end of your throw with your torso still rotating, the throwing arm going down and in toward your front leg, and your opposite arm extending to the back.

Once you have good control over this technique in a standing position (or if you have enough space behind you to do so), you may add momentum by shuffling sideways before the throw, which is explained later with the single-arm throws with heavier objects.

TECHNIQUE TIP

Although it's always good practice to train both arms, most of us have a dominant arm. You can use the weaker arm in practice, but in real-life situations, always use the stronger, more skillful arm.

Single-Arm Throws with Heavier Objects

You can throw heavier objects with a single arm, although there is a point where something becomes so heavy that it's not sustainable to throw with a single arm, and you must use both arms to support the object. As a matter of fact, it's possible to use both hands to hold the load using any of the single-arm/one-handed techniques shown here.

You can't throw medium-weight objects at great distances, but you can throw them short to medium distances with sufficient enough precision and impact.

With greater weight often comes greater bulk, which means objects become too voluminous to be held with the fingers and must be supported with an open-hand grip. While it may still be possible to open the arm (the photo in which the object is extended to the back and side) to add range of motion and power to the throw, it can be tricky and counterproductive for two reasons: It might pull your arm down and even make your upper body lean down with it (as in the middle photo), and it might roll off your hand as you try to balance it while going through a wide-arm motion.

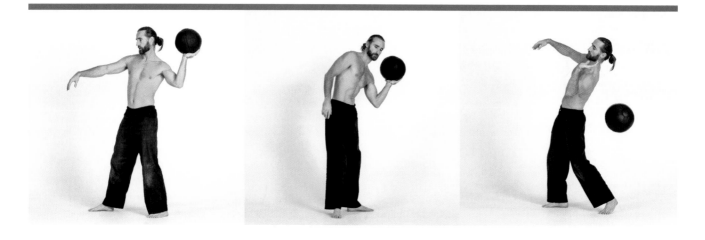

The solution is the One-Handed Rack, which is shown in the next set of photos. In this position, you fully flex your arm with your hand just in front of the shoulder, so the object is close to the body for efficient combined center of gravity. This position prevents the weight of the object from pulling the forearm down, which would either pull the object off support or alter the intended trajectory of the throw. Optionally, you can raise your elbow and shrug your shoulder to press the object against the side of your neck and face, which facilitates keeping the load steady before you release it. Another important detail is that since the grip is more supportive than grasping, you want to keep your fingers spread to widen the gripping surface and maximize grip control.

Obviously, though, if you rely on only the arm to produce force, you'll have very little power and won't throw very far. The following strategies generate much greater levels of acceleration, mainly through body-weight shifting and rotation. Although you can combine the two, it's preferable to dissociate them in the beginning because it can be tricky and counterproductive to associate them without having mastered each method separately first.

Single-Arm, Back-to-Front Push-Press Throw

One of the two main ways to generate power when throwing with a single arm from the Rack hold is to use body-weight shifting, with the body leaning backward at the beginning of the throw and forward at the end.

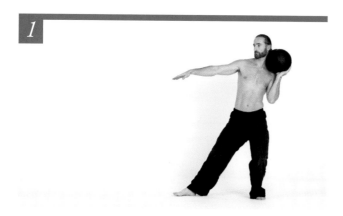

1 From a Split Stance with the object held firmly in the Rack, bend your rear leg that's on the same side as the load-bearing arm; your knee is bent, and your thigh is perpendicular to your torso. Your lead leg is straight with the foot pointing in a forward direction. If the weight is significant, maintain a vertical torso; otherwise, you may allow a slight backward lean to add to the forward momentum. You may optionally extend your free arm forward or at an angle to add a better sense of alignment with the intended target.

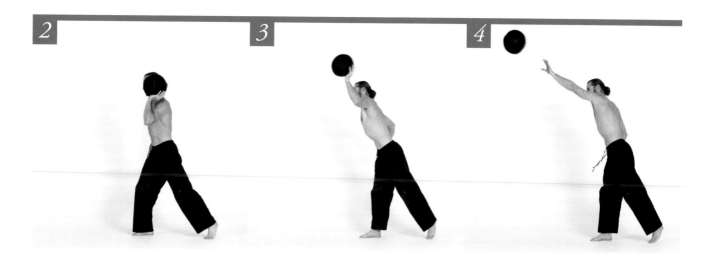

2 Strongly push off your back leg to generate power, which shifts your body weight to your front foot. Keep maintaining a stable Rack at this point. Your hips rotate to enable your back foot to keep shifting body weight to your front foot rather than trying to produce additional force through rotational hip motion.

3 Just before you finish shifting all body weight onto your lead foot, begin to extend your arm to throw the object while staying focused on the intended trajectory and point of impact.

4 Propel the object in the air by powerfully extending your arm. The angle of your arm determines the airborne trajectory of the object. Depending on how much momentum you've produced, you may follow through with a forward step.

Single-Arm Rotational Press Throw

This method relies exclusively on the power that you generate through hip rotation. This throw is wonderful training if you lack rotational hip power, especially because you do it with the resistance of the load. To learn to harness rotational hip power, you must refrain from adding power from body-weight shifting as in the back-to-front method; you avoid leaning backward and forward (or at least you don't lean in any significant way). Regardless of the amplitude of your hip rotation, your body weight should remain equally distributed on both feet from start to end.

Start to learn to control rotational hip power with a partial, 90-degree rotation in the beginning, progress to a complete 180-degree hip rotation, and finish with a rotational stepping motion of the rear leg. The one-arm Rack hold remains the same regardless of the amount of rotation. Ultimately, you can do all techniques that use rotational hip power with varying degrees of amplitude and velocity, depending on how much force you need to produce.

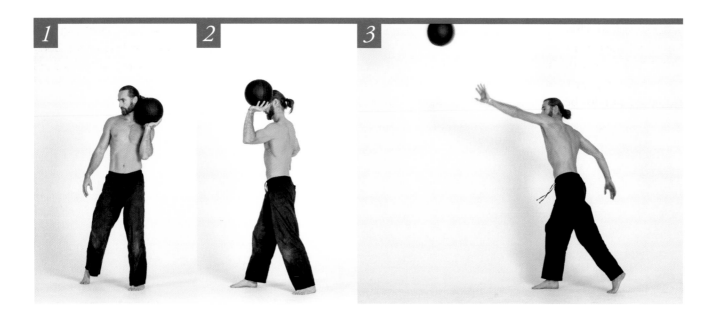

1   Start in a Side Standing position with your hips aligned with the direction where you intend to throw and your feet pointing perpendicularly to that direction. The ball of your lead foot ideally aligns with the heel of your back foot.

TECHNIQUE TIP

I like to lift the heel of the lead foot to remove some friction and facilitate complete hip rotation.

2   Swiftly initiate a strong hip rotation that turns your back hip all the way toward the front to its end range of motion. Start extending your arm just before you reach the full rotation. Both your feet must simultaneously pivot to pointing forward in the direction of the throw to enable hip rotation.

3   Fully extend your arm and throw. You may slightly lean forward at the end of hip rotation, although the rotation rather than the lean generates most of the power.

Push-Press Throw and Catch

The Push-Press Throw and Catch are similar in pattern to the Push-Press Lift. The difference lies in the fact that you release your grip in the throw, and you extend your arms at diverse angles depending on the trajectory you intend rather than extending them vertically overhead. If the object isn't too heavy, you can hold it at chest level rather than shoulder level, usually when you intend a power throw in a straight horizontal line.

Like the Push-Press Lift, the throw relies mostly on lower-body strength, but upper-body strength plays an important role, especially if the object is relatively light and must be thrown forward horizontally at a great speed, in which case the throw may rely mostly (or sometimes exclusively) on upper-body strength.

While pushing through your legs at an angle may add power to your throw, it also shifts the combined center of gravity beyond your base of support and forces you off balance into a step forward, which might not always be possible. You must learn to Push-Press Throw first while maintaining standing balance in one spot upon release before you learn to use body angle and forward stepping to maximize power output.

The Push-Press Catch is the reverse sequence, with your arms starting to decelerate the object before your lower body does. Physiologically the muscular effort in the arms is like the downward motion of the Press-Up, and in the legs it's like the downward motion of the Squat Get-Up; so, you're not actually pressing and pushing because the effort involves eccentric contraction. Ultimately, you can do both throwing and catching movements using more or less lower-body range of motion and power, depending on how much force you need to produce.

Throw

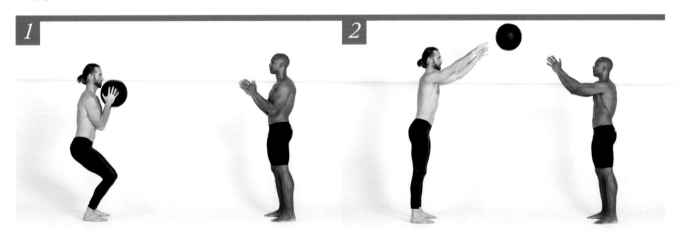

(continued on next page)

1 Begin with a hip width stance in front of your partner and hold the object you intend to throw in the Rack at shoulder level with your elbows tight to your body. Flex at the hips and knees to wind up for the throw. Squat about a one-quarter of the way down and move quickly.

2 Stand up explosively and extend your arms to direct the path of the object toward your partner's hand. In a partnership practice, you should aim at an elliptical trajectory that ends at the hip level of your partner, so your partner can raise their arms to catch it at about head level.

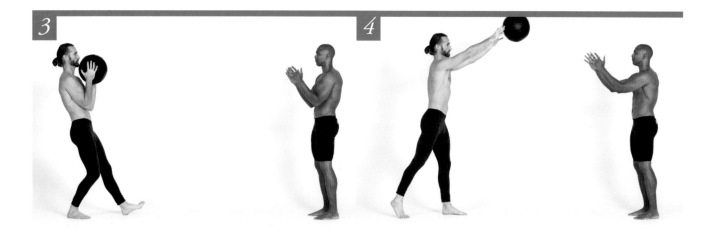

3   Alternatively, begin in a Staggered Stance and wind up by flexing your rear knee and shifting your weight behind you. Allow the ball of your lead foot to lift as you shift.

4   Shift your weight onto the lead foot and extend your rear leg explosively while extending your arms to direct the object toward your partner's extended arms. Allow your weight to shift more onto your lead foot by flexing your lead knee, which affords you more distance to absorb the energy of your partner's return throw.

Catch

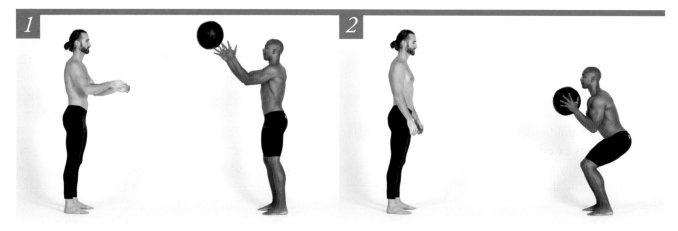

1   Prepare to catch the object by standing with good alignment and extending your arms. Watch the object as its trajectory nears, and prepare to maximize the gripping surface area by spreading your fingers and slightly bending your elbows. You want to progressively train yourself to stay relaxed with your arms down so that you raise your arms only at the last moment.

2   After grasping the object, decelerate progressively by flexing your arms, hips, and knees.

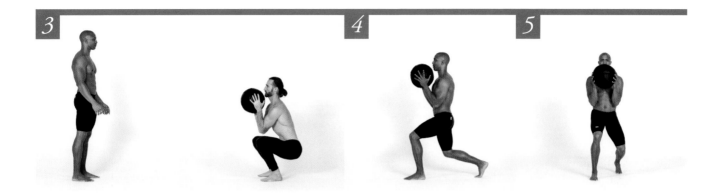

3 If the object is significantly heavy, or for practice, you may fully flex your hips and knees to finish in a Deep Squat.

4 When the forward force of the object is great, you may step backward with either foot to a Split Stance to lengthen the distance and time between the moment you grasp the object and the moment its velocity is brought down to zero. Conversely, when the trajectory is too short, you may step forward to catch it.

5 Be sure to maintain hip width alignment for stability if you catch in a Split Standing position.

Front Swing Throw and Catch

The Front Swing pattern is when you use a Hip Hinge pattern to generate power through hip extension (or "hip swing") and accelerate an object, which usually aims at throwing it but can also be used as a way to lift an object to a Chest Carry, a Shoulder Carry, or even a Head Carry. When you do the Hip Hinge with a load—that is, you're holding a heavy object in your hands with your arms extended—the Front Swing becomes a highly potent way to harness and develop power output at the hips, with benefits to any skills involving the Hip Hinge.

You use the same pattern to catch a moving object and decelerate it only if you perform the movements in reverse motion. Both acceleration and deceleration actions can be done independently as a throwing or catching action. In the absence of a training partner, you can maintain constant grip on the object (usually thanks to a handle) and repeat the Front Swing pattern repetitively and without a pause. This exercise, well known as the "kettlebell swing" (which can obviously be done with diverse types of objects), is a very effective way to develop power endurance. However from a practical movement standpoint, what you're actually doing is no less than replicating a throwing and catching action minus the grip release upon hip extension or the grasping moment before hip flexion.

The downside is that it doesn't help develop the precision required for accurate throws at a distance or help develop the grasping accuracy and timing, eye-hand coordination, alertness, and responsiveness essential to catch effectively and efficiently.

Another important aspect of this movement pattern is that the load travels dynamically over a relatively long distance—from the front of your body at about chest level to behind it at about knee level, or the other way around—so you can effectively accelerate and/or decelerate the load. There are several consequences to this.

- Managing the combined center of gravity requires impeccable positional control throughout the movement, as it shifts faster over a greater range of motion.
- The accelerating or decelerating forces tend to pull the load away from your hands, which requires that you have more friction and strength in your grip than you need with other throwing and catching movements, which helps you develop them.

No Handle Versus Handle and Progression

Both working with an object with a handle and working with an object without a handle have value. It's more challenging to ensure gripping on objects that don't have a handle, which develops your ability to create and maintain efficient grip regardless of the object; this is more realistic and better for real-world physical competency. However, objects with a handle enable greater grip friction and make it possible for you to manipulate heavier loads, which benefits the development of power output. Another difference is that although a handle doesn't lengthen the range of motion the body goes through (or minimally so), it does lengthen the distance traveled by the combined center of gravity because the center of mass of the object stands farther away from the body; the effect is that acceleration and deceleration are maximized. The last advantage of the handle is that you can swing with a single arm, which is impossible otherwise (except if the object is really small, in which case it's also relatively light and should be thrown or caught using a different pattern).

The Front Swing pattern is a complex movement that becomes inefficient under heavy load or when the grip is challenging. It's quite difficult to learn efficient form when you practice with a partner who's also learning.

I recommend you first learn efficient mechanics by practicing the movement on your own with a light load that has a handle, so you can maintain a constant grip and practice the front swing several times in a row; replicate both the throwing and the catching patterns each time with no pause in between. This way you can focus on efficient pattern rather than struggling to secure your grip at the expense of proper form.

When you've established efficient form, first increase the load of the object with a handle before practicing with an object that doesn't have a handle. If you start with an object that doesn't have a handle, make sure that it's relatively light.

First, let's consider aspects of the movement that must remain constant throughout both the throwing and catching actions:

- This is a Hip Hinge pattern with full hip flexion and slight knee flexion, not a Squat, which involves maximum hip and knee flexion.

- Maintain a neutral spine, abdominal tension, and breathing. Avoid lower back flexion at the bottom of the backward swing, or lower back hyperextension when you reach the lockout position as you stand. A slight extension of the neck to maintain a forward line of vision is necessary for efficient accuracy and timing in both throwing and catching.

- Keep your shoulder blades retracted with your arms fully extended. Depending on the object, you also might need to exert additional inward pressure on the object perpendicular to its trajectory to help grip friction.

- Your arms contribute, but not excessively.

- Keep your shins vertical.

- Manage the combined center of gravity with close to equal weight distribution at the center of your feet. Don't shift it to your heels when you Hip Hinge, or you might fall off balance backward. Don't let your weight shift to the balls of your feet when you extend your hips unless you want to triple extend (which means including the ankles) to throw with maximum power with the body at a forward angle.

If you don't need to produce maximum force at a given time, you should do the technique with less amplitude and velocity. To produce power, the velocity of your movement matters more than the amplitude of it; of course, maximum power production stems from both velocity and amplitude.

Throw

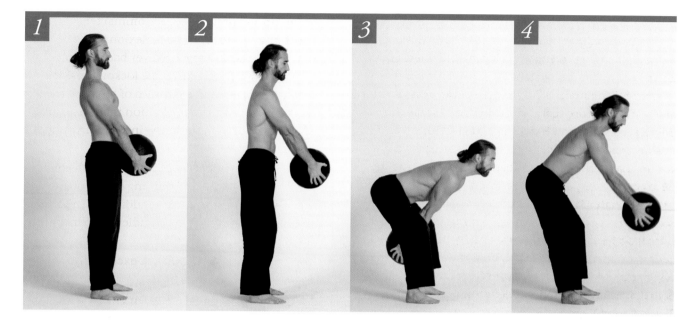

1   Begin with the object in front of you by grasping it with both hands on the sides of the object and standing up fully with good alignment. Mentally check out the aspects of your movement that must remain constant throughout the motion.

2   Initiate the swing motion by either pushing and slightly lifting the object forward through the shoulders or bumping the object forward by thrusting your hips forward, then immediately hinge at the hips while you fully extend your arms. Without the distance created between the object and your body, your arms and the load lower straight down as you Hip Hinge. The forward distance enables a backward swinging motion of your arms following the Hip Hinge and the backward acceleration of the object following an arc trajectory.

3   Flex at the hips first and then slightly flex at the knees as the object descends and passes through your knees. If you're seeking maximum deceleration or acceleration force possible, flex your hips to the maximum to drive your rear as far backward as you can, so the object can travel as far behind you as possible. With the proper amount of hip and knee flexion, at the bottom range of motion your shoulders should not be overly forward relative to your knee position as

your forearms reach the inside of your thighs and your torso position is nearly parallel to the ground. (In the photo, the forward swing has already started). The whole action sets you up for a more powerful forward swing and acceleration. If you intend to throw with accuracy, keep your neck slightly extended to maintain a forward gaze and line of vision; tilting your head as you swing forward may be too late to anticipate your trajectory, angle, and point of release, and the result could be that you become destabilized. Otherwise, you may keep your neck neutral and maintain forward eye position.

4   Immediately after reaching maximum backward range of motion and distance (load), explosively drive your hips forward, allowing the object to follow the same arc trajectory in reverse. To effectively translate the kinetic energy of your extension into the object, be sure to keep your arms straight and relaxed as the object accelerates to chest level. Strongly contracting your glutes enables a more powerful forward hip drive. Finish fully extending your knees and hips to a locked-out position with additional tension in the abdominal and glute muscles to ensure a neutral spine, vertical body position, and balance. As your arms elevate, release your grip on the

object at an angle and point that depends on the trajectory you intend it to follow, usually around shoulder level if you train with a partner. If you're throwing a relatively heavy object to the maximum distance, the first Front Swing might not reach peak velocity or height and produce enough acceleration to throw an effective distance. In this case, don't release your grip yet, and use the existing momentum created by the first swing to generate even greater momentum for the next swing. If you're training solo with constant grip, let the object elevate to about chest height. Because you're not releasing it to a throw, you should experience a "floating" moment as the object's velocity drops down to zero. Wait until you feel gravity starting to pull the load back down to resume backward swinging motion.

Catch

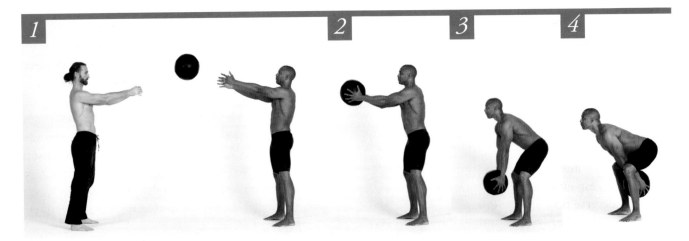

1   To catch the object, fully extend your arms forward to lengthen the distance between grasping and decelerating. Because of the elliptical shape of the object trajectory, the force upon impact is not as high as with a horizontally straight trajectory.

2   Ensure a smooth grasping moment by slightly bending at the elbows when the object contacts your hands and before you initiate the Hip Hinge.

3   Push the object back to full arm extension; then immediately Hip Hinge to swing the object down.

4   Load your hips and legs through the Hip Hinge as you also decelerate the object through the upper body until the object comes to a stop. If you intend to throw back or swing back (solo practice with constant grip), push the load as far behind you as possible while maintaining spinal alignment to wind up for your return throw or swing.

Throw *and* Catch Progressions

Progressions involve varying the intensity and complexity (or both).

To increase intensity, use heavier objects or throw for greater distance, height, speed, or impact—or combine several of these variables. For instance, intensity in terms of speed may have to do with how many throws you can perform in a limited amount of time or how fast you run toward the object to grasp it; intensity in terms of impact may have to do with how powerfully you can slam an object or strike a tool. As a rule of thumb, when an object becomes too heavy to throw or to be caught by someone else at a certain distance, it's wise to consider carrying it or displacing it by other means.

To increase complexity, manipulate objects with an uneven shape or weight distribution or that challenge grip. Throwing for accuracy, including hitting a target, reaching over or through a given surface, or throwing so that the object lands and stays on top of a surface. When throwing for accuracy, you may use sharp objects such as a knife, ax, or spear. (You would never try to catch these objects.) When you're practicing with a single arm, you can increase complexity by switching sides. You can throw objects toward or catch objects coming from multiple directions. You can throw the object with a spin that makes it rotate while airborne and makes it more challenging for the catcher to grasp efficiently. Last, throwing and catching from diverse positions (ground, hanging, balancing positions), in between positional transitions, or as mixed-skills movements (running, swimming, jumping, and so on while throwing or catching) elevates complexity to the greatest level.

Complexity in throwing and catching can become addictive. However, make sure to keep a certain level of realism in the diverse drills and challenges you come up with. High levels of complexity can be very fun—such as with complex juggling drills—but there's a point where high levels of manipulation complexity become very time-consuming and detrimental to the attention developing actual practical skills requires, yet without adding to your capability relative to realistic real-world demands or scenarios.

Although combining a certain level of intensity and complexity in throwing and catching is sustainable to a point, it can easily reach a threshold above which practice becomes overly challenging as well as unsafe. The heavier an object becomes, the more difficult to throw or catch it becomes. However, variables other than weight, such as how complex the movement pattern is, how difficult to grasp the object is, and how complex the environment where you're doing the movement is, contribute to increasing the challenge. There's a point where you must make a choice between increasing intensity with heavier objects while not increasing complexity and increasing the diverse aspects of complexity while reducing the weight of the object manipulated, as high intensity and high complexity manipulation do not go hand in hand.

Acknowledgments

To my predecessors Georges Hébert, Amoros, Mercurialis, who are just a few in the long line of people who have been transmitting the mindset and practice of real-world physical capability through history.

To the diverse teachers I have met in my life and who have contributed in one way or another to some area of my movement skills, education, and knowledge.

To Christopher McDougall, who discovered my work when nobody knew about it and who went on a mission to help me bring my Natural Movement "gospel" to the world.

To Gray Cook, Lee Saxby, and the many coaches and functional movement experts who have been supporting and believing in my work for years. You know who you are.

To my amazing team of MovNat instructors, who are relentlessly traveling the land, sky, and seas to teach new practitioners how to move as well as the other team members who handle equally essential tasks.

To our wonderful international MovNat/Natural Movement community of amateur practitioners, certified teachers, and licensed gyms around the globe.

To Danny Clark, our MovNat Performance director, for providing valuable feedback during the editing process, Mark Bixby for helping me finalizing many of the position names in the book, Dylan Chatain for his design insights, Anton Brkic for his photography skills and patience during our demanding-yet-epic multiday photo shoot.

To Ross and Tracy Alloway for gifting the MovNat method with its first scientific study and establishing its superior benefits on working memory.

To the countless journalists, bloggers, and podcasters who have helped me spread the word about MovNat and Natural Movement for nearly a decade.

To MMA champion Carlos "Natural Born Killer" Condit and to my Special Forces friends in the SEAL community who have been training MovNat and helped spread the word about it.

To Jessika, who is last on the list but first in my heart—my true companion, soul sister, and guardian angel. To my children Feather, Eagle, and Sky—my most precious diamonds. And to Creator, my ultimate spiritual guide and support system.

DISCARDED
Worthington Libraries